A PRACTICAL APPROACH
TO PULMONARY MEDICINE

A PRACTICAL APPROACH TO PULMONARY MEDICINE

Editors

Ronald H. Goldstein, M.D.
Professor of Medicine
Pulmonary Center
Boston University School of Medicine
Boston Medical Center, and
Boston Veterans Administration Medical Center
Boston, Massachusetts

James J. O'Connell, M.D.
Assistant Professor of Medicine
Department of Medicine
Boston University School of Medicine
Boston Medical Center
Boston, Massachusetts

Joel B. Karlinsky, M.D.
Associate Professor of Medicine
Pulmonary Center
Boston University School of Medicine, and
Assistant Chief, Medical Service
Chief, Pulmonary Outpatient Clinic
Boston Veterans Administration Medical Center
Boston, Massachusetts

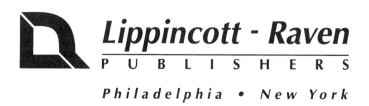

Lippincott - Raven
P U B L I S H E R S

Philadelphia • New York

Acquisitions Editor: Joyce-Rachel John
Developmental Editor: Julia Benson
Manufacturing Manager: Dennis Teston
Production Editor: Jodi Borgenicht
Cover Designer: Karen K. Quigley
Indexer: Jayne Percy
Compositor: Compset
Printer: Maple Press

Printed in the United States of America

9 8 7 6 5 4 3 2 1

Library of Congress Cataloging-in-Publication Data

A practical approach to pulmonary medicine / editors, Ronald H.
    Goldstein, James J. O'Connell, Joel B. Karlinsky.
        p.   cm.
    Includes bibliographical references and index.
    ISBN 0-7817-1237-8
    1. Respiratory organs—Diseases. I. Goldstein, Ronald H.
II. O'Connell, James J. (James Joseph), 1948-   III. Karlinsky,
Joel B.
    [DNLM: 1. Respiratory Tract Diseases—therapy. WF 140 P895 1997]
    RC731.P625 1997
    616.2'06—dc21
    DNLM/DLC
for Library of Congress

Care has been taken to confirm the accuracy of the information presented and to describe generally accepted practices. However, the authors, editors, and publisher are not responsible for errors or omissions or for any consequences from application of the information in this book and make no warranty, express or implied, with respect to the contents of the publication.

The authors, editors, and publisher have exerted every effort to ensure that drug selection and dosage set forth in this text are in accordance with current recommendations and practice at the time of publication. However, in view of ongoing research, changes in government regulations, and the constant flow of information relating to drug therapy and drug reactions, the reader is urged to check the package insert for each drug for any change in indications and dosage and for added warnings and precautions. This is particularly important when the recommended agent is a new or infrequently employed drug.

Some drugs and medical devices presented in this publication have Food and Drug Administration (FDA) clearance for limited use in restricted research settings. It is the responsibility of the health care provider to ascertain the FDA status of each drug or device planned for use in their clinical practice.

To Andrea, Cassie, and Hayley, for all their love

RHG

To the BHCHP staff, heros one and all

JJOC

To Cynthia, who had to do it the hard way and did

JBK

Contents

Contributing Authors

Khaled Al-Asad, M.D. *Senior Fellow, Pulmonary Center, Boston University School of Medicine, Boston, Massachusetts 02118*

Frank S. Becker, M.D. *Assistant Professor of Medicine, Pulmonary and Critical Care Medicine, Northwestern University Memorial Hospital, Chicago, Illinois 60611*

Dennis J. Beer, M.D. *Associate Professor of Medicine, Tufts University School of Medicine; Chief, Pulmonary and Critical Care, Newton-Wellesley Hospital, Newton, Massachusetts 02162*

Joshua O. Benditt, M.D. *Associate Professor of Medicine, Division of Pulmonary and Critical Care Medicine, University of Washington Medical Center, Seattle, Washington 98195*

John L. Berk, M.D. *Assistant Professor of Medicine, Pulmonary Center, Boston University School of Medicine, 80 East Concord Street, Boston, Massachusetts 02118*

Jeffrey S. Berman, M.D. *Associate Professor, Pulmonary Center, Boston University School of Medicine, Boston, Massachusetts 02118*

John Bernardo, M.D. *Associate Professor of Medicine, Pulmonary Center, Boston University School of Medicine, Boston, Massachusetts 02118*

Brian B. Bloom, M.D. *Senior Fellow, Pulmonary Center, Boston University School of Medicine, Boston, Massachusetts 02118*

Bartolome R. Celli, M.D. *Professor of Medicine, Tufts University, and Chief, Pulmonary and Critical Care Medicine, St. Elizabeth Medical Center, Boston, Massachusetts 02135*

David M. Center, M.D. *Professor of Medicine and, Chief, Pulmonary and Critical Care Medicine, Boston University School of Medicine, Boston Medical Center, Boston, Massachusetts 02118*

Geoffrey L. Chupp, M.D. *Senior Fellow, Pulmonary Center, Boston University School of Medicine, Boston, Massachusetts 02118*

David Ciccolella, M.D. *Assistant Professor of Medicine, Division of Pulmonary and Critical Care Medicine, Temple University School of Medicine, Philadelphia, Pennsylvania 19148*

Kevin R. Cooper, M.D. *Professor of Medicine, Pulmonary Disease and Critical Care, Virginia Commonwealth University, Medical College of Virginia, Richmond, Virginia 23298*

Francis Cordova, M.D. *Assistant Professor of Medicine, Division of Pulmonary and Critical Care Medicine, Temple University School of Medicine, Philadelphia, Pennsylvania 19140*

Gerald J. Criner, M.D. *Professor of Medicine, Director of Pulmonary and Critical Care Medicine, Temple University School of Medicine, Philadelphia, Pennsylvania 19140*

Gary R. Epler, M.D., M.P.H. *Clinical Associate Professor of Medicine, Harvard Medical School, and Chairman, Department of Medicine, New England Baptist Hospital, Boston, Massachusetts 02120*

Scott K. Epstein, M.D. *Assistant Professor of Medicine and, Associate Director, Medical Intensive*

Care, Pulmonary and Critical Care Division, New England Medical Center, Tufts University School of Medicine, Boston, Massachusetts 02111

Harrison W. Farber, M.D. *Professor of Medicine, Pulmonary Center, Boston University School of Medicine, Boston, Massachusetts 02118*

Alan Fine, M.D. *Assistant Professor of Medicine and Biochemistry, Pulmonary Center, Boston University School of Medicine, Boston, Massachusetts 02118*

Daniel R. Gale, M.D. *Assistant Professor of Radiology, Boston Veterans Administration Medical Center, Boston, Massachusetts 02130*

M. Elon Gale, M.D. *Associate Professor of Radiology, Department of Radiology, Boston University School of Medicine, Boston Veterans Administration Medical Center, Boston, Massachusetts 02130*

Rachel J. Givelber, M.D. *Senior Fellow, Pulmonary Center, Boston University School of Medicine, Boston, Massachusetts 02118*

Jeffrey Glassroth, M.D. *Thomas Vischer Professor and Chairman, Department of Medicine, Hahnemann School of Medicine, Philadelphia, Pennsylvania 19129*

Bernadette R. Gochuico, M.D. *Senior Fellow, Pulmonary Center, Boston University School of Medicine, Boston, Massachusetts 02118*

Ronald H. Goldstein, M.D. *Professor of Medicine, Pulmonary Center, Boston University School of Medicine, Boston Medical Center, and Boston Veterans Administration Medical Center, Boston, Massachusetts 02118*

Daniel M. Goodenberger, M.D. *Associate Professor of Medicine and, Director, Residency Training Program, John Milliken Department of Medicine, Barnes-Jewish Hospital, Washington University School of Medicine, St. Louis, Missouri 63110*

Daniel J. Gottlieb, M.D., M.P.H. *Assistant Professor of Medicine, Pulmonary Center, Boston University School of Medicine, Boston, Massachusetts 02118*

Krista K. Graven, M.D. *Assistant Professor of Medicine, Pulmonary Center, Boston University School of Medicine, 80 East Concord Street, Boston, Massachusetts 02118*

Samuel I. Hammerman, M.D. *Senior Fellow, Pulmonary Center, Boston University School of Medicine, Boston, Massachusetts 02130*

Helen M. Hollingsworth, M.D. *Associate Professor of Medicine, Pulmonary Center, Boston University School of Medicine, Boston, Massachusetts 02118*

Martin F. Joyce-Brady, M.D. *Associate Professor of Medicine, Pulmonary Center, Boston University School of Medicine, Boston, Massachusetts 02118*

Joel B. Karlinsky, M.D. *Associate Professor of Medicine, Pulmonary Center, Boston University School of Medicine, Boston, Massachusetts 02118 and; Assistant Chief, Medical Service and Chief, Pulmonary Outpatient Clinic, Boston Veterans Administration Medical Center, Boston, Massachusetts 02130*

Lawrence D. Klima, M.D. *Attending Physician, Pulmonary and Critical Care Medicine, West Palm Beach Veterans Administration Medical Center, West Palm Beach, Florida 33410-6400*

Hardy Kornfeld, M.D. *Associate Professor of Medicine and Pathology, Pulmonary Center, Boston University School of Medicine, Boston, Massachusetts 02118*

Peter S. Kussin, M.D. *Associate Professor of Medicine and, Director of Medical Staff Operations, Duke University School of Medicine, Durham, North Carolina 27710*

Fernando J. Martinez, M.D. *Associate Professor of Medicine, Department of Pulmonary and Critical Care Medicine, University of Michigan Medical Center, Ann Arbor, Michigan 48109*

Anne Menenghetti, M.D. *Senior Fellow, Pulmonary Center, Boston University School of Medicine, Boston, Massachusetts 02118*

James J. O'Connell, M.D. *Assistant Professor of Medicine, Department of Medicine, Boston University School of Medicine, Boston Medical Center, Boston, Massachusetts 02118*

George T. O'Connor, M.D. *Associate Professor of Medicine, Pulmonary Center, Boston University School of Medicine, Boston, Massachusetts 02118*

Robert Paine III, M.D. *Associate Professor of Internal Medicine, Department of Pulmonary and Critical Care Medicine, University of Michigan Medical Center, Ann Arbor Veterans Administration Medical Center, Ann Arbor, Michigan 48109-0360*

Nereida A. Parada, M.D. *Assistant Professor of Medicine, Department of Internal Medicine, Pulmonary Center, Boston University School of Medicine, Boston, Massachusetts 02118*

Charles Andrew Powell, M.D. *Instructor of Medicine, Pulmonary Center, Boston University School of Medicine, Boston, Massachusetts 02118*

Donna M. Poyant, R.R.T *Respiratory Therapy, Pulmonary and Critical Care Medicine, Department of Veterans Affairs Medical Center, 150 South Huntington Avenue Boston, Massachusetts 02130*

Christine C. Reardon, M.D. *Assistant Professor of Medicine, Pulmonary Center, Boston University School of Medicine, Boston, Massachusetts 02118*

Jeffery B. Rubins, M.D. *Associate Professor of Medicine, Department of Pulmonary Diseases, University of Minnesota, Minneapolis Veterans Administration Medical Center, Minneapolis, Minnesota 55417*

Jussi J. Saukkonen, M.D. *Assistant Professor of Medicine, Pulmonary Center, Boston University School of Medicine, Boston Medical Center, Boston, Massachusetts 02118*

Victor F. Tapson, M.D., F.C.C.P. *Associate Professor of Medicine, Division of Pulmonary and Critical Care Medicine, Duke University Medical Center, Durham, North Carolina 27710*

Arthur C. Theodore, M.D. *Assistant Professor of Medicine, Pulmonary Center, Boston University School of Medicine, Boston, Massachusetts 02118*

Margaret A. Vallen-Mashikian, M.D. *Senior Fellow, Pulmonary Center, Boston University School of Medicine, Boston, Massachusetts 02118*

Randall P. Wagner, M.D. *Assistant Professor of Medicine, Division of Pulmonary Diseases and Allergy, George Washington University School of Medicine, Washington, D.C. 20037*

David M.H. Wu, M.D. *Senior Fellow, Pulmonary Center, Boston University School of Medicine, Boston, Massachusetts 02118*

Leslie H. Zimmerman, M.D. *Assistant Professor of Medicine, Pulmonary and Critical Care Medicine Section, University of California San Francisco, San Francisco Veterans Administration Medical Center, San Francisco, California 94121*

Foreword

A Practical Approach to Pulmonary Medicine is a clearly written, well-organized text dealing with issues pertaining to the care of patients with respiratory illnesses and is intended for use by the busy internist or primary care physician, as well as by practicing pulmonary physicians. All chapters are presented in a logical sequence; therefore the book should quickly become a resource for basic, practical information referable to respiratory diseases. While remaining simple enough for use as course material for students or house officers, the depth of the insights into pulmonary diseases will also be useful for the fully trained pulmonologist.

The reader will note that the senior authors for all of the chapters were the faculty and graduates of the Boston University Pulmonary and Critical Care Medicine and related training programs over the past 25 years. Many of our graduates are now Boston University Faculty members, while others have emigrated to distinguished careers at other institutions. In many ways, this text represents the approach to pulmonary medicine that has been developed at Boston University. It is derived from a combination of knowledge obtained from an understanding of the basic disease mechanisms that have evolved over the past quarter century and from practical lessons learned at the bedside and in the outpatient clinics. Most of all, this book contains the experience of individuals who have devoted decades of their lives to understanding, practicing, and teaching the "bread and butter" of respiratory diseases. As a participant in this process, I am struck by the dynamic changes that have occurred in our approaches over time.

There are two unique aspects to our approaches at Boston University. The first is a historical perspective of pulmonary disease. In certain diseases, like chronic bronchitis and lung cancer, this perspective is sometimes sobering because our therapeutic approaches have changed little during the past 25 years. While in other diseases, like asthma and certain infectious diseases, the progress in our understanding of pathogenesis have been translated into many new therapeutic options that require continuing education for today's pulmonary physicians. The second aspect involves our application of the knowledge gained from basic science directly into practical bedside and outpatient approaches to diagnosis and treatment of respiratory illnesses. Perhaps the latter comes from the fact that our academic faculty is comprised of clinicians who share a common interest in both the theoretical and practical aspects of pulmonary medicine.

While reading the text, I particularly felt the presence of Jerome Brody, Gordon L. Snider, and Edward Gaensler. Their quest for knowledge and desire to apply the best medicine to benefit our patients has taught us to never be complacent. They have been our teachers at Boston University School of Medicine, and this text is a testimony to what we have learned from them.

David M. Center, M.D.
Professor of Medicine
Chief, Pulmonary and Critical Care Medicine
Boston University School of Medicine
Boston Medical Center
Boston, Massachusetts

Preface

A Practical Approach to Pulmonary Medicine provides guidelines for practicing primary care physicians and clinicians in the diagnosis and management of a broad array of pulmonary problems as viewed from the perspective of pulmonary specialists. The structure of this book accords with that of other books in this series, in the respect that information is provided in a readily accessible format and each chapter deals with a separate aspect of pulmonary medicine. We have tried to give realistic recommendations for the diagnosis and management of pulmonary diseases. Information about potential complications and treatment options associated with certain diseases is also provided.

While it is likely that this book will be useful to fully trained pulmonary specialists, it was specifically written to provide the internist and primary care physician with the means to treat certain pulmonary problems in an era of managed care. In most cases, indications for appropriate subspecialist referral are provided. As authors, our perspective as pulmonary subspecialists was tempered by one of the Editors, who is a primary care physician not specially trained in pulmonary disease. His influence has helped us to address the particular concerns of general health care providers.

Although the most common pulmonary problems are discussed individually in discrete chapters, some overlapping exists, and some topics are explored from a different viewpoint in other chapters. For example, conditions resulting from airway hypersensitivity are discussed in the chapters on asthma, hypersensitivity pneumonia, and the sick building syndrome. Other chapters deal with less common, but often problematic, conditions such as pulmonary fibrotic disorders or pulmonary vasculitides. Some rare disorders, such as certain congenital pulmonary problems, are not likely to be seen by the primary care physician and are either only briefly mentioned or excluded from discussion.

All the contributors to this book have shared common training experiences in the Pulmonary Division at Boston University School of Medicine. Many are current or past faculty members in the Pulmonary Division. This commonality of background and management philosophy provides the thread that weaves this book together into a comprehensive and coherent approach to general pulmonary problems.

We hope that this book serves its intended purpose as an aid to those primary care physicians taking on greater responsibility for patients with pulmonary disorders.

Acknowledgments

We would like to thank all the contributors for their efforts and our teachers and patients, from whom we continually learn and who always remind us to be humble. Thank you to our friends at Little, Brown and Co. and Lippincott-Raven Publishers, who have helped us focus our efforts to structure and complete this book.

A PRACTICAL APPROACH
TO PULMONARY MEDICINE

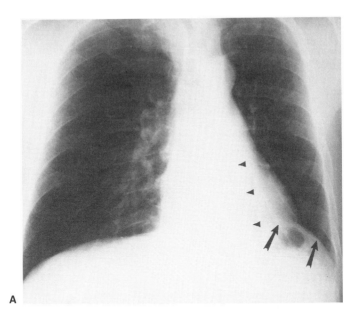

A

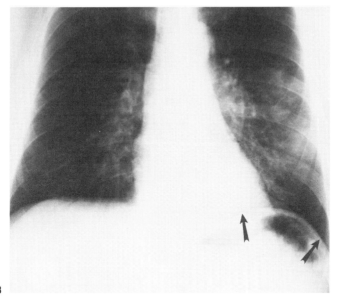

B

Fig. 1-1. A: This chest film illustrates the classic radiographic findings of left lower lobe collapse. These include volume loss as demonstrated by shift of the mediastinum, heart, and trachea to the left, a triangular opacity in a retrocardiac location (*black arrow heads*), and silhouetting of the medial portions of the left hemidiaphragm. Only the lateral portion of the hemidiaphragm (*black arrows*) is delineated. **B:** After chest physical therapy, the chest film shows resolution of the left lower lobe collapse. The shift of the mediastinum and the triangular retrocardiac opacity are no longer present. The left hemidiaphragm is identified medially.

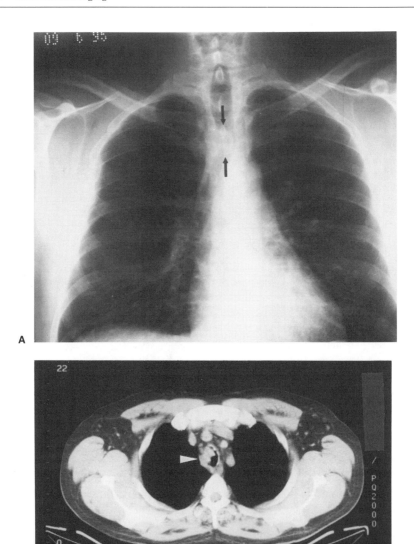

Fig. 1-2. A: Chest radiograph demonstrates a subtle mass (*black arrows*) projected in the tracheal air column. **B:** A chest CT confirms the presence of a large fungating mass (*white arrow head*) within the trachea. The vast majority of tracheal neoplasms are either squamous cell or minor salivary gland in origin. The pathologic specimen revealed adenoid cystic carcinoma.

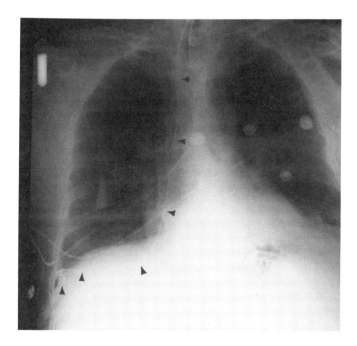

Fig. 1-3. Portable chest film demonstrates abnormal placement of a nasogastric tube (*black arrow heads*) into the right costophrenic angle. Feeding tubes are much more likely to be inappropriately placed than nasogastric tubes because of their smaller diameter and more pliable composition.

C. **Utility of the old chest film**
   1. An old chest x-ray is one of the most important resources in the diagnostic process because of two factors. First, by serving as a baseline examination, detection of change is possible. Second, a measure of the relative acuity or chronicity of an observation is possible, an invaluable aid in the development of a differential diagnosis.
   2. When abnormalities are detected, old films should be obtained for comparison whenever possible. Costs are minimized by reducing the need for additional imaging, and quality of care is improved by an expedited evaluation.
D. **Portable chest radiograph**
   1. After conventional chest radiographs, portable anteroposterior chest radiographs are the next most frequent radiographic examination of the chest. Unlike a typical PA and lateral chest x-ray, no commonly accepted standards or techniques are available for performing portable chest radiographs. As a result, the quality and reproducibility of a portable chest x-ray are extremely variable. The repeat rates for portable chest radiographs are from two to four times greater than for conventional radiographs. Portable chest x-rays are often obtained on the sickest and medically most unstable patients. The variabilities of exposure, penetration, and positioning make interpretation of portable chest x-rays more difficult. Standard protocols that maximize consistent and reproducible high-quality portable films should be used.
   2. The most commonly employed portable chest x-ray technique uses manually

selected low kV and exposure times, without a grid. This technique results in portable films of relatively high contrast that are often degraded by scatter radiation. The mediastinal structures or lung parenchyma may not be optimally visualized because the films are either under- or overexposed. Overexposure may be done intentionally to improve visualization of a monitoring line or tube. However, this is an unnecessary practice that contributes to poor overall film quality.

   3.   Portable chest x-rays should be obtained using a fixed high-kV technique (approximately 110 kv) with a grid and phototiming. Phototiming devices are not available in many hospitals, and manually selected exposure times are required. This protocol is preferred because portable films can be produced that consistently approximate the quality of a conventional chest x-ray. An important added benefit is decreased radiation exposure to the patient and surrounding personnel. The decrease in exposure time more than compensates for the higher kV used.

E.   **Decubitus films** can delineate the presence and quantity of a free-flowing pleural effusion prior to performance of a diagnostic or therapeutic thoracentesis. Views are obtained with the patient lying recumbent; both hemithoraces should be alternately visualized in the dependent position. An important advantage of obtaining bilateral decubitus views is that as fluid shifts, the underlying lung parenchyma can more adequately be evaluated for potential abnormalities that might have been hidden by the pleural fluid and associated compressive atelectasis. In unusual circumstances, a decubitus view of the chest can demonstrate a tiny pneumothorax not necessarily seen on a expiratory upright chest film.

F.   **Oblique films**

   1.   Oblique films of the chest are obtained by rotating the patient with respect to the film to ascertain whether an opacity in the lung represents a parenchymal abnormality rather than an overlap of bronchovascular markings or an abnormality originating in the ribs. These views are usually requested by a radiologist when the level of suspicion is not particularly high that an abnormality seen on a chest x-ray represents a true parenchymal abnormality or when the availability of a CT scan is limited.

   2.   Oblique chest radiographs have been used to improve the identification, documentation, and characterization of pleural abnormalities, such as pleural plaques. This function has largely been replaced by CT scanning. With the availability of chest CT, diagnostic ultrasound, and MR imaging, the indications and use of oblique films are limited.

   3.   Rib films, also obtained with the patient positioned obliquely with respect to the film, differ from oblique chest films in that radiographic techniques used for a rib series are designed to improve identification of bone abnormalities such as fractures and metastatic disease at the expense of visualization of lung parenchyma.

G.   **Apical lordotic films**, obtained with patient standing erect and the x-ray angled 15° cephalad of the chest, are of limited use. These views, along with apical kyphotic views, had been used to improve visualization of lung apices, thoracic inlet, and superior mediastinum. However, apical lordotic views rarely provide sufficient additional information to arrive at a diagnosis that is not available using conventional radiographs. Questionable thoracic inlet or mediastinal abnormalities that previously were evaluated by apical lordotic views should be imaged with chest CT or MR scans.

H.   **Chest fluoroscopy**

   1.   The use of chest fluoroscopy has declined in the evaluation of thoracic abnormalities because of chest CT scanning. Unlike routine chest radiography, fluoroscopy of the chest is usually performed with around 70 kV. The low-kV technique enhances the ability to detect calcium within a thoracic lesion.

   2.   Current indications for chest fluoroscopy include:

      a.   Diagnosis of diaphragmatic paralysis.

      b.   Distinguishing between a possible rib or pleural abnormality and a parenchymal lung abnormality (pleural plaques versus a pleural-associated small parenchymal lung nodule).

    c. Guiding needle placement during invasive procedures involving the chest (percutaneous needle biopsies of lung, pleural, rib, and mediastinal masses and percutaneous drainage of fluid collections within the chest).

    d. Guiding and assuring correct positioning of a bronchoscope and needle prior to transbronchoscopic biopsy.

  I. **Digital chest radiography.** The ability to acquire and display radiographs including chest films in a digital format should improve efficiency and decrease radiation exposure to patients and medical personnel (12-15).

III. **Computed tomography of the chest.** CT scans have two very significant advantages over routine chest radiographs: superior contrast sensitivity to help differentiate among fat, water, air, and calcium; and the ability to display cross-sectional anatomy and thereby eliminate superimposing adjacent anatomic structures. Although images are usually obtained and displayed in a transverse fashion, multiplanar displays now allow sagittal and/or coronal reconstructions. With the advent of spiral CT scans, three-dimensional displays and holography may be obtained. All of these additional reconstructed display formats are designed to simplify complex anatomic relationships. Decreased spatial resolution is the one significant disadvantage of CT scanning compared to conventional chest radiography. The identification of small pulmonary nodules is easier on a chest CT scan, not because of enhanced spatial resolution but rather because of enhanced contrast sensitivity between essentially black normal lung parenchyma and the soft tissue density characteristic of pulmonary nodules, and also because relevant anatomy is displayed without superimposition of normal structures seen on chest x-ray.

  A. **Technique**

    1. CT scans are usually obtained in end-inspiratory volume with the patient lying supine. Two basic designs of commercial CT scanners are currently available. In one design, the x-ray tube and detectors rotate simultaneously around the patient; and in the other, the detector wing is stationary and the x-ray tube rotates. Either design will produce high-quality images. Routine scanning of the chest is usually done with slices 8-10 mm thick, obtained contiguously from the lung apex to include the entire lungs through the diaphragm and often the adrenal glands as well. This basic scanning protocol may be modified depending on the specific clinical problem.

    2. In general, the use of intravenous contrast material should be limited to evaluations of suspected vascular lesions (pulmonary arteriovenous malformation [AVM], pseudoaneurysm), or to whenever precise vascular anatomy is needed (invasion of a pulmonary artery by a lung neoplasm). Intravenous contrast material can also be used to resolve a central lung mass from associated lung collapse or to identify a pleural effusion as transudative versus exudative (16).

  B. **Indications**

    1. All possible indications for a chest CT are too numerous to review here. The more common indications include:

      a. Staging of common primary malignancies of the thorax (bronchogenic carcinoma, esophageal carcinoma) (17).

      b. Staging of intrathoracic lymphoma.

      c. Evaluation of suspected vascular abnormalities (AVM, venous varices, pseudoaneurysms, aneurysms with or without dissection).

      d. Evaluation of extrapulmonary processes:

        i. Pleural lesions (mesothelioma) (18) (Fig. 1-4).

        ii. Rib lesions (primary bone tumor, Ewing's sarcoma).

        iii. Pleural space processes (empyema).

        iv. Chest wall lesions.

        v. Diaphragmatic lesions (diaphragmatic hernias, congenital or post-traumatic).

      e. Detailed evaluation of hilar and mediastinal structures and of abnormalities arising from these structures, including thymic neoplasms (thymolipoma, thymoma), esophageal abnormalities (duplication cysts),

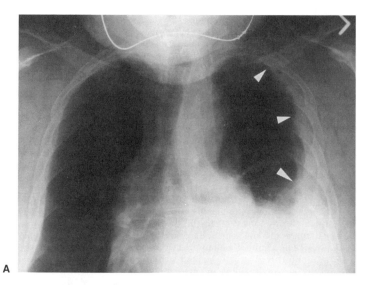

A

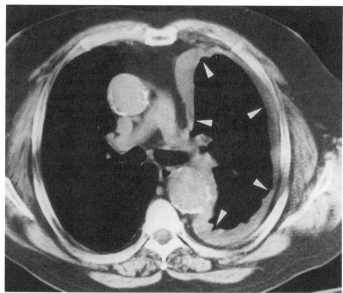

B

Fig. 1-4. A: Chest radiograph reveals a blunted costophrenic angle with a lobular configuration (*white arrow heads*) along the lateral pleural surface. This is atypical for a simple transudative pleural effusion, which would have a smooth interface between the lung and pleura and not surround the entire lung. The appearance of this film is very suggestive of a mesothelioma, which was confirmed on the chest CT scan. **B:** A single image from a chest CT scan showed an encased left lung with associated constriction of the hemithorax.

pericardial or cardiac abnormalities (pericardial effusions, pericardial cysts), tracheal neoplasms (primary squamous cell carcinoma, salivary gland tumors), mediastinal or hilar adenopathy, and neoplasms that originate in or invade the mediastinum (germ cell tumors, goiter) (19).

   f. Staging of malignant neoplasms with a propensity to metastasize to the lung such as melanoma or renal cell carcinoma.

   g. Characterizing more completely an abnormality of uncertain etiology detected on a chest CT (Fig. 1-5).

C. **High-resolution chest CT** (HRCT) scans employ a modification of the standard acquisition and display protocol to produce thin-section (1.0-1.5 mm) cuts that enhance spatial resolution of lung parenchyma with sharper-edge enhanced images and shorter scan times (20-25).

   1. HRCT can detect abnormal lung when the chest x-ray and conventional CT scan are both normal. **This modality is used in the evaluation of early interstitial lung disease;** active disease is characterized by ground-glass opacities and interstitial or air-space nodules, and inactive disease by scarring. Areas of lung deemed active by HRCT can be biopsied or followed as a marker during therapy.

   2. Certain specific diagnoses may be made by HRCT without need for biopsy of a parenchymal abnormality in the appropriate clinical setting. The entities most confidently diagnosed include lymphangiomyomatosis, histiocytosis X, lymphangitic carcinomatosis, sarcoidosis, silicosis, and idiopathic pulmonary fibrosis.

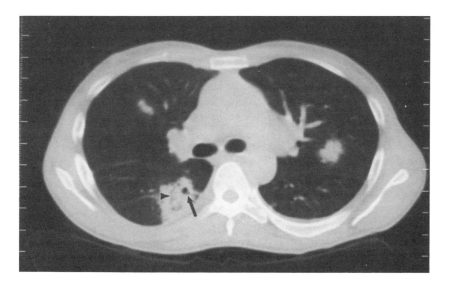

Fig. 1-5. Chest CT scan reveals three poorly defined nodular infiltrates. In one of the nodular opacities, air bronchograms (*black arrow head*) and cavitation (*black arrow*) are visible. The differential diagnosis includes diverse clinical conditions such as non-Hodgkin's lymphoma, bronchoalveolar cell carcinoma, and Wegener's granulomatosis. With the appropriate clinical history, for example, a patient with fever and a new systolic murmur, then the differential diagnosis is narrowed to septic emboli.

D. **Helical CT scanning** is an important recent technologic innovation in which the patient is continuously fed through the scanner gantry as the x-rays are being taken. This technique generates volumetric information that can be displaced in a conventional axial plane or in a variety of orthogonal planes (26,27).

   1. Helical CT offers three significant advantages over conventional scans. First, scan times are reduced to 30-60 seconds, effectively increasing productivity. Second, less intravenous contrast is required to achieve high-quality scans, and misregistration artifacts are significantly reduced. Third, multiplanar reformation is possible with less degradation of the image.

   2. Clinically, detection and quantification of **suspected pulmonary nodules** is enhanced over conventional CT scan. **Vascular imaging** is vastly improved so that helical CT can replace angiography in the evaluation of aortic dissection and trauma and may eventually replace coronary angiography and pulmonary arteriography. Multiplanar reformatting capabilities have been used to display complex mediastinal and tracheobronchial anatomy (28).

IV. **Nuclear imaging of the thorax.** Nuclear imaging of the thorax is performed for a variety of clinical indications. By far the most common indication is to evaluate a patient with suspected pulmonary embolus.

   A. **Technique**

   1. A radionuclide, usually coupled to a pharmaceutical, is administered intravenously. Technetium Tc 99m is the most commonly used radionuclide in diagnostic imaging because it has no particulate emission, a relatively short half-life (6 hours), and emits almost entirely 40-keV photons. This makes it a relatively ideal nuclear medicine imaging agent.

   2. After administration, the relevant organ or organs are imaged with a gamma camera. The gamma camera measures the number of photons emitted by the radionuclide and displays these counts as dots, with the intensity of the display proportional to the amount of activity.

   3. The choice of the particular radionuclide or radiopharmaceutical to be used is guided by its pharmacology. For example, the radionuclide xenon Xe 133 gas is used almost exclusively for lung ventilation studies, while the radiopharmaceutical agent Tc 99m macroaggregated albumin (Tc 99m MAA) is used to detect pulmonary emboli and right-to-left shunting.

   B. **Indications**

   1. The most common and important use of nuclear imaging is in the workup of a suspected pulmonary embolus (ventilation-perfusion [V/Q] scans).

   a. A radionuclide is inhaled, and a radiopharmaceutical agent is injected intravenously so as to simultaneously assess both pulmonary ventilation and perfusion. The most commonly used radiopharmaceutical in a ventilation examination is xenon Xe 133 gas. Images obtained during inhalation, steady-state breathing, and exhalation provide information about regional and overall dynamics of the ventilation.

   i. Radiolabeled aerosols are sometimes used instead of radioactive gases. Studies using these radioactive aerosols are technically more difficult to perform and may not detect small ventilation defects, but they provide the important advantage of ease in obtaining images in views corresponding to the perfusion abnormalities.

   ii. Perfusion is assessed using a radiolabeled pharmaceutical, usually Tc 99m MAA. The majority of the particles are in the 10-30-µm range and after injection mix in the right atrium and ventricle. The particles then enter the pulmonary circulation and become trapped in the pulmonary capillary vascular bed. Due to the relatively small numbers of particles compared to the number of pulmonary capillaries, functional vascular obstruction does not occur. Nevertheless, in patients with known pulmonary hypertension or suspected right-to-left shunts, the quantity of Tc 99m MAA injected is usually reduced.

   b. Images from the ventilation and perfusion portions of the examination are interpreted using criteria and guidelines developed from the Prospective Investigation of Pulmonary Embolus Diagnosis (PIOPED) study. Small but important modifications and refinements to the criteria have recently been made (29-32).

   i. The size and number of matched and mismatched defects, as well as concurrent chest x-ray, are assessed in order to determine the relative probability of pulmonary embolus. Scans are rated as either high, intermediate, low, or very low probability, or normal. In revised PIOPED criteria, four categories have arbitrarily been assigned numerical values: high (80% to 100%), intermediate (20% to 79%), low (<19%), and normal, respectively.

  ii. The classic nuclear imaging characteristic of pulmonary embolus is a high-probability V/Q scan (normal ventilation scan with multiple peripheral perfusion defects corresponding to lobar or segmental anatomy). High-probability V/Q scans have a specificity for pulmonary embolus of approximately 97%.

 iii. Although the specificity of a V/Q scan is high, the sensitivity is low. Only about 41% of the patients demonstrated to have pulmonary embolus by angiography also had a high-probability V/Q scan. Angiography studies have shown that a clinically high suspicion for pulmonary embolus and a high probability on V/Q scan strongly correlate with the presence of pulmonary embolus, and likewise a clinically low suspicion of pulmonary embolus and a low-probability V/Q scan correlate strongly with the absence of pulmonary embolus.

  2. **Perfusion lung scans** are also used preoperatively to estimate the amount of remaining lung function in patients with poor lung function prior to lobectomy or pneumonectomy (see chapter 2) and to detect and quantify right-to-left shunting (hepatopulmonary syndrome). To document right-to-left shunting, images of the brain or kidney are usually obtained to identify the abnormal location of radioactivity and document the arteriovenous shunt. By measuring the amount of activity in these organs and the amount of activity trapped in the lungs, the percentage of shunting can be calculated (33).

  3. **Nuclear imaging is also used to evaluate occult or suspected pulmonary infection, to assess hilar and mediastinal adenopathy secondary to metastatic disease or lymphoma, and to detect inflammation in the lung parenchyma secondary to adverse drug reactions or alveolitis.**

     a. Gallium citrate Ga 67 is used to detect lung injury from drugs such as bleomycin prior to any abnormality on chest x-ray, occult lymphoma in mediastinal lymph nodes of normal size on CT, and occult infections affecting the interstitium, such as pneumocystis. Gallium has also been used in conjunction with angiotension-converting enzyme (ACE) levels to estimate the activity of sarcoidosis in the lung (34).

     b. Gallium Ga 67 and thallium-201 scans in combination have been shown to be extremely useful in distinguishing among Kaposi's sarcoma, mycobacterial infection, and lymphoma. This is a common problem in patients with the acquired immune deficiency syndrome (AIDS). Matched patterns of uptake on gallium and thallium scans indicate a non-Hodgkin's lymphoma, while a gallium-negative and thallium-positive pattern indicates Kaposi's sarcoma. Finally, a gallium-positive and thallium-negative scan is very suspicious for mycobacterial infection, although other granulomatous infections such as cryptococcosis, histoplasmosis, or coccidioidomycosis cannot be completely ruled out (35).

V. **Angiography.** Angiography is the least common of the radiographic studies employed to investigate chest abnormalities. Nevertheless, angiography is an important diagnostic and potentially therapeutic tool used in the evaluation of specific pulmonary abnormalities.

  A. **Technique**

     1. Access to the arterial or venous system is gained by catheterization using the Seldinger technique or one of its variations, either in the groin or in the upper extremity. Contrast material is injected into the vascular system via a catheter, and rapid-sequence films are obtained. Angiography is associated with minor and major complications that may be divided into systemic, local, and catheter-related occurrences. Complication rates are low.

  a. Systemic complications include the development of contrast-induced nephropathy or severe allergic reaction with cardiovascular collapse.

  b. Examples of local, puncture-site related complications are development of a groin hematoma or pseudoaneurysm.

  c. Examples of catheter-related complications are distal embolization or intimal dissection.

2. Before any interventional procedure is undertaken, the relative benefits versus risks need to be clearly understood by the radiologist, the referring clinician, and the patient. To prevent complications and assess risk, a complete history should be taken (diabetes, contrast allergy, previous bleeding diatheses), and the coagulation status (platelet count, prothrombin time, partial thromboplastin time) and the serum creatinine should be determined.

B. Indications

1. Pulmonary arteriography is the most common angiographic procedure involving the thorax and is usually performed to rule out pulmonary embolus. Other indications for pulmonary angiography include assessing chronic thromboembolic disease as a suspected cause of pulmonary hypertension and evaluation of small pulmonary AVMs. Large malformations are more easily diagnosed using contrast-enhanced chest CT.

2. In the workup of pulmonary embolus, pulmonary arteriography is almost always preceded by a nuclear medicine V/Q scan. If the scan is abnormal, findings can be used to guide the catheterization of the pulmonary arteries. If the V/Q scan demonstrates a segmental defect in the left lower lobe, then the left lower lobe pulmonary artery is catheterized first to expedite the diagnosis of pulmonary embolus and obviate the need for additional angiographic runs. However, a negative study of the left lower lobe pulmonary artery does not in turn obviate the need to image the entire pulmonary artery system. Documented pulmonary embolus by angiography does not necessarily correspond to defects observed on a V/Q scan.

  a. The classic angiographic findings with pulmonary embolus include intraluminal filling defects and abrupt arterial cutoffs (Fig. 1-6). Since intraluminal clot begins to dissolve after 24 hours and 80% of the clot has lysed by 7 days, pulmonary arteriography should be performed as close in time to the suspected clinical event as possible.

  b. Elevated pulmonary artery pressure and left bundle branch block are relative contraindications to pulmonary arteriography. An increase in mortality (<0.5%) is associated with right ventricular end-diastolic pressures greater than 20 mm Hg, and a left bundle branch block may progress to complete heart block during the procedure. These relative contraindications can be addressed by modifying the angiographic technique and placing a temporary transvenous pacing wire.

3. Angiography is also used in the evaluation of the systemic circulation, the thoracic aorta (thoracic aortography), and the bronchial circulation (Fig. 1-7). The indications for thoracic aortography vary from institution to institution; at the present time, CT and MR scanning have begun to replace thoracic aortography. These diagnostic techniques have the particular advantage of being noninvasive, less labor intensive, and more cost effective.

  a. Thoracic aortography is performed in the evaluation of three possibilities: thoracic aortic aneurysm, thoracic aortic dissection, and traumatic injury to the thoracic aorta.

  b. Bronchoarterial arteriography is usually performed to identify the site of bronchial artery bleeding in patients with life-threatening hemoptysis from a known etiology who cannot undergo surgical resection (Fig. 1-8). After identification of the bleeding site, the vessel is embolized. Bronchi-

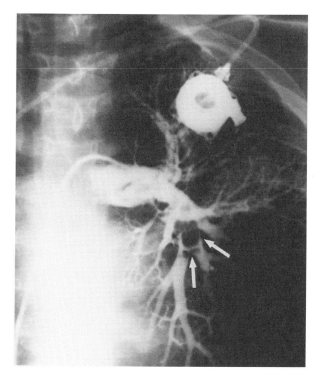

Fig. 1-6. Pulmonary arteriogram illustrates multiple pulmonary emboli. A large filling defect (clot) (*white arrows*) is depicted in the left lower lobe pulmonary artery. Anticoagulation therapy does not immediately take effect in preventing additional emboli. Fibrinolytic therapy has limited indications in the treatment of pulmonary embolus.

ectasis, aspergillosis, or cystic fibrosis are the most frequent etiologies of this type of hemoptysis.

4. **Venography** of the central veins in the chest, such as the superior vena cava, left and right innominate veins, or the azygos vein, is performed rarely. Patients with problems related to thrombosis of these vessels due to mediastinal neoplasm, mediastinitis, or iatrogenic instrumentation are more easily diagnosed noninvasively with either a CT, MR, or ultrasound examination. Occasionally, vascular stents have been deployed in the treatment of superior vena cava syndrome.

VI. **Magnetic Resonance imaging.** This relatively new imaging technique produces images without the use of ionizing radiation. In an MR image, each voxel is a gray-scale representation of the relative intensity of a radio-wave signal emanating from tissue that has been perturbed by a characteristic radiofrequency (RF) pulse. The radio-wave signal emanating from each tissue is dependent on several factors, the most important of which is time. T1 and T2 relaxation times originate from this principle. Cardiac gating and respiratory-motion suppression are essential components in producing diagnostic-quality images. At this time, poor spatial resolution, respiratory motion, and the lack of sufficient hydrogen protons in lung makes MR imaging of the lung parenchyma impractical for most indications.

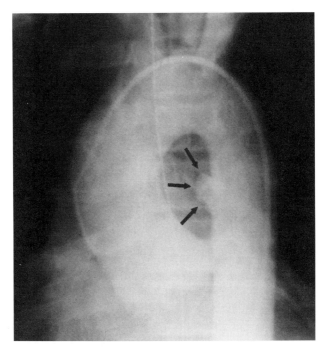

Fig. 1-7. Thoracic aortogram demonstrates an abnormal collection of contrast (*black arrows*) outside the normal wall of the descending thoracic aorta at the level of the ligament of the ductus arteriosus, diagnostic of an aortic laceration. Aortic lacerations are almost always associated with a deceleration injury, especially in automobile accidents.

A. Advantages

1. While the information in CT scans is acquired in a transverse plane through the chest, MR scans are capable of imaging the chest in any plane. Another advantage of MR imaging over CT is the ability to identify vascular structures without the use of intravenous iodinated contrast. Gadolinium-based contrast agents have a better safety profile than iodinated contrast and can be used to further delineate vascular structures. Although neither CT nor MR scanning can detect neoplastic invasion of tissues at the microscopic level, the superior contrast resolution of MR offers an advantage in the diagnosis of subtle invasion of fat or soft tissues.

2. Current applications of MR imaging include evaluation of both central venous and central pulmonary vasculature. Suspected superior vena cava syndrome, either from malignancy or mediastinitis, is easily imaged and diagnosed with MR scanning. Suspected invasion of pulmonary arteries or even the heart by a large central mass is also easily studied. Thoracic aneurysms and pseudo-aneurysms, as well as aortic dissections, are readily identified on MR scans (Fig. 1-9A,B). Mediastinal masses originating from any compartment may be imaged (36,37).

3. The ability to study anatomic structures in sagittal or coronal planes and the excellent contrast resolution make MR imaging the modality of choice when investigating abnormalities related to the diaphragm, lung apex, chest wall,

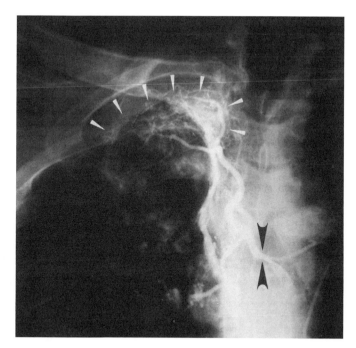

Fig. 1-8. Bronchial arteriogram in a patient with life-threatening hemoptysis from a right upper lobe aspergilloma shows cannulation of the artery (*black arrowheads*) just prior to embolization. Abnormal neovasculature (*white arrow heads*) is shown.

and mediastinum (Fig. 1-10). Diaphragmatic abnormalities, such as post-traumatic or congenital hernias, are displayed to advantage. Similarly, abnormalities originating within the lung apex, such as a superior sulcus neoplasm, are optimally staged with an MR scan as confined to the thorax or invading the brachial plexus. Chest-wall or mediastinal masses originating in any compartment are also easily imaged and studied.

4. MR is also extremely useful in evaluating perihilar and pericardial abnormalities (38-40). However, it is presently only used as an adjunct to CT scanning in evaluation of nonvascular abnormalities of the mediastinum and hilar regions, primarily because of expense. Unfortunately, MR signal characteristics cannot reliably distinguish between benign and malignant adenopathy in patients with lung carcinoma. However, residual fibrosis and active disease can be distinguished following radiation therapy for lymphoma. Likewise, MR imaging is capable of distinguishing between rebound thymic hyperplasia and recurrent disease (41-43).

VII. **Interventional procedures. Interventional procedures of the chest that require imaging guidance and are nonangiographic** fall into two general categories: percutaneous biopsy (parenchymal lesions, mediastinal mass, pleural abnormalities) using either a skinny or cutting needle, and percutaneous aspirations and/or drainage of fluid collections located within the pleural space or lung parenchyma and the mediastinum. Imaging guidance for interventional procedures is provided by fluoroscopy, CT, or ultrasound. The choice of imaging guidance depends on availability, expertise, and experience of the operator.

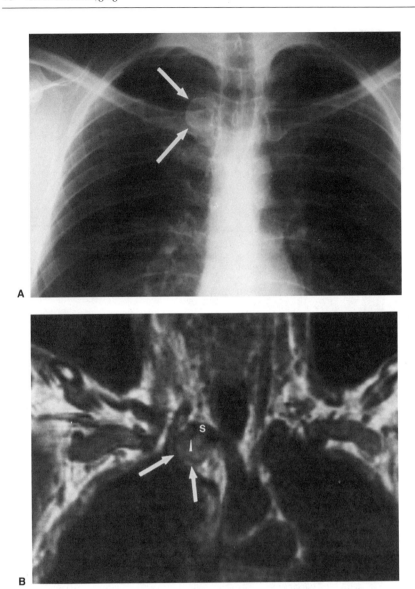

Fig. 1-9. A: Chest radiograph demonstrates a 2-cm, peripherally calcified mass in a right para-tracheal location. A vascular origin should be suspected in any chest lesion with peripheral curvilinear calcification. **B:** Coronal MR image displays a pseudoaneurysm (*white arrows*) of the right subclavian artery (S) (*white arrow head*) in a patient with a remote history of a pene-trating knife wound.

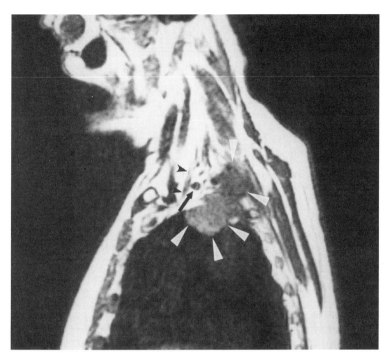

Fig. 1-10. A superior sulcus neoplasm (*white arrow heads*) extending through the parietal pleura into the supraclavicular fossa is depicted on a sagittal MR image. The cancer spares the subclavian artery (*black arrow*) and brachial plexus, immediately cephalad to the artery.

A. **Complications**
   1. Significant intrapulmonic hemorrhage is an avoidable complication associated with interventional procedures. If adequately functioning platelets are greater than 75,000 and the INR less than 1.4, then the risk of significant hemorrhage is greatly reduced. Patients with known bleeding disorders or abnormal coagulation parameters require a detailed hemostatic evaluation to avoid morbidity associated with these procedures. In addition, the needle route should be chosen to avoid larger vessels such as the internal mammary, intercostal, central hilar, and mediastinal vessels. Significant morbidity has occurred when these vessels have been punctured.
   2. **Pneumothorax** is the most common complication of percutaneous biopsy of the chest, with a reported rate between 5% and 60% of all biopsies (average rate approximately 25% to 30%). Several factors increase the risk of pneumothorax (44,45).
      a. The rate of pneumothorax correlates with underlying lung disease, especially when adjacent to the biopsied lesion (emphysema), and the number of needle passes, especially when passes transgress multiple pleural surfaces (crossing a fissure when biopsying mediastinum).
      b. The percutaneous biopsy route should avoid crossing multiple pleural surfaces. Up to half of patients who experience a pneumothorax as a result of a percutaneous biopsy require chest tube drainage. A small pneu-

mothorax that does not affect hemodynamics or respiration may be treated with a small catheter and Heimlich valve. If the pneumothorax is large and affects hemodynamics and/or respiration, a large-bore chest tube should be placed.

   3. Frank hemoptysis is almost always self-limiting.

B. Percutaneous lung biopsy

   1. Percutaneous lung biosy has a relatively high safety profile and is usually performed with needles less than 19 gauge, although larger needles are required for core biopsies.

   2. The diagnostic yield for lesions that are malignant is approximately 95%. The diagnostic yield is not as high for nonmalignant lesions. The appropriate handling of a specimen is crucial in assuring an accurate diagnosis and requires cooperation between the radiology, laboratory, and clinical services. For example, malignant cytologies are more likely to be obtained from a percutaneous biopsy specimen directly prepared by the cytopathologist or pathologist. Some specimens require special handling (flow cytometry); this will necessitate special preparation of the aspirate to be successful.

C. Percutaneous drainage of fluid collections. Although large pleural effusions are usually managed without imaging guidance, percutaneous drainage of smaller pleural, parenchymal, or mediastinal fluid collections requires imaging. Small and loculated pleural effusions are most conveniently aspirated under ultrasound guidance. Uncomplicated empyemas are characterized by lack of loculations, early clinical presentation, relatively nonviscous purulent material, and the absence of a thick pleural peel, and they may be drained successfully with a percutaneously placed catheter. Postoperative or loculated empyemas or those associated with bronchopleural fistulas are less likely to be drained successfully by the percutaneous technique. Fibrinolytic agents have been introduced into the pleural space to aid in the drainage of loculated empyemas. Percutaneous drainage of lung abscesses and mediastinal abscesses has a limited role (46-48).

VIII. Approach to interpretation of radiographic studies. The approach to the interpretation of radiographic studies discussed here utilizes a series of simple but informative questions applicable to simple and sophisticated radiologic techniques and most clinical problems. The answers to these questions assist in characterizing an abnormality identified on a radiographic examination and thereby build a differential diagnosis. After a radiologic differential diagnosis has been constructed, a clinical decision can be made as to further diagnostic work-up.

A. An accurate clinical history is a critical component in the diagnostic process of identifying and characterizing an observed radiologic abnormality and developing a differential diagnosis. While a clinical history aids in the interpretation of an examination, the radiologic history (previous film) is also an important tool that improves and contributes to the accuracy of observations. For example, a clinical history of dyspnea, cough, wheezing, pedal edema, and jugular venous distention would suggest a likelihood of signs of congestive heart failure on a chest radiograph. Or a prominent hilum that might otherwise be dismissed as a normal variant will be understood as a probable mass when an old film is available that shows a change in configuration.

B. Is the abnormality old or new? A widened mediastinum on a chest radiograph has a large differential diagnosis, but knowing the chronicity or acuity of the finding will limit the differential diagnosis. A chronically widened superior mediastinum unchanged over many years suggests a benign etiology, such as mediastinal lipomatosis. A newly widened superior mediastinum suggests a more acute process, such as lymphoma or metastatic adenopathy. An acutely widened mediastinum indicates a probable mediastinal hematoma, especially with the confirmatory clinical history of a recent line placement or an automobile accident.

C. Is the abnormality solitary, multifocal, or diffuse? A solitary pulmonary nodule on chest x-ray has a vast differential diagnosis, but in a specific clinical situation as in a patient with a long smoking history and occupational exposure to asbestos, a primary lung carcinoma is very likely. However, if on a subsequent chest CT scan, this solitary pulmonary opacity is demonstrated to be one of three pulmonary nodules, the differential diagnosis is dramatically altered to suggest metastatic disease to the lung. Similarly, if a follow-up chest x-ray in 3 days demonstrates multiple nodular cavitating opacities, the differential diagnosis would change again to perhaps multiple septic emboli or cavitating granulomatous disease.

D. What is the composition (density) of an abnormality?

   1. Although the internal composition of a lesion can sometimes be determined on a chest radiograph, chest CT or MR scanning can accomplish this task more accurately and are therefore indicated for this purpose. There are five important internal tissue types that may be easily identified on CT or MR scans:

      a. Gas (cavitation)

      b. Low-density material (lipid) (Fig. 1-11)

      c. High-density material (hemorrhage)

      d. Intermediate-density material (soft tissue)

      e. Calcification.

   2. A cavitating lesion may represent a lung abscess, a cavitating carcinoma, or mycetoma. A calcified lesion might represent a calcified granuloma if located centrally, or a lung carcinoma engulfing an adjacent calcified granuloma if located eccentrically. A solitary lesion containing material of several types of density by CT suggests a hamartoma.

E. What are the shape, size, and margins of the lesion?

   1. A defect that conforms to the shape of a segment of lung on a perfusion scan has considerably more significance than the shape of a perfusion defect that is either subsegmental or round in appearance. Combining an earlier principle

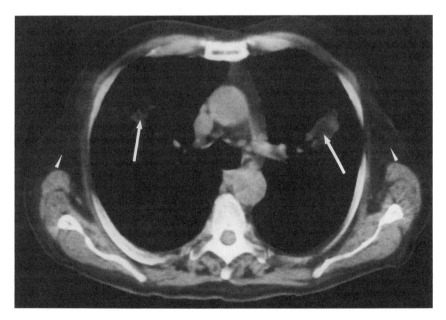

Fig. 1-11. Chest CT scan was done to further characterize abnormalities, multiple nodular fleeting infiltrates, identified on a series of chest radiographs (not shown). The chest CT shows that the internal composition of the nodular infiltrate (*white arrows*) had low attenuation similar to subcutaneous fat (*white arrow heads*) consistent with lipid pneumonitis. It is difficult to differentiate radiographically exogenous and endogenous lipid pneumonia. In this case, the lipid originated from aspirated nasal lipid drops.

(solitary vs. multiple) with the principle of shape and size, then multiple seg-mental defects on a perfusion lung scan without corresponding matches on a ventilation scan changes the interpretation of the examination to high proba-bility for pulmonary embolus.

2. Similarly, the differential diagnosis for multiple bilateral rounded opacities is vastly different depending on the size of the opacities. When the radiologic dif-ferential diagnosis is broad, the clinical history becomes very important. A fine nodular pattern on a chest radiograph in a febrile patient suggests a differ-ential diagnosis that includes fungal, tuberculous, nocardial, or viral infec-tions, whereas in an afebrile patient the differential diagnosis includes sar-coidosis, inhalational disease, metastasis, or less common entities such as eosinophilic pneumonia (Fig. 1-12).

3. It is also important to determine whether the margins of a lesion are sharply or poorly demarcated. A sharply demarcated lesion suggests encapsulation, whereas indistinct and fuzzy margins suggest a lesion that may be infiltrating into adjacent structures (Fig. 1-13A,B). For example, multiple bilateral rounded opacities with poorly defined margins on a chest x-ray suggest a differential di-agnosis that includes inflammatory, neoplastic, connective tissue, vascular, oc-cupational, iatrogenic, and idiopathic entities. Additional information, such as that the opacities wax and wane, occasionally cavitate, and are not associated with febrile episodes, restricts the differential diagnosis to etiologies such as Wegener's or lymphomatoid granulomatosis (Fig. 1-14A,B). Violation of anatomic boundaries usually suggests an aggressive process, although not necessarily a neoplasm. An abnormality located in the periphery of the lung with evidence of

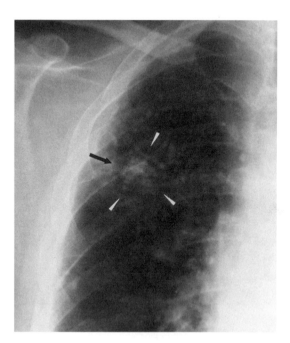

Fig. 1-12. Chest radiograph demonstrates numerous <1-cm pulmonary nodules. Some of the nodules are calcified, and in the right upper lobe the nodules (*white arrow heads*) are more confluent. This area represents a developing conglomerate mass in a patient with silicosis. Cyst formation occurs peripheral to the contracting nodules (*black arrow head*).

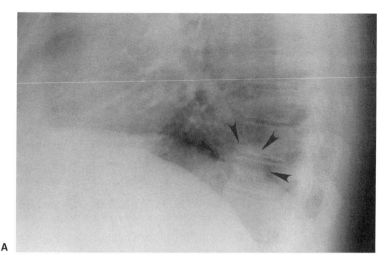

A

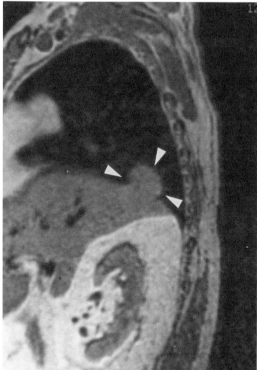

B

Fig. 1-13. A: Lateral chest radiograph demonstrates an approximately 2-cm rounded opacity (*black arrow heads*) adjacent to the right hemidiaphragm. Since the inferior margin of the lesion was silhouetted by the diaphragm, it was suspected that the abnormality originated from or below the diaphragm. **B:** Sagittal MR image of the chest shows liver herniation through the diaphragm (*white arrow heads*).

pleural reaction and rib destruction might be due to actinomycosis rather than carcinoma of the lung.

F. From what tissue does the abnormality originate?

1. Specifically, does the lesion arise from the rib or pleura, or from the lung parenchyma, or from within a mediastinal structure? The characteristics of the margin of the lesion also contain important information. For example, a peripherally situated mass forming acute angles with the pleural surface suggests that the mass originates within the lung parenchyma, whereas the same mass forming obtuse angles suggests a pleural or chest-wall origin.

2. Sometimes the anatomic location of an abnormality is easily determined from the chest radiograph, as in the case of rib destruction (implying that the abnormality is located in part in the pleural space and also in the chest wall). Imaging with CT or MR scanning is usually required to obtain this information (Fig. 1-15A,B).

3. Localizing an abnormality within a specific anatomic compartment is also extremely valuable when constructing a differential diagnosis. For example, if a mediastinal mass can be localized to the posterior mediastinum or interstitial lung disease is confined to the lung bases, then the differential diagnosis is further narrowed.

G. Communication between the primary care physician and the radiologist is of prime importance in planning a diagnostic and therapeutic work-up and in discussing the interpretation of test results. The primary care physician and radiologist should work together to organize the type and order of necessary studies to achieve the most cost-efficient plan.

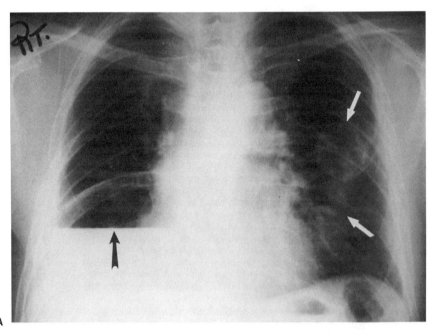

A

FIG. 1-14 A: Postoperative chest radiograph demonstrates an air fluid level (black arrow) in the right pleural space following an open lung biopsy. In the left lung, two cavitary masses *(white arrows)* are identified.

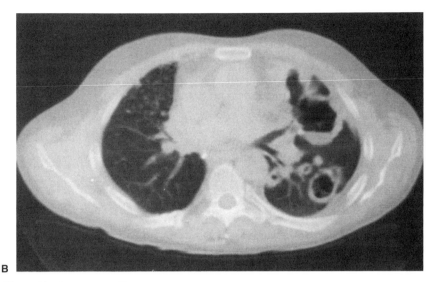

B

Fig. 1-14. *(Continued)* **B:** Chest CT demonstrates several cavitary masses. These masses, which waxed and waned over a period of months, were pathologically proven to be Wegener's granulomatosis.

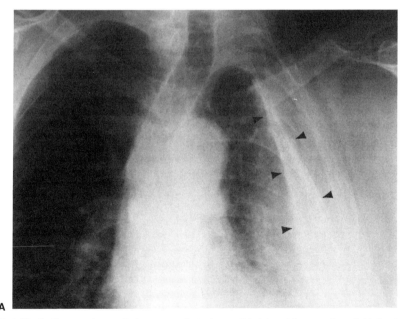

A

FIG. 1-15 A: Chest radiograph depicts a relatively small left hemithorax, pleural thickening, and extensive pleural calcification.

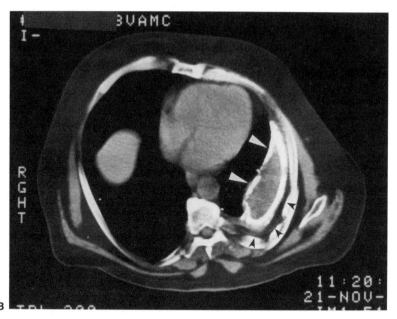

Fig. 1-15. *(Continued)* **B:** A subsequent chest CT scan reveals calcification of the visceral *(white arrow heads)* and parietal pleura surrounding a high-density pleural effusion. The apparent pleural thickening on the chest radiograph is shown to be extensive subpleural fat *(black arrow heads)*. Increased asymmetric subpleural fat associated with a pleural effusion is almost always indicative of an empyema, in this case a tuberculous empyema.

References

1. Harris JH: Referral criteria for routine screening chest x-ray examinations. *Am Coll Radiol Bull* 1982;38:17. (Report from the Chairman of the Board.)
2. Forman HP, Fox LA, Glazer HS, et al.: Chest radiography in patients with early-stage prostatic carcinoma. *Chest* 1994;106:1036–1041.
3. Rucker L, Frye EB, Staten MA: Usefulness of screening chest roentgenograms in preoperative patients. *JAMA* 1983;250:3209–3211.
4. Sagel SS, Evens RG, Forrest JV, Bramson RT: Efficacy of routine screening and lateral chest radiographs in a hospital-based population. *N Engl J Med* 1974;291:1001–1004.
5. Schneider RL, Hansen NI, Rosen MJ, et al.: Lack of usefulness of radiographic screening for pulmonary disease in asymptomatic HIV infected adults. *Arch Intern Med* 199x;156:191–195.
6. Benacerraf BR, McLoud TC, Rhea JT, et al.: An assessment of the contribution of chest radiography in outpatients with acute chest complaints: a prospective study. *Radiology* 1981;138:293–299.
7. Butcher BL, Nichol KL, Parenti CM: High yield of chest radiography in walk-in clinic patients with chest symptoms. *J Gen Intern Med* 1993;8:114–119.
8. Heckerling PS, Tape TG, Wigton RS, et al.: Clinical prediction rule for pulmonary infiltrates. *Ann Intern Med* 1990;113:664–670.
9. Jochelson MS, Altschuler J, Stomper PC: The yield of chest radiography in febrile and neutropenic patients. *Ann Intern Med* 1986;105:708–709.
10. Henschke CI, Yankelevitz DF, Wand A, et al.: Accuracy and efficacy of chest radiography in the intensive care unit. *Radiol Clin North Am* 1996;34:21–31.

11. Wandtke JC: Bedside chest radiography. *Radiology* 1994;190:1–10.
12. van Heesewijk H, Neitzel U, van der Graaf Y, et al.: Digital chest imaging with a selenium detector: comparison with conventional radiography for visualization of specific anatomic regions of the chest. *AJR* 1995;165:1635–1640.
13. Thaete FL, Fuhurman CR, Oliver JH, et al.: Digital radiography and conventional imaging of the chest: a comparison of observer performance. *AJR* 1994;575–581.
14. Frank MS, Jost RG, Molina PL, et al.: High-resolution computer display of portable, digital, chest radiographs of adults: suitability for primary interpretation. *AJR* 1993;160:473–477.
15. Correa J, Souto M, Tahoces P, et al.: Digital chest radiography: comparison of the unprocessed and processed images in the detection of solitary pulmonary nodules. *Radiology* 1995;195:253–258.
16. Acquino SL, Webb WR, Gushiken BJ: Pleural exudates and transudates: diagnosis with contrast-enhanced CT. *Radiology* 1994;192:803–808.
17. Friedman PJ: Lung cancer staging: efficacy of CT. *Radiology* 1992;182:307–309.
18. McLoud TC, Flower CDR: Imaging the pleura: sonography, CT, and MR imaging. *AJR* 1991;156:1145–1153.
19. Brown LR, Aughenbaugh GL: Masses of the anterior mediastinum: CT and MR imaging. *AJR* 1991;157:1171–1180.
20. Corcoran HL, Renner WR, Milstein MJ: Review of high-resolution CT of the lung. *RadioGraphics* 1992;12:917.
21. Muller NL: Differential diagnosis of chronic diffuse infiltrative lung disease on high-resolution computed tomography. *Semin Roentgenol* 1991;26:132–142.
22. Muller NL: Computed tomography in chronic interstitial lung disease. *Radiol Clin North Am* 1991;29:1085–1093.
23. Padley SG, Brendan A, Muller NL: High-resolution computed tomography of the chest: current indications. *J Thorac Imaging* 1993;8:189–199.
24. Bessis L, Callard P, Gotheil C, et al.: High-resolution CT of parenchymal lung disease: precise correlation with histologic findings. *RadioGraphics* 1992;12:45.
25. Webb WR: High-resolution lung computed tomography. *Radiol Clin North Am* 1991;29:1051–1063.
26. Naidich DP: Helical computed tomography of the thorax. *Radiol Clin North Am* 1994;32:759–774.
27. Touliopoulos P, Costello P: Helical (spiral) CT of the thorax. *Radiol Clin North Am* 1995;33:843–861.
28. Trerotola SO: Can helical CT replace aortography in thoracic trauma? *Radiology* 1994;197:13-15.
29. PIOPED investigators: Value of the ventilation/perfusion scan in acute pulmonary embolism. *JAMA* 1990;263:2753-2759.
30. Gottschalk A, Sostman HD, Cloeman RE, et al.: Ventilation-perfusion scintigraphy in the PIOPED study. Part II. Evaluation of the scintigraphic criteria and interpretations. *J Nucl Med* 1993;34:1119-1126.
31. Ralph DD: Pulmonary embolism. The implications of prospective investigation of pulmonary embolism diagnosis. *Radiol Clin North Am* 1994;32:679-687.
32. Worsley DF, Alvai A, Aronchick JM, et al.: Chest radiographic findings in patients with acute pulmonary embolism: observations from the PIOPED study. *Radiology* 1993;189:133-136.
33. Wernly JA, Kirchner PT, Oxford DE: Clinical value of quantitative ventilation-perfusion lung scans in the surgical management of bronchogenic carcinoma. *J Thorac Cardiovasc Surg* 1980;80:535-543.
34. Line BR: Scintigraphic studies of inflammation in diffuse lung disease. *Radiol Clin North Am* 1991;29:1095-1114.
35. Lee VW, Fuller JD, O Brien MJ, et al.: Pulmonary Kaposi sarcoma in patients with AIDS: scintigraphic diagnosis with sequential thallium and gallium scanning. *Radiology* 1991;180:409-412
36. Link KM, Samuels LJ, Reed JC, et al.: Magnetic resonance imaging of the mediastinum. *J Thorac Imaging* 1993;8:34-53.
37. Mayo JR: Magnetic resonance imaging of the chest. *Radiol Clin North Am* 1994;32:795-809.
38. Fortier M, Mayo JR, Swensen SJ, et al.: MR imaging of chest wall lesions. *RadioGraphics* 1994;14:597.
39. Kuhlman JE, Bouchardy LM, Fishman EK, Zerhouni EA: CT and MR imaging evaluation of chest wall disorders. *RadioGraphics* 1994;14:571.
40. Padovani B, Mouroux J, Seksik L, et al.: Chest wall invasion by bronchogenic carcinoma: evaluation with MR imaging. *Radiology* 1993;187:33–38.
41. Brown MJ, Miller RR, Muller NL: Acute lung disease in the immunocompromised host: CT and pathologic examination findings. *Radiology* 1994;190:247–254.

42. Grover FL: The role of CT and MRI in staging of the mediastinum. *Chest* 1994;106:391S–396S.
43. Quint LE, Francis IR, Wahl RL, et al.: Preoperative staging of non-small-cell carcinoma of the lung: imaging methods. *AJR* 1995;164:1349–1359.
44. Shepard JO: Complications of percutaneous needle aspiration biopsy of the chest. *Semin Intervent Radiol* 1994;11:181–186.
45. van Sonnenberg E, Casola G, Ho M, et al.: Difficult thoracic lesions: CT-guided biopsy experience in 150 cases. *Radiology* 1988;167:457–461.
46. Klein JS, Schultz S, Heffner JE: Interventional radiology of the chest: image-guided percutaneous drainage of pleural effusions, lung abscess, and pneumothorax. *AJR* 1995;164:581–588.
47. van Sonnenberg E, D Agostino HB, Casola G, et al.: Lung abscess: CT-guided drainage. *Radiology* 1991;178:347–351.
48. Zerbey AL, Dawson SL, Mueller PR: Pleural interventions and complications. *Semin Intervent Radiol* 1994;11:187–197.

2

Pulmonary Function Testing

Khaled Al-Asad and Joel B. Karlinsky

I. **Definition.** Pulmonary function testing involves evaluating the overall gas exchange and mechanical functions of the lung parenchyma and airways. Overall gas exchange function may be evaluated by measuring the arterial Pao_2, $Paco_2$, and pH, as well as the efficacy of gas diffusion across the lung parenchyma (diffusing capacity, conductance). The mechanical function of the lung may be evaluated by measurements of lung compartment sizes, airflows, transpulmonary pressures, and inspiratory and expiratory muscle strength.

II. **Normal physiology (1–3)**

A. The physiologic factors that determine gas flow are the mechanical properties of the lung parenchyma (elastic recoil) and the resistance of the conducting airways. The elastic recoil pressure of the lung parenchyma is defined as the difference between pleural and alveolar pressures as a function of lung volume. Airway resistance depends on the lung volume, the contractility of bronchial smooth muscles, and the presence or absence of mucus—all factors that determine airway size.

B. Airflow equals transpulmonary pressure divided by the airway resistance. The resistance of the respiratory system is mainly due to the lobar bronchi and is about 2 cm H_2O/L/sec.

C. **Physiology of normal breathing**

1. At the end of expiration, the pleural pressure is negative (-5 cm H_2O). The amount of air remaining in the lungs at this point is defined as the functional residual capacity (FRC). The FRC is set by a balance of forces, where the tendency of the lung to collapse due to elastic recoil pressure is balanced by the tendency of the chest wall to move out. With inspiration (caused by the contraction of diaphragm and intercostal muscles), the pressure in the pleural space becomes more negative, and air moves into the lung (tidal volume).

2. During expiration, the pleural pressure returns to its baseline value, alveolar pressure becomes positive, and expiratory flow occurs till FRC is again reached.

III. **Simple spirometry (3–5)**

A. **The forced vital capacity (FVC), the forced expiratory volume in 1 second (FEV_1), and the FEV_1/FVC ratio are the simplest measurements of mechanical function available.** They are measures of overall volumes that may be obtained during a forced expiratory maneuver and may be used to decide whether an individual has obstructive or restrictive lung disease. Values are generally reported as a percentage of predicted values. Predicted values have been generated from healthy nonsmoking populations and are based on height and age (5).

1. **Obstructive lung disease** is likely if both the FVC and FEV_1 are reduced to levels <80% predicted, along with an FEV_1/FVC ratio that is <75% predicted. In obstructive lung disease, airway resistance is increased so that the FEV_1 is reduced out of proportion to reductions in FVC.

2. **Restrictive lung disease** is likely if both the FVC and FEV_1 are reduced to levels <80% predicted, but the FEV_1/FVC ratio is normal.

B. The **$FEF_{25\%-75\%}$**, the volume delivered between 25% and 75% of the FVC, is often reported as part of simple spirometric testing. This number is also reported as a percentage of a predicted value and is reduced if small-airways disease is present. It is more sensitive to small-airways disease than is the FEV_1, which is highly dependent on the resistance associated with large central airways.

C. **Flow-volume loops** are also often reported as part of simple spirometric testing. These curves contain little additional information over that contained in the FVC, FEV_1, and FEV_1/FVC ratio measurements; the shape of the expiratory limb of the curves may be characteristic of obstructive or restrictive disease. An additional value of the flow-volume loop lies in its ability to detect patient-induced artifacts caused by improper inspiratory and/or expiratory maneuvers, such as coughing during expiration.

   1. **Obstructive expiratory flow-volume curves** are coved with respect to the x (volume) axis, and the vital capacity is reduced.
   2. **Restrictive expiratory flow-volume curves** appear compressed relative to normal curves, and the vital capacity is also reduced.
   3. The shape of the flow-volume curve and values of flows in inspiration and expiration can be used to make a presumptive diagnosis of upper airway obstruction (6). A flat expiratory limb in association with a reduced peak flow and normal inspiratory limb is suggestive of an intrathoracic airway obstruction, as might occur with an intratracheal neoplasm. A flat inspiratory limb in association with reduced inspiratory flow is suggestive of an extrathoracic obstruction, as might be seen with a vocal cord neoplasm. Patients with these disorders will usually have a consistent history and additional work-up will be required.

D. Increases in FVC, FEV_1, and FEV_1/FVC ratio >20% after two inhalations of bronchodilator is good evidence that reversible bronchoconstriction is present and is consistent with a diagnosis of asthma.

E. **Bronchoprovocation testing** may be performed to help diagnose general and specific bronchial hyperreactivity; these tests must be performed in a laboratory experienced with the techniques (7). They are performed by exposing individuals to increasing doses of inhaled methacholine (general hyperreactivity) or histamine or to specific antigens or chemicals (toluene diisocyanate) and measuring the dose at which airway resistance increases and flows decrease (FEV_1). Measurements are made every 3–5 minutes after the inhalation. The results are compared to flow decrements noted after inhalational challenges of saline. Generally, a 20% to 30% decrement in flow at a dose of <0.1 µmol should occur for a test to be positive. The position of the dose–response curve is useful in determining the severity of the hyperreactivity. These responses are somewhat nonspecific in that patients without symptoms of asthma will respond to methacholine by decreasing flow. The test should be interpreted with caution. Crash carts should be available in case of anaphylaxis. Patients being considered for bronchoprovocation testing should be seen by a pulmonologist or allergist/immunologist.

F. **Outpatient peak-flow monitoring.** The outpatient treatment of patients with asthma is based on self-monitoring of peak flow using hand-held devices that patients are taught to use. The usual best value must be determined as a baseline from which lower values will determine treatment. The peak-flow measurement is effort dependent and is the highest value reached on a maximum expiration.

IV. **Lung volumes and diffusing capacity (3,8).** Measurement of lung volumes and lung diffusing capacity can be used to confirm a diagnosis of lung obstruction or restriction, if questions remain after simple spirometry has been performed. Volume measurements are also useful in detecting the deleterious effects on normal lung parenchyma of certain medications (chemotherapeutic agents) or in monitoring the beneficial effects of agents being used to treat lung diseases. The usual methods used for measuring lung volumes include helium dilution, nitrogen washout, and body plethysmography. Most pulmonary function laboratories employ computerized equipment that is capable of making simple spirometric, lung volume, and diffusing-capacity measurements and providing a computer-generated interpretation (see Table 2-1 for definitions of impairment).

A. **Lung volumes**
   1. The volume of air that is exchanged in normal quiet breathing is the tidal volume (TV), which is approximately 500 mL of air (dead space, 150 mL; alveolar

Table 2-1. Definitions of impairment

	VC (%pre)	FEV_1 (%pre)	FEV_1/FVC (%)	TLC (%pre)	D_LCO (%pre)
Normal	>80	>80	>70	>80	>80
Impairment					
Mild	60–80	60–80	55–70	60–80	60–80
Moderate	50–60	50–60	40–55	50–60	35–60
Severe	<50	<50	<40	<50	<35

VC =vital capacity; FEV_1 =forced expiratory volume in 1 sec; FVC =forced vital capacity; TLC =total lung capacity; D_LCO =diffusing capacity for carbon monoxide.

volume, 350 mL). TV is loosely but directly related to body weight (TV = 5–7 mL/kg during spontaneous breathing). Minute ventilation is TV multiplied by the respiratory rate over 1 minute. The inspiratory reserve volume (IRV) is the lung volume at the peak of maximum inspiratory effort minus the peak point of TV. The expiratory reserve volume (ERV) is the volume exhaled with further maximum expiratory effort after end-tidal volume. The residual volume (RV) is the volume remaining in the lung after subtraction of the ERV from the FRC; it is an indirect measurement. The FRC is usually measured by helium dilution and the ERV by having the patient make a further forced expiratory effort from FRC.

2. **Lung capacities** are also reported as part of these tests:
   a. Total lung capacity (TLC).
   b. Vital capacity (VC).
   c. Inspiratory capacity (IC).
   d. Functional residual capacity (FRC).
3. In lung obstruction, VC may be normal but will often be reduced; the RV and RV/TLC ratio will be significantly increased (>0.45) as a result of air trapping due to the increased airway resistance. In patients with bullous emphysema, the FRC should be measured by both the helium dilution and body plethysmographic techniques. The latter technique measures the volume of all gas within the thorax at FRC; the former technique measures the volume of all gas in communication with the mouth at FRC. The volume of gas within noncommunicating bullae may be estimated by subtracting the former from the latter measurement.
4. In lung restriction, all lung volumes will be reduced as a percentage of the predicted values by about the same amount. The TLC is most often reduced.
5. Certain diseases are characterized by both obstructive and restrictive features. These conditions include sarcoidosis, lymphangiomyomatosis, and eosinophilic granuloma.

B. **Diffusing capacity** is a measure of the conductance of the alveolar-capillary membrane for the test gas, which almost always is carbon monoxide. This gas is used because its partial pressure in blood is zero due to its high affinity for hemoglobin, whereas Po_2 in the pulmonary capillaries varies. The diffusing capacity (D_L) for carbon monoxide (D_LCO) is the amount of carbon monoxide (mL/min/mm Hg driving pressure) that diffuses across the alveolar-capillary membrane. The technique most often used is the single-breath test, requiring a 10-second breath hold. The gas used is a mixture of 0.3% carbon monoxide, 10% helium, 21% oxygen, and the balance nitrogen. Patients with severe chronic obstructive pulmonary disease (COPD) cannot hold their breath for the required 10 seconds, and the test results are not reliable. The D_LCO is dependent on age, body size, lung volume, hemoglobin concentration, the presence of carboxyhemoglobin, and changing body position.
   1. The D_LCO is reduced in diseases that affect the interstitium of the lung because the alveolar-capillary membrane is reduced in total area and/or because

the thickness of the membrane increases. The test is more sensitive to mild interstitial lung disease than are measurements of lung volumes, making the test useful for confirming the diagnosis and following the progression of disease on or off therapy.

2. The D_LCO is reduced in patients with alveolar wall destruction from any cause (emphysema) and helps to confirm this diagnosis in an individual with the appropriate clinical history, physical and chest radiographic findings, and other pulmonary function abnormalities (obstructive function tests). The D_LCO is also reduced by disease processes that affect the vasculature (pulmonary emboli).

3. **This test is very sensitive and is often the first measurable functional indication of lung disease.** It may be followed in patients with interstitial lung disease on therapy to demonstrate improvement (or lack of improvement) or in patients who are to receive bleomycin chemotherapy to confirm that lung disease has not developed. Patients must be able to breath-hold for 10 seconds.

V. Tests of respiratory muscle function (9)

A. **Pimax.** This test measures the strength of diaphragmatic contraction. It is performed by having the subject inhale to TLC and perform a forced expiration to RV and then by measuring the pressure developed at the mouth while inspiring against an occluded valve. Healthy subjects will generate a pressure >-60 cm H_2O; patients with diaphragmatic impairment will generate pressures in the -20 to -60-cm H_2O range. The pressure generated also depends on sex, age, height, and weight.

B. **Pemax.** This test measures the strength of the muscles of expiration and is performed by having the subject inspire from RV to TLC and then measuring the pressure developed at the mouth while a forced expiration is performed against an occluded valve. The same factors affecting Pimax also affect PEmax, and it is abnormal in patients with decreased diaphragm and accessory muscle strength from any cause (hypothyroidism).

C. **Transdiaphragmatic pressure (Pdi$_{max}$)** measurement is the definitive technique used to assess diaphragmatic function. The technique is invasive and necessitates the placement of an intraesophageal balloon to measure pleural pressure and the simultaneous placement of a gastric balloon to measure intra-abdominal pressure. The difference between these pressures is the Pdi. The measurement is usually made at FRC. If the diaphragm is not contracting normally, as might occur in phrenic nerve injuries or in several rare muscle disorders (eg, phosphorylase deficiency), then the Pdi$_{max}$ will be close to zero.

1. **The Pdi/Pdi$_{max}$** ratio as a function of breathing load (breathing through exogenously added resistances) can be used to measure the endurance of the diaphragm. This is mainly a research tool.

VI. Other tests of mechanical function

A. **Maximum voluntary ventilation (MVV)** is a test of overall respiratory system endurance and is performed by asking the subject to maximally ventilate for 15 seconds. The volume produced is multiplied by 4 to obtain the liters produced over 1 minute. Normal values may be estimated by the equation $MVV = FEV_1 \times 35$. Individuals with restrictive lung disease will have a relatively normal MVV, but those with obstructive lung disease will have markedly diminished MVV (<50% predicted value). The test requires a good deal of patient cooperation; results obtained from patients who cannot follow instructions will not be interpretable.

B. **Closing volume (3)**

1. Measurement of nitrogen concentration in a sample of gas expired after a single deep inhalation of 100% oxygen yields information regarding gas distribution in the lung. Four characteristic phases are noted:

   a. Phase I—no nitrogen in the first portion of the analyzed sample, as this reflects dead space and inspired gas (first out = last in).

   b. Phase II—start of alveolar exhalation, where the percentage of nitrogen in the collected sample rapidly increases.

   c. Phase III—the "steady state" alveolar sample, where the nitrogen concentration plateaus.

   d. Phase IV—a sharp increase in nitrogen concentration from expired air located in the apical alveoli that received no oxygen during the inspiration. The lung volume at which the intersection between phase III and IV occurs is the closing volume, and it is that lung volume below which alveoli are closed.

2. Radioactive ventilatory studies have revealed the preferential ventilation of different segments of the lung depending on lung volume. From RV to FRC, the apical alveoli are ventilated more than the basilar, while from FRC to TLC the basilar alveoli are more ventilated, reflecting the differential change in the pleural pressure from basilar to apical segments at different lung volumes.

3. The closing volume increases with age, smoking, chronic obstructive lung diseases, some forms of restrictive lung disorders, neuromuscular diseases, and obesity. Some believe that an increased closing volume plays a major role in the pathogenesis of hypoxia in such diseases.

4. This test is generally not available and is rarely used because it requires special equipment. In addition, the point of closing volume is difficult to identify, especially in patients with severe COPD; it is almost never necessary to obtain this test.

C. **Static deflation volume–pressure curve (2,3)**

1. Body plethysmography and placement of an esophageal balloon are necessary to measure the deflation volume—pressure curve of the lung, from which measurements of lung compliance are derived. Lung compliance is the ratio of the change in volume to change in pressure ($\frac{\Delta V}{\Delta P}$), and normal values are between 0.12 and 0.25 L/cm H_2O elastic recoil (transpulmonary) pressure.

2. Patients with emphysema will have increased compliance (big, floppy lungs), and patients with interstitial lung disease (or any disease that fills interstitium with cells, connective tissue, or water) will have reduced compliance (small, stiff lungs).

3. Because this measurement requires construction and placement of an esophageal balloon, it is not generally performed except for research purposes. Measurements of static lung compliance are not generally useful except in intubated, ventilated patients with adult respiratory distress syndrome or pulmonary edema from cardiac causes.

VII. **Arterial blood gases.** Measurement of P_{O_2}, P_{CO_2}, and pH is the gold standard for measuring respiratory system function, because it assesses the adequacy of oxygen uptake and carbon dioxide removal.

A. **The alveolar-arterial oxygen gradient (A-a)Do_2.**

1. There is a normal difference between the alveolar and arterial (end-capillary) P_{O_2}, because every human being has a right-to-left shunt of 3% to 5%, so that about 3% to 5% of the right ventricular cardiac output does not traverse the lungs. This normal difference amounts to between 10–15 Torr (for details regarding calculations see chapters 21 and 36).

2. If the difference between PA_{O_2} and Pa_{O_2} ($PA_{O_2} - Pa_{O_2}$) exceeds 15 Torr when the patient is breathing room air, then a pulmonary disease is present that is interfering with gas exchange, even if the chest x-ray or CT scan is normal.

B. **Causes of hypoxemia**

1. Ventilation–perfusion (V/Q) mismatch (bronchitis, infections, asthma, congestive heart failure).

2. Anatomic right-to-left shunt (V/Q = 0) [atrial septal defect (ASD) pulmonary arteriovenous malformations].

3. Diffusion abnormality [interstitial lung disease, sarcoidosis, idiopathic pulmonary fibrosis (IPF)].

4. Low inspired oxygen tension (high altitude).

5. Central hypoventilation (central sleep apnea).

C. **Use of the (A-a)Do_2.** The last two causes above may be ruled out by checking the fraction of inspired oxygen (FI_{O_2}) and by measuring the (A-a)Do_2; if the gradient is normal and the P_{CO_2} is high, then the diagnosis is hypoventilation or a low inspired oxygen tension. If the (A-a)Do_2 is elevated and the P_{CO_2} is high, then pulmonary disease is present. True anatomic shunt may be ruled out by measurement of the (A-a)Do_2 and/or Pa_{O_2} while the patient is breathing 100% oxygen. If true shunt is present, then the reduction in the gradient and increases in Pao_2 will be minimal. If hypoxemia is due to V/Q mismatch, breathing 100% oxygen will result in an improved gradient and a large increase in Pao_2. Isolated diffusion abnormalities occur rarely and do not cause substantial hypoxemia except with exercise; such conditions are interstitial and will be recognized on chest radiographs.

D. Hypercapnea. When hypercapnea is present along with hypoxemia, the minute ventilation should be measured. If the minute ventilation is low, then conditions affecting respiratory center function (strokes, drug ingestions, tumors) or the primary hypoventilation syndrome (Pickwickian syndrome) are likely. Other causes of low minute ventilation include spinal cord disease, neuromuscular diseases (myasthenia gravis), or muscular disorders (muscular dystrophy). If hypercapnea is present and the minute ventilation is increased, then conditions affecting gas transport (asthma, COPD exacerbation, emphysema) need to be considered.

E. pH. The pH, the negative log of hydrogen ion concentration, is a reflection of the overall acid-base status of the body. The normal range of body pH is 7.35–7.45. Acidosis is defined as a pH <7.35, and alkalosis as a pH >7.45. The Pco_2 may be estimated by the equation $Pco_2 = 1.5 \times [HCO_3] + 8$.

1. **Acidosis**
   a. Metabolic acidosis = low serum $[HCO_3]$ and low Pco_2.
   b. Respiratory acidosis = high serum $[HCO_3]$ and high Pco_2.
2. **Alkalosis**
   a. Metabolic alkalosis = high serum $[HCO_3]$ and low Pco_2.
   b. Respiratory alkalosis = normal to high serum $[HCO_3]$ and low Pco_2.
3. To determine if the acidosis or alkalosis is acute or chronic and compensated:
   a. Acute change in pH by one point = $Pco_2 \times 0.008$.
   b. Chronic change in pH by one point = $Pco_2 \times 0.003$.
   c. For acute increases in Pco_2 of 10 points, bicarbonate increases by one mEq/L.
   d. For acute decreases in Pco_2 of 10 mm Hg, bicarbonate decreases by 2 mEq/L.
   e. For chronic increases in Pco_2 of 10 mm Hg, bicarbonate increases by 4 mEq/L.
   f. For chronic decreases in Pco_2 of 10 mm Hg, bicarbonate decreases by 5 mEq/L.

VIII. Pulmonary exercise testing (10,11)
A. Normal physiologic response to exercise
1. Muscle contraction is an active process requiring adenosine triphosphate (ATP) for the interaction between actin and myosin. Muscles are classified according to their time to peak tension following stimulation. Type I muscle fibers take a long time to reach peak tension and are known as slow-twitch fibers. Type II fibers are fast twitch, as they rapidly reach peak tension following stimulation. Type I fibers contain a large amount of myoglobin, which acts as an oxygen store and aids oxygen release; these fibers also contain high concentrations of oxidative enzymes and are rich in capillaries; they are also fatigue resistant. In contrast, type II fibers lack myoglobin and have low concentrations of oxidative enzymes and are relatively deficient in capillaries, making them fatigue susceptible. These fibers are subclassified into type IIa (fast-oxidative glycolytic), and type IIb (fast glycolytic) fibers.
2. Skeletal muscles utilize energy sources (mainly carbohydrate and fat) to form pyruvate and produce ATP. As workload increases, more oxygen will be required, placing demands on the cardiovascular system to increase cardiac output (heart rate × stroke volume) and catecholamines, leading to increases in both blood pressure and cardiac output. Ventilation and tidal volume will increase as well, and the arteriovenous oxygen content will widen. As the demand for oxygen exceeds the ability of the body to supply oxygen, the anaerobic threshold will occur (at which time three molecules of ATP/glucose will be produced rather than the 38 produced during aerobic metabolism). Lactic acid and carbon dioxide output will increase, pH will fall, and ventilation will significantly increase, if possible.
3. The normal exercise response requires a normal interaction among the circu-

latory system, the ventilatory system, and the muscular system. Ventilation will assure oxygen intake by the lung (reflecting consumption). The circulatory system will ensure the delivery of oxygen to the muscles, which will be utilized in the mitochondria to produce energy.

B. The abnormal response to exercise

   1. Abnormalities in the circulatory (oxygen delivery) system, ventilatory (oxygen consumption, carbon dioxide release) system, or muscular system will lead to suboptimal performance and early fatigue.

   2. The basic exercise test measurements listed below should be obtained. Patterns of measurements will be consistent with defects in the cardiovascular, pulmonary, or muscle systems.

C. Patients are required to exercise according to standard bicycle or treadmill protocols that provide graded increases in workload, and the following variables will be obtained as a function of time and workload.

D. Basic exercise test measurements

   1. $\dot{V}_2$ is a measure of oxygen consumption (mL/kg/min). It depends on the cardiac output, the extraction of oxygen by tissues, and the ventilatory efficiency. It cannot be used to determine the cause of exercise limitation; its maximum value ($\dot{V}o_2$max) reflects whether the patient can achieve normal aerobic function. Its relation to the work rate during exercise can be used to confirm the presence of cardiac or systemic or pulmonary vascular disease.

   2. $\dot{V}co_2$ is a measure of carbon dioxide production (mL/kg/min) and is related to the oxygen consumption (respiratory quotient) and the acid-base status (buffering of lactic acid by bicarbonate). The amount of ventilation required to clear carbon dioxide is reflected by the alveolar carbon dioxide. Knowing these values allows calculation of the dead space/tidal volume ratio (VDS), which is increased in certain diseases.

   3. **Heart rate.** The predicted maximum heart rate is calculated as $220 -$ age. The heart rate reserve (predicted maximum $-$ observed maximum) calculation is useful because it is increased due to poor effort, claudication, and angina, as well as in certain lung diseases.

   4. **Breathing reserve.** The breathing reserve is calculated as the difference between the predicted maximum voluntary ventilation and the observed maximum ventilation. Low values are observed in primary lung diseases, while high reserve is seen in cardiovascular diseases.

   5. **Anaerobic threshold (AT).** The AT is the level of $\dot{V}o_2$ at which anaerobic energy production begins to supplement aerobic production. It is characterized by an increase in lactate production and is affected by the size of the muscle exercised. The value of AT is commonly obtained from the plot of $\dot{V}o_2/\dot{V}co_2$ at the point where $\dot{V}co_2$ begins to increase at a more rapid rate. The AT is important in diagnosing the primary process leading to exercise limitation, as it is mainly affected by factors decreasing perfusion of exercising muscle.

   6. **Blood pressure before, during, and after exercise.** A drop in blood pressure during exercise can be due to coronary artery disease, intrinsic myocardial pathology (cardiomyopathy), or drugs that prevent an appropriate increase in heart rate in order to maintain cardiac output.

   7. **Respiratory quotient.**

   8. **Arterial blood gases prior to and at maximum exercise.** With exercise, the dead space (Vd) tends to decrease in healthy individuals. An increase in Vd in an otherwise normal individual unassociated with any other pulmonary function abnormalities may be due to pulmonary vascular disease.

   9. **ECG before, during, and after exercise.**

IX. Indications for pulmonary function and exercise testing (12–15) (see Table 2-2). Pulmonary function and exercise testing are used in conjunction with the clinical history and physical examination to determine whether obstructive or restrictive pulmonary disease is present, to objectively measure the degree of functional impairment associated with lung disease, and to obtain values that can be followed in patients on therapies that are designed to improve function. Specific clinical conditions in which pulmonary function and exercise testing are especially useful are discussed below. Pulmonary func-

Table 2-2. Indications for pulmonary function and exercise testing

Diagnostic	Follow-up
Evaluation of dyspnea	Defining asthma and reversibility
Defining obstructive airway physiology	Monitoring the response to therapy (sarcoidosis)
Defining restrictive lung physiology	Following the progression of disease
Preoperative assessment	Predicting prognosis
Disability evaluations	

tion standards have been developed from study of healthy individuals and are based on age and height. Predicted values normally decline with increasing age.

A. Evaluation of dyspnea. Pulmonary function testing is used as part of the work-up to determine whether dyspnea is due to diseases of the lung and/or respiratory muscles. The work-up of dyspnea generally includes evaluation of the cardiac, hematologic, metabolic, and central nervous systems, as well as of the pulmonary system. Measurements of arterial blood gases and spirometric, lung volume, and diffusing capacity should be obtained as initial tests to determine whether obstructive or restrictive lung disease is present and to quantitate the degree of impairment. If tests of mechanical function are within normal limits, further evaluation should be done to rule out pulmonary vascular or neuromuscular disease; such an evaluation might include pulmonary exercise testing and measurements of diaphragmatic strength and endurance.

B. Characterization of obstructive versus restrictive lung disease
   1. Obstructive lung diseases include COPD (components of emphysema, bronchitis, asthma), chronic bronchitis, emphysema, asthma, and bronchiolitis and its subtypes, cystic fibrosis and bronchiectasis. These conditions are characterized by decreased expiratory airflow secondary to increases in airway resistance (a preferable term is *airflow limitation,* since other causes than obstruction can decrease flow). Pulmonary function testing typically reveals reductions in airflow consistent with one of these diagnoses. Other functional parameters are variably affected by the different disease processes. Patients may become hypoxemic as a result of V/Q mismatch. Lung volumes may increase from hyperinflation. The diffusing capacity may decrease in emphysema and increase in asthma. Exercise testing may be indicated in this group of patients, if lung resectional surgery is being considered. See Table 2-3 for differential diagnoses of obstructive lung disease.
   2. Restrictive lung diseases are those in which the TLC is decreased. Restriction may be caused by infiltration of the lung by cells or water or by increases in connective tissue (collagen, elastin). There will usually be no compromise in airflow adjusted for the reductions in lung volume. Interstitial lung disease is a prototype disease producing restriction. Other causes of restrictive physiologies include obesity, neuromuscular disorders, and pleural disease. See Table 2-4 for differential diagnoses of restrictive lung disease.

Table 2-3. Differential diagnoses of obstructive lung disease

Intrapulmonic airway	Extrapulmonic airway	Parenchyma
Asthma	Upper airway tumors	Emphysema
Acute and chronic bronchitis	Aspiration of foreign body	
Bronchiectasis	Tracheal stenosis	
Mixed disorder	Other	

Table 2-4. Differential diagnoses of restrictive lung disease

Interstitial	Pleural	Chest wall	Other
Interstitial pneumonitis	Effusion	Kyphoscoliosis	Obesity
Congestive heart failure	Pneumothorax	Neuromuscular	
Occupational	Hemothorax		
Granulomatous	Fibrothorax (trapped lung)		
Fibrotic lung disease			

C. **Diagnosis of asthma.** Asthma may be diagnosed by pulmonary function testing by demonstrating increases in flow rates of 20% or more after several inhalations of bronchodilator medications (16–19).

D. **Following effect of therapies.** If patients are being treated with drugs that influence airway size (inhaled steroids or bronchodilators) or parenchymal inflammation (steroids for sarcoid or eosinophilic pneumonia), the effectiveness of therapies may be monitored by repetitive pulmonary function testing (16–19). A true baseline set of numbers is required in order to make judgments of the effectiveness of therapy.

E. **Preoperative assessment.** Pulmonary function testing is used to assess whether patients are low or high risk for resectional thoracic surgery.

F. **Indications for exercise testing.**
   1. Differentiating cardiac, pulmonary, and neuromuscular causes of dyspnea (20,21).
   2. More extensive preoperative assessment of high-risk patients being considered for potential resectional lung surgery.
   3. Early diagnosis of interstitial lung disease and pulmonary vascular disease.
   4. Determination of functional impairment.
   5. Evaluation of patients for pulmonary rehabilitation (22).
   6. Following effects of therapies.

G. **Abnormal patterns of exercise.** Generally, patients requiring pulmonary exercise testing should be evaluated by a pulmonary specialist to help with the design of the tests and the interpretation of the results. General patterns of measurements consistent with common conditions are listed in Table 2-5.

H. **Contraindications to pulmonary function and pulmonary exercise testing.**
   1. There are few contraindications to routine pulmonary function and pulmonary exercise testing. Patients must be able to understand and follow instructions. The main contraindications to routine pulmonary function testing include:
      a. Active pulmonary tuberculosis.
      b. A tracheostomy preventing a good seal.
   2. The main contraindications to pulmonary exercise testing include:
      a. Unstable or untreated coronary artery disease.

Table 2-5. Exercise test values in various diseases

Disease	$\dot{V}o_2$ max	Anaerobic threshold	Breathing reserve	V_D/V_T	$(A\text{-}a)Do_2$
Heart*	Low	Low	Increased		Increased
Pulmonary Vascular	Low	Low	Increased	Increased	Increased
COPD	Low	Undetermined	Decreased	Increased	Increased
Interstitial Lung Disease	Low	Decreased	Decreased	Increased	Increased

$\dot{V}o_2$ =oxygen consumption per unit time; V_D/V_T = ratio of dead-space volume to tidal volume; $(A\text{-}a)Do_2$ = alveolar-arterial oxygen gradient.
*In heart disease, there are usually accompanying ECG and blood pressure changes or chest pain.

    b. Rheumatologic problems (cannot walk on treadmill or ride bicycle).

    c. Active medical or pulmonary diseases (patient not in stable state).

X. Basic principles of preoperative assessment (23–26). The extent to which preoperative assessment of patients is necessary depends on the history and physical examination. In patients without evidence of cardiopulmonary disease by history or physical examination, further testing is not indicated. Patients who smoke or have evidence of cardiac or pulmonary disease by history or physical examination require further testing to determine whether they are at risk for development of postoperative pulmonary complications. Cardiac problems will not be discussed here. Pulmonary complications generally include postoperative pneumonia and prolonged ventilator dependence, both of which lead to long hospitalizations and the development of other complications. The variables to be considered in a patient with lung disease include the type of surgery (thoracic vs. nonthoracic) and the type and severity of pulmonary disease and obesity. Age is generally not a consideration. Necessary emergency life-saving procedures should be undertaken without further work-up, regardless of pulmonary function.

A. General

    1. **The basic work-up of all patients with pulmonary disease should include simple spirometry and determination of arterial blood gases.**

    2. Patients with mild obstructive disease and no carbon dioxide retention at rest have little risk for the development of postoperative complications. Patients whose FEV_1 is <40% predicted and/or baseline Pco_2 is >50 Torr are at risk for the development of complications and death (see chapter 16 for further details).

    3. Patients with restrictive lung disease generally tolerate surgery well, unless the disease is far advanced. Because they have little difficulty with carbon dioxide retention, they can usually be extubated quickly after the procedure. Oxygenation is also not usually a problem in these individuals.

B. Nonthoracic procedures in patients at risk

    1. The farther the procedure is from the diaphragm, the less the probability of a postoperative complication. Thus, upper abdominal procedures are more risky than those performed on the extremities. This is because upper abdominal procedures may reduce the effectiveness of diaphragmatic contraction, and this will be magnified in patients receiving narcotics postoperatively whose respiratory rates and level of consciousness will be diminished.

    2. Laparoscopic procedures are less risky than laparotomies.

    3. The use of narcotic and sedative medications should be kept to a minimum in patients at risk.

C. Thoracic procedures in patients at risk

    1. If pulmonary tissue is to be resected in a patient with diminished function, further assessment must be done to determine whether the patient will have sufficient function to support daily activities postoperatively. The minimum amount of function necessary is generally 800 mL of FEV_1.

    2. The amount of function remaining after surgery may be estimated by obtaining a perfusion or ventilation scan prior to surgery and multiplying the amount of perfusion or ventilation that will remain after surgery (in percent) by the preoperative FEV_1. For example, the expected postoperative FEV_1 following a right upper lobectomy when the baseline FEV_1 is 1.5 L and the right upper lobe is receiving 20% of the total cardiac output is $1.5 - (1.5 \times 0.2) = 1.2$ L.

    3. Patients at risk should undergo an intensive course of pulmonary rehabilitation (smoking cessation, bronchodilators, antibiotics, corticosteroids, incentive spirometry) for 2 weeks prior to elective surgery. This may be done as an outpatient if the patient is willing. Spirometry should be performed again to document improvement. All such patients should be seen by a pulmonary specialist prior to surgery, since more sophisticated testing may be necessary and these patients may require prolonged ventilatory support postoperatively (27,28).

XI. Pulmonary function testing in the office (29–31). Office-based spirometers may be used to screen and identify individuals who have lung disease in a matter of minutes. Office-based spirometers should be portable, should not require a lot of training or maintenance, and should yield results that are reproducible and free from error. Parameters usually available from these devices include FVC, FEV_1, FEV_1/FVC ratio, and mid–maximum flow rates. Volume and diffusing capacity measurements are generally not available. Individuals who smoke should be tested at least once a year to measure flows; decrements in flows may spur quitting. These devices may also be used to follow patients on therapy for obstructive diseases (asthma) and are also useful to follow patients with interstitial lung disease on steroid therapy.

References

1. Mead J: Mechanical properties of the lung. *Physiol Rev* 1961; 41:281–330.
2. Comroe JH, Forster RE, Dqubois AB et al: *The lung: clinical physiology and pulmonary function tests*, 2nd ed. Chicago: Year Book Medical Publishers, 1962:7–23,111–137,162–196.
3. Bates DV: *Respiratory function in disease*, 3rd ed. Philadelphia: WB Saunders, 1989:106–152.
4. American Thoracic Society: Lung function testing: selection of reference values and interpretive strategies. *Am Rev Respir Dis* 1991;144:1202–1218.
5. Clausen JL: Prediction of normal values in pulmonary function testing. *Clin Chest Med* 1989; 10:135–143.
6. Lunn WW, Sheller JR: Flow volume loops in the evaluation of upper airway obstruction. *Otolaryngol Clin North Am* 1995;28:721–729.
7. Rosenthal RR: Approved methodology for methacholine challenge. *Allergy Proc* 1989;10:301–312.
8. Beck K, Offord K, Scanlon P: Comparison of four methods for calculating diffusing capacity by the single breath method. *Chest* 1994;105:594–600.
9. Celli B: Clinical and physiologic evaluation of respiratory muscle function. *Clin Chest Med* 1989; 10:199–214.
10. Wasserman K, Hansen JE, Sue DY et al: *Principles of exercise testing and interpretation*, 2nd ed. Philadelphia: Lea and Febiger, 1994:1–78.
11. Messner-Pellenc P: Cardiopulmonary exercise testing. *Chest* 1994;106:354–360.
12. Stoller JK: Spirometry: a key diagnostic test in pulmonary medicine. *Cleve Clin J Med* 1992;59: 75–78.
13. Crapo RO: Pulmonary-function testing. *N Engl J Med* 1994;331:25–30.
14. Crapo RO, Morris AH: Pulmonary function testing: sources of error in measurement and interpretation. *South Med J* 1989;82:875–879.
15. McKay RT, Lockey JE: Pulmonary function testing: guidelines for medical surveillance and epidemiological studies. *Occup Med* 1991;6:43–57.
16. Brown LK: Pulmonary function testing in bronchial asthma: standard and emerging techniques. *Mt Sinai J Med* 1991;58:507–520.
17. Li JT, O'Connell EJ: Clinical evaluation of asthma. *Ann Allergy Asthma Immunol* 1996;76:1–13.
18. Weiss SM, Petty TL: Physiologic evaluation of bronchial asthma. Why objective testing is essential. *Postgrad Med* 1995;97:56–58,61–63,66–67.
19. Siefkin AD: Using pulmonary function testing in the diagnosis and treatment of asthma. *Clin Rev Allergy* 1990;8:179–196.
20. Manning H, Schwartzstein R: Pathophysiology of dyspnea. *N Engl J Med* 1995;333:1547–1553.
21. Mahler DA: Dyspnea: diagnosis and management. *Clin Chest Med* 1987;8:215–230.
22. Casaburi R: Exercise for pulmonary rehabilitation. *Contemp Intern Med* 1994;6:36–46.
23. Wait J: Southwestern Internal Medicine Conference: preoperative pulmonary evaluation. *Am J Med Sci* 1995;310:118–125.
24. Zibrak JD, O'Donnell CR: Indications for preoperative pulmonary function testing. *Clin Chest Med* 1993;14:227 236.
25. Dunn WF, Scanlon PD: Preoperative pulmonary function testing for patients with lung cancer. *Mayo Clin Proc* 1993;68:371–377.
26. Cottrell JJ, Ferson PF: Preoperative assessment of the thoracic surgical patient. *Clin Chest Med* 1992;13:47–53.
27. Boysen PG, Clark CA, Block AJ: Graded exercise testing and postthoracotomy complications. *J Cardiothorac Anesth* 1990;4:68–72.
28. Bechard D, Wetstein L: Assessment of exercise oxygen consumption as preoperative criterion for lung resection. *Ann Thorac Surg* 1987;44:344–349.

29. Heffner JE: Pocket computer for interpretation of office spirometry. *South Med J* 1988;81: 354–356.
30. Kotses H, Stout C, McConnaughy K et al: Evaluation of individualized asthma self-management programs. *J Asthma* 1996;33:113–118.
31. Jones KP, Mullee MA: Lung function measurement in general practice: a comparison of the Escort spirometer with the Micromed turbine spirometer and the mini-Wright peak flow meter. *Respir Med* 1995;89:657–663.

3   Pulmonary Procedures

Lawrence D. Klima and Joshua O. Benditt

Several medical procedures are routinely performed in the evaluation of pulmonary diseases. Some may be handled by the primary care physician, whereas others are more safely performed by a specialist. In this chapter, procedures will be described with an emphasis not only on the indications, risks, and contraindications but also on the appropriate timing of a consultation. Six procedures will be discussed: (a) thoracentesis, (b) pleural biopsy, (c) transthoracic needle biopsy, (d) radial artery cannulation, (e) pulmonary artery catheterization, and (f) flexible fiberoptic bronchoscopy.

I. **Thoracentesis.** Thoracentesis samples fluid from the pleural space via a small-bore needle or catheter passed through the chest wall. This common procedure can easily be performed by most physicians on an awake patient.

    A. **Indications.** Thoracentesis can be both a diagnostic and a therapeutic procedure. Its most common indication is the evaluation of a pleural effusion of unknown etiology. The procedure is also used to determine whether further drainage procedures are necessary for infectious or parapneumonic pleural effusions. Thoracentesis is an important part of the work-up of pleural effusions associated with lung cancer, as well as a therapeutic method to reduce dyspnea in patients with large effusions.

    B. **Equipment.** The following are generally necessary for this procedure:

        1. Material to cleanse and sterilize the skin over the insertion site.

        2. 1% or 2% lidocaine for local anesthesia in a syringe with a small-bore needle (20–22 gauge).

        3. Aspirating needle or catheter (16–19 gauge). Recent studies indicate that use of a short pliable plastic catheter or metal needle (1.5 inches and 20 gauge) is safer than using longer needle catheter systems (1) by reducing the incidence of pneumothorax.

        4. 20–30-mL syringe to be attached to the aspirating needle.

        5. Vacuum bottles and flexible connecting tubing needed for the removal of large volumes of fluid.

    C. **Patient preparation.** A directed history should be obtained, focusing on bleeding disorders, use of anticoagulant medications, and reactions to local anesthetic agents. Percussion of the posterior chest wall should be performed to assess the level of the pleural effusion and identify the appropriate intercostal space for insertion of the needle. Ultrasound is useful to mark the site of the effusion and guide needle placement for effusions that are difficult to localize (2), particularly for patients who are mechanically ventilated (3).

    D. **Technique.** The patient should be seated upright on the hospital bed or examining table and leaning forward over a comfortable supporting device (Fig. 3-1A). Localization of the effusion and appropriate entry site are identified, and the skin is sterilized and anesthetized. The skin is entered with the sampling needle and syringe, and the needle is carefully advanced through the inferior margin of the intercostal space immediately over the rib (Fig. 3-1B). This avoids injury to the neurovascular bundle in the superior portion of the intercostal space. Once the fluid is localized, a sample of 20–50 mL is withdrawn for diagnostic tests. If larger volumes of fluid are to be withdrawn, vacuum bottles and flexible plastic connecting tubing are employed at this time.

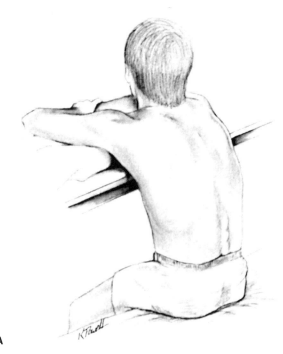

A

Fig. 3-1. A: Standard position for patient undergoing thoracentesis. The patient is comfortably positioned, sitting up, and leaning forward over a pillow-draped, height-adjusted bedside table. The arms are crossed in front of the patient to elevate and spread the scapulae.

E. **Contraindications.** The most frequent contraindications include inability of the patient to consent to and/or cooperate with the procedure, patient anatomy that precludes identification of the appropriate landmarks, and the lack of an operator skilled in the procedure.

F. **Complications**

1. **Pneumothorax** reportedly occurs in approximately 10% of cases, although some series have found an incidence as high as 39% that is closely related to operator experience (1). Other risk factors for pneumothorax include a small effusion, loculated fluid, a thick chest wall, and an uncooperative patient.

2. **Hemothorax** is a rare complication that can occur in a patient with an abnormal coagulation status or may result from laceration of an intercostal artery.

3. **Reexpansion pulmonary edema** may be more common than previously recognized and has been observed in 14% of thoracenteses in one series (4). The etiology of reexpansion pulmonary edema is unknown, but it appears to occur more commonly with large effusions, especially with the removal of more than 1 L (5). Therefore, no more than 1 L of fluid should be removed at one time during the thoracentesis procedure.

G. **Specimens.** Analysis of the thoracentesis specimen is critical for the differentiation of the possible causes of pleural effusion. (A thorough discussion of the chemical and cytologic characteristics of different types of pleural effusions is found in chapter 12.)

1. **Appearance.** The pleural fluid should be examined directly. Frank pus may have a putrid odor and suggests an empyema. A cloudy appearance is consis-

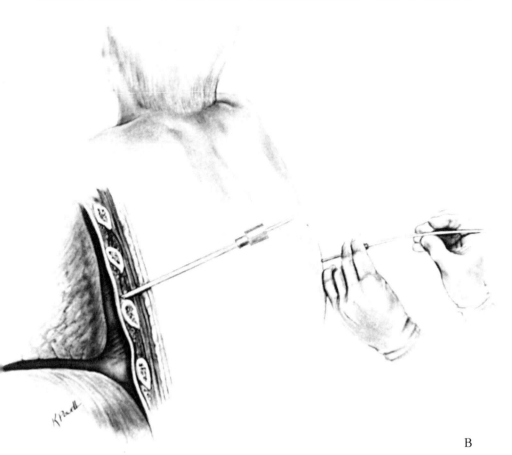

B

FIG. 3-1. *Continued* **B:** Catheter technique for thoracentesis of freely flowing pleural field. The catheter is gently advanced after the needle has crossed the surface of the rib. It will not advance if it meets the resistance of soft tissue. The catheter is not forced into the soft tissue. (From Rippe JM. *Intensive care medicine.* Boston: Little, Brown, 1994:159–160.)

tent with either chylothorax or empyema. Grossly bloody fluid, with an hematocrit >50% of the peripheral value, indicates a traumatic hemothorax (6).

2. **Chemistry values** to be obtained from pleural fluid include protein, lactate dehydrogenase (LDH), and glucose. Pleural fluid LDH and protein values differentiate exudative from transudative effusions (see chapter 12).

   a. The **glucose level** of the pleural fluid can help define the cause of pleural effusion. Diagnoses associated with low glucose levels include malignant, tuberculous, or parapneumonic effusions; empyema; rheumatoid pleural effusion; and hemothorax.

   b. **Other chemistries** may be ordered when specific etiologies of the effusion are suspected. Measurement of pleural fluid amylase, triglycerides, and cholesterol, lipoprotein electrophoresis, and studies for rheumatoid factor and antinuclear antibodies are usually not necessary in the initial evaluation of a pleural effusion.

3. **Cell count.** A complete cell count and differential should be obtained on pleural fluid samples. The differential cell count is particularly helpful in limiting the diagnosis (see chapter 12).

4. **Cultures and microbiologic smears.** Most pleural fluid samples should be Gram- and acid-fast-stained and cultured for tuberculosis as well as for aerobic and anaerobic organisms. The most cost-effective approach utilizes these bacteriologic tests only with a second thoracentesis sample obtained whenever the initial fluid is an exudate.

5. **Cytology.** Cytologic analysis of spun samples of pleural fluid can be diagnostic in 40% to 90% of malignant effusions. The yield of this procedure increases with the volume of fluid received by the cytology laboratory (7), and repeated sampling may further increase the diagnostic yield.

II. **Pleural biopsy.** Three common methods can be used to biopsy the pleura: (a) closed needle technique, (b) thoracoscopic biopsy, and (c) open pleural biopsy requiring a thoracotomy. Only closed needle biopsy will be discussed in detail since it is the only procedure routinely performed by the pulmonologist or generalist. Thoracoscopy and open biopsy are in general performed by thoracic surgeons.

A. **Closed needle pleural biopsy**

1. **Indications**

a. Closed needle pleural biopsy is indicated for exudative pleural effusions of unknown etiology whenever tuberculosis or malignancy is suspected clinically. Pleural biopsy is particularly helpful for tuberculous pleural effusions because cultures of the pleural fluid are only 25% sensitive in detecting infection. Cultures of both pleural biopsy and pleural fluid increase the sensitivity for detecting tuberculosis to 90% (8).

b. Pleural biopsy is less effective in the diagnosis of malignancy, with a reported sensitivity of only 46% (9). The combination of pleural fluid cytology with histology of biopsy specimens increases the sensitivity to greater than 65% (7,10). Pleural fluid should be sampled during the pleural biopsy procedure whenever malignancy is suspected (9).

2. **Equipment**

a. One of the following closed pleural biopsy needles:

   i. Cope.

   ii. Abrams.

   iii. Tru-cut.

b. Material to cleanse and sterilize the skin (alcohol and/or iodine solution).

c. 15 mL of 1% or 2% lidocaine for local anesthesia in a syringe with a small-bore needle (20–22 gauge) and a 1.5-inch 19-gauge needle for anesthesia of the rib periosteum.

d. Aspirating needle or catheter (16–19 gauge).

e. 20–30-mL syringe that can be attached to the pleural biopsy needle.

f. #11 Scalpel.

g. Suture material.

h. Specimen containers with formalin and saline for histology and culture of tissue specimens, respectively.

i. Vacuum bottles and flexible connecting tubing will also be needed if larger volumes of fluid are to be withdrawn.

3. **Patient preparation.** Patient preparation for pleural biopsy is essentially the same as that for thoracentesis as noted above.

4. **Technique.** The approach to the closed pleural biopsy is similar to that for thoracentesis.

a. **Anesthesia.** After an appropriate site on the wall of the posterior thorax has been located and cleansed, anesthesia to the skin is applied and followed by deeper anesthesia to the periosteum of the lower rib and the parietal pleura. This is best done with a large volume of 2% lidocaine administered in multiple radial passes to anesthetize a large area of the parietal pleura (11).

b. **Insertion of the biopsy needle.** A 0.5-cm incision in the skin with the #11 scalpel allows easier passage of the blunt biopsy needle through the skin and subcutaneous tissues. Prior to application of the biopsy needle, the pleural effusion is located with a smaller aspiration needle. The biopsy needle is then inserted through the incision with the cutting edge placed inferiorly to avoid damage to the neurovascular bundle of the superior rib. Multiple samples (5–10) are obtained. If needed for analysis, pleural fluid may be drained through the biopsy needle into a syringe or vacuum bottle. The incision site is closed with suture material, and a clean dressing placed over the site.

5. Contraindications are the same as those for thoracentesis.
6. Complications. The major risks of closed pleural biopsy are hemorrhage due to damage to an intercostal vessel, and pneumothorax. In addition, malignant cells can be seeded along the needle biopsy tract when the effusion is malignant (12).
7. **Specimens.** Pleural fluid specimens are usually sent in the same manner as that described under thoracentesis. Two or three tissue specimens should be sent for culture in 0.9% saline, with the remainder placed in 10% formalin for histologic evaluation.

B. **Thoracoscopic pleural biopsy.** Endoscopic evaluation of the visceral and parietal pleural surface is possible with fiberoptic instruments allowing directed biopsy of the pleural surface. In a series of 150 patients with malignant effusions and negative results on a closed pleural biopsy, thoracoscopic biopsy resulted a diagnosis in 87% compared with 36% for a repeated closed needle biopsy (13).

C. **Open pleural biopsy.** This procedure involves thoracotomy and direct visualization of the pleura with biopsy. This is rarely necessary for the evaluation of malignant pleural effusion, given the other modalities currently available.

III. **Transthoracic needle biopsy (TNB).** This technique, also known as percutaneous needle aspiration biopsy, is used in the assessment of infectious and malignant lesions of the lung. Biopsies can be performed either with a narrow-gauge (20–25 gauge) aspiration needle to obtain samples for cytologic and culture analysis or with larger-bore needles (16–19 gauge) designed to obtain histologic samples. Only specialists trained in the procedure (radiologist, pulmonologist, or thoracic surgeon) should perform TNB.

A. **Indications.** TNB should be reserved for lung lesions whose etiology remains unclear after other diagnostic procedures such as bronchoscopy have been performed. This procedure is appropriate for infectious or noninfectious lesions, both focal and diffuse. Examples of lesions appropriate for TNB include peripheral coin lesions or masses, as well as focal or diffuse infiltrates. TNB has also been shown to be effective in the diagnosis of human immunodeficiency virus (HIV)-related pulmonary infections. The sensitivity of the procedure is dependent on the type of lesion involved; TNB has been reported to be 90% sensitive in the case of malignancy. The overall diagnostic accuracy appears to be in the range of 85%, with a specificity of nearly 100% (14,15). A positive diagnosis on TNB is very helpful in the overall diagnostic work-up. A negative biopsy calls for further evaluation.

B. **Equipment**
1. Material to cleanse and sterilize the skin over the insertion site (alcohol and/or iodine solution).
2. 1% or 2% lidocaine in syringe with a small-bore needle (20–22 gauge) for local anesthesia.
3. TNB aspiration needle (16–25 gauge) with several 20–30 mL syringes.
4. Cytology technician on site or specimen containers with formalin and saline for histology and culture specimens.
5. Fluoroscope or CT scanner for localization of focal lesions.

C. **Patient preparation.** The patient should have nothing by mouth for at least 6–8 hours prior to TNB. Premedications usually include 0.6 mg atropine IM or IV and codeine to suppress cough.

D. **Procedure.** The patient is positioned appropriately on the instrument table in the fluoroscopy or CT suite. The skin over the lesion is sterilized and anesthetized. The lesion is entered under visual guidance (fluoroscope) or by measurement (CT scan). A syringe containing 5 mL of sterile saline is attached and suction is applied, while the needle is gently advanced and retracted in the lesion to macerate tissue.

The needle is then removed, and the specimen ejected onto a microscope slide or into an appropriate container. More than one pass of the biopsy needle is usually required. The patient should be observed for several hours and an expiratory chest x-ray obtained to exclude a pneumothorax. If none is present, the patient may be safely discharged.

E. **Specimens** are sent for cytologic evaluation with Papanicolaou stain, as well as for smears and culture for bacteria, mycobacteria, and fungi. With the larger biopsy needles, core tissue samples are usually obtained and sent for pathologic examination. The presence of a cytology technician capable of identifying malignant cells in the procedure suite is invaluable in the work-up of malignancy. On-site collection, preparation, and rapid cytologic interpretation allow repeated passes of the needle to be undertaken until a positive identification of tumor cells is made, thus avoiding false-negative results.

F. **Contraindications.** Contraindications to TNB include the inability of the patient to consent to and/or cooperate with the procedure and the absence of a skilled operator. Significant coagulation abnormalities and the need for mechanical ventilation are also contraindications.

G. **Potential complications.** The major complications of TNB are pneumothorax and intraparenchymal pulmonary hemorrhage. The risk varies with the size of the aspiration needle used. Small-bore (23–26 gauge) needles for cytology have a 10% risk of pneumothorax and a 5% risk of bleeding (16). The larger-bore (16–20 gauge) histology needles have a much higher risk of pneumothorax (30%) and bleeding (10%) (16,17).

IV. **Radial artery cannulation.** Radial arterial cannulation is the insertion of a catheter into the radial artery to provide hemodynamic monitoring and/or access to arterial blood in the critically ill patient. It is best performed by physicians with training and ongoing practice with the procedure.

A. **Indications**

1. Radial artery cannulation allows for continuous arterial pressure monitoring in patients requiring intravenous vasopressors or vasodilators. At the extremes of blood pressure, sphygmomanometric cuff pressures may be misleading, causing errors in therapy (18). Patients with impending respiratory failure or undergoing mechanical ventilation require frequent arterial sampling.

2. Radial artery cannulation prevents repeated trauma to the artery from frequent punctures and allows for multiple laboratory determinations in critically ill patients with limited venous access (19). Arterial cannulation can be avoided in some patients who have central venous access. In such patients, central venous blood can be used to estimate pH and Pco_2, and oximetry can be used to assess oxygen saturation, provided that a blood gas determination demonstrates close correlation between the measurements.

B. **Equipment**

1. Mechanoelectric transducer with dome, connecting cable, and monitor.
2. Constant flush device.
3. Fluid-filled noncompliant tubing with stopcocks.
4. Arm board and roll of gauze.
5. Povidone-iodine solution and ointment.
6. 1% lidocaine without epinephrine and 3-mL syringe with 25-gauge needle.
7. Sterile gloves and drapes.
8. 1¼-2-inch 20-gauge nontapered Teflon angiocatheter.
9. 3-0 silk suture with needle.

C. **Patient preparation.** Prior to the insertion of a radial artery catheter, a modified Allen's test (compression of the radial artery to assure adequate perfusion of the hand by the ulnar artery) should be performed to assure that adequate collateral blood flow is present.

D. **Technique**

1. Radial artery cannulation is accomplished by inserting a plastic angiocatheter into the radial artery at an approximately 30° angle to the skin, 2–3 inches proximal to the distal wrist crease, using the radial pulse as a guide. The volar surface of the wrist should be cleansed and sterilized, and the arm attached to

a supporting arm board with the wrist extended. Both sides of the artery should be injected with 0.5 mL of lidocaine to minimize patient discomfort and decrease the likelihood of arterial vasospasm (19).

2. Once placed, the arterial line is connected to preflushed pressure tubing and sutured in place to prevent accidental removal. Gauze from underneath the wrist should be removed as prolonged dorsiflexion may lead to neurologic injury of the hand (18). The wrist should be fixed in the neutral position on the arm board to prevent flexion and kinking of the catheter. Povidone-iodine ointment should be applied to the skin at the insertion site, and the line should be covered with a sterile dressing.

E. **Contraindications.** Absolute contraindications include overlying skin breakdown or infection or the presence of an arterial graft. Relative contraindications include poor collateral circulation, a bleeding diathesis, or thrombocytopenia.

F. **Complications**

1. While thrombosis occurs in 5% to 25% of patients (19), symptomatic occlusion occurs in fewer than than 1% (18). Predisposing factors include cannulas larger than 20 gauge, with tapered ends, or made of non-Teflon material, as well as hypotension/circulatory failure, use of vasopressors, multiple puncture attempts, and placement for longer than 4 days. If evidence of ischemia is present, the catheter should be removed immediately. If ischemia persists after catheter removal, treatment includes thrombolytics or surgical/radiologic embolectomy.

2. Distal embolization can occur with the fragmentation of catheter-related thrombus. Cerebral embolization, even from a radial arterial catheter, can result from retrograde flow secondary to overaggressive flushing.

3. Local infection of the catheter site occurs in 10% to 15% of patients, whereas catheter-related bacteremia occurs in 0.2% to 5% (20). Predisposing factors include breaks in the sterile technique of insertion, catheter care, or blood draws; infusate that contains dextrose or hangs for greater than 48 hours; placement exceeding 4 days; and placement by surgical cut-down.

4. Other complications include development of pseudoaneurysms up to 2 weeks after catheter removal, median nerve neuropathy caused by prolonged wrist hyperextension or blood compression of the nerve in the carpal tunnel, diagnostic blood loss secondary to frequent sampling (with 3–5 mL of blood discarded with each sample), and the formation of arteriovenous fistulas.

G. **Proper handling of blood specimens.** Specimens for arterial blood gas analysis should be drawn into heparinized syringes. All air bubbles should be expelled from the syringe to prevent equilibration of gas tensions between air and the sample. The specimen should be immediately placed on ice and sent to the laboratory for analysis as soon as possible.

V. **Pulmonary artery (PA) catheterization.** PA catheterization is the insertion of a catheter through the right heart into the PA to accurately measure hemodynamics. The procedure is usually performed in critically ill patients whose hemodynamic situation may be unstable or in question. Clinical assessment and indirect measures can often be misleading and cause errors in management in these individuals. PA catheterization should be performed only by individuals trained in a supervised setting who place the catheters on a frequent basis.

A. **Indications (Table 3-1)**

B. **Equipment**

1. Equipment for a percutaneous catheter sheath insertion.
2. Pressure-monitoring lines, transducer, and monitor.
3. PA catheter, sheath, and syringe for balloon inflation.
4. Sterile gowns, drapes, and gloves.
5. Mask and hair cover.

C. **Patient preparation.** A careful history should be obtained with an emphasis on potential contraindications to the procedure, particularly past or current bleeding disorders, anticoagulant medications, and cardiac disorders (particularly conduction block). Informed consent is required for this procedure.

D. **Technique**

Table 3-1. Indications for pulmonary artery catheterization

Assessment of the cause of hypotension
  Hypovolemic
  Septic
  Cardiogenic
Assessment of the cause of respiratory distress
  Cardiac
  Noncardiac (ARDS) pulmonary edema
Assessment of cardiac function/hemodynamic status in
  Myocardial infarction
  Severe left ventricular failure
  Ventricular septal rupture
  Acute mitral regurgitation
  Cardiac tamponade
  Valvular heart disease
  Undiagnosed tachyarrhythmias
  Pulmonary hypertension (primary or secondary)
Assessment of fluid status in
  Acute renal failure
  Gastrointestinal bleeding
  Sepsis
Assessment of the results of therapeutic intervention in the above conditions

ARDS = adult respiratory distress syndrome.

1. A percutaneous 8 French catheter sheath should be placed into an internal jugular, subclavian, or femoral vein using standard sterile techniques.
2. The PA catheter is then visually inspected with the balloon inflated. The balloon should not leak and should extend just beyond the catheter tip, which prevents endovascular damage and ectopy during passage through the right ventricle (21). The catheter should be flushed with sterile saline solution to remove all air and prevent air embolization. While being watched on the monitor, the catheter should be shaken briefly to assure that a pressure tracing is displayed.
3. The catheter is placed through the introducer sheath into the vein. At 15 cm, the balloon is inflated and the catheter advanced until a right atrial (RA) tracing appears with appropriate respiratory changes, indicating intrathoracic placement (Fig. 3-2). The catheter is carefully advanced until a right ventricular (RV) pressure tracing appears (Fig. 3-2) and then is further advanced until the diastolic pressure rises above RV diastolic pressure. This is a PA tracing. The pulmonary capillary wedge pressure (PCWP) waveform appears as the pressure falls when the catheter is advanced slightly beyond the PA (Fig. 3-2).
4. Deflating the balloon results in to a PA waveform. If the PA tracing does not reappear, the catheter should be pulled back (with the balloon deflated) into the PA. No more than two-thirds of the manufacturer's recommended balloon volume should be necessary to produce a PCWP tracing. Less volume suggests that the catheter is too distal, placing the patient at risk for pulmonary infarction. If >15 cm from the point of entry into the RV are required before a PA waveform appears, the catheter may be coiling in the RV, and the balloon should be deflated and the catheter withdrawn to the RA.
5. The catheter is sutured in place and the sterile sleeve secured when the catheter is properly positioned.
6. The balloon should be deflated at all times except for intermittent PCWP readings. The empty syringe should be left on the balloon port to ensure that fluid is not accidentally infused.

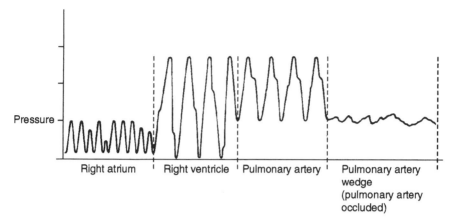

Fig. 3-2. Characteristic pressure recording observed during insertion of pulmonary artery flow-directed catheter. (From Gore JM, Alpert JS, Benotti JR et al. *Handbook of hemodynamic monitoring.* Boston: Little, Brown, 1985:36.)

    7. A chest radiograph is necessary to confirm that the catheter tip is within 3–5 cm of the midline. Daily chest x-rays should be obtained to ensure the catheter has not migrated distally. Continuous waveform monitoring assures that the catheter neither retracts into the RV nor advances into a PCWP position, as the catheter can soften with warming from body temperature.

E. Contraindications

    1. Patients who are anticoagulated or receiving thrombolytic therapy should undergo central venous catheterization and right heart catheterization only from sites directly accessible to direct pressure, such as the basilic or internal jugular vein (21).

    2. Patients with preexisting left bundle branch block (LBBB) should only undergo right heart catheterization with external or transvenous pacemaker equipment on immediate standby (22). In this situation, there is a small risk of a right bundle branch block (RBBB) developing, resulting in complete heart block (22,23).

F. Complications

    1. Pneumothorax has a 1% to 6% incidence with the subclavian approach, compared with <1% with the internal jugular approach (24).

    2. Ventricular arrhythmias, including premature ventricular contractions, nonsustained and sustained ventricular tachycardia, and ventricular fibrillation, occur frequently (30% to 60%) with the insertion of the PA catheter. However, treatment is required in only 3% of cases (24), and most of these respond favorably to therapy (25). Patients at risk appear to be those with myocardial ischemia, acidosis, hypoxia, and electrolyte abnormalities (22).

    3. Pulmonary infarction is caused by the occlusion of the small branches of the PA because of distal migration of the catheter tip. Careful monitoring of waveforms has lowered the incidence of this complication to <2% (25).

    4. Local thrombosis can occur around the catheter and in the central vein; the incidence has decreased with the introduction of heparin-bonded catheters. Minimizing the amount of time the catheter is left in place also reduces the frequency of this complication.

    5. Transient RBBB occurs in approximately 3% of cases (23). In patients with preexisting LBBB, complete heart block is a potential complication. External and transvenous pacemaker equipment should be on immediate standby for the procedure.

6. Catheter-related septicemia has been reported in <1% of catheterizations, with the incidence rising when the catheter is left in place for more than 3–4 days (24).
7. PA rupture is the most feared complication of PA catheterization. While the incidence is very low (<0.2%), the mortality is high (26). Risk factors include pulmonary hypertension, anticoagulation, hypothermia, and recent cardiopulmonary bypass (27). The balloon should always be carefully inflated and never left inflated while the catheter is in the wedge position. Balloon rupture occurs if more than the recommended inflation volume is used. Rupture can result in the embolization of balloon fragments to the pulmonary circulation and/or an air embolus gaining access to the arterial circulation (28).
8. Intracardiac knotting of the PA catheter has been reported (29). This complication can be eliminated with careful attention to the distance the catheter is inserted.

G.   Measurements (Table 3-2)
1. Pressures. All pressures should be measured at end-expiration.
   a. Right atrium: normal is 0–6 mm Hg. The two positive pressure waves are the a wave (atrial contraction) and the v wave (venous filling of the right atrium).
   b. Right ventricle: normal is 17–30/0–6 mm Hg. The RV systolic pressure should equal the PA systolic pressure.
   c. Pulmonary artery: normal is 15–30/5–13 mm Hg.
   d. Pulmonary capillary wedge: normal is 2–12 mm Hg. An a wave and a v wave can be identified. The pressure correlates well with the left ventricular (LV) diastolic pressure in those patients with a normal mitral valve and LV function.
2. Cardiac output is measured by the thermodilution technique. A known amount of cold solution is injected into the RA port, and the thermistor near the end of the catheter measures the temperature change, with the calculation of the cardiac output made from the average of at least three measurements. The measurement is inaccurate in low cardiac output states, tricuspid regurgitation, and atrial or ventricular septal defects (21).
3. Mixed venous blood is obtained by slow aspiration (<3 mL/min) from the distal port of a nonwedged catheter after the first 2.5 mL is discarded as dead space. Saturation of this blood is an indirect measure of cardiac output but should be interpreted cautiously, as several conditions (adult respiratory distress syndrome, cardiac surgery) alter its reliability.

VI.   Flexible fiberoptic bronchoscopy (FOB). Developed in 1964 by the Japanese physician Ikeda, FOB has been an invaluable tool in the diagnosis and therapy of pulmonary problems. It has largely replaced rigid bronchoscopy, except in the evaluation and treatment of massive hemoptysis, the removal of large foreign bodies from the lower airways, and in some types of laser therapy.
A.   Indications. The suggested diagnostic and therapeutic indications for fiberoptic bronchoscopy are numerous and have been published by the American Thoracic Society (30) (Table 3-3).
1. **Assessment of lung cancer**
   a. FOB is an essential tool in the diagnosis of lung cancer. The diagnostic yield for central mass lesions with an endoscopically visible component is over 90% with standard brush and forceps biopsies (31). The yield for peripheral mass lesions without endoscopically visible components is 10% to 30% or less (32,33). In this latter situation, lavage samples, brushing samples, and multiple transbronchial lung biopsies under fluoroscopic guidance may increase the yield (34,35).
   b. Staging of lung cancer prior to curative resection. Tumor invading the main carina or the presence of a second lung cancer in a separate location preclude curative surgical therapy in most cases. Metastatic disease in mediastinal lymph nodes can be accessible with FOB in some cases using transbronchial needle aspiration (see description below). The sensitivity of the procedure in the setting of suspected lymph node metastases

Table 3-2. Hemodynamic parameters in commonly encountered clinical situations

Clinical setting	Pressures (mm Hg)				Saturation (%)			CI
	RA	RV	PA	PCW	RA	PA	Art	
Normal	0–6	25/0–6	25/6–12	6–12	60	60	98	2.1
Cardiac tamponade	18	30/18	30/18	18	60	62	98	2.0
Chronic obstructive lung disease	10	70/10	70/35	<12	60	60	88	2.1
Cardiogenic shock	8	50/8	50/35	35	50	50	98	1.5
Ventricular septal defect	6	60/8	60/35	30	55	75	92	1.9
Primary right ventricular failure	16	35/18	35/18	≤14	60	60	98	2.1
Left ventricular failure	4–6	45/4–6	45/>18	>18	60	60	98	1.8
Acute pulmonary embolism	8–12	50/12	50/12–15	≤12	60	60	88	1.9
Congestive heart failure (biventricular)	6–8	65/6	65/25	25	55	55	98	1.9
Hypovolemic shock	0–2	15–20/0–2	15–20/2–6	2–6	65	65	98	2.5
Septic shock								
Warm	0–2	20–25/0–2	20–25/0–6	0–6	65	65	98	2.5
Cold	0–4	25/0–4	25/4–10	4–10	50	50	98	1.5

RA = right atrial; RV = right ventricle; PA = pulmonary artery; PCW = pulmonary capillary wedge; Art = arterial; CI = cardiac index.
From Gore JM, Alpert JS, Benotti JR et al. *Handbook of Hemodynamic Monitoring.* Boston: Little, Brown, 1985:156.

Table 3-3. Indications for fiberoptic bronchoscopy

Diagnostic evaluation
Therapeutic indications
Persistent cough
Removal of foreign bodies
Hemoptysis
Removal of retained secretions
Local wheeze on physical examination
Laser therapy of obstructive airway lesions
Nonresolving pneumonia
Difficult intubations
Atelectasis
Placement of endobronchial radiation therapy devices (brachytherapy)
Abnormal sputum cytology
Therapeutic lung lavage in patients with pulmonary alveolar proteinosis
Vocal cord paralysis
Paralyzed hemidiaphragm
Abnormalities on chest x-ray
Mass lesions
Infiltrates: diffuse or focal
Staging and evaluation of lung cancer
Airway injury in inhalation and burn injuries
Tracheobronchial injury in chest trauma
Obtaining material for microbiologic studies in suspected pulmonary infections

is reportedly as high as 76% (36), although the critical factor appears to be the experience of the bronchoscopist.

2. **Evaluation of pulmonary infections**

   a. Pneumonia in the nonimmunocompromised host. FOB is potentially useful in the diagnosis of pulmonary infection when adequate samples cannot be obtained by other methods. The techniques of quantitative culture of specimens obtained by bronchoalveolar lavage (BAL) and protected-specimen brush (PSB) biopsy have been developed to circumvent the problem of contamination of the lower respiratory tract with bacteria from the nasopharynx and oral cavity. Although there is significant debate, a specific pathogen can be identified by the finding on PSB biopsy of >103 colony-forming units (CFU) per milliliter of one organism or >105 CFU/mL on BAL in a patient who has not received antibiotics previously (37–39). Reports of sensitivity and specificity of these tests vary widely.

   b. Pneumonia in the mechanically ventilated patient. Ventilator-associated pneumonia caries a high mortality rate (40). PSB biopsy with quantitative culture may provide a method of identifying patients with pneumonia in this situation (41), although extensive data are currently lacking.

   c. Pneumonia in the patient with acquired immune deficiency syndrome (AIDS). Bronchoscopy has been highly effective in the diagnosis of infectious and noninfectious causes of lung diseases in patients with HIV infection (see chapter 26 for further details). The sensitivity for diagnosing *Pneumocystis carinii* pneumonia with BAL alone is 90% and, when combined with transbronchial lung biopsy, is near 100% (41).

B. **Equipment**

1. Bronchoscope.
2. Light source.
3. Video system (optional).
4. Biopsy brushes and forceps.
5. Pulse oximeter.
6. Continuous electrocardiogram (ECG) monitor.
7. Blood pressure monitoring device.
8. Anesthetic and sedating agents.
   a. 2% and 4% lidocaine solution.
   b. Atropine for IV administration.
   c. Optional: IV benzodiazepine (midazolam preferred).
   d. Optional: IV narcotic agent (meperidine preferred).
   e. Optional: topical cocaine solution.
9. Suction equipment.
10. Cardioverter-defibrillator and advanced life-support equipment.
11. Availability of fluoroscopy for procedure.

C. **Patient preparation**
1. A thorough history of coagulation abnormalities, arrhythmias, reactive airways disease, hypoxemia, and drug allergies should be obtained and recorded.
2. Laboratory data obtained prior to the procedure should include platelet count, prothrombin and partial thromboplastin times, arterial blood gases, chest x-ray, and an ECG in patients with a history of cardiac disease.
3. Informed consent is mandatory for this procedure, given the potential for life-threatening complications.
4. Patients should be instructed to abstain from eating for 8 hours before the procedure to minimize the risk of aspiration.
5. Local anesthesia is generally used for this procedure. Having the patient gargle with 4% lidocaine allows further anesthesia of the posterior pharynx, vocal cords, and lower airway with atomized 2% lidocaine. Once in the airway, 2–3-mL boluses of 1% to 2% lidocaine can be given locally for control of cough. The nasal passage is anesthetized with lidocaine in spray and jelly form. In some rare cases, bronchoscopy may be performed under general anesthesia, although this approach carries significantly more risk of complications.
6. Sedation. The use of sedation with IV benzodiazepines and/or narcotics is controversial. Many of the side effects of this procedure relate to premedications given, and so some authors have suggested that sedatives and IV analgesics not be given routinely (42). If conscious sedation is given, most institutions require monitoring by a nurse.

D. **Technique**
1. Bronchoscopy is frequently performed on an outpatient basis in a day surgery or procedure area. Patients should be driven to and from the procedure, as sedatives may be given. Three approaches are available to the bronchoscopist: (a) transnasal, (b) transoral, and (c) transendotracheal. Transnasal is the preferred approach and provides greater patient comfort in most cases. Transoral is generally reserved for patients with bleeding disorders or difficult nasal anatomy.
2. Anesthesia is performed as noted above. With the patient adequately anesthetized, the scope is inserted through the nose and advanced to the pharynx. After an inspection of the structures of the throat, the scope is advanced beyond the vocal cords, and all carinae and airways are visually examined. Cytologic and biopsy specimens are taken via instruments passed through a channel within the bronchoscope as indicated. The procedure generally lasts between 15 minutes and 1 hour.

E. **Specimens.** Bronchoscopy can yield specimens for cytologic, microbiologic, and histologic analysis. Four methods are utilized to obtain samples during bronchoscopy.
1. Brush biopsy. Small, 3–5 mm brushes are passed through the suction channel in the bronchoscope to obtain cytologic or microbiologic samples from visible endobronchial lesions or from distal airways that cannot be visualized. Specimens for culture can also be obtained in this way, although contamination from upper airway organisms aspirated into the suction channel is a signifi-

cant problem (43). Protected-specimen brushes (PSB) have been developed to avoid this problem (44). These devices consist of a retractable brush within a double set of polyethylene catheters.

2. Forceps biopsy utilizes pincer forceps attached to the end of a flexible cable that can be passed through the suction channel of the bronchoscope. Samples of endobronchial lesions, bronchial wall, alveoli, and lung parenchyma may be obtained. Sensitivity for the diagnosis of endoscopically visible cancers is as high as 90%, if multiple samples are obtained (32). Fluoroscopic guidance can be used to aid in the biopsy of peripheral lesions. Transbronchial biopsy utilizes the forceps instrument to sample alveolar tissue beyond the point of airway visualization for histologic examination. This technique is particularly useful in the diagnosis of diffuse lung diseases, including infections and malignancies as well as sarcoidosis or pulmonary fibrosis.

3. Bronchoalveolar lavage is a technique used to sample the alveolar space. Aliquots of normal saline to a total of 100–150 mL are instilled into the distal airway with the bronchoscope in the wedge position (inserted as far distally as airway diameter will allow). Gentle suction is used to withdraw the instilled fluid, which is then sent for differential cell count, cultures, and special stains as necessary.

4. Transbronchial needle aspiration is a technique for sampling tissue outside the airway with the use of a fine-bore needle passed through the bronchial wall. Saline is usually instilled and drawn back for cytologic analysis. This technique is most useful for sampling lymph nodes for the staging of lung cancer.

F. **Contraindications and complications**
1. Absolute contraindications to bronchoscopy include lack of patient consent; lack of an experienced operator; lack of facilities available to handle the potential complications of cardiac arrest, significant bleeding, pneumothorax; and inability to adequately oxygenate the patient during the procedure.
2. A number of conditions can increase the risk of adverse complications. These include:
   a. Angina or recent myocardial infarction.
   b. Asthma.
   c. Respiratory insufficiency with hypoxemia and hypercarbia.
   d. Pulmonary hypertension.
   e. Coagulation disorders.
   f. Uremia.
   g. Unstable cardiac arrhythmia.

G. **Potential complications**
1. With appropriate screening for high-risk patients, bronchoscopy can be a safe procedure, even in elderly patients (45). Major complications have been reported in 0.08% to 5% of bronchoscopic procedures, with death occurring in 0.01% to 0.5% (46–48). The risk of major complications is highest in those patients with active ischemic heart disease.
2. Since the arterial oxygen level generally falls about 20 mm Hg during the procedure, especially if BAL is performed, supplementary oxygen should be given to all patients and hemoglobin saturation monitored continuously with pulse oximetry (49). Fever following bronchoscopy is not uncommon, although this is infrequently associated with significant infection (50). Potentially life-threatening complications of bronchoscopy include:
   a. Bronchospasm and or laryngospasm.
   b. Allergic reactions to medications.
   c. Hypoventilation secondary to sedating medications.
   d. Hypoxemia.
   e. Myocardial ischemia and or infarction.
   f. Hemorrhage.
   g. Cardiac arrhythmia.
   h. Pneumothorax.
   i. Infection.

References

1. Grogan DR, Irwin RS, Channick R et al: Complications associated with thoracentesis: a prospective randomized study comparing three different methods. *Arch Intern Med* 1990;150:873–877.
2. Kohan JM, Poe RH, Israel RH, et al.: Value of chest ultrasonography versus decubitus roentgenography for thoracentesis. *Am Rev Respir Dis* 1986;133:1124–1126.
3. Godwin JE, Sahn SA: Thoracentesis: a safe procedure in mechanically ventilated patients. *Ann Intern Med* 1990;113:800–802.
4. Matsuura Y, Nomimura T, Murakami T, et al.: Clinical analysis of reexpansion pulmonary edema. *Chest* 1991;100:1563–1566.
5. Mahfood S, Hix WR, et al.: Re-expansion pulmonary edema. *Ann Thorac Surg* 1986;45:340–345.
6. Light RW: Pleural diseases. *Dis Mon* 1992;38:266–271, 273–331.
7. Bueno CE, Clemente MG et al: Cytologic and bacteriologic analysis of fluid and pleural biopsy specimens with Cope's needle: study of 414 patients. *Arch Intern Med* 1990;150:1190–1194.
8. Leslie WK, Kinasewitz GT: Clinical characteristic of the patient with nonspecific pleuritis. *Chest* 1988;94:603–608.
9. Prakash UBS, Reiman HM: Comparison of needle biopsy with cytologic analysis for the evaluation of pleural effusion: analysis of 414 cases. *Mayo Clin Proc* 1985;60:158–164.
10. Poe RH, Israel RH, Utell MJ, et al.: Sensitivity, specificity, and predictive values of closed pleural biopsy. *Arch Intern Med* 1984;144:325–328.
11. McLeod DT, Ternouth I, Nkanza N: Comparison of the Tru-cut biopsy needle with the Abrams punch for pleural biopsy. *Thorax* 1989;44:794–796.
12. Law MR, Hodson ME, et al.: Malignant mesothelioma of the pleura: clinical aspects and symptomatic treatment. *Eur J Respir Dis* 1989;65:162–168.
13. Boutin C, Viallat JR,Cargnino P, Farisse P: Thoracoscopy in malignant pleural effusions. *Am Rev Respir Dis* 1981;124:588–592.
14. Poe RH, Tobin RE: Sensitivity and specificity of needle biopsy in lung malignancy. *Am Rev Respir Dis* 1980;122:725 729.
15. Zavala DC, Schoell JE: Ultrathin needle aspiration of the lung in infectious and malignant disease. *Am Rev Respir Dis* 1981;123:125–131.
16. Stevens GM, Lillington GA, et al.: Needle aspiration biopsy of localized pulmonary lesions. *Calif Med* 1967;106:92–97.
17. Fontana RS, Miller WE,Beabout JW, Payne WS, Harrison EG Jr: Transthoracic needle aspiration of discrete pulmonary lesions. *Med Clin North Am* 1970;54:961–971.
18. Kaye W: Invasive monitoring techniques: arterial cannulation, bedside pulmonary artery catheterization, and arterial puncture. *Heart Lung* 1983;12:395–427.
19. Seneff M: Arterial line placement and care. In: Rippe JM, Irwin RS, Alpert JS, Fink MP, eds. *Intensive care medicine*, 2nd ed. Boston: Little, Brown, 1991:37–47.
20. Venus B: Vascular cannulation. In: Civetta JM, Taylor RW, Kirby RR, eds. *Critical care*, 2nd ed. Philadelphia: JB Lippincott, 1992:149–169.
21. Wiedemann H, Matthay M, Matthay R: Cardiovascular-pulmonary monitoring in the intensive care unit (part 1). *Chest* 1984;85:537–549.
22. Sprung C, Rozen R, Rozanski J, et al.: Advanced ventricular arrhythmias during bedside pulmonary artery catheterization. *Am J Med* 1982;72:203–208.
23. Sprung C, Elser B, Schein R, et al.: Risk of right bundle-branch block and complete heart block during pulmonary artery catheterization. *Crit Care Med* 1989;17:1–3.
24. Matthay M, Chatterjee K: Catheterization of the pulmonary artery: risks compared with benefits. *Ann Intern Med* 1988;109:826–834.
25. Boyd K, Thomas S, Gold J, Boyd A: A prospective study of complications of pulmonary artery catheterizations in 500 consecutive patients. *Chest* 1983;84:245–249.
26. McDaniel D, Stone J, Faltas A, et al.: Catheter-induced pulmonary artery hemorrhage: diagnosis and management in cardiac operations. *J Thorac Cardiovasc Surg* 1981;82:1–4.
27. Barash P, Nardi D, Hammond G, et al.: Catheter-induced pulmonary perforation: mechanisms, management, and modifications. *J Thorac Cardiovasc Surg* 1981;82:5–12.
28. Voyce S, Urbach D, Rippe J: Pulmonary artery catheters. In: Rippe JM, Irwin RS, Alpert JS, Fink MP, eds. *Intensive care medicine*, 2nd ed. Boston: Little, Brown, 1991.

29. Lipp H, O'Donoghue K, Resnekou L: Intracardiac knotting of a flow-directed balloon catheter. *N Eng J Med* 1971;284:220.
30. Sokolowski JW, Burgher LW, Jones FL: Guidelines for fiberoptic bronchoscopy in adults. *Am Rev Respir Dis* 1987;136:1066.
31. Popovich JJ, Kvale PA, Eichenhorn EA: Diagnostic accuracy of multiple biopsies from flexible fiberoptic bronchoscopy: a comparison of central versus peripheral carcinoma. *Am Rev Respir Dis* 1982;125:521–523.
32. Gellert AR, Rudd RM, Sinha G, et al.: Fiberoptic bronchoscopy: effect of multiple bronchial biopsies on diagnostic yield in bronchial carcinoma. *Thorax* 1982;37:684–687.
33. Zavala D: Diagnostic fiberoptic bronchoscopy: techniques and results of biopsy in 600 patients. *Chest* 1975;68:12–19.
34. Richardson RH, Zavala DC, Mukerjee PK, et al.: The use of fiberoptic bronchoscopy and brush biopsy in the diagnosis of suspected pulmonary malignancy. *Am Rev Respir Dis* 1974;109:63–66.
35. Cortese DA, McDougall JC: Biopsy and brushing of peripheral lung cancer with fluoroscopic guidance. *Chest* 1979;75:141–145.
36. Wang KP, Terry P: Transbronchial needle aspiration in the diagnosis of bronchogenic carcinoma. *Am Rev Respir Dis* 1983;127:344–347.
37. Wimberley NW, Bass JB Jr, Boyd BW, et al.: Use of a bronchoscopic protected catheter brush for the diagnosis of pulmonary infections. *Chest* 1982;81:556–562.
38. Pollock HM, Hawkins EL, et al.: Diagnosis of bacterial pulmonary infections with quantitative protected catheter cultures obtained during bronchoscopy. *J Clin Microbiol* 1983;17:255–259.
39. Glanville AR, Marlin GE, et al.: The use of fiberoptic bronchoscopy with sterile catheter in the diagnosis of pneumonia. *Aust N Z Med* 1985;128:309–319.
40. Chauncey JB, Lynch JP,Hyzy RC, Toews GB: Invasive techniques in the diagnosis of bacterial pneumonia in the intensive care unit. *Semin Respir Infect* 1990;5:215–224.
41. Fagon JY, Chastre J,Hance AJ, et al.: Detection of nosocomial lung infection in ventilated patients. *Am Rev Respir Dis* 1988;138:110–116.
42. Shelley MP, Wilson P, Norman J: Sedation for fiberoptic bronchoscopy. *Thorax* 1989;44:769–775.
43. Bartlett JG, Alexander J, Mayhew J, Sullivan-Sigler N, Gorbach SL: Should fiberoptic bronchoscopy aspirates by cultured? *Am Rev Respir Dis* 1976;114:73–78.
44. Wimberley N, Faling LJ, Bartlett JG: A fiberoptic bronchoscopy technique to obtain in contaminated lower airway secretions for bacterial culture. *Am Rev Respir Dis* 1979;119:337–343.
45. O'Hickey S, Hilton AM: Fiberoptic bronchoscopy in the elderly. *Age Aging* 1987;16:226–233.
46. Pereira W, Kovnat DM, Snider GL: A prospective cooperative study of complications following flexible fiberoptic bronchoscopy. *Chest* 1978;73:813–816.
47. Credle WF Jr, Smiddy JF, Elliott RC: Complications of fiberoptic bronchoscopy. *Am Rev Respir Dis* 1974;109:67–72.
48. Dreison RB, Albert RK, et al.: Flexible fiberoptic bronchoscopy. *Chest* 1978;74:144–149.
49. Albertini RE, Harrell JH, Kurihara N, Moser KM: Arterial hypoxemia induced by fiberoptic bronchoscopy. *JAMA* 1974;230:1666–1667.
50. Pereira W Jr, Kovnat DM, Snider GL: Fever and pneumonia after flexible fiberoptic bronchoscopy. *Am Rev Respir Dis* 1975;112:59–64.

4

Allergy

Dennis J. Beer

Allergy refers to tissue inflammation and organ dysfunction caused by immune responses to environmental antigens. The clinical features of each allergic disease reflect the immunologically mediated inflammatory response in the affected organ(s) or tissue(s).

I. **Allergy.** The diversity of allergic disease expression arises from different immunologic effector mechanisms evoking specific patterns of tissue injury.
   A. For IgE antibody–mediated allergy, the sequential factors that determine expression of disease include **allergen** (an antigen capable of inducing an allergic response), **exposure and sensitization** (generation of an immune response), **reintroduction** of the sensitizing antigen, and **target-organ response.** Implicit in this sequence is the precept that a clinical state of allergy develops only in susceptible individuals encountering particular allergens.
   B. In the context of the IgE–mast cell mediator pathway of immunologically induced inflammation, the term **atopy** refers to a genetically determined state of **IgE-antibody production directed against common environmental allergens.** Atopy affects 10% to 30% of the population; allergic rhinoconjunctivitis and allergic asthma are the most common clinical manifestations. Atopic dermatitis is less common, and allergic gastroenteropathy is rare. IgE antibodies also may be pathogenetic in nonatopic allergic diseases, namely, anaphylaxis and urticaria/angioedema. The disease processes causally associated with IgE antibodies lack the genetically determined propensity and the target-organ hyperresponsiveness of atopy and have no special predilection for the atopic individual. Lastly, rhinitis, asthma, eczematous dermatitis, anaphylaxis, and urticaria/angioedema all may occur through pathogenic mechanisms that do not involve IgE antibodies.

II. **General diagnostic and therapeutic principles**
   A. **History and physical examination**
      1. **The most important portion of the clinical evaluation of diseases suspected of being mediated by IgE allergy is the expertly obtained history.** The history not only provides diagnostic information, but it also directs further diagnostic testing and subsequent therapies. Once the details of the chief complaint are ascertained, questions relating to other symptoms of allergic origin should be posed. Further history should focus on the presence of **skin eruptions, headache, nasal pruritus, sneezing, rhinorrhea, postnasal drip, nasal congestion, nasal polyposis, eye irritation, hearing loss, dyspnea, cough, wheezing, and aspirin sensitivity.** Even though the patient may not associate multiple allergic symptoms with a common etiology, such symptom complexes often coexist. Once a strong suspicion that IgE-mediated allergic disease is present, further allergy history is necessary to allow a correlation of symptoms with the known site and time of exposure to various allergens (Table 4-1). It is crucial to establish when and where the individual has symptoms. The history should include questions related to severity and functional consequence of symptoms, exact yearly timing of symptoms, and fluctuation of symptoms in relation to geographic or specific environmental circumstances (barns, fields, damp basements, factories).
      2. Sneezing, rhinorrhea, and nasal congestion without nasal pruritus or ocular ir-

Table 4-1. Inhaled aeroallergens causing rhinitis, conjunctivitis, and asthma

Pollens (tree, grass, weed)
Dust mite (*Dermatophagoides*)
Animal proteins (cat, dog, horse, guinea pig, gerbil, rat)
Fungal spores (*Alternaria, Aspergillus, Cladosporium, Penicillium*)
Pyrethrum and pyrethroids
High-molecular-weight organic compounds derived from plants, bacteria, and insects
Inorganic and organic chemicals of low molecular weight

ritation suggest that the symptoms are probably not allergic in origin. Likewise, unilateral nasal or ocular symptoms are rarely manifestations of allergy. Allergic symptoms are usually intermittent in character; even when continuous, periods of waxing and waning intensity are common.

3. The propensity to generate IgE antibody upon exposure to allergens is genetically determined, and most allergic patients will have a **positive family history of atopy.**

4. **A prior medication history** revealing a salubrious clinical response to antihistamines, cromolyn, corticosteroids, or allergen-injection therapy suggests an allergic diathesis. Furthermore, a full medication history may suggest that an individual's symptoms are secondary to a given drug.

   a. Alpha-sympathomimetic nasal sprays, rauwolfia, oral contraceptives, β-blockers, tricyclic antidepressants, and other medications may be the primary cause of nasal obstruction. Various forms of β-blockers, including topical ocular preparations, may result in dyspnea, cough, or wheezing. Angiotensin-converting enzyme (ACE) inhibitors can result in angioedema or cough. **Failure to obtain the medication history may lead to unnecessary allergic evaluations.**

5. **Allergens**

   a. **Pollens.** Protein-rich pollen grains (the male gametes of plants) are among the most important seasonal allergens (1). In general, allergenic pollens must be antigenic, produced in large quantities by a common plant, and dispersed primarily by the wind. In the United States, most trees and grasses as well as certain weeds produce large quantities of highly allergenic, wind-borne pollen. The seasonal occurrence of these pollens varies with geographic location and accounts for the seasonality of allergic symptoms. Transfer of pollen between flowering plants is accomplished by insects and not by wind dispersal; therefore, these flowering plant pollens are not major allergens. Goldenrod, popularly considered to cause hay fever, has little clinical significance because the pollen rapidly falls to the ground. In contrast, ragweed pollenates at the same time of year as goldenrod but is a major allergen because the pollen is abundant, small, light-weight, and dispersed by the wind.

   b. **Fungi.** *Alternaria, Aspergillus, Cladosporium,* and *Penicillium* species are the most common allergenic fungi (1), colonizing many habitats and prolifically producing spores. Although these allergens can result in perennial symptoms, certain environmental circumstances (warmth and humidity followed by windy weather) result in large numbers of airborne spores and fluctuating seasonal exacerbations of symptoms in susceptible individuals. Likewise, certain habitats such as damp basements, food storage areas, and compost heaps provide optimal conditions for spore production.

   c. **Mites.** The excreta of house dust mites (*Dermatophagoides* species) are the major source of allergens in house dust (1). A major food source for dust mites is human dander, and these vermin are quite plentiful in bedding. Dust mite—sensitive individuals have perennial symptoms exacerbated when dust mites proliferate with increased indoor warmth and humidity and when dust becomes aerosolized during house cleaning and bed making.

   d.   Pets. In the allergic individual, sensitivity to animals must always be suspected. Household pet serum proteins found in urine or pelts are easily transferred to furniture, bedding, and rugs and are another source of perennial indoor allergens (1). Although cats and dogs are the most common animals involved, many other animals are often culprits, including hamsters, gerbils, rabbits, and mice. Similarly, certain occupational groups such as veterinarians, farmers, ranchers, and laboratory workers may be exposed to a wide variety of allergenic animals. Because of emotional attachments, patients often underestimate the importance of this type of exposure. A patient with inhalant allergy whose symptoms begin to flare after a period of good pharmacologic control may have had the recent introduction of a pet into the home.

6.   Physical examination. In evaluating an individual with known or suspected IgE-mediated allergic disease, particular attention should be paid to the skin, eyes, nose, throat, and chest.

   a.   The **skin lesions** of atopic dermatitis are variable and consist of erythematous patches, papules, vesicles, scaling, crusting and/or lichenification. The distribution of the skin lesions varies with the age of the patient. In the adolescent/adult phase of atopic dermatitis, lesions are usually pruritic, erythematous, papular, scaly patches that tend to involve the forehead, periorbital areas, neck, antecubital and popliteal fossae, and hands.

   b.   **Allergic rhinoconjunctivitis** causes erythema and edema of the conjunctiva bilaterally, a watery ocular discharge, and occasionally periorbital edema with a bluish discoloration about the eyes. In the acute stages of allergic rhinitis, examination of the nasal cavity demonstrates a pale, wet, boggy mucosa. Clear thin nasal secretions are often present, and swollen turbinates may completely occlude the nostrils, resulting in mouth breathing. Nasal polyps may be noted. The nasal obstruction of allergic rhinitis may be accompanied by fluid accumulation in the middle ear.

   c.   Depending on the severity of an asthmatic attack, **chest examination** in an asthmatic may be entirely normal or reveal the use of accessory muscles of respiration, diffuse inspiratory and expiratory wheezing, a prolonged expiratory phase of respiration, and cyanosis. Under extreme circumstances, the acutely ill asthmatic patient may appear somnolent, and no breath sounds will be heard on auscultation.

7.   A detailed survey of the patient's home, school, and/or work environment is often useful in identifying the source of allergens.

B.   Laboratory investigation. Both *in vivo* and *in vitro* assays may be useful in the evaluation of atopic disease.

1.   *In vivo* assay of IgE. Immediate hypersensitivity skin testing is a convenient, inexpensive, safe, and expeditious way to detect the presence of allergen-specific IgE (2). For reliable testing, the subject must not be receiving antihistamines (astemizole and other long-acting agents can alter skin test results for 6–8 weeks after their discontinuation), must be capable of developing a wheal-and-flare response upon stroking of the skin (dermatographism), and must not be so exquisitely sensitive to a given allergen that there is a high risk of skin testing–induced anaphylaxis. In addition, the skin to which the allergens are to be applied must be free of disease.

   a.   **Prick and intradermal skin test** methods are most commonly employed. In prick testing, the size of the histamine-induced wheal is assessed 20 minutes after a single drop of allergen in solution (concentrated allergen extract typically 20,000–100,000 allergy units [AU]/mL, 1:10 weight/volume [w/v], or 20,000 protein nitrogen units [PNU]/mL) is applied to the skin by a needle prick. The size of the wheal is compared to the size of wheals at positive (histamine) and negative (saline) control sites. Wheal size is graded and reported as 1 to 4+. The flare (erythema) component of the cutaneous response to allergen is an evanescent axonal reflex that is not a major element of the grading in most scoring systems.

    b. Intradermal skin testing with a 1:10 or 1:100 dilution of the concentrated allergenic extract should be performed for allergens suspected of contributing to an atopic diathesis and not eliciting a positive response by prick application. With intradermal testing, the controls and the scoring system are identical to that of prick testing. The interpretation of a properly performed skin test result requires a comprehensive knowledge of the history and physical findings.

        i. A positive skin test is only a demonstration of the presence of IgE antibody directed against a given allergen and does not mean that a subject has an allergic disease or that an atopic person has had a clinically significant reaction to the specific allergen. To incriminate an allergen in the pathogenesis of an allergic diathesis requires integration of clinical and testing data.

        ii. With inhalant antigens, correlating positive skin tests with a history that suggests clinical sensitivity strongly incriminates an allergen. Conversely, a negative skin test and a negative history exclude the allergen as being clinically relevant. If a skin test to a particular allergen is positive but no history suggests clinical sensitivity to that allergen, then the patient should be reevaluated using a natural exposure to the allergen. If no disease is present, then the individual's positive skin test result should be viewed as a risk factor for the subsequent development of allergen-induced disease.

  2. *In vitro* assay of IgE

    a. Serum total IgE is usually measured by solid-phase noncompetitive radioimmunoassays and expressed as International Units (IU) of IgE per milliliter (IU/mL; 1 IU = 2.4 ng) (3). IgE concentrations vary with age, sex, family history of allergic disease, and the presence of allergy. The mean IgE level is higher in atopic than nonatopic individuals, but values overlap widely.

    b. The *in vitro* measurement of allergen-specific IgE is clinically more important than quantitation of serum total IgE. Such testing is useful in patients who cannot undergo immediate hypersensitivity skin testing because of continued use of long-acting antihistamines, extensive dermatitis, dermatographism, or risk of anaphylaxis. Assays are modifications of noncompetitive, solid-phase immunoassay techniques.

        i. The **radioallergosorbent test (RAST)** or a variant of RAST is most commonly employed (4). Allergen-bearing solid phase is incubated with serum to permit binding of serum-specific IgE. After washing, the solid-phase allergen–antibody complex is incubated with radiolabeled antihuman IgE and washed again. The measured quantity of radioactivity bound to the solid phase is proportional to the quantity of serum allergen-specific IgE. Through standardization measurements, exact amounts of allergen-specific IgE can be determined. **The RAST correlates well with a variety of *in vivo* provocation tests for allergy, including skin testing, nasal or bronchial challenge, and *in vitro* allergen-induced histamine release. However, RAST results are less sensitive than immediate hypersensitivity skin testing. Similar to *in vivo* skin testing, the interpretation of RAST results must be done in the context of the patient's history and physical examination.**

C. Therapeutic principles

  1. The three principles of treatment of IgE-mediated allergic diseases are allergen avoidance, pharmacotherapy, and immunotherapy (allergen injection). Because IgE-mediated allergic disease requires interaction between allergen and antibody, **the first tenet of allergy management is allergen avoidance** (Table 4-2). Agents that elicit IgE responses and clinical sensitivity (foods, drugs) should be avoided. For optimal management, those animals causing allergic symptoms should be removed from the indoor environment. In dust

Table 4-2. Environmental control

General measures
1. Keep relative humidity at 50% or less by using air conditioning and dehumidifier.
2. Eliminate irritants from home, especially cigarette smoke.

Specific measures for

1. Pollens:	Use air conditioner and keep the windows of the house and car closed. During the peak of the pollen season, avoid outside activities.
2. Molds:	Outdoor molds can be excluded by keeping the windows closed. Use exhaust fan in bathroom and kitchen to keep humidity <50%.
3. Dust mite:	Cover mattresses, box spring, and pillows with an impermeable encasing. All bedding should be washed in hot water (temperature greater than 130°F) once a week. Use synthetic pillows. If possible, remove carpet. Keep the humidity <50%.
4. Feathers:	Replace feather pillow with Dacron (washable) pillow, and wash regularly.
5. Pets:	Remove the pet from the home. If the patient does not agree to remove the pet, the pet should not be permitted in the bedroom. In addition, to decrease antigen shedding, the pet should be bathed once a week.

mite–sensitive individuals, a diminished degree of exposure can be attained by the use of synthetic bedding with zippered plastic encasement of the pillows, mattress, and box spring; maintenance of <50% indoor humidity and an ambient temperature of <68° Fahrenheit; and removal of upholstered furniture and curtains from the bedroom. To limit exposure to mold spores, barns, mowed grass, and raked leaves should be avoided. Damp areas within the home, especially the basement, should be equipped with a dehumidification system. In order to prevent the growth of mold, dehumidifier filters should be changed or cleaned regularly. For other inhalant allergens such as grass, tree, and weed pollens, complete avoidance is practically impossible; however, air conditioners and air-filtration systems can reduce aeroallergen load (5).

    2. **Systemic and local pharmacotherapy** consisting of epinephrine, bronchodilators, antihistamines, decongestants, corticosteroids, cromolyn, and/or nedocromil may be administered to control allergic symptoms. Specific pharmacologic interventions are discussed in the subsequent sections relating to specific diseases.

    3. **Allergen immunotherapy,** the subcutaneous injection of increasing doses of allergen over time, is designed to prevent allergic symptoms that occur in the sensitized individual upon exposure to allergen. Rigorous, double-blind trials have validated the efficacy of conventional high-dose immunotherapy (first introduced by Noon in 1911 as a treatment for pollen-induced rhinitis) in the treatment of specific-inhalant-induced allergic rhinitis and asthma over the last 35 years (6).

        a. **Conventional high-dose immunotherapy** utilizes a variety of immunization schedules with the goal of reaching a maintenance dose (0.1 to 0.5 mL of a 1:10 or 1:100 dilution of the most concentrated allergen extract) given every 3–5 weeks for several years.

        b. With the exception of poorly controlled asthmatics, candidates for inhalant-allergen immunotherapy should have significant allergen-induced (pollens, molds, spores, dust mites, and well defined animal dander) disease that is not adequately controlled with environmental measures and pharmacotherapy. Although certain foods, chemicals, drugs, and unusual environmental substances can result in IgE-mediated allergy, sensitivity to these agents should not be treated with immunotherapy. Several other techniques of allergen immunotherapy, including skin titration testing and treatment (Rinkel method), subcutaneous provocation and neutralization testing, and sublingual provocation testing, have been employed but have not been validated by rigorous controlled trials (7).

III. **Allergic rhinitis.** Allergic rhinitis is an IgE-mediated inflammatory disease involving the mucous membranes of the nose. Symptoms usually begin in childhood or early adulthood but can occur at any age. Allergic rhinitis often occurs seasonally, when pollen comes into direct contact with the respiratory mucosa, but it can also occur perennially. Specific interactions between antigen and IgE occur on the surface of submucosal mast cells, leading to the release of mediators and the production of symptoms (8).

A. Clinical manifestations

1. Mild symptoms of allergic rhinitis include nasal pruritus, rhinorrhea, and sneezing; more severe symptoms include violent paroxysms of sneezing and total obstruction of airflow caused by copious amounts of mucus (9). Other symptoms are lacrimation and soreness of the eyes, irritability, fatigue, lethargy, and anorexia. These symptoms may be aggravated by nonspecific irritants such as cigarette smoke, aerosols, strong odors, perfumes, and insecticides. Complicating inflammatory or infectious sinusitis results in maxillofrontal headache, postnasal discharge, and persistent nasal stuffiness. Occasionally, mild obstructive disease of the lower airways may be demonstrable without overt clinical symptoms of bronchial asthma.

2. **Nasal physical findings** include pale blue mucous membranes, edematous turbinates coated with thin, clear secretions, dark circles under the eyes, and mouth breathing necessitated by nasal obstruction. Some patients may have erythematous nasal mucosa. Nasal polyps are uncommon in uncomplicated rhinitis. Lacrimation, scleral and conjunctival injection, periorbital edema and fluid, or retraction of the tympanic membrane may also be observed. Enlarged tonsils and adenoids, cervical lymph node swelling, and fever are not typically associated with allergic disease, and their presence should prompt a search for complicating infection or other disease.

B. Diagnosis

1. The diagnosis of allergic rhinitis depends on a careful medical history and identification of IgE directed against the responsible allergen (2,10). Most patients have a family history of atopy. Seasonal patterns of symptoms should be noted and related to the local pattern of plant pollenation. Determination of specific IgE antibodies against various allergens is usually documented by skin testing or sensitive *in vitro* radioimmunoassay.

2. The direct scratch, prick, or intradermal skin test, using appropriate allergens, is the quickest and least expensive test currently available (2,11). However, in some patients (eg, those who have extensive eczema or marked dermatographism or take medications that may interfere with skin reactivity), the *in vitro* RAST, which measures specific serum IgE levels, may be more useful (3,12).

3. Normal or increased numbers of eosinophils may be found in the peripheral blood and/or nasal secretions of individuals with either allergic or nonallergic rhinitis. Examination of nasal secretions for eosinophils is often more useful than examination of peripheral blood. **Positive nasal smears (>20% eosinophils) are obtained in approximately 50% of patients with proven allergic rhinitis but are rarely found in normal persons or in those with rhinitis due to other causes** (13). Large numbers of neutrophils in the nasal smear suggest infection. The serum total IgE level is elevated in only 30% to 40% of patients with allergic rhinitis. In allergic rhinitis, unless infectious sinusitis is present, roentgenograms of the paranasal sinuses are usually normal and unnecessary.

C. Differential diagnosis

1. Conditions and causes to consider in the differential diagnosis of seasonal allergic rhinitis include upper respiratory viral infection, excessive use of alpha-sympathomimetic nasal drops or sprays, hormonally related rhinitis that occurs premenstrually or during pregnancy, and use of specific drugs such as oral contraceptives, reserpine derivatives, β-blocking agents (propranolol, etc), ACE inhibitors (captopril, etc), hydralazine, aspirin, and other nonsteroidal anti-inflammatory drugs (NSAIDs). The manifestations of upper respiratory tract infection usually last no longer than a week and may include fever, pain, and neutrophils in secretions (14).

2. Conditions that must be ruled out in cases of perennial allergic rhinitis include structural nasal abnormalities such as septal deviation, endocrine abnormali-

ties such as hypothyroidism, nasal mastocytosis, nonallergic rhinitis with nasal eosinophilia, use of specific drugs (see above), or perennial nonallergic rhinitis of unknown cause (vasomotor rhinitis). Structural abnormalities of the nose usually can be differentiated by physical examination; mastocytosis is detected by examination of a biopsy of the nasal mucosa. The symptoms of perennial nonallergic rhinitis of unknown cause often occur with changes in temperature or humidity and after exposure to irritants or air pollution (14).

D. Treatment

  1. Three strategies are used to treat allergic rhinitis: avoidance of offending aeroallergens, use of antihistamines and other drugs, and allergen-specific immunotherapy (9,14,15). Although allergens usually cannot be completely avoided, measures to reduce exposure generally provide some relief (see Table 4-2). Exposure to dust can be reduced by the use of dust-proof covers on pillows, mattresses, and box springs. Avoiding outdoor activities during the height of the pollen season can reduce exposure to these allergens. Patients sensitive to mold spores should avoid contact with hay and should not rake leaves or mow grass. Air conditioners and electrostatic filters are often helpful. Many nonspecific irritants that aggravate symptoms (eg, smoke, pollution, or dust) should also be avoided (5).

  2. The judicious use of drugs may eliminate most symptoms in the majority of patients.

   a. The most frequently used medications are **H₁-blocking antihistamines.** These agents effectively control the acute symptoms of nasal itching, watery rhinorrhea, and sneezing. Terfenadine, or its safer derivative (fexofenadine) are long-acting antihistamines with little or no sedative effect, are administered orally in a dosage of 60 mg BID. Astemizole and loratidine are two other long-acting, nonsedating antihistamines administered orally in a dosage of 10 mg once daily. Potentially life-threatening cardiac arrhythmias (ventricular tachycardia of the "swinging" variety or torsades de pointes) may result from pharmacokinetic changes of terfenadine or astemizole clearance induced by concomitant administration of macrolide antibiotics (eg, erythromycin, troleandomycin, clarithromycin, and azithromycin), ketoconazole, or itraconazole (15–18).

   b. Antihistamine therapy alone is often insufficient, especially for nasal congestion (15,16). In such cases, the oral administration of sympathomimetic drugs, including phenylpropanolamine and pseudoephedrine hydrochloride, is recommended. Care must be taken when sympathomimetics are given to patients with cardiovascular disease because these agents can cause blood pressure and the heart rate to rise. The long-acting sympathomimetic pseudoephedrine sulfate, taken orally in a dosage of 120 mg BID, may be useful. Preparations containing combinations of antihistamines and decongestants also may be used.

   c. For cases in which avoidance of allergens and the use of antihistamines and decongestants do not reduce symptoms, intranasal application of 4% cromolyn sodium solution, which prevents the release of mast cell mediators, or topical corticosteroids (beclomethasone dipropionate, flunisolide acetate, budesonide, or triamcinolone acetonide) is recommended. The dosage of cromolyn sodium is usually one spray to each nostril TID to QID. Corticosteroids are usually given in a dosage of two inhalations to each nostril BID to TID; once-daily dosing is often possible after symptoms have been controlled. Clinical improvement is usually apparent within several days, but maximal clinical benefit may not be achieved for as long as 2 weeks. These topically administered corticosteroid preparations do not cause the side effects associated with systemic administration of corticosteroids. Local nasal irritation is the principal side effect of intranasal steroids, and about 10% of patients will sneeze or experience some burning or irritation after corticosteroid administration. Systemic corticosteroids are rarely indicated; in very severe cases, however, a short course (up to 1 week) can dramatically reduce symptoms (14).

   d. **Patients with allergic rhinitis who are not attaining satisfactory clinical improvement with environmental control and symptomatic drug treatment can be treated with allergen-specific immunotherapy.** Extracts of the specific allergens are injected subcutaneously, usually at weekly intervals. Small amounts are injected initially, and the dose is gradually increased until a maintenance level is achieved. In most cases, 6 months to a year after immunotherapy is begun, a decrease in symptoms and in the need for medication becomes apparent; maximum efficacy is reached in 2–3 years. In controlled, double-blind studies, immunotherapy has been shown to be effective for allergic rhinitis caused by ragweed, grass, and tree pollens. Efficacy has been correlated with the total dose administered, but relapses can occur, even after maintenance therapy of 3–5 years' duration is discontinued. The results are specific for the particular allergens that are employed in the therapy (6). Although allergen-injection therapy induces many alterations in both humoral and cellular allergen-specific immune responses (19), the development of a specific IgG response is the only immunologic change consistently correlated with the clinical efficacy of immunotherapy.

IV. **Allergic conjunctivitis.** Allergic conjunctivitis is the most common ocular disorder seen in the practice of allergy. The ocular analogue of allergic rhinitis, allergic conjunctivitis occurs in 30% to 40% of patients with seasonal allergic rhinitis and also is caused by an IgE-mediated mast cell and basophil response. As a result of allergen–IgE interaction on the surface of mast cells in the conjunctiva, histamine and other mediators are liberated. Patients with acute allergic conjunctivitis have an increased amount of IgE in their tears and increased numbers of eosinophils in ocular scrapings. A consequence of the IgE–allergen interaction is local conjunctival vasodilation and edema (20).

   A. **Clinical manifestations.** Pruritus is always a prominent feature in patients with allergic conjunctivitis. Both eyes are usually involved, but only one eye may be affected when the cause is manual contamination by allergens such as food or animal dander. The conjunctiva generally appears injected and edematous. In severe cases, the eyes may be swollen shut. Allergic conjunctivitis rarely occurs without allergic rhinitis; however, in some patients, ocular symptoms may be more prominent than nasal symptoms. The condition is unlikely to be allergic conjunctivitis if symptoms or signs of allergic rhinitis are absent.

   B. **Diagnosis**
      1. The diagnosis of allergic conjunctivitis is based on the history and physical examination. Symptoms usually occur seasonally and are accompanied by a personal and/or family history of atopy. Skin testing may confirm suspected seasonal allergy. **Hansel stain of conjunctival secretions usually reveals numerous eosinophils.**
      2. The **differential diagnosis** includes other forms of acute conjunctivitis, particularly those of viral etiology, specific forms of bacterial conjunctivitis, contact dermatitis from the instillation of drugs or from airborne irritants, keratoconjunctivitis sicca, and vernal conjunctivitis (20).

   C. **Treatment**
      1. Treatment of allergic conjunctivitis is the same as that of allergic rhinitis and other allergic diseases: avoidance of the allergen, medication, and, if necessary, immunotherapy. **When allergic conjunctivitis is associated with respiratory allergic disease, the course of treatment is dictated by the more debilitating respiratory condition.** Avoidance of ubiquitous aeroallergens is difficult; however, effective therapy for symptoms can usually be achieved with topical medications such as vasoconstrictors, antihistamines, and corticosteroids. Many preparations used to treat allergic conjunctivitis contain a combination of an antihistamine and a vasoconstrictor. The usual dosage is two drops in each eye every 3–4 hours as needed. If this combination is not effective, ophthalmic cromolyn sodium should be tried next, before corticosteroids.
      2. **Corticosteroid therapy usually should be limited to a period of 1 week. If longer therapy is necessary, intraocular pressure should be measured**

before therapy is started and every 3–4 weeks thereafter. Medrysone, an effective corticosteroid, is poorly absorbed and is less likely to cause changes in intraocular pressure than the more readily absorbed corticosteroids. The dosage is one drop of 4% solution in each eye QID.

    a. Before a patient is given topical corticosteroids, **varicella-zoster blepharoconjunctivitis should be excluded** because corticosteroids will exacerbate and spread the infection. Hyperemia and an infiltrative conjunctivitis, associated with the typical vesicular eruption along the dermatomal distribution of the ophthalmic branch of the trigeminal nerve, are characteristic of herpes zoster infection. If a diagnosis of allergic conjunctivitis cannot be made with certainty prior to institution of specific therapy, an ophthalmologic consultation should be obtained.

    3. No controlled, double-blind studies of allergen-specific immunotherapy have been done in patients with allergic conjunctivitis, but immunotherapy for associated allergic respiratory disease has often been observed to partially relieve ocular symptoms.

V. Allergic asthma

  A. Definition

    1. Asthma is a clinical syndrome characterized physiologically by hyperresponsiveness of the tracheobronchial tree to allergens, irritants, ingestants, exercise, infections, and nonspecifc chemical bronchoconstrictors producing variable symptoms of breathlessness, chest tightness, wheezing, cough, and eosinophil-laden sputum that resolve spontaneously or with treatment.

    2. Underlying this clinical description of the asthmatic diathesis and central to its pathogenesis is a multicomponent cellular and mediator spectrum of airway inflammation (21). A comprehensive discussion of asthma and its treatment is provided in chapter 5. A brief review of asthma from the perspective of allergy follows.

  B. Clinical manifestations

    1. Allergic asthma (extrinsic, atopic, or immunologic) generally develops early in life. Other manifestations of atopy, namely, allergic rhinoconjunctivitis and atopic dermatitis, often coexist, and a family history of atopic disease is common. Asthmatic flares occur upon exposure to relevant aeroallergens. Immediate hypersensitivity skin tests show wheal-and-flare reactions to the causative allergens, and serum total IgE levels are frequently, but not always, elevated.

    2. The controlled laboratory inhalation of relevant allergens in allergic asthma **(allergen bronchoprovocation)** causes acute airflow obstruction **(early response)** that reverses with or without bronchodilators. This sequence is often followed by a second bronchospastic response 4–8 hours later **(late response)** associated with cellular and humoral inflammation. Clinically, this late response tends to be difficult to treat. In the laboratory, pretreatment with NSAIDs can attenuate the late response (22).

  C. Treatment

    1. Four treatment modalities are available for allergic asthma: patient education, environmental control, pharmacotherapy, and allergen-injection immunotherapy. The goals of effective asthma management include the maintenance of normal activity levels, maximization of pulmonary function as measured by spirometry, prevention of chronic troublesome symptoms, prevention of recurrent exacerbations, and avoidance of adverse effects of therapy. Once offending allergens have been identified by history and *in vivo* or *in vitro* measurement of specific IgE, reducing allergen exposure is the first therapeutic option (see Table 4-2) (5).

    2. Pharmacotherapy for asthma is a dynamic endeavor and must be tailored to the individual in a graded fashion (23).

      a. Mild episodic asthma, characterized by occasional intermittent disease flares with prolonged symptom-free periods associated with normal pulmonary function, may be treated as needed with an inhaled β-agonist (albuterol, metaproterenol, or pirbuterol). Proper instruction in the use of the inhaler and demonstrated patient compliance with optimal technique are essential. For those individuals with poor hand–lung coordination, the use of a spacer may optimize drug delivery.

b. **Moderate asthma,** characterized by frequent symptoms, especially at night, and chronic spirometric impairment, implies the presence of significant airway inflammation and therefore should be treated with regular use of an inhaled anti-inflammatory agent such as a corticosteroid, nedocromil, or cromolyn or an oral leukotriene antagonist. Of these agents, corticosteroids are the most consistently effective. Depending on the clinical circumstances, inhaled β-agonist therapy is continued either on a regular or an as-needed basis. If nocturnal symptoms remain problematic, a long-acting theophylline preparation (anhydrous theophylline sustained-action or extended-release tablets/capsules) or a long-acting inhaled β-agonist (salmeterol) can be added.

c. In **severe asthma,** characterized by an inadequate response to high doses of inhaled corticosteroids and intensive bronchodilators, treatment should include systemic corticosteroids in addition to the above. Some patients require only bursts of systemic corticosteroids, while others require continuous daily or every-other-day therapy. Because of the associated toxicities of prolonged systemic corticosteroid administration, the use of corticosteroid-sparing drugs such as methotrexate, gold, and cyclosporine should be considered.

d. Involvement of patients with moderate to severe asthma in the management of their disease is crucial. Patient self-monitoring with morning and evening measurement of peak expiratory flow rates (PEFR) may be most beneficial in helping to make therapeutic adjustments (24). Use of specific medications is reviewed in chapter 5.

3. **Immunotherapy** may be useful in the treatment of some patients with allergic asthma caused or aggravated by certain pollens (ragweed and grass), mold spores (*Alternaria*), house dust mites, or animals (cats) (25). **Indications include documented specific IgE antibody and clinical allergy to the allergen with an inadequate response to environmental control measures and limited pharmacotherapy.** Because of the increased risk of a fatal reaction, poorly controlled asthma is an absolute contraindication to immunotherapy (6).

VI. **Upper airway inflammation and asthma**

A. **Definition.** Recognition that acute attacks of asthma could follow aspirin ingestion dates back to the early part of this century (26). Aspirin sensitivity frequently is characteristic of patients with asthma accompanied by vasomotor rhinitis, sinusitis, and/or nasal polyposis. In 1967, Samter and Beers (27) first suggested that the triad of asthma, nasal polyposis, and sensitivity to aspirin and related compounds was the clinical manifestation of an inflammatory disease of the upper and lower airways.

B. **Clinical manifestations**

1. The prevalence of this syndrome in all asthmatics is 2% to 3%, with a higher rate in the severe asthmatic population (28). The typical patient with the classic Samter's syndrome is a middle-aged individual with vasomotor rhinitis (with or without sinusitis and/or nasal polyps), perennial asthma, blood and/or respiratory secretion eosinophilia, negative immediate hypersensitivity skin tests, and intolerance to aspirin (but not sodium salicylate, salicylic acid esters, and choline salicylate) and related compounds (NSAIDs). Whether aspirin-sensitive patients are also more sensitive than aspirin-nonsensitive asthmatics to the yellow dye tartrazine remains controversial. The onset of an aspirin-induced reaction is generally within 30 minutes after ingestion and may include rhinorrhea and gastrointestinal distress in addition to asthma.

2. Classically, the onset of asthma most often occurs after the upper airway symptoms have been present for some time. Intolerance to aspirin and related compounds is usually noted after the rhinosinusitis and asthma are well established. This classic sequence of disease manifestations is not absolute, and pa-

tients may occasionally develop two or three of the clinical features simultaneously or over several weeks.

C. **Diagnosis and treatment.** The diagnosis is easily established on the basis of history and physical examination. Treatment of this syndrome is avoidance of respiratory irritants, aspirin, and NSAIDs, as well as the use of pharmacologic measures designed to control rhinosinusitis and asthma. Because aspirin-sensitive patients can tolerate acetaminophen, this agent can be used for mild analgesia. If aspirin or related compounds are needed for the treatment of other medical conditions, aspirin or NSAID desensitization can be performed (29).

VII. **Occupational asthma**
   A. **Definition**
   1. Occupational asthma is defined as symptomatic variable airflow obstruction and airway hyperresponsiveness induced by a specific substance in the workplace (30). In the fourth century BC, Hippocrates described asthma in horsemen, fishermen, tailors, and metal workers. Occupational asthma may arise from IgE-mediated mechanisms or from nonimmunologic sensitivity. This disorder is distinct from airway hyperresponsiveness acquired *de novo* following acute inhalation of toxic chemical fumes or smoke (reactive airways dysfunction syndrome).
   2. The causative substances of occupational asthma are either high-molecular-weight proteins derived from plants or animals or low-molecular-weight reactive chemicals such as certain anhydrides (phthalic or trimellitic anhydride), dyes (methyl blue), diisocyanates (toluene diisocyanate), or antibiotics (penicillin or tetracycline) (30).
   B. **Clinical assessment and treatment**
   1. Evaluation of the patient with suspected occupational asthma begins with a detailed medical and occupational history. A diagnosis must be confirmed by a decrement in lung function parameters (PEFR or forced expiratory volume in 1 second [FEV_1]) at work associated with exposure to the putative offending substance. If uncertainty persists as to the relation of asthma to the work environment even after these measures, controlled bronchoprovocation studies may be performed.
   2. Once the diagnosis has been established, cessation of exposure is the preferred treatment. New cases may be prevented by institution of industrial engineering or process modification that reduces airborne exposure to previously identified causative agents. Although pharmacotherapy administered according to the same principles that direct the therapy of nonoccupational asthma is indicated for the acute management of occupational asthma, pharmacotherapy is not considered a suitable alternative for the reduction of exposure to causative agents. Immunotherapy for occupational asthma has not been studied adequately and therefore is not a recommended treatment option (6,30).

VIII. **Multiple chemical sensitivity syndrome**
   A. **Clinical and immunologic profile**
   1. Multiple chemical sensitivity syndrome (also called environmental illness, clinical ecological illness, total allergy syndrome, and chemical AIDS) is a puzzling clinical entity that has emerged in the latter half of this century as an illness of ostensible allergy or sensitivity to almost all organic and synthetic chemicals (31–33). Typically, previously healthy individuals present either because of upper respiratory symptoms or ill-defined central nervous system dysfunction related to living or working in a tightly sealed building served by a closed system of ventilation or because of similar symptomatolgy following an accidental exposure to an established toxin. Despite removal from the initial offending environment or toxin, symptoms recur and intensify over time and eventually generalize to involve virtually all organ systems.
   2. The most prominent symptoms are typically constitutional, cardiorespiratory, neuropsychologic, and gastrointestinal. The symptoms, initially caused by a single or limited number of offending substances, are eventually precipitated by a vast array of chemically unrelated compounds at doses far below those

established in the general population to cause harmful effects. In extreme cases, patients become recluses from everyday life. Despite a wide array of subjective complaints, physical examination discloses no abnormalities.

3. Immunologically, these patients are functionally intact (31–34). As a group, they display no deficiency or excess in their ability to mount appropriate immune responses, nor do they suffer an excess prevalence of allergic reactions, autoimmune diseases, unusual opportunistic infections, or cancer (34). Likewise, no data have substantiated an infectious or toxicologic etiology for this malady. A psychiatric foundation for this illness has been proposed, but there is no unifying psychiatric diagnosis.

B. **Therapeutic approach**

1. Although the mechanism(s) underlying the pathogenesis of multiple chemical sensitivity syndrome is unknown and despite the controversy regarding whether or not this entity is an organic disease process, physicians should be prepared to manage the significant numbers of individuals with the above outlined clinical profile. A subgroup of practitioners, namely, clinical ecologists or environmental physicians, armed with untested theories of disease and unvalidated diagnostic testing (33), have instructed patients on substance-avoidance strategies, often reaching extremes of social isolation and severe dietary restriction.

   a. For purposes of eliminating contaminating chemicals from the body and creating proper balance of immune function, the clinical ecologists' approach to therapy includes nutritional supplementation, detoxification programs, anticandidal medication or desensitizing injections of *Candida albicans* extract, intradermal or subcutaneous administration of neutralizing doses of putative offending substances, and periodic administration of intravenous gamma globulin (33). The efficacy of any of these therapies is unproven.

   b. Until more scientific understanding of multiple chemical sensitivity syndrome is obtained, individuals manifesting this illness should be counseled on short-term, modest, workable goals aimed at reducing disability and a reorientation toward health rather than focusing on specific symptoms, obtaining a series of diagnostic tests, or embarking on unvalidated therapies.

References

1. Solomon WR, Platts-Mills TAE: Aerobiology and inhalant allergens. In: Middleton E Jr, Reed CE, Ellis EF et al, eds. *Allergy: principles and practice*, 4th ed. St. Louis, MO: Mosby-Year Book, 1993:469.
2. Bousquet J, Michel FB: In vivo methods for study of allergy. In: Middleton E Jr, Reed CE, Ellis EF et al, eds. *Allergy: principles and practice*, 4th ed. St. Louis, MO: Mosby-Year Book, 1993:573.
3. Lopez M, Fleisher T, deShazo RD: Use and interpretation of diagnostic immunologic laboratory tests. In: deShazo RD, Smith DL, eds. *Primer on allergic and immunologic diseases. JAMA* 1992; 268:2970.
4. Kelso JM, Yunginger JN: Laboratory test for IgE-mediated diseases. In: Lockey RF, Bukantz SC, eds. *Allergen immunotherapy.* New York: Marcel Dekker, 1991:145.
5. Fernandez-Caldas E, Fox R: Environmental control of indoor air pollution. *Med Clin North Am* 1992;935.
6. Ohman JL Jr: Allergen immunotherapy: review of efficacy and current practice. *Med Clin North Am* 1992;76:977.
7. Reisman RE: American Academy of Allergy: position statements—controversial techniques. *J Allergy Clin Immunol* 1981;67:333.
8. Wasserman SI: Mediators of immediate hypersensitivity. *J Allergy Clin Immunol* 1983;72:101.
9. Mathews K: Allergic and non-allergic rhinitis, nasal polyposis, and sinusitis. In: Kaplan AP, ed. *Allergy.* New York: Churchill Livingstone, 1985:323.
10. Norman PS, Lichtenstein LM, Ishizaka K: Diagnostic tests in ragweed hay fever. *J Allergy Clin Immunol* 1973;52:210.

11. Norman PS: Skin testing. In: Rose NR, Friedman H, Fahey JL, eds. *Manual of clinical laboratory immunology.* Washington, DC: ASM, 1986:660.
12. Barbee RA, Halonen M, Lebowitz M et al: Distribution of IgE in a community population sample: correlations with age, sex, and allergen skin test reactivity. *J Allergy Clin Immunol* 1981;68:106.
13. Mullarkey MF, Hill JS, Webb DR: Allergic and nonallergic rhinitis: their characterization with attention to the meaning of nasal eosinophila. *J Allergy Clin Immunol* 1980;65:122.
14. Badhwar AK, Druce HM: Allergic rhinitis. *Med Clin North Am* 1992;76:789–803.
15. Naclerio RM: Allergic rhinitis. *N Engl J Med* 1991;325:860–869.
16. Simons FER, Simons KJ: Antihistamines. In: Middleton E Jr, Reed CE, Ellis EF et al, eds. *Allergy: principles and practice*, 4th ed. St. Louis, MO: Mosby-Year Book, 1993:856.
17. Monahan BP, Ferguson CL, Killeavy ES, et al.: Torsades de pointes occurring in association with terfenadine use. *JAMA* 1990;264:2788
18. Simons FER, Kesselman MS, Giddins NG, et al.: Astemizole-induced torsades de pointes. *Lancet* 1988;2:624.
19. Gurka G, Rocklin R: Immunologic responses during allergen-specific immunotherapy for respiratory allergy. *Ann Allergy* 1988;61:239.
20. Friedlaender MH: Ocular allergy. In: Middleton E Jr, Reed CE, Ellis EF et al, eds. *Allergy: principles and practice*, 4th ed. St. Louis, MO: Mosby-Year Book, 1993:1649.
21. Djukanovic R, Roche WR, Wilson JW, et al.: Mucosal inflammation in asthma. *Am Rev Respir Dis* 1990;142:434.
22. Lemanske RF Jr: The late phase response: clinical implications. In: Stollerman GH, Lamont JT, Leonard JJ, Siperstein MD, eds. *Advances in Internal Medicine.* St. Louis, Mo: Mosby-Year Book, 1991;36:171.
23. *Guidelines for the diagnosis and management of asthma. Expert panel report.* Bethesda, Md: National Heart, Lung and Blood Institute, National Institutes of Health, 1992; publication 91-3042.
24. Cross D, Nelson HS: The role of the peak flow meter in the diagnosis and management of asthma. *J Allergy Clin Immunol* 1991;87:120.
25. Ohman JL: Allergen immunotherapy in asthma: evidence for efficacy. *J Allergy Clin Immunol* 1989;84:133.
26. Gilbert GB: Unusual idiosyncrasy to aspirin. *JAMA* 1911;56:1262.
27. Samter M, Beers RF Jr: Concerning the nature or intolerance to aspirin. *J Allergy* 1967;40:281.
28. Farr RS: The need to re-evaluate acetylsalicylic acid (aspirin). *J Allergy* 1970;45:321.
29. Stevenson DD, Simon RA: Sensitivity to aspirin and nonsteroidal antiinflammatory drugs. In: Middleton E Jr, Reed CE, Ellis EF et al, eds. *Allergy: principles and practice*, 4th ed. St. Louis, Mo: Mosby-Year Book, 1993:1747.
30. Bernstein DI: Occupational asthma. In: deShazo RD, Smith DL, eds. *Primer on allergic and immunologic diseases. JAMA* 1992;268:917.
31. American College of Physicians: Position paper: clinical ecology. *Ann Intern Med* 1989;111:186.
32. Cullen MR, Cherniack MG, Rosenstock L: Occupational medicine. *N Engl J Med* 1990;322:675.
33. Council on Scientific Affairs, American Medical Association: Clinical ecology. *JAMA* 1992;268: 3465.
34. Simon GE, Daniell W, Stockbridge H, et al.: Immunologic, psychologic and neuropsychological factors in multiple chemical sensitivity: a controlled study. *Ann Intern Med* 1993;119:97.

5

Asthma

Rachel J. Givelber and
George T. O'Connor

Asthma is a chronic inflammatory disease of the bronchial tree characterized by hyperresponsiveness to bronchoconstricting stimuli with episodic airflow limitation that is reversible either spontaneously or with therapy. The recognition that asthma is an inflammatory disorder has profound implications for management and prevention.

I. **Presenting signs and symptoms**
   A. **Spectrum of disease severity.** Some individuals with asthma may be entirely asymptomatic between rare attacks provoked by specific exposures. Other asthmatics may have nearly continuous symptoms and frequent severe attacks. Episodic exacerbations of asthma range in severity from mildly bothersome wheezing to life-threatening bouts of respiratory failure. Clinicians must be able to distinguish acute asthmatic exacerbations that can safely be treated in the outpatient setting from those requiring hospitalization and intensive care.
   B. **The cardinal symptoms of asthma** include episodic wheezing, dyspnea, chest tightness, cough, and sputum production. The symptoms of asthma are frequently bothersome during the late-night and early-morning hours, with disruption of sleep a common problem. Episodes of wheezing and dyspnea provoked by inhalation of airborne irritants or allergens, especially if relieved by use of an inhaled bronchodilator, constitute an essentially pathognomonic history. Other presentations of asthma, such as isolated persistent unexplained cough (cough-variant asthma) or exertional chest tightness and dyspnea, may be impossible to diagnose with certainty on the basis of symptoms alone (1).
   C. **Signs**
      1. Patients with asthma may have entirely normal physical examinations during intervals between exacerbations.
      2. **During acute asthma exacerbations,** tachypnea, tachycardia, wheezing, and expiratory prolongation are usually present. Airflow may be so impaired in severe attacks that breath sounds are diminished and no wheezing is heard. Cyanosis, accessory muscle use, and an elevated pulsus paradoxus (systolic blood pressure in expiration exceeding that in inspiration by >10 mm Hg) may be observed in severe attacks. Evidence of pneumothorax or subcutaneous emphysema on physical examination indicates a severe, life-threatening episode.
      3. **In chronic asthma,** patients may have wheezing on auscultation of the chest. Coughing may be observed during the examination, and clear or yellow sputum may be expectorated. Asthma is often associated with atopy, and physical examination evidence of allergic rhinitis or conjunctivitis, nasal polyposis, or eczema may be seen.

II. **Etiology and pathogenesis**
   A. The etiology and pathogenesis of asthma are **not fully understood** and are areas of intensive scientific investigation (2). Asthma appears to be a **multifactorial** disorder with both genetic and environmental causes and is likely to be a common clinical manifestation with **diverse causes and pathogenic mechanisms**. For example, childhood-onset atopic asthma, adult-onset asthma in a middle-aged ex-smoker without apparent allergies, and asthma developing in the setting of occupational ex-

posure to toluene diisocyanate are likely to result from different cellular and molecular abnormalities despite their common characteristics of airway hyperresponsiveness, airway inflammation, and variable airflow obstruction.

B. Genetic factors. Asthma is familial but does not occur in a pattern consistent with a single major Mendelian gene. Recent genetic epidemiologic studies have mapped a gene for asthma to a locus on chromosome 5, where numerous genes encoding inflammatory cytokines are located (3). Asthma is frequently associated with clinical manifestations of atopy (familial allergy to common aeroallergens) and elevated serum total IgE concentration, but some evidence suggests that asthma and allergy may be inherited independently (4).

C. Epidemiologic data suggest that exposure to certain **environmental factors**, especially early in life, such as allergens derived from dust mites, cats, and other common environmental aeroallergens, may play a causal role in allergic sensitization and the development of atopic asthma (5–7), but more research is needed to confirm and quantitate the risk associated with such exposures. Exposure to inhaled or ingested allergens can clearly aggravate asthma chronically and precipitate life-threatening exacerbations (8). Passive exposure to environmental tobacco smoke appears to be a risk factor for the development of childhood asthma (9,10), but whether this is a risk factor for asthma that persists into adulthood is less clearly understood. A variety of chemicals encountered in the workplace can cause asthma by mechanisms that apparently do not involve IgE-mediated hypersensitivity (11).

D. Pathophysiology. The **eosinophil** is a major effector cell in asthmatic airway inflammation, but the mast cell and T lymphocyte also play crucial roles (12,13). **Cytokines** mediate the interactions between these cells and appear to play important roles in the pathogenesis of asthma.

    1. Leukotrienes are a class of arachidonic acid–derived mediators released by airway mast cells and eosinophils that have inflammatory and bronchoconstricting effects.

    2. Neuropeptides released by the autonomic and sensory neurons in the bronchial tree also appear to influence airway inflammation. Ongoing research on the cellular and molecular mechanisms underlying the bronchial mucosal inflammation of asthma may ultimately hold the key to finding better therapies for this disease.

III. Relevant physiology

A. Variable airflow limitation. Generalized airflow obstruction that varies spontaneously or in response to treatment over time is a defining characteristic of asthma. During intervals between exacerbations, spirometry may be normal or may indicate an isolated reduction in the mid–expiratory flow rate ($FEF_{25\%–75\%}$) consistent with slight limitation of airflow in the bronchioles ("small" airways). In moderate-to-severe chronic asthma, as well as during an asthmatic exacerbation, spirometry reveals airflow obstruction. The airflow obstruction characteristically improves following administration of an inhaled rapidly acting bronchodilator. An improvement in forced expiratory volume in 1 second (FEV_1) or forced vital capacity (FVC) of 12% or greater following administration of an inhaled bronchodilator is considered a significant response, that is, a response greater than that observed in the majority of nonasthmatic persons.

B. Nonspecific bronchial hyperresponsiveness may be detected by bronchoprovocation tests with an inhaled pharmacologic bronchoconstrictor such as methacholine or histamine. Spirometry is performed at baseline and after each incremental dose. Patients with asthma display greater nonspecific bronchial responsiveness than persons without asthma, although some overlap exists between the distributions of responsiveness of asthmatic and normal persons (14,15). Persons with asthma also display increased bronchial responsiveness to exercise, inhalation of cold air, and other physical stimuli.

C. Bronchial responsiveness to a specific inhaled allergen may be measured for research purposes, although this testing entails some risk of a severe asthma attack and is rarely done in clinical practice. Spirometry is performed at baseline and after incremental doses of an aerosolized allergen. A characteristic dual asthmatic response to inhaled allergen may be elicited: a rapid but short-lived airflow limitation (early response) followed by the gradual onset of more prolonged airflow limitation (late response) (16). The early response is caused by bronchial smooth muscle contraction produced by the allergen-induced release of bronchoconstricting mediators from bronchial mucosal mast cells. The late response is caused by bronchial mucosal inflammation induced by the proinflammatory cytokines also released by mast cells in response to allergen. The delay in the development of this response relates to the time required for the recruitment and influx of eosinophils and other inflammatory cells.

IV. **Differential diagnostic possibilities.** A classic history may be so suggestive of asthma that other diagnostic possibilities are excluded. The diagnosis may be less straightforward in many cases, and alternative diagnoses may need to be considered. The elderly and those with chronic symptoms may be especially problematic in this regard. **The differential diagnostic possibilities for adults presenting with asthma-like symptoms are listed in Table 5-1, along with helpful diagnostic clues.** Asthma-like symptoms that fail to improve with bronchodilator and corticosteroid therapy should suggest the possibility of a diagnosis other than asthma.

Table 5-1. Differential diagnosis for patients with symptoms suggesting asthma

Condition	Clues that help distinguish the condition from asthma
Localized anatomic lesion(s) obstructing airways, eg, tumor, foreign body	Unilateral or monophonic wheezing on physical examination Chest x-ray or chest CT abnormality Flow-volume loop consistent with central airway obstruction Fiberoptic bronchoscopy is definitive test
Laryngeal dysfunction	Inspiratory stridor on physical examination during acute episode Fiberoptic laryngoscopy during acute episode is definitive test
Pulmonary emphysema	History of exertional dyspnea, sometimes with wheeze, that is constant over time, as opposed to the variable and episodic nature of asthma; middle-aged or older patient with smoking history Spirometry indicating airflow obstruction with relatively little reversibility to bronchodilator Reduced diffusing capacity Chest x-ray revealing hypovascularity or bullae consistent with emphysema
Chronic bronchitis	History of chronic cough and sputum in a tobacco smoker or worker with occupational dust exposure; no history of episodic dyspnea or wheezing
Congestive heart failure	History of ischemic heart disease or other cardiac problems; complaint of edema, orthopnea Crackles on chest auscultation; edema, cardiomegaly on examination Cardiomegaly, pulmonary congestion on chest x-ray ECG abnormalities; echocardiographic evidence of left ventricular dysfunction
Pulmonary infiltration with eosinophilia, either idiopathic or related to parasite infestation	Immigration from or travel to endemic area for parasites Marked blood eosinophilia (although eosinophilia is common in atopic asthma) Pulmonary infiltrates on chest x-ray
Cough secondary to ACE inhibitors or other drugs	History of cough beginning with institution of ACE inhibitor
Pulmonary embolism	Acute presentation in patient with no prior history of asthma and evidence of deep venous thromboembolism

ACE = angiotensin-converting enzyme.

V. Long-term management. For convenience, the management of asthma can be divided into long-term management and the management of exacerbations.

A. **In order to formulate the long-term management plan for a patient with asthma,** the clinician should assess the frequency and severity of asthma symptoms, the frequency of nocturnal symptoms interfering with sleep, the degree of disruption of school or work by asthma, and the number of hospitalizations or emergency department visits for asthma attacks.

1. In addition, **peak expiratory flow rate (PEFR) or spirometry should be performed to assess the severity of airflow obstruction.** These data, as well as physical examination findings, permit the classification of the severity of asthma in a patient seen in the outpatient setting (Table 5-2). Symptom frequency and lung function data should be followed over time at follow-up visits to assess the response to therapy.

2. **The patient must be taught to monitor asthma severity to know when to escalate medical therapy, contact a clinician, or seek emergency care.** Patients can monitor asthma severity by paying close attention to symptom frequency and duration. The frequency of bronchodilator use is especially useful in this regard. In addition, current guidelines recommend that many asthmatics perform home PEFR monitoring with a simple inexpensive peak-flow meter and follow an action plan based on symptoms as well as PEFR measurements (17). Many clinicians reserve home PEFR monitoring for asthma patients who have required hospitalization, emergency department visits, or prolonged oral corticosteroid therapy.

B. **Asthma therapy** should be tailored to the severity of asthma in each individual patient. Pharmacologic agents available in the United States that have established value for the long-term management of asthma are listed in Table 5-3.

C. **Specific agents**

1. **Inhaled corticosteroids** are the most effective inhaled anti-inflammatory agents for asthma and are the cornerstone of long-term management for most asthmatic adults. Corticosteroids exert numerous actions on the immune system that result in reduced airway inflammation. Airway hyperresponsiveness and the frequency of asthma exacerbations are reduced (18,19). Inhaled corticosteroids appear to be a safe therapy (20).

   a. Oral thrush and hoarseness may occur but are uncommon when these agents are inhaled with a spacer or chamber, as recommended, and administration is followed by rinsing the mouth. Transient cough and wheezing provoked by inhalation of these agents are uncommon and, when necessary can be prevented by pretreatment with a β_2-agonist bronchodilator.

   b. Regular use of inhaled corticosteroids has measurable effects on the hypothalamopituitary axis, although only rare cases of adrenal insufficiency have been reported. It has been suggested that patients receiving ≥ 1000 µg/d of inhaled beclomethasone, or the equivalent, should be given hydrocortisone to prevent adrenal insufficiency at times of severe illness or surgery (21).

   c. Easy bruising as a complication of inhaled corticosteroid use has been reported. Long-term use of inhaled corticosteroids may be a risk factor for osteoporosis, but prospective longitudinal data supporting this hypothesis are not available.

2. **Cromolyn sodium** and **nedocromil sodium** are inhaled medications that reduce bronchial responsiveness to inhaled allergen, reduce airway inflammation, and prevent asthma symptoms and exacerbations (22,23). Although the mechanisms of action are not fully understood, these medications appear to inhibit the release of bronchoconstricting and proinflammatory mediators and cytokines by mast cells, eosinophils, and other cells important in the pathophysiology of asthma. These agents do not help all patients with asthma and are less effective than inhaled corticosteroids. Thus, cromolyn and nedocromil are used less often and have received less emphasis in recent practice guidelines for adult asthma than have inhaled corticosteroids.

3. **Inhaled short-acting β_2-agonist bronchodilators** are recommended as rescue therapy to provide immediate relief of symptoms and airflow obstruction

Table 5-2. Long-term management of asthma (excluding infants and young children)

Severity of asthma	Clinical features				Therapy		
	Daytime symptoms	Nocturnal symptoms	Peak flow or FEV_1	Short-acting beta agonist prm	Long-acting bronchodilator[a]	Long-term oral corticosteroid
Step 1: Intermittent	≤2 times/wk	≤2 times/mo	≥80% predicted	Yes	No	No
Step 2: Mild persistent	>2 times/wk but not daily	>2 times/mo	≥80% predicted	Low dose (or cromolyn or nedocromil, or zafirlukast or zileuton)	Usually not	No
Step 3: Moderate persistent	Daily	>1 time/wk	>60% to <80% predicted	Medium to high dose	Sometimes	No
Step 4: Severe persistent	Continuous	Frequent	≤60% predicted	High dose	Yes	Yes

[a]Long acting bronchodilators available in the U.S. include inhaled salmeteral, oral theophylline, and oral sustained-release beta-agonists.
Adapted from National Asthma Education Program. Expert panel report II. Guidelines for the diagnosis and management of asthma. U.S. Department of Health and Human Services, Washington DC; 1997. NIH publication 97–4051.

Table 5-3. Asthma medications

Medication	Dose range or usual dose	How supplied
Anti-inflammatory agents		
Inhaled corticosteroids (MDI)		
Beclomethasone dipropionate		
42 μg/inhalation	6 to >20 inhal/day	200 inhal/cannister
84 μg/inhalation	3 to >10 inhal/day	120 inhal/cannister
Flunisolide (250 μg/inhalation)	2 to >8 inhal/day	100 inhal/cannister
Fluticasone		
44 μg/inhalation	2-6 inhal/d - low dose	60, 120 inhal/can
110 μg/inhalation	2-6 inhal/d - med dose	120 inhal/cannister
220 μg/inhalation	>3 inhal/d - high dose	120 inhal/cannister
Triamcinalone acetonide (100 μg/inhal)	4 to >20 inhal/day	240 inhal/cannister
Inhaled cromolyn sodium		
MDI (800 μg/inhalation)	2 inhal. QID	200 inhal/cannister
Solution for nebulization	1 ampule QID	20 mg/ampule'
Inhaled nedocromil sodium		
MDI (1.75 mg/inhalation)	2 inhal QID	104 inhal/cannister
Oral corticosteroids	5–60 mg/day (prednisone or equivalent)	Various strengths
Leukotriene modifiers		
Zafirlukast	20 mg q12h	20 mg tablets
Zileuton	600 mg QID	300, 600 mg tabs
Inhaled bronchodilators (short-acting)		
Inhaled beta-2 agonists		
Albuterol		
MDI (90 μg/inhalation)	2 inhal q4h prn	200 inhal/cannister
solution 0.5%	0.5 mL q4h prn	Mix with 2.5 mL saline; 20 mL bottle
solution 0.083%	1 ampule q4h prn	Unit dose vial
Bitolterol		
MDI (0.37 mg/inhalation)	2 inhal q4h prn	300 inhal/cannister
solution 0.2%	0.5–1.0 mL q6h prn	Mix with 1–3 mL saline; 10, 30, 60 mL bottles
Isoetharine		
MDI (340 μg/inhalation)	2 inhal q4h prn	200 or 300 inhal/vial
solution 1%	0.5 mL q4h prn	Dilute 1 : 3 with saline; 30 mL bottle
Metaproterenol		
MDI (650 μg/inhalation)	2 inhal q4h prn	200 inhal/cannister
solution 5%	0.3 mL q4h prn	Mix with 2.5 mL saline; 10, 30 mL bottles
Pirbuterol MDI (200 μg/inhalations)	2 inhal q4h prn	400 inhal/cannister
Terbutaline MDI (200 μg/inhalation)	2 inhal q4h prn	300 inhal/cannister
Inhaled anticholinergic agent		
Ipratropium		
MDI (18 μg/inhalations)	2–3 inhal QID	200 inhal/cannister
solution 0.02%	1 ampule QID	Unit dose vial

Table 5-3. (continued)

Medication	Dose range or usual dose	How supplied
Oral bronchodilator (short-acting)		
Oral beta-2 agonists		
Albuterol		
tablets	2–4 mg TID–QID	2 mg, 4 mg tablets
suspension 2 mg/tsp	2–4 mg TID–QID	16 oz. bottle
Metaproterenol		
tablets	20 mg TID–QID	10 mg, 20 mg tablets
suspension 10 mg/tsp	20 mg TID–QID	16 oz. bottles
Terbutaline tablets	2.5–5.0 mg TID	2.5 mg, 5.0 mg tablets
Bronchodilators (long-acting or sustained release)		
Theophylline tablets	400–900 mg/day (not exceeding 13 mg/kg/day ideal body weight)	Various size tablets
Salmeterol MDI (21 μg/inhalation)	2 inhal q12h	120 inhal/cannister
Albuterol extended-release tablets	4–8 mg q12h	4 mg tablets

MDI = metered-dose inhaler; prn = as needed; QID = four times a day; q4h = every 4 hours; TID = three times a day.

caused by asthma (24). By stimulating bronchial smooth muscle β-adrenergic receptors, these agents cause smooth muscle relaxation and bronchodilation within several minutes of administration. The duration of action of these agents is 4–6 hours, although this duration declines with frequent repeated use. Oral preparations are available for patients who cannot use inhalers (with appropriate instruction, such patients should be unusual), but they cause more side effects than inhaled forms.

a. **Side effects** relate to the imperfect β_2-adrenergic specificity of these agents. Tremor, palpitations, and anxiety may occur. Despite earlier concerns, the use of currently used inhaled preparations at recommended doses does not appear to be an important cause of clinically significant dysrrhythmias or hypokalemia. The use of these agents should be minimized in patients with paroxysmal atrial fibrillation or recurrent supraventricular tachycardia.

b. The possibility that regular daily use of these agents, as opposed to "as-needed" use as rescue therapy, may worsen asthma and even be a risk factor for fatal asthma remains controversial (25,26). This possibility has been raised by findings of increased nonspecific bronchial responsiveness and increased responsiveness to inhaled allergen among patients taking a regular QID regimen of an inhaled β_2-agonist compared to patients taking only rescue therapy on an "as-needed" basis (27). Although more research will be needed to resolve this controversy, current guidelines suggest that these agents be used on an as-needed basis. One concrete advantage of such use of these agents is that the frequency of use can be monitored as a marker of asthma control.

c. With appropriate instruction, most patients can master the correct technique for using the metered-dose inhaler (MDI) preparations of these agents. When necessary, the use of a spacer or chamber may help assure adequate MDI technique. For the patient who cannot learn the technique of using a MDI, an electric-powered air compressor and nebulizer can be prescribed for use at home to administer a β_2-agonist solution.

4. **Long-acting and sustained-release bronchodilators.** Each of the three choices available in this category has its own advantages and disadvantages. No consensus has yet emerged regarding the best long-acting bronchodilator, so the clinician must weigh the advantages and disadvantages of these agents for each patient. Some severe asthma patients not controlled on regular anti-inflammatory therapy may require both a long-acting β_2-agonist and theophylline.

   a. **Oral theophylline** causes bronchodilation by uncertain mechanisms. A major advantage is the ease of oral administration of once- or twice-a-day preparations. Disadvantages include potential gastrointestinal, central nervous system, and cardiac toxicity, the need to monitor serum levels, and the potential for drug interactions (eg, with erythromycin, ciprofloxacin, and cimetidine) (28).

   b. **Oral extended-release β_2-agonists** (eg, albuterol) have the advantage of BID oral administration. Disadvantages include β_2-agonist side effects (tremor, anxiety, palpitations), which are more common with oral than inhaled preparations (29), and concerns in the literature noted earlier that the regular daily use of a β_2-agonist might lead to worsening asthma control.

   c. **Inhaled salmeterol** is the only long-acting inhaled β-agonist available in the United States. It is postulated that the long lipophilic side chain of the salmeterol molecule leads to persistence in the cell membrane and prolonged stimulation of the β-adrenergic receptor. Salmeterol has a 12-hour duration of action following inhalation, and few side effects have been reported in clinical trials (30). Once again, the controversial hypothesis that regular daily use of a β_2-agonist might lead to worsening asthma control remains a possible disadvantage to the use of salmeterol.

5. **Oral corticosteroids.** Because of powerful anti-inflammatory effects, oral (and parenteral) corticosteroids play a central role in treating exacerbations of asthma. By reducing bronchial mucosal inflammation and perhaps also by other actions (eg, increasing expression of β-adrenergic receptors), corticosteroids lead to improved airflow, fewer symptoms, and reduced airway responsiveness (31).

   a. **Seven- to 14-day bursts** of oral corticosteroid therapy for exacerbations are a vital element of outpatient asthma management. Such bursts usually begin with 40–60 mg of prednisone per day, or its equivalent. No data have convincingly demonstrated whether a constant daily dose or tapering schedule is better. Early recognition of exacerbations and prompt treatment with oral corticosteroids can help prevent progression to more severe, dangerous, and costly attacks. Oral corticosteroids have significant and serious side effects, and long-term use is reserved for severe persistent asthma refractory to other therapies. When prescribed for long-term use, the dosage of oral corticosteroid should be kept as low as necessary to control the asthma, and an alternate-day regimen should be used whenever possible. In addition, high-dose inhaled corticosteroid should be continued to help keep the required dose of oral steroid to a minimum.

   b. **Short courses of an oral corticosteroid** are generally well tolerated, although weight gain, edema, and insomnia may occur. Even a relatively short course of oral corticosteroid may lead to adrenal insufficiency if severe illness or surgery occurs soon afterward, so stress coverage with hydrocortisone is recommended at these times for any patient who has received a course of oral prednisone within the past year. Long-term therapy may lead to substantial weight gain, immunosuppression, osteoporosis, cataracts, skin fragility and bruising, aseptic necrosis, adrenal insufficiency upon discontinuation or at times of stress, and Cushing's syndrome. Peptic ulcer disease may be a complication, but this remains controversial.

6. **Cytotoxic agents** (eg, methotrexate, azathioprine, cyclosporine) have been employed in severe asthma requiring long-term high-dose oral corticosteroids.

Their benefit is unproven and their use remains controversial (32). At this time, the use of these agents is probably best limited to research protocols.

7. **Leukotriene modifiers. Zileuton,** a leukotriene synthesis inhibitor, and **zafirlukast,** a leukotriene receptor antagonist, are oral medications which have recently been approved for the treatment of asthma in the U.S. In patients with mild-to-moderate asthma, zileuton has been reported to have bronchodilator and anti-inflammatory effects and to reduce the frequency of asthma exacerbations (33). The regular use of zafirlukast has been reported to improve asthma symptoms, modestly reduce the use of as-needed short-acting bronchodilators and improve FEV_1 (34). The effectiveness of either agent relative to inhaled corticosteroid as a preventive anti-inflammatory therapy remains to be established. The potential "steroid-sparing" activity of these agents also remains to be established, although a related leukotriene antagonist has recently been reported to permit reduction in the dosage of inhaled corticosteroid without worsening of asthma control (35). Both zileuton and zafirlukast increase the half-life of warfarin, and zileuton also inhibits metabolism of terfendine and theophylline. Because liver toxicity has been found in some subjects taking zileuton, monitoring of liver function tests is recommended when this medication is used.

D. **Strategy for using asthma medications in long-term management.** The Expert Panel Report II: Guidelines for the Diagnosis and Management of asthma, published by the National Institutes of Health in 1997 (36), is a set of practice guidelines that provides a clear approach to the use of medications for the long-term management of asthma (see Table 5-2).

1. Initiation of treatment is recommended at the step most appropriate to the initial severity of asthma. If control is sustained for at least 3 months, then a gradual reduction in treatment may be possible. A rescue course of oral corticosteroid may be needed at any time and at any step.

2. In practice, the inhaled corticosteroid dosage recommendations listed in Table 5-2 must be translated into a specified number of inhalations for a given preparation. Agents available in the United States are listed in Table 5-3. The relative potency, bioavailability and drug delivery device influence clinical efficacy, thus the different medications are not equivalent on a per inhalation or microgram basis. The recommendations of the National Asthma Education and Prevention Program for estimating low, medium and high doses of each inhaled corticosteroid are reflected below and in Table 5-3 (37); however, the most important determinant of appropriate dosing is the clinician's judgement of the patient's response to therapy. "Low dose" inhaled corticosteroid referes to dosages from the bottom to the middle of the listed range; "medium dose' refers to doses from the middle to the upper end, and "high dose" to daily inhalations exceeding the highest listed value. Thus, for beclomethasone (42 µg/inhalation), 4-12 inhalations/day would be considered low dose, 12–20 inhalations/day would be considered medium dose, and >20 inhalations/day would be high dose.

E. **Avoidance and control of asthma triggers (38).** Inhalation of airborne allergens and irritants may aggravate asthma and precipitate exacerbations, so a careful history is crucial to identifying such exposures. A history that a particular exposure provokes asthma (or nasal) symptoms should be taken as evidence that the exposure is capable of aggravating asthma by either an allergic or irritant mechanism and should be avoided. A history of a seasonal asthma pattern or seasonal rhinoconjunctivitis is important in determining the role of allergy and specific outdoor allergens.

1. Some exposures may aggravate asthma without the individual's awareness (eg, dust mite and cockroach allergens). In addition, some aggravating exposures that are quite evident to many patients may not be evident at all to other patients; for example, cat allergens may not be recognized by a patient who has been living with a cat for many years and has become used to chronic asthma.

2. **Testing for allergy** or determination of serum specific IgE levels by radioallergosorbent test (RAST) may help the clinician decide whether clinically important allergy to a specific allergen is present. Some of the allergens known to aggravate asthma are listed in Table 5-4, along with the control measures that can be undertaken to reduce exposure to them.

3. **Avoidance measures.** Many household chemicals release irritant fumes that can aggravate asthma by nonallergic mechanisms. Some of these are listed in Table 5-5, along with some alternative products that can be used more safely by persons with asthma.

4. Evidence suggests that exposure to tobacco smoke can exacerbate asthma (39). All asthmatics should be educated to avoid any active and passive exposure to tobacco smoke.

F. **Action plans for managing asthma exacerbations.** A detailed, written action plan for managing asthma exacerbations is a vital component of long-term management.

Table 5-4. Strategies for household allergen mitigation

Exposure	Control measures
Cockroach	Cleaning; sealing stored food; fixing water leaks; improving ventilation; using boric acid or hydramethylnon bait stations, or professional extermination.
Dust mite	Impermeable mattress and pillow covers; hot water washing of bedding; eliminating stuffed animals, down comforters, wool blankets; removing carpets or treating with acaracide or tannic acid; avoiding (or treating or covering) upholstered furniture
Cat	Eliminating; if impossible, banishing from bedroom and eliminating carpets, upholstery from bedroom; weekly washing of cat; double-thickness vacuum filter bags
Pollen	Keeping windows closed and using air conditioning; drying clothes indoors (not on outdoor clothes line)
Mold	Maintaining low humidity in home (<50%); improving ventilation; fixing leaks; removing plants; washing floors, walls, and moist surfaces with dilute bleach; removing water-damaged items

Table 5-5. Common household chemicals that can aggravate asthma

Products to avoid	Suggested substitutes
Ammonia, floor cleaners	Wash floor with vinegar and hot water
Air deodorizers and sprays	Avoid altogether
Bleach	Wash bathroom with baking soda and water
Deodorants and antiperspirants	Unscented stick or roll-on
Hairsprays	Hair gels
Harsh detergents	Chlorine-, dye-, and perfume-free detergents
Disinfectants	Borax and hot water
Fragranced products, especially pine scented	Unscented products, when available
Gasoline, kerosene	Store outdoors in well ventilated area; use electric heater indoors
Oven cleaner	
Paint and turpentine	Have someone else handle these products; leave household when they are in use
Pesticides	
Solvents	

Early recognition of and prompt response to incipient exacerbations can help prevent life-threatening episodes and avoid costly consequences such as hospitalization or absence from school or work. Action plans may be based on symptoms alone or may be based on both symptoms and home PEFR measurements. Home peak flow–based action plans have been emphasized in recent guidelines, although firm evidence of the superiority of such plans to symptom-based action plans is lacking. An example of a PEFR-based action plan for managing exacerbations of asthma at home is shown in Fig. 5-1.

G. **Patient education.** The successful long-term management of asthma demands that the patient be an active participant in the treatment plan. The patient must understand the need for maintenance medications, the correct technique for using the inhalers, the early warning signs of an asthma attack, the use of home PEFR monitoring, environmental control measures, and the steps to take in case of an exacerbation. Considerable effort must be devoted to patient education if this material is to be mastered. Nurses and health educators are playing an increasingly important role in the education of patients with asthma.

H. **Regular follow-up care.** Asthma severity often varies greatly over time as a result of variation in environmental exposures, compliance with medications, respiratory infections, and other factors that may be difficult to identify. To maintain optimal asthma control and avoid preventable complications, patients with asthma should have periodic outpatient visits with a clinician experienced in long-term asthma.

VI. **Management of acute exacerbations.** Depending on the severity and response to therapy, exacerbations may be managed at home or in the emergency department or may require hospitalization. Recent practice guidelines published by the NIH and other organizations are reflected in the following recommendations (36,37). Acute asthma exacerbations may be fatal, and patients presenting with this condition must be treated aggressively and monitored with great care (40).

A. **Initial assessment** of a patient presenting with an acute exacerbation should include a history (focusing on previous asthma hospitalizations, intubations, steroid use, and symptoms suggesting infection), physical examination (focusing on vital signs, breath sounds, use of accessory muscles, and cyanosis), measurement of PEFR or FEV_1, oximetry, and, in more severe cases, arterial blood gases.

B. **Initial treatment** includes an inhaled short-acting β-agonist (eg, albuterol). This is typically administered by nebulization, although administration by MDI with the use of a chamber device has been shown to be equally effective in the acute setting. A common regimen is to administer albuterol solution 3 mL of a 0.083% solution by nebulizer every 20 minutes for three doses. Supplemental oxygen should be administered to maintain an oxygen saturation of at least 90%. If a rapid and complete response to inhaled β-agonist is not obtained, then corticosteroid therapy is warranted. A typical initial dose for treating an acute asthma exacerbation is prednisone 60 mg orally or the equivalent dose of a parenteral corticosteroid.

1. Patients who present with severe airflow obstruction that does not respond promptly to inhaled β-agonists may be treated with subcutaneous epinephrine; however, this therapy is associated with greater risk of cardiovascular complications, particularly in older patients who may have underlying ischemic heart disease, and should generally be avoided in favor of inhaled β-agonists.

C. **After this initial therapy, the patient should be reevaluated.** Subsequent therapy will depend on the response of the patient to the initial treatment.

1. **Good response to initial therapy.** If the symptoms resolve, the physical examination normalizes, and the PEFR improves to >70% of the patient's baseline or predicted value, than the patient can generally be discharged safely to home. Discharge instructions should generally include a 1–2 week course of prednisone, as-needed β-agonist by inhalation, and outpatient follow-up within the next few days.

2. **Incomplete response to initial therapy.** Patients who improve partially in response to the initial treatment with a PEFR of 50% to 70% of baseline or predicted value may also require hospitalization, especially those with a history

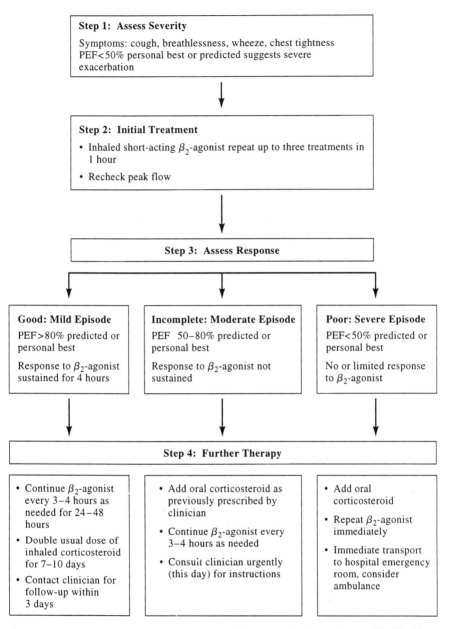

Step 1: Assess Severity

Symptoms: cough, breathlessness, wheeze, chest tightness
PEF<50% personal best or predicted suggests severe
exacerbation

Step 2: Initial Treatment

- Inhaled short-acting β_2-agonist repeat up to three treatments in 1 hour
- Recheck peak flow

Step 3: Assess Response

Good: Mild Episode

PEF>80% predicted or personal best

Response to β_2-agonist sustained for 4 hours

Incomplete: Moderate Episode

PEF 50–80% predicted or personal best

Response to β_2-agonist not sustained

Poor: Severe Episode

PEF<50% predicted or personal best

No or limited response to β_2-agonist

Step 4: Further Therapy

- Continue β_2-agonist every 3–4 hours as needed for 24–48 hours
- Double usual dose of inhaled corticosteroid for 7–10 days
- Contact clinician for follow-up within 3 days

- Add oral corticosteroid as previously prescribed by clinician
- Continue β_2-agonist every 3–4 hours as needed
- Consult clinician urgently (this day) for instructions

- Add oral corticosteroid
- Repeat β_2-agonist immediately
- Immediate transport to hospital emergency room, consider ambulance

Fig. 5-1. PEFR-based plan for management of asthma exacerbations at home. (Modified from *National Asthma Education Program: Expert Panel Report II. Guidelines for the diagnosis and management of asthma.* Washington DC: U.S. Department of Health and Human Services, 1997. NIH publication 97-4051.

of severe asthma in the past, a current exacerbation of long duration, psychosocial problems, or the absence of supportive family members at home.

3. **Poor response to initial therapy.** Patients who fail to respond to therapy, whose PEFR remains <50% of baseline or predicted, who appear drowsy or confused, or who have hypoxemia or hypercapnia should be admitted to the hospital.

D. **Treatment during hospitalization.** When hospitalization is necessary, the patient should be treated with an inhaled short-acting beta$_2$-agonist (albuterol), and a systemic corticosteroid (methylprednisolone 60 mg IV q6h, or the equivalent). Some evidence suggests that the addition of nebulized ipratropium bromide enhances the recovery of patients with acute asthma exacerbations admitted to the hospital. Oral theophylline or intravenous aminophylline may offer additional bronchodilation, but reports are conflicting whether this therapy confers any additional benefit to patients already receiving a β-agonist and corticosteroid. The use of theophylline or aminophylline may be warranted in patients hospitalized for acute asthma who fail to respond quickly to therapy with β-agonist and corticosteroid therapy.

E. **Indications for admission to intensive care unit (ICU).** Patients with drowsiness, confusion, hypercapnia, or severe hypoxemia should be admitted to an ICU. Patients experiencing asthmatic exacerbations typically hyperventilate and have low arterial P_{CO_2}. Thus, a "normal" P_{CO_2} of approximately 40 mm Hg in this setting is worrisome and constitutes grounds for admission to an ICU. Intubation and mechanical ventilation may be life-saving in a severe asthma exacerbation complicated by respiratory failure unresponsive to initial therapy (status asthmaticus).

VII. **Problems and complications of therapy**

A. **Inadequate patient adherence** to the prescribed maintenance regimen of medications is a major problem encountered by all clinicians providing long-term asthma care. A major barrier to adherence is the fact that an inhaled anti-inflammatory medication, unlike inhaled β-agonists, causes no immediate symptomatic improvement when used. Thus, a symptomatic patient may mistakenly conclude that the anti-inflammatory inhaler is not helping and stop using it, while relying on more frequent use of a β-agonist instead. Alternatively, a patient currently experiencing few symptoms may conclude that the inhaled anti-inflammatory agent is no longer needed because the asthma is better, and stop using it. The clinician faces a major challenge in educating the patient about the importance of daily inhaled anti-inflammatory medications, in changing the patient's behavior to achieve regular use of such medications, and in monitoring adherence.

B. **The difficulty many patients have mastering the technique of using the MDI** is another major problem encountered in asthma care. Patient education efforts and repeated reexamination of a patient's inhaler technique during office visits are essential to success. The use of spacers and chambers may help patients who otherwise cannot use the inhalers adequately. Occasional patients may benefit from nebulizers at home because of the inability to master the use of the MDI due to cognitive or physical limitations.

C. **Patients may be unable or unwilling to make home environmental modifications** needed to reduce exposure to an allergen that aggravates asthma. The classic example is the patient who continues to keep a cat despite evidence that cat allergy is aggravating his or her asthma. It may be impossible to adequately control the asthma if such allergen exposure continues. The clinician should persist in efforts to convince the patient to make the necessary changes in the home environment, and specific and practical assistance should be given as necessary.

D. **Oral thrush and hoarseness may occur as a side effect of inhaled corticosteroid use.** These can usually be prevented by prescribing spacers or chambers with instructions to rinse the mouth after each use. Thrush should be treated by rinsing the mouth and then swallowing nystatin oral suspension (5 mL QID) or dissolving clotrimazole lozenges (10 mg) slowly in the mouth five times daily for 14 days or until asymptomatic for longer than 48 hours.

E. **Complications of long-term oral corticosteroid therapy** include Cushing's syndrome, osteoporosis, opportunistic infections, cataracts, aseptic necrosis, and adrenal insufficiency if corticosteroids are discontinued. These complications are discussed in detail in chapter 35.

   F. Complications of acute status asthmaticus
   1. Pneumothorax may occur spontaneously during severe acute asthmatic attacks. The treatment of respiratory failure with positive-pressure mechanical ventilation may also result in pneumothorax, including tension pneumothorax, as a manifestation of barotrauma. Emergency chest tube insertion is required when pneumothorax occurs in the mechanically ventilated patient.
   2. **Excessively rapid ventilatory rates in patients requiring mechanical ventilation** may result in inadequate expiratory time for the degree of airflow obstruction present. This can lead to excessive positive end-expiratory pressure (auto-PEEP), high intrathoracic pressure, diminished venous return, and life-threatening hypotension (41). Relatively low ventilatory rates and "permissive hypercapnia," with intravenous sodium bicarbonate infusion if necessary to maintain arterial pH, are often required (42). Patients requiring mechanical ventilation for acute asthma should be managed by physicians skilled in ventilator management and critical care.

VIII. Special considerations
   A. **Rhinitis/sinusitis** (43). Upper airway disease can increase asthmatic symptoms in some patients. Although the mechanisms underlying this association have not yet been established, treatment of allergic sinusitis with topical corticosteroids or cromolyn sodium can decrease the severity of concomitant bronchospasm. Both acute and chronic sinusitis can worsen symptoms of asthma, and conversely the treatment of associated sinusitis in some severe therapy-resistant asthmatics may significantly improve asthmatic symptoms. The diagnosis of sinusitis requires x-ray or CT scan confirmation. Medical therapy should include at least 3 weeks of appropriate antibiotics and topical nasal corticosteroids, as well as an optional shorter course of topical nasal decongestants. Surgical therapy of chronic sinusitis should rarely be required but may be warranted for patients with severe asthma in whom sinusitis does not improve after prolonged conventional treatment.
   B. **Gastroesophageal reflux disease (GERD)** (44). Although the incidence of GERD in adult patients with asthma ranges from 35% to 75%, the relationship between reflux and increased symptoms of asthma remains unclear. Most patients with GERD have a suggestive history, including heartburn, effortless regurgitation, dysphagia

Table 5-6. Occupational allergens

Agent	Occupations at risk
Animal dander and urine	Laboratory animal workers, veterinarians
Enzymes	Detergent users, pharmaceutical workers, food processors
Latex	Health care workers
Wood dust	Sawmill workers, carpenters
Mites	Granary workers, poultry workers
Soybean dust	Farmers
Wheat and rye flour dust	Bakers
Cotton dust	Cotton textile workers
Anhydrides	Users or manufacturers of plastics or epoxy resins
Isocyanates	Auto painters, foundry workers, polyurethane foam workers
Colophony resins	Electronics workers, solderers
Persulfate	Hairdressers
Disinfectants (formaldehyde, glutaraldehyde)	Hospital workers
Metallic salts	Refinery workers, metal plating workers, diamond polishers

Table 5-7. Tolerance of nonsteroidal anti-inflammatory drugs (NSAIDs) in aspirin-sensitive asthma

Well tolerated NSAIDs	Drugs reported to precipitate exacerbations
Sodium salicylate	Salicylates
Choline salicylate	Aspirin
Choline magnesium trisalicylate	Diflunisal
Salicylamide	Salicylsalicylic acid
Dextropropoxyphene	Polycyclic acids
Benzydamine	Indomethacin
Cholorquine	Sulindac
	Diclofenac
	Ketorolac
	Proprionic acids
	Ibuprofen
	Naproxen
	Fenoprofen
	Ketoprofen
	Pyrazolones
	Aminopyrine
	Sulfinpyrazone
	Phenylbutazone
	Fenemates
	Mefenamic acid
	Flufenamic acid
	Cyclofenamic acid
	Enolic acids
	Piroxicam

or hoarseness, or asthma symptoms that worsen after eating, drinking alcohol, at night, or when supine. Esophageal pH monitoring is the best test to make a diagnosis of GERD when reflux symptoms are atypical or to correlate episodes of reflux with pulmonary symptoms.

 1. Medical therapy of GERD is often effective and should include both lifestyle changes (small frequent meals, avoiding eating for several hours before bedtime, elevating the head of the bed, and elimination of foods known to aggravate reflux, including fats, alcohol, chocolate, and peppermint) and acid-reducing medications. Improvement in the control of asthma after treatment with H_2-antagonists or omeprazole may take longer (7–12 weeks) than improvement in esophageal symptoms. Oral β_2-agonists and theophylline may decrease lower esophageal sphincter tone and should be avoided when possible.

 2. Surgery is not always effective and should be reserved for severely symptomatic patients with documented esophagitis who have failed medical management.

C. **Occupational asthma** (11). Exposures in the workplace are estimated to cause or exacerbate 4% to 15% of asthma in the United States. The asthma history should always include an occupational history and questions about the relation of respiratory symptoms to work. Some of the numerous organic and chemical agents reported to cause occupational asthma are listed in Table 5-6. Most cause or aggravate asthma by IgE-mediated hypersensitivity; for some agents, the mechanisms are unknown. Therapy for occupational asthma usually requires substitution of an alternative agent in the workplace or transfer to a different job whenever possible. Improved ventilation or personal respiratory protection devices are often inadequate because of the minute amount of exposure needed to provoke symptoms once sensitization has occurred. Referral to a physician specializing in occupational medicine and/or an industrial hygienist may be necessary to help identify the offending agent and remedy the exposure.

D. **Sensitivity to aspirin and other nonsteroidal anti-inflammatory drugs (NSAIDs)**
    (45). Sensitivity to aspirin and NSAIDs, the most common cause of drug-induced
    asthma, is reported in 4% of adult asthmatics by history and up to 20% if the diagnosis
    is based on aspirin challenge. These patients have a characteristic clinical syndrome:
    symptoms usually appear in the third to fourth decade of life and begin with intense vasomotor rhinitis, followed over several months by chronic nasal congestion and polyposis; sinusitis occurs in >90% of patients. Aspirin intolerance
    and asthma, often severe and protracted, develop subsequently. In sensitive individuals, ingestion of aspirin leads to wheezing that may be life-threatening, flushing of the
    head and neck, rhinorrhea, and conjunctival irritation. Avoidance of aspirin does not
    affect the course of the underlying asthma. In aspirin-induced asthma, cross-reactivity to other NSAIDs varies with each drug's ability to inhibit cyclooxygenase and the
    individual patient's sensitivity. Table 5-7 lists NSAIDs reported to have aggravated
    asthma and those believed to be safe in patients with aspirin-induced asthma.

E. **Treatment with β-adrenergic blocking agents** may worsen bronchospasm in
    asthma. These agents are commonly prescribed for hypertension, heart disease,
    glaucoma, or migraine headaches. Asthma exacerbation has been reported even
    with the cardioselective agents (those blocking primarily β_1 receptors) and may occur shortly after the β-blocker is introduced or after months of use. Severe reactions, including death, have been reported. Because it is not possible to predict
    which asthmatics will develop severe airway obstruction, these agents should be
    administered with extreme caution.

F. **Specialist referral** should be obtained for any difficult-to-control asthmatic patient, including those requiring daily oral steroids. Patients with frequent emergency department visits or ICU admissions for treatment of asthma require evaluation by a pulmonary specialist. In addition, patients with diagnostic problems
    related to asthma should have a specialist referral.

References

1. Corrao WM, Braman SS, Irwin RS: Chronic cough as the sole presenting manifestation of bronchial asthma. *N Engl J Med* 1979;300:633–637.
2. Drazen JM, Turino GM: Progress at the interface of inflammation and asthma. Report of an ATS-sponsored workshop, November, 1993. *Am J Respir Crit Care Med* 1995;152:386–387.
3. Postma DS, Bleecker ER, Amelung PJ, et al.: Genetic susceptibility to asthma-bronchial hyper-responsiveness coinherited with a major gene for atopy. *N Engl J Med* 1995;333:894–900.
4. Sibbald B: Genetic basis of asthma. *Semin Respir Med* 1986;7:307–315.
5. Cockcroft DW: Mechanism of perennial allergic asthma. *Lancet* 1983;2:253–255.
6. Bush RK: The role of allergens in asthma. *Chest* 1992;101:378S–380S.
7. Sporik R, Holgate ST, Platts-Mills TAE, Cogswell JJ: Exposure to house-dust mite allergen (der p I) and the development of asthma in childhood. *N Engl J Med* 1990;323:502–507.
8. O'Hollaren MT, Yunginger JW, Offord KP, et al.: Exposure to an aeroallergen as a possible precipitating factor in respiratory arrest in young patients with asthma. *N Engl J Med* 1991;324:359–363.
9. Cunningham J, O'Connor GT, Dockery DW, Speizer FE: Environmental tobacco smoke, wheezing, and asthma in children in 24 communities. *Am J Respir Crit Care Med* 1996;153:218–224.
10. Martinez FD, Cline M, Burrows B: Increased incidence of asthma in children of smoking mothers. *Pediatrics* 1992;89:21–26.
11. Chan-Yeung M, Malo J: Occupational asthma. *N Engl J Med* 1995;333:107–112.
12. Barnes PJ: Cytokines as mediators of chronic asthma. *Am J Respir Crit Care Med* 1994; 150:S42–S49.
13. Goldstein RA, Paul WE, Metcalfe DD, et al.: Asthma. NIH conference. *Ann Intern Med* 1994; 121:698–708.
14. O'Connor GT, Sparrow D, Weiss ST: Normal range of methacholine responsiveness in relation to prechallenge pulmonary function. *Chest* 1994;105:661–666.
15. Cockcroft DW, Hargreave FE: Airway hyperresponsiveness. Relevance of random population data to clinical usefulness. *Am Rev Respir Dis* 1990;142:497–500.
16. Malo J, Cartier A: Late asthmatic reactions. In: Weiss EB, Stein M, eds. *Bronchial asthma: mechanisms and therapeutics*, 3rd ed. Boston: Little, Brown, 1993:135–146.

17. Clark N, Evans D, Mellins RB: Patient use of peak flow monitoring. *Am Rev Respir Dis* 1992; 145:722–725.
18. Rutten-Van Molken M, Van Doorslaer E, Jansen M, et al.: Costs and effects of inhaled cortico-steroids and bronchodilators in asthma and chronic obstructive pulmonary disease. *Am J Respir Crit Care Med* 1995;151:975–982.
19. Barnes PJ: Inhaled glucocorticoids for asthma. *N Engl J Med* 1995;332:868–875.
20. Hanania NA, Chapman KR, Kesten S: Adverse effects of inhaled corticosteroids. *Am J Med* 1995; 98:196–207.
21. Toogood JH: What are the clinically relevant risks, and what to do? Making better—and safer—use of inhaled steroids. *J Respir Dis* 1993;14:221–238.
22. Cherniack RM, Wasserman SI, Ramsdell JW, et al.: A double-blind multicenter group comparative study of the efficacy and safety of nedocromil sodium in the management of asthma. *Chest* 1990; 97:1299–1306.
23. Petty TL, Rollins DR, Christopher K, et al.: Cromolyn sodium is effective in adult chronic asth-matics. *Am Rev Respir Dis* 1989;139:694–701.
24. Nelson HS: B-adrenergic bronchodilators. *N Engl J Med* 1995;333:499–506.
25. Barrett TE, Strom BL: Inhaled beta-adrenergic receptor agonists in asthma: more harm than good? *Am J Respir Crit Care Med* 1995;151:574–577.
26. Burrows B, Lebowitz M: The B-agonist dilemma. *N Engl J Med* 1992;326:560–561.
27. Cockcroft DW, O'Byrne PM, Swystun VA, Bhagat R: Regular use of inhaled albuterol and the al-lergen-induced late asthmatic response. *J Allergy Clin Immunol* 1995;96:44–49.
28. Weinberger M, Hendeles L: Theophylline in asthma. *N Engl J Med* 1996;334:1380–1388.
29. Larsson S, Svedmyr N: Bronchodilating effect and side effects of beta$_2$-adrenergic stimulants by different modes of administration (tablets, metered aerosol, and combinations thereof). A study with salbutereol in asthmatics. *Am Rev Respir Dis* 1977;116:861–869.
30. Pearlman DS, Chervinsky P, Laforce C, et al.: A comparison of salmeterol with albuterol in the treatment of mild-to-moderate asthma. *N Engl J Med* 1992;327:1420–1425.
31. McFadden ER Jr: Dosages of corticosteroids in asthma. *Am Rev Respir Dis* 1993;147:1306–1310.
32. Moss RB: Alternative pharmacotherapies for steroid-dependent asthma. *Chest* 1995;107:817–825.
33. Israel E, Cohn J, Dube' L, Drazen JM: Effect of treatment with zileuton, a 5-lipoxygenase in-hibitor, in patients with asthma. *JAMA* 1996;275:931–936.
34. Spector SL, Smith LJ, Glass M: Effects of 6 weeks of therapy with oral doses of ICI 204,219 a leu-kotriene D4 receptor antagonist, in subjects with bronchial asthma. *Am J Respir Crit Care Med* 1994;150:618–623.
35. Tamaoki J. Kondo M, Sakai N, et al. Leukotriene antagonist prevents exacerbation of asthma dur-ing reduction of high-dose inhaled corticosteroid. *Am J Respir Crit Care Med* 1997;155: 1235–1240.
36 National Asthma Education Program: *Expert panel report II. Guidelines for the diagnosis and management of asthma.* Washington, DC: U.S. Department of Health and Human Services, 1997: NIH publication 97-4051.
37. Global Initiative for Asthma: *Global strategy for asthma management and prevention. NHLBI/WHO workshop report.* Bethesda, Md: National Heart, Lung, and Blood Institute, 1995; publication 95-3659.
38. Duff AL, Platts-Mills TAE: Allergens and asthma. *Pediatr Clin North Am* 1992;39:1277–1291.
39. Chilmonczyk BA, Salmun LM, Megathlin KN, et al.: Association between exposure to environ-mental tobacco smoke and exacerbations of asthma in children. *N Engl J Med* 1993;328: 1665–1669.
40. McFadden ER Jr, Hejal R: Asthma. *Lancet* 1995;345:1215–1220.
41. Tuxen DV: Detrimental effects of positive end-expiratory pressure during controlled mechanical ventilation of patients with severe airflow obstruction. *Am Rev Respir Dis* 1989;140:5–9.
42. Tuxen DV: Permissive hypercapnic ventilation. *Am J Respir Crit Care Med* 1994;150:870–874.
43. Friday GA Jr, Fireman PH: Sinusitis and asthma: clinical and pathogenic relationships. *Clin Chest Med* 1988;9:557–565.
44. Harding SM, Richter JE: Gastroesophageal reflux disease and asthma. *Semin Gastrointest Dis* 1992;3:139–150.
45. Hunt LW Jr, Rosenow EC III: Drug-induced asthma. In: Weiss EB, Stein M, eds. *Bronchial asthma: mechanisms and therapeutics,* 3rd ed. Boston: Little, Brown, 1993:621–631.

6 Community-Acquired Pneumonia

Margaret A. Vallen-Mashikian and
Anne Menenghetti

I. **Definition.** In the United States, pneumonia is the leading cause of death from infection and ranks sixth as a cause of all deaths (1). Community-acquired pneumonia (CAP) is defined as a lower respiratory tract infection of the lung parenchyma occurring either in the community or within the first 3 days of hospitalization or institutionalization. Controversy persists concerning the validity of diagnosis, the significance of certain microbiologic isolates, and the optimal therapy. Treatment is often empiric, since even intensive diagnostic efforts fail in identifying a pathogen in more than half of cases. The outpatient mortality rate remains low at 1% to 5% despite the lack of consensus within the medical community regarding management (2).

II. **Epidemiology and risks.** CAP is not a reportable illness, and information about its incidence is based on crude estimates. As many as four million cases occur annually. The attack rate in the United States is currently estimated at 12 per 1,000 adults, resulting in approximately 600,000 hospitalizations annually (3,4).

    A. Major changes have occurred in the **epidemiology of CAP** since the 1930s, when almost all cases were due to *Streptococcus pneumoniae*. The etiology of almost 50% of current cases is unknown (5). Infection with a variety of newly identified or previously unrecognized pathogens has become more frequent. CAP is increasingly common among older patients, as well as those with coexisting illnesses, including chronic obstructive pulmonary disease (COPD), diabetes, congestive heart failure (CHF), renal insufficiency, and chronic liver disease (6).

    B. Immunosuppressive therapy for an expanding list of indications has changed the epidemiology of CAP to include numerous opportunistic pathogens. Persons older than 65 years are the fastest growing segment of the United States population, and the increasing number of cases in this at-risk group has been a major factor in the changing epidemiology of CAP.

III. **Common pathogens**

    A. Pneumococcus is the most common pathogen in patients 60 years and younger who are without comorbid illness and are treated out of the hospital. The next most common pathogens are listed in Table 6-1. Organisms within the miscellaneous group are present in about 1% of patients. Mortality of patients in this category is between 1% and 5% (2).

    B. Table 6-2 lists the common agents causing mild-to-moderate pneumonia treated out of the hospital who have a comorbid illness and/or are older than 60 years. While mortality in this setting is <5%, about 20% of patients initially treated as outpatients may require hospitalization (2).

IV. **Host immune status**

    A. **Knowledge of the immune status** is key to the formulation of a working diagnosis and the determination of empiric therapy. *S. pneumoniae* may infect any host, while other pathogens such as gram-negative rods (GNR), *Legionella pneumophila*, and some viruses are more likely to invade certain populations at risk. The precise nature of any immune defect will determine the risk for various pathogens (Table 6-3).

Table 6-1. Common organisms causing community-acquired pneumonia in patients under age 60 without comorbidity

Organisms

Streptococcus pneumoniae
Mycobacterium pneumoniae
Respiratory viruses
Chlamydia pneumoniae
Haemophilus influenzae

Therapy

Macrolide antibiotic (use a newer macrolide for smokers)
Tetracycline (S. pneumoniae may be resistant)

Table 6-2. Common organisms causing community-acquired pneumonia in patients with comorbidity or over age 60

Organisms

Streptococcus pneumoniae
Respiratory viruses
Haemophilus influenzae
Aerobic gram-negative rods
Staphylococcus aureus
Miscellaneous: *Moraxella catarrhalis, Legionella spp., Mycobacterium tuberculosis, endemic fungi*

Therapy (not for HIV patients)

Second-generation cephalosporin
Trimethoprim/sulfamethoxazole
Beta-lactam antibiotic + beta-lactamase inhibitor
Macrolide antibiotic (if *Legionella* is a concern)

HIV = human immunodeficiency virus.

Certain vocations, avocations, and environments predispose to infection by specific agents, even in the immunocompetent individual (Tables 6-4 and 6-5).

B. **Normal host defense mechanisms.** Although the lungs are accessible to the external environment, checkpoints along the bronchopulmonary tree intercept microbes before invasion occurs. Understanding which checkpoint is compromised gives clues to the causative agent of pneumonia in an individual.

1. In the upper airways, aerodynamic filtration, mucociliary clearance, cough, and neurologic reflexes prevent aspiration of bacteria from the oropharynx. The nasal mucosa is bathed in secretions containing IgA immunoglobulins, the first line of humoral defense.

2. The tracheobronchial epithelium is equipped with a mucociliary transport system that sweeps foreign material away from the lower airways.

3. Organisms that reach the lower airways encounter bactericidins such as lysozyme, opsonins (IgA, IgG, complement), as well as surfactant.

4. The last line of defense prior to bacterial invasion of lung tissue involves complex cellular interactions between bacteria and resident alveolar macrophages and circulating cells such as monocytes and polymorphonuclear (PMN) leukocytes that are attracted by extracellular chemotactic factors. These cells can phagocytose bacteria. Pathogen-specific immune responses may involve dendritic cells and T and B lymphocytes.

Table 6-3. Impaired host defenses and community-acquired pneumonia

Risk group	Alteration in defense	Likely organisms
Smokers	Impaired mucociliary clearance, alterations in local immunity	*H. flu, M. cat, S. pneu, Legionella* sp.
COPD (emphysema and bronchitis)	Tracheobronchial colonization, structural lung abnormalities, ciliary dyskinesia, mucus forms a culture medium, cellular and humoral immune defects (11)	*S. pneu, H. flu, M. cat, Legionella* sp, GNR (if exposed to multiple antibiotics or hospitalizations), fungi (if on steroids) *Strongyloides*, MAI
Alcoholics	Aspiration risk, ethanol effect on marrow, malnutrition	*S. pneu*, GNR (including *Klebsiella*), anaerobes, *H. flu, M. cat, S. aureus*
Altered mental status	Aspiration	Anaerobic, GNR, mixed infections
Intravenous drug abusers	Risk for endocarditis/septic pulmonary emboli, skin infections	*S. aureus*
Diabetes mellitus	Uncertain, possibly microangiopathic changes, neurologic changes predisposing to aspiration, factors associated with renal and cardiac disease, altered PMN and T-cell function (IDDM) (21)	GNR, *H. flu, S. aureus* (30% are nasal carriers), TB, fungus including mucormycosis Increase mortality from: Group B streptococci, *Legionella*, Influenza (21)
Renal disease (end stage)	Impaired cellular immunity	*E. coli, S. aureus, Legionella* sp.
Immunosuppressive drugs (steroids, cytotoxics), transplants, hematologic malignancies prior to therapy (lymphomas, myeloma, Hodgkin's disease)	Altered cell-mediated immunity, (T and B cell, macrophage)	Viruses (CMV, HSV, VZV, RSV, Adeno), *Legionella* spp., PCP, fungi, *Nocardia*, TB, *Strongyloides*
Malnutrition (eg, malignancy)	Depressed cellular immunity	Bacteria, fungi, TB
Chemotherapy, inherited and acquired neutropenias, myeloproliferative diseases	Leukopenia, impaired phagocytosis and inflammatory response	*P. aerug, E. coli, Klebsiella*, other GNR, *S. aureus, S. epi, Candida, Aspergillus*
IgA deficiency	Altered humoral immunity, increased bacterial adherence	Recurrent bacterial organisms, viruses *(or may be normal)*

Table 6-3. (continued)

Risk group	Alteration in defense	Likely organisms
IgG deficiency (myeloma, CLL, nephrotic syndrome, congenital deficiencies, splenectomy, hypogammaglobulinemia)	Altered humoral immunity, abnormal B-cell function, impaired opsonization and inefficient phagocytosis	*S. pneu, S. pyog, H. flu, P. aerug*
Sickle-cell anemia, splenectomy	Impaired B-cell function	*S. pneu, H. flu, E. coli, S. aureus*
Complement deficiencies (congenital, SLE, other rheumatologic disorders)	Altered humoral immunity, impaired opsonization, and inefficient phagocytosis	*S. pneu, H. flu, P. aerug, Neisseria* spp.
Bullous or cystic lung disease, old tuberculosis, previous radiation	Abnormal lung structure may impair clearance	fungi, MAI
Cystic fibrosis, immotile cilia	Abnormal mucus clearance, bronchiectasis	*Staphylococcus*, resistant *Pseudomonas*, other GNR
Postobstructive pneumonia (foreign body, cancer, previous radiation, tuberculosis, or surgery sequestration)	Abnormal clearance	*S. pneu, H. flu, M. cat*, anaerobes
Postinfluenza	Altered epithelial defenses and mucociliary clearance	*S. pneu, S. aureus*, mixed bacterial infection, *H. flu*

Adeno = adenovirus; CLL = chronic lymphocytic leukemia; CMV = cytomegalovirus; COPD = chronic obstructive pulmonary disease; *E. coli* = *Escherichia coli*; GNR = gram-negative rods; *H. flu* = *Haemophilus influenzae*; HSV = *Herpes simplex virus*; IDDM = insulin-dependent diabetes mellitus; *M. cat* = *Moraxella catarrhalis*; MAI = *Mycobacterium avium-intracellulare*; *P. aerug* = *Pseudomonas aeruginosa*; PCP = *Pneumocystis carinii* pneumonia; PMN = polymorphonuclear leukocytes; RSV = Respiratory syncytial virus; *S. aureus* = *Staphylococcus aureus*; *S. epi* = *Staphylococcus epidermidis*; SLE = systemic lupus erythematosus; *S. pneu* = *Streptococcus pneumoniae*; *S. pyog* = *Streptococcus pyogenes*; TB = *Mycobacterium tuberculosis*; VZV = Varicella-zoster virus.

Table 6-4. Less common causes of community-acquired pneumonia

Risk group	Organism	Features	Chest x-ray	Diagnosis	Treatment
After pharyngitis or viral illness, or in outbreaks	*Streptococcus pyogenes* (group A hemolytic)	Abrupt, rigors, productive cough, pharyngitis, pleuritic chest pain, may cause ARDS	Segmental infiltrates in lower lobes, large pleural effusion, cavities may occur, empyema in 40% (20)	GPC chains, PMNs, sputum and pleural fluid Cx; blood Cx positive in 10–15% (20)	PCN, macrolide, 1st-generation cephalosporin; complications: pleural thickening, glomerulonephritis
Elderly or debilitated patients (DM, CVA, dementia, cancer, neonates, pregnancy)	Group B streptococci, often poly-microbial (20)	High fever, tachycardia, SBP <100 (20)	Variable	High WBC	Pen G 12–18 mill U/day IV, cephalosporins; mortality 30–85%
Sporadic, postviral, or in military outbreaks	*Neisseria meningitidis*	Abrupt/gradual, sore throat, pleural pain; rare: meningitis/skin symptoms	Patchy alveolar infiltrates, often in lower lobes (effusions, cavities are rare)	GP diplococci in cytoplasm of PMN, blood Cx typically negative	PCN, cefuroxime, 3rd-generation cephalosporin, chloramphenicol
Military recruits, outbreaks	Adenovirus	Cough, conjunctivitis, rhino/pharyngitis	Patchy lower lobe consolidation	Viral culture, serology	Supportive care
Military recruits, outbreaks	Measles (rubeola)	Before, with, or after rash; cough, purulent sputum, occasionally pleural pain	Diffuse, bilateral reticular pattern, hilar LN (segmental pattern: consider bacterial super-infection)	WBC normal/low, isolation from secretions is cumbersome, serology	Supportive care

ARDS = adult respiratory distress syndrome; CVA = cerebral vascular accident; Cx = culture; DM = diabetes mellitus; GP = gram-positive; GPC = gram positive cocci; LN = lymph node; PCN = penicillin; Pen G = penicillin G; PMNs = polymorphonuclear leukocytes; SBP = systolic blood pressure; WBC = white blood cell count.

Table 6-5. Zoonoses

Risk group	Organism	Features	Chest x-ray	Diagnosis	Treatment
Exposure to infected bird droppings, pet shops, ducks, parrots; veterinarians, turkey farmers	*Chlamydia psittaci* (psittacosis)	Sudden high fever, pharyngitis, headache, myalgias, nonproductive or mucoid cough, occasional epistaxis or splenomegaly, rash (Horder's spots)	Variable: normal in 30% (22), worse than exam; homogeneous or patchy, segmental, lobar nodules, or miliary, hilar lymph nodes may occur; lower lobes often involved (22)	Usually normal WBC, proteinuria; liver tests may be abnormal; single titer of >1 : 16, or fourfold CF rise; x-reactivity may occur (*Brucella*, *Coxiella burnetti*, *Legionella*)	Tetracycline 2 g/d *Radiographic resolution may be delayed; relapses may occur; mortality is 1%. Refer to department of public health*
Tick/insect bites, infected-small-animal exposure, lab workers, southern U.S. and elsewhere, Canada, Scandinavia	*Francisella tularensis* (tularemia)	Abrupt, headache, non-productive cough, sore throat, cutaneous ulcer, regional lymphadeno-pathy, pleural rub	Variable: consolidations, often hilar lymphadeno-pathy, effusions, "ovoid bodies," cavitation is rare	PMNs, no organisms (GNR), laboratory workers at risk; single titer of 1 : 160 suggestive, titers peak at 4–8 wk. X-reactivity with brucellosis	Tetracyclines, chloramphenicol, streptomycin 15–20 mg/kg/d divided into 2 doses
Exposure to animal tissues and fluids, sheep, goats, cattle, parturient cats, dust, tick bites, raw milk; biting flies; lab workers	*Coxiella burnetti* (Q fever)	Abrupt fever, rigors, severe headache, chills, myalgias, pleuritic chest pain, nonproductive cough; 1–5-wk incubation	Variable: segmental consolidation, usually lower lobes, occasionally effusions	Usually normal WBC; serologic titres (acute and convalescent CF, ELISA); coccobacillary bodies in AM on TBBx	Tetracyclines 2 g/d ×2 weeks, doxycycline, chloramphenicol; mortality <1%
Wild and domestic animal bite or scratch, underlying respiratory disease	*Pasturella multocida*	Purulent bronchitis, suppurative pleural effusions	Nonspecific	Small GNR, bipolar staining, easily grown	Penicillin, tetracycline
Animal fur, hides-wool sorters, combers	*Bacillus anthracis* (23)	Acute bronchitis, acute dyspnea, shock can occur	Mediastinal lymphadenopathy, patchy opacities, bilateral effusions	GNR; culture blood and sputum, but micro lab workers at risk	Therapy may precede cytology results in high-risk patients

Organism	Epidemiology/Source	Clinical symptoms	Radiographic findings	Diagnosis	Treatment
Yersinia pestis (plague)	Asia, Africa, South America, southwestern U.S., fleas, rodents (airborne or bites), mammals	Bubonic (buboes with regional lymph nodes) and pneumonic forms (bloody sputum, pleural pain)	Nonsegmental, homogenous consolidation, no cavities, hilar/paratracheal lymphadenopathy, effusions	Bipolar-staining GNR; culture blood, sputum, or lymph node by routine cytology, serology	Aminoglycoside and tetracycline or chloramphenicol
Leptospirosis	Family pets and wild animals; farmers, veterinarians, water	Nonproductive cough, headache, muscle pain, chills, GI and GU symptoms	Peripheral nonsegmental patchy or diffuse consolidation	Serologies, special culture media, ELISA, titres	
Brucella sp.	Abattoir: via skin or respiratory or oral tracts	Cough, wheezing, hoarseness	Granulomas may calcify; lymphadenopathy; may not see infiltrates	small GN coccobacilli, ELISA	Doxycycline + rifampin for 4–6 wk
Pseudomonas pseudomallei (melioidosis)	Southeast Asian foods, animals, rodent-contaminated water and soil	Abrupt cough, chills, bloody sputum, pleuritic chest pain, diarrhea; may also reactivate years later	Acute: irregular nodules bilaterally; may cavitate Chronic: similar to TB	Bipolar-staining GNR; cytology: sputum, urine, blood, CSF; grows readily, serology	ticarcillin, trimethoprim/sulfamethoxazole
Rocky Mountain spotted fever	Arthropods, North American, esp. mid-Atlantic states	Constitutional symptoms, severe headache, rash, nonproductive cough	Diffuse interstitial infiltrate, patchy pneumonia	Serology, fluorescent antibody of skin lesions	Tetracycline, chloramphenicol

AM = alveolar macrophage; CF = cystic fibrosis; CSF = cerebrospinal fluid; ELISA = enzyme-linked immunosorbent assay; GNR = gram-negative rods; PMNs = polymorphonuclear leukocytes; TB = tuberculosis; TBBx = transbronchial biopsy; WBC = white blood cell count.

V. Clinical features of typical vs. atypical CAP

  A. Clinicians have relied on the distinction between typical and atypical clinical presentations to predict the etiology of CAP. Recent studies suggest limitations to this approach. The clinical features of CAP (signs, symptoms, radiographic findings) cannot reliably establish an etiology with adequate sensitivity and specificity for two reasons. First, *Legionella* and *Chlamydia psittaci* are typical of certain pathogens that may present with a clinical picture exhibiting features of both syndromes. Second, abnormal hosts with comorbid illnesses or advanced age may present with atypical clinical features, even when disease is caused by a typical bacterial pathogen (7–9). Nonetheless, these historical distinctions serve to separate the pathogens into two groups that share some basic features.

   1. **Typical CAP is most commonly caused by** *S. pneumoniae* (60%). Other causes of typical pneumonia include *Haemophilus influenzae* (15%), aerobic GNR (6% to 10%) (15), and *Staphylococcus aureus* (2% to 10%) (10). Information about specific pathogens may be found later in this chapter.

   a. **Symptoms.** Classically, CAP presents with the sudden onset of fevers and shaking chills followed by cough productive of mucopurulent sputum and pleuritic chest pain. Streaky hemoptysis is not uncommon in pyogenic infections. Hypothermia may be seen in elderly or debilitated patients. Sputum production is less likely in the setting of dehydration, neutropenia, or respiratory muscle weakness. Dyspnea and lassitude may be present.

   b. **Signs.** Tachycardia, fever, and tachypnea may be present. The physical examination of the chest usually reveals evidence of consolidation, including decreased breath sounds, dullness to percussion, increased fremitus, and egophony ("e" to "a" change). A pleural friction rub may be heard.

   c. **Chest roentgenogram.** The chest x-ray usually confirms the presence of consolidation with a lobar or multilobar infiltrate, a radiologic pattern nonspecific for any pathogen.

   d. **Laboratory findings.** The peripheral white blood cell (WBC) count is usually elevated but may be normal or low, and the differential usually reveals an increased number of immature PMN leukocytes (>5%) (11,12).

   e. **Sputum Gram's stain.** If a quality specimen (described below) is obtained and stained correctly, a predominant morphologic type of bacteria should indicate the causative organism.

   2. **Atypical CAP is caused by a variety of agents, the most common of which is** *Mycoplasma pneumoniae.* Less common causes of atypical disease include *C. pneumoniae, C. psittaci* (psittacosis), and *Coxiella burnetti* (Q fever). The most common viral agents associated with atypical pneumonia in adults include influenza A and B, adenovirus types 3,4, and 7, and parainfluenza virus. Legionnaires' disease may present as either an acute typical or atypical CAP (10). The clinical presentation of atypical pneumonia differs from that of typical pneumonia in several respects.

   a. **Symptoms.** The onset is usually insidious, consisting of headache, sore throat, myalgias, and fatigue. A persistent dry cough is usually reported; sputum production is seen in up to a third of patients.

   b. **Signs.** A pulse–temperature dissociation may be noted. The physical examination reveals scattered wheezing, rhonchi, or rales, but evidence of pulmonary consolidation is minimal or absent. Fever is present but chills are uncommon.

   c. **Laboratory.** Mild leukocytosis is present but is <15,000/mm^3 in most of the cases. Sputum Gram's stain reveals neutrophils but few organisms

   d. **Chest roentgenogram.** Chest x-ray reveals diffuse reticulonodular infiltrates that may be unilateral or bilateral poorly marginated peripheral densities or may appear diffuse and patchy.

VI. **Diagnosis.** The responsible pathogen escapes detection in 50% of patients with CAP despite extensive diagnostic testing (5). No single test can identify all potential pathogens, and each diagnostic test has limitations. The chest x-ray, with few exceptions, does little to guide the clinician to a specific pathologic conclusion. Since sputum is contaminated with oral flora, definitive confirmation of a specific pathogen requires culture from a normally sterile site, such as blood or pleural fluid. The nonspecificity of clinical and radiographic findings and the limitations of laboratory diagnostic testing often require initial therapy to be empiric.

A. Laboratory studies

   1. Sputum Gram's stains

      a. Sputum may contain organisms that come from the normal flora of the upper respiratory tract, since collected sputum exits the mouth. A properly performed Gram's stain of expectorated sputum (>25 neutrophils and <5–10 squamous epithelial cells per low-power field) provides a diagnostic sensitivity of between 60% and 85% and is therefore useful in the initial evaluation of patients with CAP. This remains controversial (10, 13,14).

         i. The presence of only one morphologic type of bacteria on Gram's stain is suggestive of the causative agent. However, the sensitivity and specificity of the Gram's stain in predicting sputum culture recovery of pneumococcus in CAP has varied widely in several studies (13). Therefore the usefulness of the Gram's stain in CAP remains uncertain.

         ii. An adequate sputum Gram's stain that fails to reveal a preponderance of staphylococci or GNR diminishes the suspicion that those agents are causative. The results may be deceptive if a patient has been on antibiotics for at least several days. Frequently encountered pathogens such as *M. pneumoniae, C. pneumoniae,* and respiratory viruses are not detectable by sputum Gram's stain (2).

      b. Specific stains of the sputum may be diagnostic for pulmonary infections due to flora that are normally not found in the normal respiratory tract (2):

         i. *Mycobacterium* sp. (acid-fast stain).

         ii. Endemic fungi (methenamine silver stain).

         iii. *Pneumocystis carinii* (silver stain or direct fluorescent antibody [DFA]).

         iv. *Legionella* sp. (DFA).

   2. Routine bacterial cultures of sputum often demonstrate pathogenic organisms, but sensitivity and specificity are poor. If heavy growth of a pathogen on sputum culture correlates with the Gram's stain findings, it is reasonable to assume that the pathogen is causing the pneumonia. Recovery of organisms that are never part of the normal respiratory flora may be meaningful. Culture and sensitivity results may not reveal any organism or may reveal a resistant organism in patients on antibiotics at the time of evaluation.

      a. Sputum should be cultured for mycobacteria, *Legionella,* and endemic fungi only in the appropriate clinical setting (patients with risk factors listed in Table 6-3). Most otherwise healthy patients do not require a sputum culture, as empiric therapy is generally effective. Viral cultures are not useful in the initial evaluation of patients with CAP and should not be routinely performed (2).

   3. Blood cultures are not indicated in the nonhospitalized patient with CAP. If the patient is likely to be bacteremic, the patient should be admitted.

   4. The WBC count is unlikely to alter management and need not be routinely obtained in otherwise healthy persons. While an elevated count is never diagnostic, one >15,000/mm^3 is more suggestive of bacterial illnesses (15).

      a. Low WBC counts may be due to underlying disease, or the deleterious effect of cytokines or other mediators on the marrow. Very low WBC counts may be a negative prognostic indicator. Lymphopenia may be caused by immunosuppressive drugs, human immunodeficiency virus (HIV) infection, or malnutrition.

   5. Anemia may be either a manifestation of underlying disease or the result of one of several infectious diseases or antibiotics capable of causing a hemolytic reaction. Cold agglutinins may be seen with *Mycoplasma,* as well as *Legionella,* adenovirus, influenza virus, and other infectious and noninfectious conditions.

   6. Chemistries. Hyponatremia and liver test abnormalities have previously been considered indicative of atypical pneumonia, *L. pneumophila* in particular. Such features are now recognized to be common associations with pneumonia caused by a variety of organisms.

   i.   Hyponatremia may be caused by dehydration or the syndrome of inappropriate antidiuretic hormone (SIADH).

   ii. Hypernatremia, an increased blood urea nitrogen/creatinine ratio, and an elevated bicarbonate level may all be found in patients with CAP and volume contraction.

   iii. Sepsis is associated with an anion gap metabolic acidosis.

7. **Serologic testing** for specific pathogens is not useful in the initial evaluation of patients with CAP and should not be performed routinely. Acute and convalescent (3–6 weeks later) titers may be useful for retrospective confirmation of suspected diagnosis and/or epidemiologic studies (1). A sample of acute serum should be frozen in perplexing cases for which a diagnostic dilemma or public health issue may be anticipated.

8. **Measurement of urinary *Legionella* antigen detects** *L. pneumophila* **serogroup 1 antigen** and is useful because the results are rapidly available and are 80% to 99% sensitive and 99% specific. Since the *L. pneumophila* serogroup 1 causes 70% to 90% of all cases of legionnaires' disease, this assay is very useful in the diagnostic work-up of patients with suspected *Legionella* (6).

B. **Thoracentesis** should be performed in individuals who have sizable pleural effusions, since cultures of pleural fluid are not likely to be contaminated with oral flora. The pH of the fluid should be measured (pleural fluid is collected in a blood gas syringe, with all bubbles tapped out and the syringe iced until measurement). Cell counts, differential, and Gram's stain should be obtained. Determinations of protein and lactate dehydrogenase (LDH) levels should be made. A large amount of fluid should be sent for culture, with particular attention paid to identifying organisms suspected by the clinical history.

C. **Transtracheal needle aspirates** performed to obtain samples uncontaminated by oral flora are no longer recommended.

1. Bronchoscopy with bronchoalveolar lavage (BAL) may be performed in cases where *Mycobacterium tuberculosis* and fungi are suspected as causative organisms. Even with this technique, samples will still be contaminated by the passage of the bronchoscope through the mouth and upper airway.

D. **The standard posteroanterior (PA) and lateral chest radiographs are an integral part of the work-up of CAP.** Radiography is useful for evaluating illness severity by identifying multilobar involvement, suggesting (but not confirming) specific etiologies such as *M. tuberculosis*, *S. aureus*, *P. carinii*, etc, and revealing coexisting conditions such as bronchial obstruction, pleural effusions, or abscess formation (2).

1. Since many different infectious agents can cause similar radiographic findings, chest x-ray patterns should not be relied on for a definitive diagnosis.

2. With the above caveat, cavitation is more suggestive of *S. aureus*, mixed anaerobic infections, tuberculosis, squamous cell cancer, or *Nocardia*. Bulging interlobar fissures are seen with intense inflammatory reactions in *Klebsiella* pneumonia. Aspiration pneumonia will occur in certain areas of the lung according to the laws of gravity (see X. Aspiration pneumonia and anaerobes below). **Reasons for a negative chest x-ray in CAP** include dehydration, inadequate inflammatory response as occurs in neutropenic individuals, and difficulty in interpreting films because of baseline abnormalities.

E. Patients with persistent disease who are immunocompromised or rapidly deteriorating require more invasive testing to obtain lung tissue or more reliable culture material. The following techniques may be used: bronchoscopy with or without transbronchial biopsy, BAL, and protected brushings; computed tomography (CT)-guided transthoracic needle biopsy of peripheral disease; thoracoscopic lung biopsy; or open lung biopsy. These procedures are rarely required in CAP.

VII. **Treatment.** Due to the wide range of potential pathogens and the limitations of diagnostic testing, broad-spectrum empiric antibiotic coverage is now used in the initial treatment of each group, based on likely etiologies (see Tables 6-1 through 6-3). Other treatment may include oxygen, hydration, and treatment of any underlying causes and comorbidities.

A. Antibiotic therapy

1. The recognition of a specific pathogen by clinical presentation or radiograph is generally not possible. Thus, a judicious estimate of epidemiologic likelihood and interpretation of laboratory data and clinical findings should be used in making a prescribing decision. More than one potential pathogen must often be targeted for therapy. The American Thoracic Society recently presented an approach to the initial empiric therapy of CAP based on disease severity, presence of coexisting diseases, age, and the need for hospitalization (2) (see Tables 6-1 and 6-2).

2. Specific information about antibiotic classes is contained in Table 6-6. All antibiotics can produce alterations in normal flora, resulting in diarrhea, yeast infections, and other problems.

3. Macrolide antibiotics. Erythromycin covers many typical and atypical agents, with the exception of some *H. influenzae*. The newer macrolides clarithromycin and azithromycin should be considered in smokers and in those with gastrointestinal intolerance of erythromycin (2).

4. **Tetracycline.** Many isolates of *S. pneumoniae* are resistant to tetracycline, and it should be used only if the patient is allergic to or intolerant of macrolides (6).

5. **Second-generation cephalosporins** include cefuroxime, cefaclor, cefprozil, and loracarbef. These agents are effective against most typical organisms but do not cover atypicals.

6. **Trimethoprim/sulfamethoxazole** has not been formally studied in patients with CAP, but its *in vitro* activity and efficacy in other infections involving the pathogens shown in Table 6-2 suggests that it might be an effective alternative for patients who meet CAP guidelines (2).

7. **β-lactam/β-lactamase inhibitor** combinations such as amoxicillin/clavulanate potassium are useful for treating the β-lactamase-producing organisms, such as *H. influenzae, Moraxella catarrhalis*, anaerobes, and others.

B. Penicillin-resistant pneumococcus has increased in incidence due to the approach of using empiric broad-spectrum antibiotics in CAP.

1. In some areas of the United States, up to 25% of *S. pneumoniae* isolates are penicillin-resistant, and resistance is even more commonplace in parts of Europe, Africa, and Australia (15,16). In addition to geography, resistant strains are more likely in patients at the extremes of age (<2 and >70 years) with a history of previous hospitalizations or β-lactam therapy, or in children who attend child daycare centers (16).

2. Most resistant strains (80%) have only intermediate resistance and respond to higher doses of penicillin or to cephalosporins (17). Some penicillin-resistant strains are also resistant to other classes of antibacterials.

3. **Vancomycin should be used to treat penicillin-resistant pneumococcus.** A recent review suggests that mortality associated with the treatment of penicillin-resistant strains may not be worse than with sensitive strains (18).

C. Bacterial pneumonia should generally be treated for 7–10 days (11,12). Cases of *M. pneumoniae* and *C. pneumoniae* require 10–14 days of antibiotic therapy.

1. Legionnaires' pneumonia requires 2–3 weeks of antibiotics (11,12). Shorter treatment courses may be possible with the new 15-member macrolide, azithromycin. The long half-life (11–14 hours) of this agent allows it to remain in the tissues for several weeks, so that its reduced length of treatment (5 days) is somewhat misleading (19). Specific agents for common organisms are listed in sections XIII through XVII.

2. The usual clinical course of CAP is detailed in Table 6-7.

D. Hydration is a necessary part of therapy because the fever and tachypnea associated with pneumonia often result in insensible fluid losses. If oral intake is poor, parenteral replacement is required and may be given in the home in selected individuals.

Table 6-6. Antibiotics and community-acquired pneumonia

Class	Drug	S. pneu	H. flu M. cat	M. pneu C. pneu L. pneu	Dosage	Comments	Cost
Penicillins	Penicillin	Fair			500 mg TID–QID	Positive anaerobic activity, hypersensitivity reaction; some S. pneu resistant	$
	Amoxicillin	OK			500 mg TID		
	Amox + clav	OK	OK		500 mg TID	Diarrhea, cholestatic hepatitis reported; covers anaerobes	$$$$
Cephalosporins	Cephalexin	OK			250–500 mg QID	Poor gram-negative and anaerobic coverage	$$
	Cefuroxime	OK	OK		500 mg BID	Covers some anaerobes	$$$$$
	Cefaclor	OK	OK		250 mg TID	Serum sickness, rash, purpura, interstitial nephritis	$$$
Macrolides	Erythromycin	OK	M. cat OK	OK	500 mg QID	Nausea, vomiting, cramps, diarrhea, hepatotoxic; noanaerobic coverage	
	Clarithromycin	OK	OK	OK	500 mg BID	Avoid in pregnancy	$$$
	Azithromycin	OK	OK	OK	500 mg, then 250 mg/d	1% CNS effects; not studied in pregnant women	$$
	Clindamycin	OK			300 mg TID	Excellent for anaerobes; associated with pseudomembranous colitis	$$
Sulfa drugs	TMP/SMX	Fair	M. cat OK	L. pneu OK	1 DS BID	Rash, anemia, CNS, hyperkalemia, falsely high creatinine; some GNR coverage	$
Tetracyclines	Doxycycline	Fair	OK	OK	100 mg BID	Avoid in pregnancy; nausea, esophagitis, photosensitivity uncommon	$
Fluoroquinolones	Ciprofloxacin		OK	L. pneu and M. pneu OK	500 mg BID	No anaerobic activity, but covers GNR; drug interactions	$$$
	Ofloxacin		OK	OK	400 mg BID	No anaerobic activity, but covers GNR; hyper- or hypoglycemia noted	$$$$

Amox + clav = amoxicillin/clavulanate potassium; BID = twice a day; C. pneu = Chlamydia pneumoniae; DS = double strength; GNR = gram-negative rod; H. flu = Haemophilus influenzae; L. pneu = Legionella pneumophila; M. cat = Moraxella catarrhalis; M. pneu = Mycoplasma pneumoniae; QID = four times a day; S. pneu = Streptococcus pneumoniae; TID = three times a day; TMP/SMX = trimethoprim/sulfamethoxazole.
Gray and black shading denotes suboptimal coverage or inadequate studies. These sensitivities are a generalization based on hospital data; sensitivity patterns will differ according to geography and prescription habits. Costs ($–$$$$$) are relative, according to actual wholesale prices, based on a usual course (10 days for most, 5 days for azithromycin).

Table 6-7. Clinical and radiographic course of community-acquired pneumonia

Organism	Clinical	Radiographic course		
		Worsening	Time to resolution	With residual (%)
S. pneu, nonbacteremic	Defervescence in 2–3 d; fever may last up to 5 d in patients on proper therapy (25)	Occasional	1–3 mo	Rare
S. pneu, bacteremic		Common	3–5 mo	25–35 (streaky pleural densities)
M. pneu	Rapid improvement in first 1–2 wk	Rare	2 wk–2 mo	Rare
Anaerobes	Most patients respond within 3–4 d and are usually afebrile by day 7–10 (22)	Cavities may develop even on correct therapy	Radiographic clearing may require 2–4 mo in some cases (22)	Data not available
Legionella	Fever may persist in first week of therapy; weakness and fatigue may persist for months	Common	2–6 mo	10–25 (linear scars)
Viral	Depends on host and virus	Variable	Variable	Common (VZV, adeno)

Adeno = adenovirus; *M. pneu* = *Mycoplasma pneumoniae*; *S. pneu* = *Streptococcus pneumoniae*; VZV = varicella-zoster virus.

    E. Oxygenation. An assessment of oxygenation should be made when tachypnea or bradypnea is present, respirations appear labored, the general appearance is poor, or the potential for respiratory compromise (multilobar involvement) is high.

       1. Impressive decrements in oxygenation may be caused by relatively small infiltrates due to severe ventilation–perfusion mismatching.

       2. Caution should be used in interpreting oxygen saturation levels (oximetry). By hyperventilating, some patients may be able to maintain a near normal Po_2 and oxygen saturation over 90% at the expense of significant respiratory exertion. Respiratory fatigue may ensue when normoxemia is achieved through hyperventilation to maintain a low carbon dioxide. **Arterial blood gases should always be measured to obtain the carbon dioxide level, and the alveolar-arterial oxygen gradient [(A-a)Do_2] should be calculated to assess severity of disease and its progression.**

    F. Isolation. Most adult patients with CAP do not require isolation. Reporting of bacterial and viral pneumonias to departments of public health, the Centers for Disease Control and Prevention, or other authorities is also not required in most cases.

       1. CAP secondary to zoonoses may require further investigation and reporting. Symptomatic CAP patients should take care to avoid close contact with immunocompromised individuals.

VIII. Decision to hospitalize. The single most important decision faced by clinicians during the evaluation and course of CAP is whether to hospitalize the patient.

    A. No strict guidelines exist for helping to make this decision. However, comorbidities increase the risk of morbidity and mortality from CAP, and hospitalization should be considered when one or more of these are present (2).

    B. The most frequent agents causing CAP that require hospitalization are *S. pneumoniae, Legionella, Pseudomonas aeruginosa,* and other GNR.

    C. The absence of a responsible caregiver in the home is another strong indication for hospitalization.

    D. In the absence of the above risk factors, if the overall appearance of the patient is unfavorable, admission to the hospital on an observational status for 24–48 hours is warranted.

IX. Persistent pneumonia. The resolution of pneumonia depends on the immunologic status of the host, the appropriateness of pharmacologic and supportive therapy, and the characteristics of the causative agent (24). The causes of persistent pneumonia may be found in Table 6-8.

    A. Otherwise healthy individuals with intact immune systems usually defervesce within 2–4 days of initiation of appropriate antibiotics. Physical examination findings may continue to be abnormal in as many as 40% of patients at 1 week (20). Changes in therapy should not be made in the first 72 hours, unless the clinical picture deteriorates or cultures show that the organism is not sensitive to empiric therapy (20).

    B. In competent hosts, fever and symptoms that have not improved after 4–5 days are a cause for concern. Progression of symptoms on therapy is another indication that further investigation or a change in antibiotics is necessary. Major risk factors for delayed resolution of CAP include: age >50 years, impaired host defense, emphysema, diabetes mellitus, CHF, and alcoholism.

       1. Chest x-ray

          a. While clinical signs and symptoms usually resolve rapidly, roentgenographic resolution may be quite slow, with chest x-rays remaining abnormal for up to 6 weeks after uncomplicated pneumonia (see Table 6-7). Repeated films in the early days of treatment are not often helpful unless the clinical situation worsens, as the chest radiograph may worsen initially even with proper therapy.

          b. Follow-up films should be obtained at 6 weeks in patients at risk for lung cancer in order to rule out mass lesions that might have produced a postobstructive pneumonia.

          c. Recurrent pneumonias in the same area should also be radiographically followed to resolution to assess possible structural causes (bronchiectasis). A CT scan of the chest may be indicated in these patients.

Table 6-8. Features of persistent "pneumonia"

Situation	Possible causes	Diagnosis
Failure of empiric therapy	Noncompliance with medications Antibiotic resistance Unsuspected organisms: atypical *H. flu*, viral, fungal, TB, MAI, unusual organisms	Careful history, observation under therapy Sputum cytology with sensitivities Sputum cytology with sensitivities, if unrevealing bronchoscopy with BAL +/−transbronchial biopsy
Persistent dry cough, otherwise improved	Cough-variant asthma	PFTs with and without bronchodilators; treat as asthma, begin therapy with inhaled bronchodilators
Smokers	Postobstructive pneumonia	CT, bronchoscopy to rule out cancer
Unsuspected immunocompromise	HIV, underlying malignancy	Consider HIV testing, CBC, etc.
Persistent or repeated right middle lobe (RML) or lingular infiltrate	RML or lingula syndrome	Bronchoscopy reveals tight anatomy and chronic inflammation
Persistent or repeated infiltrates in one location	Foreign body or anatomic obstruction	History, bronchoscopy to rule out structural abnormality
Noninfectious interstitial infiltrates	CHF, inflammatory diseases (SLE, RA, sarcoidosis, hypersensitivity pneumonitis, eosinophilic pneumonia), lymphangitic spread of malignancy, pulmonary fibrosis, pneumoconioses	Bronchoscopy and biopsy; thorough search for systemic disease
Noninfectious alveolar infiltrates	Inflammatory diseases (BOOP, drug reactions, rheumatic diseases, Wegener's), sarcoidosis, pulmonary emboli, hypersensitivity pneumonitis, ABPA, alveolar hemorrhage, lipoid pneumonia, bronchoalveolar cell carcinoma	History of prescription and OTC medications, recent viral infection; biopsy, if necessary
Recent viral infection	Impaired mucociliary clearance, superinfection with pneumococcus, or rarely S. aureus	History, observation under continued therapy
Impaired mucociliary clearance	COPD, structural lung diseases, CF, bronchiectasis, bronchopulmonary sequestration, neurologic disease impairing cough	Chest x-ray and CT, history, and exam for neurologic causes

ABPA = allergic bronchopulmonary aspergillosis; BAL = bronchoalveolar lavage; BOOP = bronchiolitis obliterans with organizing pneumonia; CBC = complete blood cell count; CF = cystic fibrosis; CHF = congestive heart failure; COPD = chronic obstructive pulmonary disease; CT = computed tomography; *H. flu* = *Haemophilus influenzae*; HIV = human immunodeficiency virus; MAI = *Mycobacterium avium-intercellulare*; OTC = over the counter; PFTs = pulmonary function tests; RA = rheumatoid arthritis; *S. aureus* = *Staphylococcus aureus*; SLE = systemic lupus erythematosus; TB = tuberculosis.

   C. Compliance with therapy should be continually assessed in patients with persistent pneumonia, until clinical and radiographic resolution has occurred. Repeated sputum cultures, chest radiographs, and blood cultures should be obtained as necessary depending on clinical factors.

   D. Generally, blood cultures should be collected in all patients with persistent pneumonia and all pleural fluid should be tapped. Consideration of *Legionella*, *M. tuberculosis*, *P. carinii*, fungi, and other pathogens may be warranted depending on the patient's risk profile. It may be necessary to obtain lung tissue for culture.

   E. **Specialists**

      1. Pulmonologists should be consulted in cases that fail to respond to therapy. The elderly and patients with underlying illnesses (eg, malignancy, significant cardiopulmonary disease, end-stage renal disease, severe diabetes, immunocompromise) often tolerate pneumonia poorly and should be referred to a specialist if there is no response to initial therapy within the first week. A specialist should also be consulted in all cases that do not show complete radiologic clearing at 6 weeks.

      2. Pulmonologists may continue observation and proceed to bronchoscopy in patients who are at risk for cancer or have possible structural lesions, and may perform additional testing for fungal or mycobacterial pathogens.

X. **Pneumonia in compromised hosts due to neutrophil dysfunction**

   A. **General considerations**

      1. Infectious and noninfectious pulmonary complications account for significant morbidity and mortality in immunocompromised hosts. Diagnosis is more complex because the differential diagnosis is large, clinical manifestations may be muted or altered by underlying disease or effects of treatment, and diagnosis more often requires invasive methods such as bronchoscopy or open lung biopsy.

      2. The typical vs. atypical dichotomy noted in immunocompetent hosts is often not useful in this population because these individuals are often infected by opportunistic pathogens, as well as the usual pathogens. Response to therapy may be delayed, casting doubts about presumptive diagnoses. The difficulties of separating colonizers from true pathogens in sputum or bronchial washings are magnified in the immunocompromised. Because of the increased potential for rapid deterioration, many immunocompromised patients with pneumonia require hospitalization (see Table 6-3).

      3. **Compromised PMN leukocyte function**

         a. Neutrophils (granulocytes, PMN leukocytes) are crucial to phagocytizing bacterial organisms, and patients with defective neutrophil function or inadequate numbers of neutrophils are at risk for infection with gram-positive and gram-negative bacteria.

         b. Absolute neutropenia (absolute neutrophil count $<1000/mm^3$) may be caused by hematologic disorders, chemotherapy, or congenital or acquired leukopenias. Many of these patients are receiving immunosuppressive therapy with corticosteroids or cytotoxic drugs and may eventually experience altered T-cell and macrophage function as well (see below).

         c. Chemotherapy is one of the most common causes of neutropenia, and CAP or nosocomial bacterial pneumonia is one of the most frequent serious infections and the leading cause of death in cancer patients (26).

         d. Frequent hospitalization and repeated courses of antibiotics may lead to oropharyngeal colonization with resistant organisms. Effects of radiation and chemotherapy may lead to breaks in normal mucosal barriers and facilitate entry of bacteria, and analgesics may increase likelihood of aspiration and decrease the cough reflex.

   B. **Signs and symptoms**

      1. Neutropenic patients with pneumonia present with fever but may or may not produce sputum or have other symptoms. Dyspnea may be present and may be exacerbated by anemia. Other symptoms may include pleuritic chest pain and constitutional complaints.

2. The physical examination may reveal hypotension with dehydration, increased respiratory rate, fever, and tachycardia. Fever may be absent if anti-inflammatory drugs were taken. Examination of the lung may reveal decreased breath sounds, rales, increased fremitus, dullness to percussion, and pleural friction rub; it may also be entirely normal.

C. **Chest radiograph**
   1. Due to low numbers of circulating WBCs, the chest radiograph may not be dramatically abnormal, especially if the patient is simultaneously dehydrated.
   2. Even common typical pathogens may present with an atypical radiographic pattern in immunocompromised patients.
      a. **Focal areas of consolidation are seen in bacterial and candidal pneumonia and in pulmonary hemorrhage (27).**
      b. **Diffuse infiltrates are seen with transfusion reactions, adult respiratory distress syndrome, pulmonary edema, or pulmonary emboli (27).**
      c. **Radiation pneumonitis classically follows a sharply demarcated line corresponding to the radiation port.**
      d. **Cavitation and abscesses may be seen in pneumonia due to GNR, *S. aureus,* or anaerobes.**

D. In addition to the infectious causes listed above, **noninfectious causes of pulmonary infiltrates must also be considered in the differential diagnosis.**

E. **Specific approach**
   1. While the differential diagnosis of CAP in immunocompromised hosts is large, the predominant concern is averting death from overwhelming gram-negative infection. **Neutropenic patients who are rapidly deteriorating should have an expeditious diagnostic evaluation, including bronchoscopy with lavage and transbronchial biopsy, especially for patients with diffuse infiltrates.**
   2. Bacterial pneumonias may often be diagnosed by sputum Gram's stain and culture, even though these patients are often chronically colonized by GNR. Fungal and viral pathogens are less likely to be diagnosed by sputum samples. Cytology may be helpful to assess cytopathologic changes and possible metastatic disease.
   3. High-resolution CT may help distinguish lymphangitic spread of tumor and pneumonitis caused by drugs or radiation. For peripheral lesions, percutaneous CT-guided biopsy may be useful.
      a. Contraindications to transthoracic needle biopsy include platelet count <30,000, bleeding diathesis, bullous lung disease, contralateral pneumonectomy, COPD, restrictive lung disease, and pulmonary hypertension (27).
      b. Open lung biopsy has a diagnostic yield of 87% to 94%, with a mortality of 1% to 1.8%. Early studies on thoracoscopic lung biopsy indicate that it is associated with a low mortality.

F. **Management**
   1. **Hospitalization is indicated for most neutropenic patients with CAP.**
   2. Individuals with hematologic malignancies are more likely to have bacteremia associated with pneumonia than are normal hosts. Febrile neutropenics require blood, sputum, and urine cultures; any pleural fluid should be tapped.
   3. Patients should be treated with two synergistic antimicrobial agents to cover *Pseudomonas.* A combination of two drugs, each from a different group (listed below), can be used for empiric therapy (eg, aminoglycoside plus antipseudomonal semisynthetic penicillin). Specific antibiotic choices can be changed when the susceptibility pattern is known.
      a. Aminoglycoside: gentamicin, tobramycin, amikacin.
      b. Antipseudomonal penicillin: piperacillin.
      c. Antipseudomonal third-generation cephalosporin: ceftazidime.
      d. Fluorinated quinolones: ciprofloxacin, ofloxacin.
      e. Imipenem.
      f. Aztreonam.

   4. The use of two β-lactams (antipseudomonal penicillin and antipseudomonal cephalosporin) has been shown to be effective in febrile neutropenic individuals.
   5. The addition of an antistaphylococcal agent is often recommended, as the clinical picture may mimic that of GNR. However, the urgency of treating staphylococcal infections does not equal that of treating GNR.
      a. The presence of staphylococci on Gram's stain or risk factors that increase the likelihood of staphylococcal bacteremia should prompt coverage for this organism.
      b. Therapy should be continued until the absolute WBC is >500/mm^3 (28), and the patient has been afebrile for 5–7 days.
   6. If patients do not respond to appropriate antibiotic therapy, granulocyte transfusion may be considered; no consensus presently exists concerning the ultimate benefit of this procedure. Granulocyte transfusion is associated with fever, allergic reactions, and other problems.
   7. The increasing use of colony-stimulating factors (CSF) (e.g., G-CSF and GM-CSF) has decreased the incidence of neutropenia in cancer and other selected patients. Whether this will diminish the overall incidence of pneumonia or improve resolution in neutropenic patients is not known.
   8. Severely immunocompromised patients should be cared for by a physician skilled in the management of pneumonia in these individuals. Patients who do not respond to initial therapy may need attention from a pulmonologist to explore more invasive diagnostic methods.
   G. Prevention. Prophylactic antibiotics should not routinely be used in neutropenic individuals, given the high probability of creation of resistant bacterial strains. Immunizations for influenza and pneumococcus should be administered according to guidelines. Neutropenic patients should avoid contact with overtly ill individuals.
XI. Pneumonia in compromised hosts due to T-cell and macrophage dysfunction
   A. Epidemiology. While neutropenic individuals are at risk primarily for GNR and staphylococcal infections, patients with compromised T-cell and macrophage function may be afflicted by a wide variety of opportunistic and intracellular pathogens including unusual bacteria, viruses, fungi, parasites, and worms.
      1. Some infections are primary, and others are due to reactivation of latent diseases.
      2. Patients with cellular immunocompromise include those on steroids and other immunosuppressive drug therapy for cancer, rheumatic disease, transplantation, asthma, or other disorders. Long-term steroid use equivalent to 20 mg prednisone daily is sufficient to impair T-cell and macrophage function.
      3. Patients with certain hematologic malignancies, malnutrition, acquired immunodeficiency syndrome (AIDS), and uremia may also suffer cellular immunocompromise (see Table 6-3 for classifications, as well as the chapters on HIV-related respiratory problems and transplantation for additional details).
   B. Signs and symptoms
      1. Patients present with a dry or productive cough; dyspnea may be present. Fever is common but may be diminished by the effects of steroids or other anti-inflammatory therapy.
      2. A thorough travel history should be obtained to rule out remote exposures to diseases that may be reactivated in the setting of immunosuppression.
      3. Because the DNA viruses—cytomegalovirus (CMV), herpes simplex virus (HSV), and varicella-zoster virus (VZV)—may reactivate systemically in the setting of immunosuppression, other organ involvement may be apparent, such as the liver (hepatitis), skin (VZV and HSV) (Table 6-9), and bone marrow.
   C. Chest x-ray
      1. In a study of pneumonia in non-HIV-immunocompromised patients, the correct pathologic diagnosis was predicted by the chest x-ray findings in only one-third of cases (29).
      2. Up to 75% of patients with nodules had an infectious cause. Large nodules were most common in invasive aspergillosis but were also seen with neoplasm (25). Multiple small nodules were seen most commonly with CMV.

Table 6-9. Dermatologic manifestations

Organisms	Skin manifestation
Chlamydia psittaci	Horder's spots (pale, raised red-brown, blanching with pressure) or EN (22)
Francisella tularensis	Maculopapular, vesicopustular, ulcerative rash, EN, EM
Varicella-zoster virus	Grouped vesicles on erythematous base at various stages of crusting
Measles (rubeola)	Maculopapular eruption, becoming confluent
Staphylococcus aureus	Erythematous pustules or bullae, ecthyma gangrenosum
Herpes simplex virus	Grouped vesicles on erythematous base at lips, nares, circumoral
Cytomegalovirus	Localized skin ulcers or maculopapular lesions (both rare)
Strongyloides	Maculopapular or urticarial eruption; cutaneous larva migrans
Pseudomonas	Ecthyma gangrenosum (erythematous lesion–bluish bulla)
Serratis marcescens	Ecthyma gangrenosum
Rocky Mountain spotted fever	Pink 1–5 mm blanching macules, becoming papular; begins on ankles, wrists, centripetal spread
Streptococcus pneumoniae, Haemophilus influenzae, Legionella	EM
Legionella	Pretibial rash
Mycoplasma pneumoniae	Maculopapular rash, urticaria, EM, EN, and Stevens-Johnson syndrome

EM = erythema multiforme; EN = erythema nodosum.

    3. Dehydrated patients may have minimal findings on chest x-ray, which become apparent after hydration.

D. Laboratory findings

    1. Patients should undergo a routine work-up as stated.

    2. Many of the likely organisms are intracellular and will not be seen on Gram's stain or grow easily in culture.

        a. Special stains for *P. carinii* and *M. tuberculosis* should be obtained in those with a compatible clinical picture.

        b. The presence of urinary antigen for *Legionella* will establish this diagnosis.

        c. Sputum cytology may detect the pathologic effects of viruses or fungi. Viral isolation and molecular biologic techniques are available, and the need for these specialized tests may be best determined by an infectious disease specialist.

E. Differential diagnosis. Infectious etiologies are listed in Table 6-3. In addition to infectious causes, there are numerous noninfectious conditions that may mimic pulmonary infection in the immunocompromised host.

F. Treatment

    1. Patients on steroids are more likely to suffer disseminated infections and increased mortality, and the threshold for initial management in the hospital setting is lower.

    2. Most patients should be treated with empiric broad-spectrum antibiotics. Those who do not respond within several days should undergo bronchoscopy or another definitive procedure designed to obtain material for stain and culture.

    3. Patients who have previously been on steroids may have suppression of the pituitary–adrenal axis, and an Addisonian crisis may be precipitated during episodes of pneumonia. When in doubt, any patient not currently on a corticosteroid should receive at least the equivalent of "stress" doses of hydrocortisone during an episode of infection.

    4. Hydration and supplemental oxygenation should be used as indicated.

    5. Severely immunosuppressed patients such as bone-marrow and solid-organ transplantation patients should be cared for by physicians familiar with the management of pneumonia in these individuals.

  G. Prevention. Prophylactic antibacterials should not be routinely administered to these individuals, since they induce a selective pressure on resident flora to produce resistant strains. Immunizations for influenza and pneumococcus should be administered according to recommended guidelines.

XII. Immunoglobulin and complement deficiencies. Humoral immunity is crucial for successful defense against pathogens with an antiphagocytic capsule, such as *S. pneumoniae, H. influenzae, Neisseria* species, and some gram-negative organisms. IgA is the major protective immunoglobulin in the upper respiratory tract, and IgG is the major protective immunoglobulin in the alveolus. Patients with isolated IgA deficiency may be normal or have recurrent sinopulmonary infections. Patients with defective antibody production include those with congenital immunoglobulin deficiencies and those with acquired defects as seen with chronic lymphocytic leukemia, multiple myeloma, and splenectomy (see Table 6-3).

XIII. Typical pneumonia: specific pathogens

  A. *Streptococcus pneumoniae.* Patients presenting with signs and symptoms suggestive of typical bacterial pneumonia should be assumed to have pneumococcal disease until proven otherwise. This organism is still the most common—but decreasingly so—cause of CAP (30).

    1. Etiology. This gram-positive, lancet-shaped diplococcus possesses a complex polysaccharide capsule that is the basis for serotyping.

    2. Epidemiology. *S. pneumoniae* can be found in all age groups and clinical settings. Infection is most common in winter and early spring. The mode of spread is usually person-to-person, but the organism commonly colonizes in the oropharynx, before leading to pneumonia. Pneumonia develops when colonizing organisms are aspirated into a lung that is unable to contain the inoculum (31).

    3. Pathogenesis. Pathogenicity and virulence are influenced by the biologic properties of the outer capsule and by host factors. Patients with CHF, chest trauma, multiple myeloma, asplenia, alcoholism, and hypogammaglobulinemia are most susceptible to pneumococcal infections (32).

    4. Clinical manifestations

      a. Symptoms. Patients with an intact immune response present with the typical pneumonia syndrome of abrupt onset of shaking chills and fever, pleuritic chest pain, and cough productive of rust-colored sputum.

      b. Signs. Patients usually appear toxic and are febrile and tachypneic with signs of consolidation on lung examination. Hypothermia is a risk factor that correlates with poor prognosis and may be a manifestation of impaired host defense (33).

    5. Chest radiograph usually demonstrates lobar consolidation, but patchy bronchopneumonia and interstitial infiltrates may be present. Pleural effusions are fairly common (25% to 60%), but are usually small in volume. Cavitation and empyema are rare. The chest x-ray may appear worse or unchanged despite clinical improvement with antibiotics. Slow radiographic resolution does not indicate treatment failure in the face of an improved clinical response (11, 12,32).

    6. Laboratory findings are nonspecific. A leukocytosis is usually present, and tests of hepatic function may be slightly abnormal. Serum bilirubin may be increased to levels not exceeding 3–4 mg/dL; the pathogenesis is multifactorial, with hypoxia, hepatic inflammation, and breakdown of red blood cells in the lung all thought to contribute (34).

    7. Diagnosis. Gram's stain of purulent sputum (20–25 WBCs per low-power field with <10 epithelial cells) revealing characteristic lancet-shaped diplococci in the absence of other predominant flora is strongly suggestive of the diagnosis.

      a. 30% of patients are unable to produce an adequate sputum sample (10,11), and the organism is recovered from sputum culture in fewer than

half of cases. Due to contamination of sputum by oropharyngeal coloniz-ers, the bacterium may be recovered from patients without infection (35).
   b. The **quellung reaction** is a well demarcated halo seen around the bac-terium produced by the interaction of the capsule with type-specific anti-capsular antibody. This test is a rapid and specific method of detecting pneumococci in clinical specimens, but it is not often required.
   c. **Counterimmunoelectrophoresis (CIE)** detects specific pneumococcal capsular antigen in sputum, cerebrospinal fluid, urine, and serum (36).
8. **Treatment.** Penicillin VK (500 mg PO QID) should be given for 7–10 days. Ery-thromycin (500 mg PO QID) for 7–10 days is suitable for patients allergic to penicillin. A cephalosporin (eg, cefazolin 1 g TID or cephalexin 500 mg TID) and clindamycin (300 mg TID) are effective alternatives (see Table 6-6).
   a. The approximately 10% of pneumococcal strains in the United States that are intermediately resistant to penicillin (defined by minimum inhibitory concentrations) can be treated with high doses of penicillin.
   b. About 1% of cases are highly resistant and should be treated with alterna-tive therapy such as vancomycin (31). Many strains of pneumococci are resistant to tetracycline, and up to 20% of isolates from children in day-care are resistant to trimethoprim/sulfamethoxazole (34).
   c. With effective therapy, clinical improvement follows within 24–48 hours, but fever may persist for 4–5 days.
9. **Complications**
   a. Pleural effusions occur in 25% of cases; they are usually small and sterile (25).
   b. Other important complications of pneumococcal pneumonia include men-ingitis, endocarditis, and septic arthritis. Rates of bacteremia vary from 13% to 40%, and individuals with bacteremia are more likely to have comorbidi-ties.
   c. Mortality is related to advanced age and to the presence and number of comorbidities (30) (Table 6-10). Mortality is high, particularly in those with positive blood cultures. The mortality rate for bacteremic patients in the 1960s was 19.5%, which is virtually the same as that reported in the 1990s (5).
   d. Of patients who die despite antibiotic therapy, 35% die within the first 24 hours of antibiotic treatment, underscoring the fulminant course this dis-ease may pursue (31).
10. **Prevention**
   a. **Patients at risk for pneumococcal infection should be receive pro-phylaxis with the 23-valent pneumococcal vaccine that is protec-tive against 85% to 90% of bacteremic strains in the United States** (37). The indications for administration of pneumococcal vaccine are listed in Table 6-11.
      i. If possible, vaccination should take place 2 weeks prior to a planned splenectomy, although good responses are found in patients post-splenectomy or with sickle cell disease (38). Following vaccination, over 80% of healthy adults develop a twofold or greater rise in anti-body titer against each antigen (37). Most subjects maintain protec-tive levels for 7–10 years.
      ii. The elderly and patients with diabetes, COPD, or alcoholic cirrhosis may generate lower antibody titers than healthy adults, but such lev-els are still considered adequate for protection (36,39).
      iii. Suboptimal antibody responses are seen in patients with leukemia, lymphoma, multiple myeloma, or HIV infection (36,40). In 1991, a large and comprehensive case–control study determined the effi-cacy of the vaccine to be 61% in immunocompetent recipients (41). Studies of the elderly show a lesser efficacy, although benefits from the vaccine are still demonstrable. Populations with a high preva-lence rate, such as Alaskan-American natives, should also be immu-nized (20).

Table 6-10. Factors associated with increased mortality from pneumococcal pneumonia

Underlying illness
    Cardiac disease
    Chronic obstructive pulmonary disease
    Cirrhosis
    Neoplasm
    Asplenia
Age > 50 years
Leukopenia (WBC < 4,000/mm^3)
Leukocytosis (WBC > 20,000/mm^3)
Multilobar involvement
Extrapulmonary involvement
Bacteremia
Hypoxemia

WBC = white blood cell count.

Table 6-11. Pneumovax recommendations: high-risk persons who should receive pneumococcal vaccine

Patients >65 years of age
Chronic cardiac disease (such as congestive heart failure)
Chronic obstructive pulmonary disease (bronchitis, emphysema)
Alcoholism
Asplenia (functional or anatomic)
Diabetes mellitus
Chronic renal failure
Chronic dialysis
Chronic liver disease
Hodgkin's disease
Chronic lymphocytic leukemia
Multiple myeloma
HIV infection

    b. All persons with medical conditions serious enough to merit influenza vaccine should also be given pneumococcal vaccine. Both vaccines can be given at different sites simultaneously without an increase in side effects or loss of antibody response (42). **Revaccination** of high-risk individuals likely to have a rapid titer decline or diminished antibody response should be considered after 6 years (42).

B. *Haemophilus influenzae*
    1. **Etiology and pathogenesis.** *H. influenzae* is a pleomorphic gram-negative, aerobic, bacillus with both a typable (encapsulated) form and a nontypable (nonencapsulated) form (5). Either can cause CAP; infection by encapsulated bacteria is more common than by nonencapsulated organisms.
        a. Organisms are typed a–f, according to the polysaccharide capsules. Type b accounts for most infections, but cases of CAP due to types c, d, e, and f have been described (43).
        b. Opsonizing antibody is needed to control both. Therefore, *H. influenzae* CAP usually occurs in the setting of impaired host defense, a defect ei-

ther in humoral immunity or in local phagocytic function (31). Spread of the organism occurs through aerosolized respiratory droplets.

2. Epidemiology

   a. The incidence of *H. influenzae* varies from 2 to 11%, and many individuals have comorbid illnesses or are elderly. Colonization of the airways by this organism is common in COPD, with the majority of isolates being nonencapsulated (5). Lower respiratory tract infections produced by nontypable organisms tend to be milder than those due to encapsulated strains (44). A small percentage of adults will sporadically harbor encapsulated strains in the oropharynx.

   b. Table 6-12 lists the type of individuals at increased risk of developing CAP from *H. influenzae* (11,12).

3. Clinical manifestations. Clinically, the presentation of *H. influenzae* CAP is indistinguishable from other bacterial CAP. In some adults, the presentation is subacute, with cough and low-grade fever for weeks prior to diagnosis (45). Hemoptysis is unusual.

4. Laboratory findings

   a. Leukocytosis is present in 75% of patients. Counts are in the range of 10,000–15,000/mm^3 (11,12).

   b. The chest roentgenogram may reveal multilobar, patchy bronchopneumonia (75%) or areas of frank consolidation (38%). Small parapneumonic effusions are common, but progression to empyema or cavitation is unusual (45).

5. Diagnosis

   a. Diagnosis of nontypable *H. influenzae* is a challenge because of the frequent presence of the organism in normal pharyngeal flora and the low incidence of bacteremia (45). Diagnosis by Gram's stain is difficult because the small, gram-negative pleomorphic coccobacilli are often overlooked or misinterpreted as *S. pneumoniae* due to poor staining.

   b. Sputum culture is useful if *H. influenzae* is recovered in the absence of other pathogens, but the organism is not detected by culture in about half of well documented cases of *H. influenzae* pneumonia (11,12). Furthermore, colonization of the bronchial tree with nontypable strains, especially in patients with COPD, complicate the interpretation of Gram's stains and cultures (11,12).

   c. CIE is used as a supplement to standard bacteriologic techniques and can detect the capsular antigen of type b *H. influenzae* in body fluids. This may be particularly helpful in the diagnosis of partially treated infections in which the organism is not recovered by culture. Since many adult infections are due to nontypable strains, the applicability of CIE is limited.

6. Treatment

Table 6-12. Risk factors for acquisition of *H. influenzae* pneumonia

Chronic obstructive pulmonary disease

Chronic alcoholism

Age >50 years

Diabetes mellitus

Hypogammaglobulinemia

Multiple myeloma

Asplenia

Sickle cell anemia

HIV infection

    a. Ampicillin was once the drug of choice, but resistance due to β-lactamase production has now been reported in 5% to 20% of nontypable *H. influenzae* isolates and 50% of type b organisms (31).

    b. Other effective antibiotics include third-generation cephalosporins, fluoroquinolones, trimethoprim/sulfamethoxazole (not every isolate is susceptible), clarithromycin, and azithromycin (31) (see Table 6-6).

7. Complications. Extrapulmonary infection is less common in adults than in children and includes meningitis, arthritis, pericarditis, and epiglottitis. Overall mortality can be as high as 30% in adults of advanced age with underlying disease. Younger patients without bacteremia have a good prognosis.

8. Prevention

    a. While untypable *H. influenzae* causes most CAP in COPD patients, the *H. influenzae* type b conjugate vaccine used commonly in children is also recommended for certain high-risk adults.

    b. Recommended recipients include those with HIV infection, Hodgkin's disease, and functional or anatomic asplenia. This vaccine may prove useful in patients with COPD; however, to date there are no prospective studies examining its effectiveness in this group of patients.

C. *Moraxella (Branhamella) catarrhalis*

    1. Etiology. This organism is an aerobic gram-negative diplococcus.

    2. Epidemiology

        a. Formerly considered a harmless commensal of the upper respiratory tract, *M. catarrhalis* is now known to cause pneumonia. Many individuals harbor the organism as part of the normal nasopharyngeal flora, and thus its recovery from sputum is not necessarily indicative of infection.

        b. The evidence for pathogenicity derives from reports of recovery of the organism in pure culture of transtracheal aspirates of patients with pneumonia (46,47).

        c. *Moraxella* pneumonia typically presents in patients with underlying medical illnesses (see Table 6-3). COPD is the single most common risk factor, although alcoholism, CHF, corticosteroid therapy, and malignancy are frequent accompaniments (11,12,46). Studies have found an increased incidence of infection during the winter months (46).

    3. Pathogenesis

        a. Studies have suggested that *M. catarrhalis* preferentially attaches to the oropharyngeal epithelial cells of patients with chronic lung disease, compared to control subjects (46). The tracheobronchial tree then becomes colonized.

        b. Factors such as smoking, intercurrent viral infection, corticosteroid use, or other forms of immunosuppression facilitate bacterial multiplication and the subsequent development of bronchitis or pneumonia.

    4. Clinical manifestations. Symptoms of dyspnea and productive cough are present several days before pneumonia is diagnosed. Pleuritic chest pain, chills, malaise, and blood-tinged sputum can also occur. Clinical signs include fever to 38.3°C or higher and physical findings compatible with either bronchopneumonia or consolidation. Extrapulmonary manifestations are rare (11,12).

    5. Laboratory findings are nonspecific. Leukocytosis generally occurs. Chest roentgenograms show bronchopneumonia or dense alveolar infiltrates. Single lobe involvement is more common than multiple. Pleural effusions are rare, and cavitation has not been described (11,12,48).

    6. Diagnosis. The diagnosis is established by culture of lower respiratory samples. A Gram's stain showing gram-negative diplococci is also helpful.

    7. Treatment

        a. 80% to 90% of strains produce β-lactamase and are resistant to penicillin (46). Appropriate initial therapy includes second- or third-generation cephalosporins, erythromycin, trimethoprim/sulfamethoxazole, ciprofloxacin, or a β-lactam/β-lactamase inhibitor combination (11,12) (see Table 6-6). Ampicillin or penicillin can be substituted when isolates are β-lactamase negative.

b. The infection should be treated for at least 10 days.

8. Complications

a. The majority of patients recover without sequelae. Empyema is rare.

b. Pneumonia has been a contributing factor in the deaths of some patients with serious underlying conditions.

D. *Staphylococcus aureus*

1. Etiology. Gram's stain demonstrates facultative, gram-positive, nonmotile cocci in clusters. The most pathogenic strains may be distinguished from the less pathogenic epidermidis strains by their ability to produce coagulase. Coagulase is important in the formation of abscesses and, along with a variety of other toxins, accounts for many of the characteristic features of *S. aureus* infections.

2. Epidemiology

a. *S. aureus* accounts for fewer than 5% of cases of CAP, producing nosocomial pneumonia much more frequently (49). It is prevalent in healthy persons.

b. Given its ubiquity and its capacity to cause a broad array of infections, an effective host response plays an important role in preventing infection (50).

c. The organism may infect the lungs by aspiration of oral secretions or through a hematogenous route. These two mechanisms account for approximately equal numbers of *S. aureus* CAP. Patients who acquire the disease from aspirated oral secretions are usually predisposed by having underlying pulmonary disease or a specific risk factor for aspiration (laryngectomy, seizure), underlying immunosuppression, or a recent viral infection (11,12).

d. *S. aureus* is second in frequency only to *S. pneumoniae* as a cause of postinfluenza bacterial pneumonia. CAP caused by hematogenous spread of *S. aureus* usually occurs in the setting of endocarditis or an infected vascular site.

3. Clinical manifestations

a. Symptoms

i. Fever, dyspnea, cough, and purulent sputum are prominent in cases caused by aspiration.

ii. In *S. aureus* CAP acquired hematogenously, signs and symptoms related to an underlying endocarditis or vascular infection predominate.

iii. Respiratory tract symptoms may be mild or absent despite radiographic evidence of multiple pulmonary infiltrates.

b. Signs

i. Prostration, fever, and respiratory distress are common physical findings.

ii. Evidence of lobar consolidation may not always be present on lung examination, as the disease process often occurs centrally (aspiration) or multifocally (emboli). Rales and diminished breath sounds are found over involved areas.

iii. When pneumonia complicates endocarditis, a murmur of tricuspid valve origin, embolic skin lesions, arthritis, splenomegaly, hematuria, and heart failure may be evident (11,12).

c. Gram's stain and laboratory findings. If an adequate specimen is stained and shows no predominance of staphylococci, then the suspicion of *S. aureus* as the etiologic agent is lowered. Leukocytosis of >15,000/mm^3 with neutrophilia and an increase in the band forms is typical.

d. Chest radiograph

i. The chest radiograph may reveal segmental or central consolidation in cases acquired by aspiration. Pleural effusion, empyema, cavities, and abscesses are common (31). Pneumothorax may occur (11,12).

ii. In staphylococcal pneumonia produced by the embolic mechanism, multiple, discrete, and often cavitary infiltrates may be seen bilaterally, predominantly in lower lobes, where blood flow is greater (50).

4. Treatment

  a. The therapy of choice is penicillinase-resistant penicillins (eg, nafcillin, oxacillin), 8–12 g/d IV.

  b. The duration of therapy should be 10–14 days in uncomplicated cases and 4–6 weeks in patients with cavitation or empyema.

  c. A first-generation cephalosporin is recommended for individuals allergic to penicillin; if the allergy is of the immediate type, vancomycin can be used.

  d. Strains of *S. aureus* resistant to methacillin, oxacillin, and nafcillin (MRSA) have become a major problem in recent years. This phenomenon is mainly observed in nosocomial infections and in community-acquired infections in IV drug users in certain geographic areas. IV vancomycin must be used to treat these highly resistant organisms (51).

 5. Complications

  a. Pleural effusions (25%), empyema (3% to 10%), and abscess formation (25%) may complicate staphylococcal pneumonia (9,11,12).

  b. Despite appropriate antibiotic treatment, mortality of this infection remains high. In a 1987 review of 61 cases of adult staphylococcal CAP, the mortality rate was 30% (52). The death rate was especially high in those older than 45 years with associated underlying medical conditions, as well as in those with associated influenza A viral infection (52).

XIV. Aspiration pneumonia and anaerobes

 A. Etiology

  1. Pulmonary manifestations of aspiration can be in one of three forms:

   a. Gastric acid or other toxic fluids can produce a **chemical pneumonitis**.

   b. Inert substances such as water or solid particles that reach the lung can lead to **drowning or airway obstruction**.

   c. Pathologic bacteria secondary to aspiration of stomach or oropharyngeal contents can cause an **infectious pneumonitis or lung abscess**.

  2. The infectious agents most likely to be aspirated and cause CAP include anaerobes that have colonized the mouth, *Prevotella* (formerly *Bacteriodes*) *melaninogenicus*, *B. fragilis*, *Fusobacterium* species, microaerophilic peptococci, and peptostreptococci (assuming aspiration occurs outside a hospital or chronic care facility) (11,12,31). Streptococci and staphylococci are the major aerobic organisms that may also be aspirated in this setting (11,12).

   a. The right lung is affected more often then the left because of the relatively straighter take-off of the right mainstem bronchus. When patients are upright during aspiration, the lower lobes are the most likely recipient of the infected inoculum because they are gravity dependent. If aspiration occurs while recumbent, the superior segments of the lower lobes and the posterior segments of the upper lobes are situated most posteriorly and are the most likely sites of pneumonia.

   b. In addition to aspiration, anaerobic organisms may also be seen in postobstructive pneumonia due to obstructing cancers or foreign bodies. Anaerobes may also be found in local tissue necrosis from cancer, bronchiectasis, or pulmonary infarction.

 B. Epidemiology

  1. Anaerobic organisms cause about 10% of CAP (53), although exact numbers are unknown because some anaerobes appear as part of mixed infections with aerobic organisms. Anaerobic isolates are recovered from 60% to 100% of patients with lung abscesses, aspiration pneumonia, and necrotizing pneumonia and are isolated from as many as 75% of patients with empyema (53).

  2. Risk factors for aspiration include seizure activity, stroke, drug or alcohol intoxication, metabolic encephalopathy, tracheoesophageal fistula, esophageal diverticulum or dysmotility, tracheostomy, intestinal obstruction, nasogastric tube, and emesis (31).

  3. Individuals with periodontal disease or gingivitis are more likely to develop aspiration pneumonia than are edentulous patients or individuals with good oral hygiene. About 45% of normal subjects aspirate during sleep (54).

C. Clinical manifestations and complications

1. **Chemical pneumonitis** secondary to gastric acid with pH <2.4 is manifested by dyspnea, bronchospasm, hypoxemia, frothy sputum, and pulmonary edema. The chest radiograph may show patchy infiltrates in dependent areas of the lung.

2. **Solid inert materials** that obstruct the airway lead to cough and atelectasis and the eventual development of symptoms associated with a secondary bacterial infection distal to the obstruction. Postobstructive pneumonia may develop into an abscess, bronchiectasis, or an empyema.

3. **Pathologic bacterial pneumonitis**
   a. Symptoms consistent with an acute infectious pneumonitis such as fever, cough (often dry), and pleuritic chest pain may develop, although the course may be indolent. Sputum is putrid-smelling in only one-half of patients (53). Progression is characterized by fatigue, low-grade fever, and purulent sputum, resulting in a necrotizing pneumonia or a lung abscess within several weeks (54). The onset of the pneumonia or abscess is usually accompanied by tachycardia, tachypnea, and temperatures well above 39°C (11,12).
   b. Empyema may be associated with an early anaerobic pneumonitis and is reported in one-third of cases of necrotizing pneumonia (11,12). However, empyema rarely occurs with lung abscesses in the absence of parenchymal lung infection. Failure to respond to therapy should prompt a search for continued aspiration, airway obstruction, or a lung abscess.

D. Chest roengtenogram

1. A bronchopneumonic infiltrate, in the absence of lobar consolidation, is generally seen within the aspiration-prone segments of the lung. A necrotizing pneumonia appears as a dense segmental infiltrate containing multiple small lucent areas of lung necrosis (<2 cm in diameter) (11,12). Necrotizing pneumonia often spreads to adjacent lobes.

2. Lung abscesses are usually single, variably sized but often approximately 2 cm in diameter, and are located in the dependent lung segments (31).

E. Diagnosis

1. The sputum Gram's stain reveals numerous polymorphonuclear leukocytes with a mix of gram-negative and gram-positive organisms of different morphologies.

2. Due to the multiple organisms involved, the sputum Gram's stain and culture are often nondiagnostic; 50% of patients with aspiration pneumonia have a mixture of aerobic and anaerobic bacteria in culture (53). Routine sputum culture of expectorated sputum is therefore not suitable for the diagnosis of anaerobic lung infections. Microbiologic confirmation of infection with an anaerobe requires recovery of the organism in a culture of a normally sterile body fluid (thoracentesis, blood culture).

F. Treatment

1. **Antibiotics**
   a. Penicillin G was previously the drug of choice for treatment of anaerobic pulmonary infection. However, penicillin resistance among anaerobes is increasing, owing to β-lactamase production. From 15% to 20% of isolates from patients with anaerobic pleuropulmonary infections are resistant to penicillin G (53).
   b. Treatment is therefore empiric and should include agents with activity against β-lactamase-producing strains of both aerobic and anaerobic organisms (clindamycin) (55).
   c. When penicillin is used in the treatment of a seriously ill patient, the addition of an agent with activity against penicillin-resistant strains, such as metronidazole, is recommended (11,12). Metronidazole alone is associated with high failure rates (53).
   d. Alternative regimens to clindamycin include ampicillin/sulbactam, amoxicillin/clavulanate, ticarcillin/clavulanate, piperacillin, and others. If susceptibility testing of anaerobes is available, therapy can be specifically tailored, but this is generally not required.

2. **Response**
   a. Most patients respond within 3–4 days and are usually afebrile by day 7–10. Treatment should continue until radiographic clearing is present. This may require 2–4 months of therapy (53).
   b. Cavities may develop despite proper therapy.
   c. Empyemas are common in aspiration pneumonia and can develop dramatically over several days. Aggressive drainage with multiple thoracenteses or chest tube placement should be done to evacuate all fluid. In one study of empyema, patients continued to be febrile for an average of 29 days, even after appropriate drainage and treatment (53).
3. **Mortality** is 5% to 12%; a worse prognosis is associated with abscesses over 6 cm in diameter, symptoms lasting 8 weeks or more, associated necrotizing pneumonia, increased age, debility, and bronchial obstruction (53). Those with unexplained anaerobic infections that fail to respond to therapy should be evaluated for cancer or airway obstruction by a foreign body.
G. **Prevention.** Prophylactic antibiotics have no proven benefit. For patients at risk of aspiration, feeding should occur in an upright position. The head of the bed should be elevated in patients receiving tube feedings. Suction should immediately follow any obvious episodes of gross aspiration. Attention to dental hygiene is recommended.

XV. **Pneumonias due to gram-negative rods**
   A. **Etiology.** *Klebsiella pneumoniae, P. aeruginosa, Escherichia coli, Proteus mirabilis, Serratia marcescens,* and other Enterobacteriaceae.
   B. **Epidemiology**
      1. GNR (bacilli) are commonly associated with nosocomial pneumonias. Given the increasing numbers of immunosuppressed and otherwise compromised patients in the community, 9% to 20% of CAP is now due to gram-negative bacilli (11,12,30,56,57).
      2. GNR are among the most deadly causes of CAP, with a median mortality of 33% (58). While rare cases of GNR pneumonia may result from bacteremic spread from a gastrointestinal or geniturinary source, the most common route is through aspiration (11,12).
      3. Approximately 18% of healthy adults may have transient oropharyngeal colonization with GNR (59). Chronically ill, frequently hospitalized, and institutionalized patients often have higher rates of chronic colonization with GNR. For example, the pharynx of one-third of ambulatory alcoholics is colonized with *Klebsiella* (11,12).
      4. **Pneumonia due to GNR should be suspected in alcoholics, diabetics, the elderly, nursing home residents, and those with underlying cardiopulmonary or renal disease, neutropenia, immunosuppression, or malignancy, as well as those who are institutionalized or frequently hospitalized** (5,11,12). GNR should be a strong diagnostic consideration, especially in the presence of chronic comorbid illnesses, in any patient warranting hospital admission.
   C. **Clinical appearance**
      1. The sudden onset of a productive cough is common. Rigors, high fever, and tachycardia are common. Endotoxin produced by GNR may result in hypotension and prostration. In very weak, dehydrated, or neutropenic patients, sputum production may be minimal or even absent. Pleuritic chest pain may be present.
      2. Sputum may be blood-tinged. *Klebsiella* pneumonia, associated with alcoholism as well as with other conditions, may be associated with production of the classic "currant-jelly" sputum (11,12). Bloody sputum may be seen in pneumonia due to other GNR as well.
   D. **Chest x-ray**
      1. Roentgenograms typically reveal consolidation.
      2. *Klebsiella* pneumonia may be associated with the classic **bulging fissure sign** due to the intense inflammatory reaction to this organism. In dehydrated patients, infiltrates may blossom with rehydration.

       3. Pleural effusions are commonly seen in GNR pneumonias, especially with *Klebsiella, Serratia,* and *E. coli.*

  E. **Diagnosis.** Diagnosis may be made by sputum Gram's stain and culture. If an adequate sputum sample is obtained, a predominance of GNR and many neutrophils may be seen. An adequate sample lacking GNR predominance lowers suspicion for GNR pneumonia, but the entire clinical picture must be considered.

  F. **Treatment**

      1. Often the comorbid illnesses and the severity of the GNR pneumonia necessitate hospitalization.

      2. Sensitivities guide therapy, but initial empiric treatment should utilize two antibiotics, anticipating possible resistance to at least one of the drugs (11,12). An antipseudomonal penicillin (eg, piperacillin or ticarcillin) should be combined with an aminoglycoside. Alternatively, an antipseudomonal third-generation cephalosporin (eg, ceftazidime) may be substituted for the penicillin derivative.

      3. Other options include ciprofloxacin, imipenem, or aztreonam (5). Double β-lactam therapy (third-generation cephalosporin with a ureidopenicillin) can also be effective.

      4. Antibiotic resistance is common, especially with organisms initially acquired in hospital or in nursing home settings. **Treatment should last a minimum of 2 weeks, or until the patient has been afebrile for 5–7 days and the neutrophil count is >500/mm³** (60).

  G. **Complications.** GNR pneumonia may be associated with lung abscesses, empyema, pericarditis, and meningitis. Regardless of the underlying susceptibility to GNR, these pneumonias are associated with a 50% mortality rate, accounting for 50,000 deaths annually (21). Prolonged antibiotic therapy may predispose to fungal infections, contribute to resistance, and increase antibiotic-related complications.

  H. **Prevention.** No accepted vaccine is currently available for GNR, and prophylactic antibiotics are not indicated.

XVI. **Atypical pneumonias**

  A. *Mycoplasma pneumoniae*

      1. **Etiology**. The mycoplasmas are free-living, nonmotile bacteria that lack a cell wall. Despite widespread occurrence in nature, few species are pathogenic for humans; *M. pneumoniae* is the most clinically significant.

      2. **Epidemiology**

         a. *M. pneumoniae* is the most commonly recognized cause of atypical CAP in the general population, accounting for approximately 20% of all cases and up to 50% in certain closed populations such as college students and military recruits (11,12,31). Transmission is person-to-person via aerosolized respiratory droplets produced by infected individuals. Mycoplasma infections occur year round, with a modest increase during the fall and winter months.

         b. Since other causes of pneumonia often have a peak incidence in winter months, *M. pneumoniae* accounts for a significant number of summertime pneumonias. The incidence varies widely and all age groups are affected. Persons under 20 years of age are most commonly affected; in those over 40 years of age, the incidence ranges from 11% to 17% (31).

      3. **Clinical manifestations.** Infection with *M. pneumoniae* is most commonly manifested as a minor respiratory infection (pharyngitis, tracheobronchitis); CAP accounts for only a small fraction of all mycoplasma-associated illness.

         a. **Symptoms**

            i. The onset of symptoms is gradual, occurring over several days to a week, which distinguishes the illness from the typically abrupt onset of influenza (61). Fever, chills, headache, malaise, and cough are early symptoms.

           ii. Cough is initially dry, often paroxysmal, and frequently worse at night. It may become productive of mucoid or mucopurulent sputum that is occasionally blood-streaked.

          iii. Pleuritic pain has been reported but is not common.

        iv. Sinus pain or fullness is reported in half of patients, and pain associated with otitis media or bullous myringitis is occasionally noted.

    b. Signs

        i. The signs of mycoplasma infection often are minimal and disproportional to the patient's complaints. Fever rarely exceeds 39°C and is likely to be much lower in the later stages of illness.

        ii. Examination of the chest may reveal diffuse rales and rhonchi over the involved site, usually a lower lobe. Not uncommonly, the chest examination is normal despite distinct radiographic abnormalities. Evidence of lobar consolidation is absent.

        iii. The posterior pharynx may be mildly erythematous, but exudate is uncommon. An erythematous immobile tympanic membrane or inflammation with formation of bulla can be seen in 10% of patients. Cervical adenopathy is encountered in 25% of cases (11,12).

    c. Chest radiographic findings are variable; often findings are more dramatic than the clinical presentation. Infiltrates may be bronchopneumonic or interstitial with Kerley's B lines (Fig. 6-1A,B). Effusions are rare.

    d. Laboratory findings

        i. The WBC count is normal in most patients, although up to 25% will show a mild to moderate leukocytosis.

        ii. Cold hemagglutinins are present in a titer of >1:32 in up to 70% of patients (31). These are IgM antibodies directed toward the I antigen on the erythrocyte membrane. Unfortunately, a positive test result is nonspecific, as cold agglutinins may be detected in patients with CAP due to *Legionella*, adenovirus, cytomegalovirus, influenza and in various other infectious and noninfectious conditions (lymphoproliferative diseases).

        iii. Coombs'-test positivity may develop in some patients with mycoplasma infection.

  4. Diagnosis

    a. Culture. *M. pneumoniae* can be cultured from sputum or throat washings using special media; 10 days are required for growth.

    b. Serology. A fourfold rise in specific *M. pneumoniae* complement fixation titer for paired acute and convalescent serum samples is confirmatory evidence of mycoplasma infection. A single titer of 1:64 is suggestive, particularly when the clinical illness is compatible with the diagnosis.

    c. A DNA probe test is now commercially available for rapid detection of *M. pneumoniae* in sputum (62).

  5. Treatment. Erythromycin and tetracycline (500 mg PO QID) are equally effective. Doxycycline, clarithromycin, and azithromycin are also effective alternatives. Two weeks is recommended as the minimum duration of treatment (11,12).

  6. Complications

    a. Autoimmune hemolysis secondary to cold agglutinins develops in some patients with mycoplasma pneumonia and can be detected by Coombs'-test positivity and mild reticulocytosis. Signs of overt hemolysis and anemia may be seen with exceptionally high titers of antibody.

    b. Mycoplasma pneumonia is associated with various exanthems in 11% to 25% of cases (see Table 6-9) (63).

    c. Other extrapulmonary manifestations include meningitis, transverse myelitis, cranial nerve palsies, myocarditis, pericarditis, hepatitis, and reversible acute renal failure secondary to fulminant intravascular hemolysis (5,31).

B. *Chlamydia pneumoniae*

  1. Etiology. *C. pneumoniae* strain TWAR is the third species of the genus *Chlamydia* and is associated with a variety of human respiratory infections including sinusitis, bronchitis, and pneumonia. TWAR is an acronym reflecting the history of the first two isolates: TW for Taiwan, the site of the first isolate; and AR for the acute respiratory disease associated with the second isolate (64).

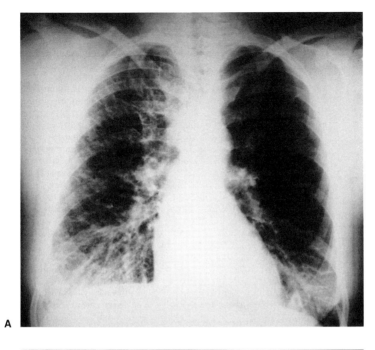

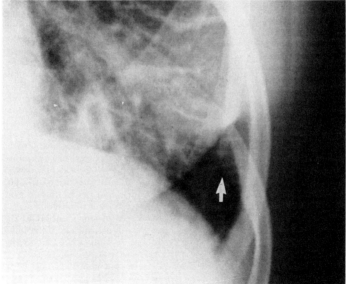

Fig. 6-1. A: PA chest x-ray in a 25-year-old patient with mycoplasma pneumonia. **B:** Detail of left lower lobe shows Kerley's B lines *(white arrow).*

2. **Epidemiology**
   a. *C. pneumoniae* has been detected in 6% to 12% of cases of CAP in the United States and Europe (31,64).
   b. A temporal periodicity has been demonstrated for this infection: High incidence rates for 2–3 years are followed by 4–5 years of lower rates. Little is known about the exact route of transmission, reservoir of infection, or incubation period. *C. pneumoniae* CAP has been identified in all age groups ranging from college students to the elderly.
3. **Clinical manifestations**
   a. Acute chlamydial infection ranges from asymptomatic to life-threatening pneumonia. No set of symptoms or signs is unique to *C. pneumoniae* CAP. While some cases have an acute onset with immediate signs and symptoms of pneumonia, a more gradual onset is typical. Upper respiratory symptoms, particularly pharyngitis with hoarseness and fever, may be seen initially without signs of pulmonary involvement.
   b. The clinical course appears to be biphasic: symptoms of upper respiratory tract infection may spontaneously regress, with cough and signs of lower respiratory infection developing several days to weeks later (65). rhonchi and rales are commonly heard on auscultation, even in the presence of relatively mild symptoms.
4. **Laboratory findings** are nonspecific. The leukocyte count is usually not elevated. Chest roentgenogram usually reveals a localized segmental or subsegmental infiltrate in the middle or lower lobe. More extensive unilateral and even bilateral pneumonitis has been found. Pleural effusions are rare. All radiographic abnormalities should resolve over the course of 2–4 weeks (11,12).
5. **Diagnosis**
   a. **Culture.** Definitive diagnosis of infection requires culture of respiratory specimens. The organism will not grow on conventional microbiologic media, and tissue culture is required to isolate the pathogen.
      i. After inoculation, tissue cultures are stained with *Chlamydia* genus–specific monoclonal antibody conjugated to fluorescein and identified with specific monoclonal antibodies by indirect fluorescent staining (11,12).
      ii. The **polymerase chain reaction (PCR)** is a promising technique for quickly demonstrating the organism in clinical specimens (66). PCR is more sensitive than isolation.
   b. **Serology.** Serum specimens can be tested for microimmunofluorescence (MIF) antibody to *C. pneumoniae* antigen to distinguish between the IgM and IgG serum fractions, and for complement-fixing (CF) antibody to *Chlamydia* species.
      i. **C. pneumoniae CAP is presumptively diagnosed with a fourfold or greater rise in MIF antibody titer (IgM or IgG) between paired serum specimens' antibody (at onset and 4–6 weeks later), as well as with an IgM titer >1:16 or an IgG titer >1:512** (11,12,64,66).
      ii. CF antibody titer >1:64 or a fourfold rise in CF antibody is considered evidence of current or recent infection (66).
6. **Treatment.** Tetracycline and erythromycin (500 mg PO QID) are equally effective. Doxycycline, clarithromycin, azithromyin, and the fluoroquinolone ofloxacin are also effective (64). Treatment for a minimum of 2 weeks is advised (11,12).
7. **Complications.** Sinusitis, laryngitis, and tonsillitis may occur with or without associated pneumonia. Complete recovery is the rule in young adults. The infection may be more severe in older adults, and fatalities have been seen in patients with preexisting illness. Persistent cough and malaise are common, even in appropriately treated patients. Bronchospasm and asthma are potential sequelae of this infection (65).

C. *Legionella* **pneumonia**
   1. **Etiology.** Organisms of the genus *Legionella* are small, weakly staining, aerobic, gram-negative bacilli. About half of *Legionella* species have been proven

to be pathogenetic in humans. *L. pneumophila* serogroup 1 is responsible for 80% of these infections (67). *L. micdadei* is the other species commonly causing human illness.

2. **Epidemiology**

   a. Legionellae are aquatic organisms, and infection is caused by inhalation of infected aerosols from contaminated water sources such as air conditioning equipment, water faucets, shower heads, and lakes.

   b. Infection by legionellae can occur in epidemic fashion, as in the 1976 Philadelphia experience involving over 200 individuals, or in an endemic outbreak when a water system becomes infected in an institution such as a hospital. Legionella infection also occurs sporadically.

   c. Those with chronic underlying lung disease, smokers, the elderly, and persons receiving immunosuppressive medications are at particular risk (31,67).

   d. Person-to-person spread has never been substantiated, nor has infection via aspiration from a colonized oropharynx (67).

   e. The incidence has ranged from 1% to 27% of all cases of CAP, but the most consistently reported figure is about 6% (30). Virulent organisms are capable of causing pneumonia in healthy individuals; however, the attack rate is much higher in individuals with the predisposing conditions listed in Table 6-3.

3. **Clinical manifestations**

   a. Nonspecific constitutional symptoms predominate early in the course and include high fever, chills, headache, myalgias, dyspnea, pleuritic chest pain, and either a productive or nonproductive cough. Symptoms are rapidly progressive, and individuals often appear quite ill at the time of presentation.

   b. Signs are also nonspecific and include mental confusion and a relative bradycardia.

4. **Chest x-ray** findings are variable, nondiagnostic, and may progress rapidly. Findings range from unilateral, poorly marginated peripheral densities, diffuse patchy infiltrates, to diffuse interstitial infiltrates. The alveolar infiltrates often spread quite rapidly. In about 30% of cases, a pleural effusion, usually of moderate volume, may be detected (67).

5. **Laboratory findings.** Blood cultures for *Legionella* are not sensitive. Hyponatremia and liver test abnormalities are suggestive but not diagnostic of legionella infection.

6. **Diagnosis**

   a. Legionellae are unlikely to be visualized on Gram's or Giemsa stain. Special culture media is required.

   b. **Urinary antigen** for *Legionella* may be measured by radioimmunoassay (RIA), enzyme-linked immunosorbent assay (ELISA), or latex agglutination. These methods offer the advantage of a rapid, noninvasive diagnosis with a sensitivity >75%. RAI is 80% to 90% sensitive (6). The specificity of both RIA and ELISA is close to 100%, and superior to the latex test (67). The primary drawbacks are that positivity may persist for months after recovery from an infection and the only commercially available RIA test restricts the diagnosis to the *L. pneumophila* serogroup 1 (68).

   c. **Direct fluorescent antibody** (DFA) test allows a rapid diagnosis (2–4 hours) but requires an experienced technician to interpret the test. Sputum DFA shows a broad sensitivity range from 18% to 33%, with a specificity of 94% (67,69). The DFA yield of bronchoalveolar lavage (BAL) is about 66% (67). The combination of DFA and culture of respiratory secretions improves the sensitivity of sputum to 78% (67). The DFA test becomes negative after 4–6 days of appropriate antibiotic treatment (69). False-positive results have been reported with tularemic pneumonia, *S. aureus*, *Bacillus cereus*, *Lactobacillus brevis*, *Pseudomonas* species, *Xanthomonas* species, and *B. fragilis* (67).

   d. **Sputum culture**, the definitive method of diagnosing legionnaires' disease, is performed on special buffered charcoal–yeast extract agar because legionellae fail to grow on standard media. The sensitivity of sputum culture ranges from 11% to 56% (67). This broad sensitivity range is probably due to differing techniques for processing specimens, as well as the lack of a diagnostic standard for comparison. Positive results from cultured respiratory samples are 100% specific (67).

  e. **Serologic tests** using immunofluorescent antibody (IFA) detection, ELISA, and microagglutination are the most readily available tests for diagnosing legionnaires' disease. However, the delay inherent in serologic diagnosis limits their clinical usefulness. In addition, 20% to 30% of patients suffering from legionnaires' disease do not develop increases in specific antibody (67). The elderly may have delayed seroconversion. All three serologic assays have a sensitivity of about 78% to 80% (67). The specificity of serologic IFA diagnosis is >95% when restricted to *L. pneumophila* serogroup 1 infection (69).

  f. **Radiolabeled DNA probe** for *L. pneumophila* RNA has recently become available. This test can be performed within a few hours and is not operator dependent. Sensitivities range from 50% to 69%, with a specificity of 99% (70). Moreover, the test may remain positive in respiratory secretions for up to 8 days after beginning proper therapy.

7. **Treatment**

  a. The treatment of choice for immunocompetent patients is erythromycin (500 mg PO QID) for 2 weeks (67). Alternatives include trimethoprim/sulfamethoxazole, tetracycline, clarithromycin, azithromycin, and ofloxacin or ciprofloxacin.

  b. In severely ill or immunocompromised patients, rifampin (600 mg q12h) should be added (67).

  c. A 3-week course of treatment is required to prevent relapse, especially in immunocompromised hosts. Cavitary disease should also be treated for a longer period of time. Patient isolation is not required, since person-to-person spread has not been documented.

8. **Complications**

  a. Fever may persist for up to 1 week after starting appropriate therapy. Mortality is <5% in normal hosts but may be as high as 25% in compromised hosts (5). Mortality may be as high as 80% in immunocompromised individuals who do not receive appropriate therapy (5). The overall mortality rate is approximately 19% (5).

  b. Although most patients have few sequelae after recovery from *Legionella* pneumonia, persistent fatigue is common. Abnormal diffusing capacities (D_LCO) have been noted as long as 2 years postinfection (71). Extensive pulmonary fibrosis has been described in several cases (67).

XVII. **Viral pneumonias**

  A. **General.** Viruses are the most common cause of pneumonia in infants and children, but relatively uncommon causes of CAP in adults (72). Documented CAP has been reported with most types of viruses; RNA-containing viruses account for the largest number of cases in normal adults (72). Cytomegalovirus (CMV) is an extremely important pathogen in patients with T-cell or macrophage immunocompromise (steroids, cytotoxic drugs). Death rates from viral pneumonia vary considerably, depending on the specific virus and host factors, but can be high in cases of influenza. Long-term morbidity has been reported in some adults. An understanding of the newer antiviral agents is essential for clinicians who care for these patients.

  1. **Etiology**

    a. The chief causes of viral pneumonia in immunocompetent adults are influenza virus types A and B, adenovirus, parainfluenza virus, and varicella-zoster virus.

    b. CMV is the most common viral pathogen in immunocompromised adults, with herpes simplex virus (HSV), adenovirus, and respiratory syncytial virus occurring less frequently.

  2. **Epidemiology**

    a. Published series of viral pneumonia have generally included individuals with recent hospitalizations; therefore, the true incidence and prevalence of viral CAP are not accurately known (72). Most viruses that cause pneumonia are spread from the upper to the lower respiratory tract by inhalation of aerosolized secretions or through person-to-person contact with infected secretions. Viral CAP occurs most commonly in the winter months and more frequently in closed populations or in those with cardiac and pulmonary diseases (72).

  b. The likelihood of viral pneumonia developing in immunocompromised individuals depends directly on the duration and degree of immunosuppression. In these patients, viral disease may represent systemic reactivation of latent disease rather than primary infection.

3. Pathogenesis. During the acute stage of respiratory viral infection, replication occurs within the ciliated cells of the airways. Subsequently, the epithelium of the tracheobronchial tree degenerates and denudes and is followed by mononuclear infiltration of the bronchial walls. When pneumonia occurs, the inflammatory process extends beyond the bronchioles and into the alveolar septa, resulting in edema and exudation. Viral infections have been found to alter bacterial colonization patterns, increase bacterial adhesion to respiratory epithelium, and reduce mucociliary clearance and phagocytosis. This impairment of host defenses allows the resident bacteria to invade normally sterile areas, such as the paranasal sinuses, middle ear, and lower respiratory tract, resulting in secondary bacterial infection. These phenomena occur most frequently with influenza infection (see Table 6-3).

4. Clinical manifestations. The clinical signs and symptoms of viral pneumonia cannot always be differentiated from those of primary bacterial CAP. When a typical viral exanthem is present, as in varicella or measles, the pneumonia is usually caused by the underlying virus (72). Otherwise, it is virtually impossible to distinguish viral from atypical bacterial etiologies of CAP on the basis of initial symptoms, physical examination, or chest x-ray (see Table 6-9).

5. Diagnosis. A definitive diagnosis is based on the isolation of virus from secretions or, retrospectively, by a rise in specific antibody titers. These tests, however, do not provide rapid diagnosis and are not clinically useful.

  a. Viral cultures. Specimens for culture can be obtained from nasopharyngeal or throat swabs, BAL, bronchial biopsy, or lung biopsy. Specimens for virus isolation should be inoculated onto several tissue-culture cell lines and observed for cytopathic effects over several weeks (72). Alerting the microbiology laboratory in advance will encourage proper specimen handling and transportation of materials.

  b. The **DFA** test can be used to diagnose infection with adenoviruses, influenza types A and B, and parainfluenza in respiratory specimens.

  c. Serology. A fourfold rise in titer between acute and convalescent sera is consistent with recent infection. Standard serologic tests for viral antibody have included complement fixation, hemagglutination inhibition, neutralization, ELISA, IFA, and RIA (72).

  d. Newer diagnostic techniques, such as PCR and *in situ* hybridization, are being applied to the detection of respiratory viruses. These techniques may provide more rapid diagnosis, allowing for earlier interventions with appropriate antiviral agents.

6. Treatment. Treatment in immunocompetent hosts is generally supportive. Vigilance must be maintained, as bacterial superinfections may occur due to alterations in host epithelial surfaces (see Table 6-3). The specific drugs for treatment are listed under each virus below.

7. Complications. As with other respiratory infections, exacerbations of reactive airways disease may be precipitated by viral pneumonia. A persistent or lingering dry cough after other signs and symptoms have resolved may be a manifestation of cough-variant asthma.

B. Influenza virus

  1. Etiology. Influenza virus is an RNA-containing enveloped virus. The envelope is studded with spikes of two types: hemagglutinin (H) and neuraminidase (N).

2. **Epidemiology.** Risk factors for influenza pneumonia include heart disease, steroid or cytotoxic therapy, pregnancy, cardiopulmonary disease, and older age (25). Influenza types A and B are the most common causes of viral CAP, accounting for >50% of all cases in adults (73). Influenza virus has the unique capability of constantly changing its viral envelope proteins as humans develop immunity, allowing for repeated cycles of infection. Influenza viral infection occurs in epidemics (called pandemics when worldwide). In a given community, an epidemic lasts 5–6 weeks and may be associated with substantial attack rates of 10% to 20% of the population in large outbreaks (74). The factors responsible for the onset and decline of an epidemic are not fully understood. The onset of influenza activity has ranged from October to April in the Northern Hemisphere but usually peaks between December and March (11,12). Alterations of antigenic structure lead to infection with variants to which little or no resistance may be present in the populations at risk. Two kinds of antigenic variation are recognized: antigenic drift and antigenic shift.

   a. **Antigenic drift** occurs in influenza A and B viruses involving relatively minor changes due to point mutations within the H or N subtype (11,12).

   b. **Antigenic shift** refers to a major change of the surface protein (the entire H, N, or both) caused by genetic recombination or reassortment (75).

3. **Clinical manifestations**

   a. **Symptoms.** Influenza virus infection commonly presents with a rapid onset of fever, chills, headache, myalgias, malaise, and anorexia. In severe cases, prostration is observed. Systemic symptoms tend to dominate the first several days of the illness, whereas respiratory symptoms, particularly dry cough or nasal discharge, predominate later in the first week of illness (11,12). Cough may be productive in some cases. Nasal obstruction, hoarseness, and dry or sore throat also may be present. Ocular symptoms, although less commonly present, are helpful diagnostically and include photophobia, tearing, burning, and pain on moving the eyes (11,12,76). Cough, lassitude, and malaise may last 1–2 weeks.

   b. **Signs.** Early in the course of illness, the patient appears toxic with flushed facies and hot, moist skin. The eyes are watery and reddened. Continuous or intermittent fever is the most important finding, usually rising rapidly to a peak of 38–41°C (100–106°F) within 12 hours of the onset of systemic symptoms (76). The fever usually lasts for 3 days but may last from 1 to 5 or more days (76). Clear rhinorrhea is common. The mucous membranes of the nose and throat are hyperemic, but exudate is not observed. Small, tender cervical lymph nodes are frequently present. Transient scattered rhonchi or localized areas of rales are found in fewer than 20% of cases (76). Chest radiographs characteristically show bilateral diffuse mid- to lower-lung infiltrates (11,12).

4. **Diagnosis**

   a. Specific diagnosis is best made by viral culture techniques or by one of the rapid diagnostic methods such as immunofluorescence or ELISA using respiratory specimens including sputum, nose and throat swabs, and nasal washes (11,12,77).

   b. Serologic studies of acute and convalescent serum can be useful in making a retrospective diagnosis. Confirmation of the diagnosis is not required in the immunocompetent host.

5. **Treatment**

   a. **Symptomatic.** Bed rest, hydration, antipyretics, and antitussives are advised for malaise, headache, fever, and cough, respectively. Patients should be warned of signs and symptoms of bacterial superinfection.

   b. **Chemoprophylaxis**

      i. When administered within 24–48 hours of the onset of uncomplicated influenza A infection, amantadine and rimantadine have been shown to reduce the duration of fever and other systemic symptoms by 1–2 days compared to placebo, as well as to reduce the duration and quantity of virus shedding in respiratory secretions (11,12,72).

    ii. The efficacy of these drugs in preventing complications of influenza when used for early treatment of infection in high-risk patients or for treatment of established complications has not been determined in controlled trials (11,12).

    iii. The usual recommended dose of amantine for adults less than 65 years old is 200 mg/d in one or two doses. Recent studies have suggested that 100 mg/d for prophylaxis provides the same protection as 200 mg/d with fewer side effects (78). Rimantidine is dosed at 100 mg BID. For persons with severe hepatic dysfunction or renal impairment and in elderly nursing home patients, the dose is reduced to 100 mg qd (78,79). Therapy should be continued until symptoms diminish, usually 3–5 days.

6. Complications. The majority of influenza cases are not associated with any significant complications.

    a. A minority of influenza cases follow a **progressive course.** Despite supportive care with artificial ventilation, progressive hypoxia ensues, and mortality is common in the setting of severe progressive disease. Autopsy findings consist of tracheitis, bronchitis, diffuse hemorrhagic pneumonia with hyaline membranes lining alveolar ducts and alveoli, and a paucity of inflammatory cells within the alveoli.

    b. **Secondary bacterial superinfection** is another complication of influenza pneumonia. Secondary bacterial pneumonia is seen more commonly than primary viral pneumonia and often presents as a distinct clinical syndrome (76). These patients, often elderly or with preexisting pulmonary disease, have a classic influenza-like illness followed by a period of improvement lasting 1–4 days and then an apparent recrudescence of illness. Recurrence of fever is associated with symptoms and signs of bacterial pneumonia such as cough, sputum production, and consolidation on examination and chest radiographs. In some cases, the interim period of improvement may not occur, and the course is quite variable. The most common infecting organisms include *S. pneumoniae, S. aureus,* and *H. influenzae* (32,79).

7. Prevention

    a. **Inactivated vaccines** are the most effective way of preventing influenza virus infection. The effectiveness of influenza vaccine in preventing or attenuating illness depends primarily on the age and immunocompetence of the host and the similarity between the virus strains included in the vaccine and those that circulate during the season (79). With a good match, influenza vaccines have been shown to prevent illness in 70% of healthy children and younger adults (80). Similar efficacy data are seen among elderly persons living in the community. Among the nursing home elderly, influenza vaccine is effective in preventing severe illness, secondary complications, and death. In this population, vaccines have been shown to be 50% effective in preventing hospitalization and pneumonia and 80% effective in preventing death (80).

    b. **Indications.** The target groups that should receive influenza vaccination are summarized in Table 6-13. Recent evidence suggests that influenza vaccination is highly cost effective in healthy working-age adults (81). Significant reductions in the rates of illness, sick leave, and visits to physicians resulted in a net estimated savings of approximately 47 dollars per person vaccinated (81). Therefore, all patients without contraindications should be encouraged to receive yearly vaccination.

    c. **Administration.** Because of continued genetic changes in the virus, immunizations must be given annually. The vaccine should be given in the autumn, before December 1 if possible. The only contraindication is allergy to chicken egg, which is used in the manufacture of the vaccine, and allergy to gentamicin. Individuals with hypersensitivity to eggs are candidates for chemoprophylaxis (see above).

    d. **Side effects.** The vaccine can cause minor local reactions. Malaise and myalgias may occur in recipients not previously exposed to vaccine anti-

Table 6-13. Target groups for influenza vaccination

Persons at risk for influenza complications

Persons >65 years of age

Residents of chronic care facilities

Chronic cardiopulmonary disease, including asthma

Those requiring medical care for chronic illness such as diabetes, renal disease, hemoglobinopathy, or immunosuppression

Persons who might transmit to high-risk persons

Health care workers, including physicians and nurses

Chronic care facility workers caring for high-risk persons

Household members and home caregivers of high-risk persons

Other groups

Anyone wishing to lessen chances of acquiring infection

Essential community service providers

Foreign travelers

Pregnant women with high risk for influenza complications

gens; these reactions begin about 6–12 hours after vaccination and subside within 48 hours (79). Recipients of the 1976 swine influenza vaccine developed Guillain-Barré syndrome at a rate of about 1 case per 100,000 persons vaccinated (79). Neurologic complications have not been reported in subsequent influenza vaccines.

8. **Rimantadine and amantadine** have both been shown to be 70% to 90% effective in preventing illnesses caused by the naturally occurring strains of influenza A, but they are not effective against type B (79). These drugs may be used prophylactically in unvaccinated people but are most effective when used in combination with the vaccine. Prophylaxis must be started at the onset of an epidemic and continued for 5–6 weeks, the usual duration of the epidemic. If the patient is simultaneously vaccinated for influenza A, treatment with rimantadine or amantadine can be stopped after 2 weeks, when protective antibody has developed.

C. **Parainfluenza virus**

1. **Etiology.** This group of enveloped viruses has a single-stranded RNA genome contained in a helical nucleocapsid. Unlike influenza type A viruses, parainfluenza viruses are antigenically stable and do not undergo genetic recombination (11,12). Four serotypes and two subtypes of parainfluenza (PI) virus have been identified: types 1, 2, 3, 4a, and 4b (82).

2. **Epidemiology.** PI viruses are important as a cause of lower respiratory tract disease in young children and are the most commonly recognized cause of croup (acute laryngotracheobronchitis). Reinfection of older children and adults is common and produces milder forms of respiratory illness. PI viruses have a worldwide distribution, and almost all persons are initially infected during childhood, usually by age 5 years (82). Subsequently, people have recurrent infections throughout life. Peak activity typically occurs between October and November, although epidemics have been identified throughout the year (11,12). Transmission occurs from person-to-person by direct contact with infectious respiratory secretions or by large-particle aerosols; the virus spreads readily among family members.

3. **Clinical manifestations.** Reinfections are frequently asymptomatic. Symptomatic infections are manifested as common colds, usually without fever, and less often as pharyngitis, tracheobronchitis, or an influenza-like illness. Pneumonia and exacerbations of chronic airways disease have been described in adults (83).

   4. **Diagnosis.** See above.
   5. **Treatment.** Management is supportive. No specific antiviral therapy or vaccine of proven value has been established.
   6. **Complications.** In up to 5% of primary infections, lower respiratory tract illnesses are severe enough to require hospitalization (11,12). Secondary bacterial infections can involve the middle ear and less frequently the larynx, trachea, or lung.
D. **Adenovirus**
   1. **Etiology.** Adenovirus is a nonenveloped virus with a genome composed of linear double-stranded DNA. The heterogeneity of the DNA of adenovirus immunotypes has been demonstrated by DNA restriction enzyme analysis. Currently, 47 antigenic types of adenovirus are associated with humans, although not all types have been associated with human disease (11,12,84).
   2. **Epidemiology.** Adenovirus can cause pneumonia in normal adults; most reported cases have been in military recruits. Only serotypes 3, 4, 7, and 21 are responsible for these cases (11,12). In military recruits, respiratory disease has been reported to occur throughout the year, although the most prominent peaks occur from late fall to late spring. In civilians, most respiratory disease has been recognized in the summer months. Various subtypes of adenovirus have been associated with fatal pneumonia in transplant and immunodeficient patients.
   3. **Clinical manifestations.** Adenovirus pneumonia is usually mild and clinically indistinguishable from mycoplasma pneumonia. Besides the usual constitutional symptoms associated with viral infections, adenovirus may be associated with pharyngitis and/or conjunctivitis. Conjunctivitis is not as common as with other major respiratory infections (11,12). Gastrointestinal involvement, including diarrhea, abdominal pain, and hepatitis, may occur. In immunocompromised patients such as those with bone marrow transplants (BMT), a nonproductive cough and high fever may predominate. Hypoxemia may occur. Chest radiographs show bilateral infiltrates, and pleural effusions are reported in up to 15% of this population. Mortality in BMT patients may be as high as 60%.
   4. **Diagnosis.** Viral isolation from an appropriate specimen is the best method for diagnosis. Viral cytopathic effects usually appear within 3–7 days but may take several weeks. Routine serology of acute and convalescent serum can be done by complement fixation. ELISA and immunofluorescence tests can more rapidly detect adenovirus antigen but are less sensitive than cell cultures.
   5. **Prevention.** An effective and safe live oral vaccine for adenovirus types 4 and 7 is used in the military (11,12). The vaccine is not licensed for civilian use.
   6. **Complications.** Fulminant cases of pneumonia have been reported that may lead to bronchiolitis obliterans, interstitial fibrosis, or death (85).
E. **Varicella-zoster virus**
   1. **Etiology.** Varicella-zoster virus (VZV) is one of the human herpes viruses. VZV infection occurs primarily as chickenpox or herpes zoster. In normal adults, VZV pneumonia is regarded as the most frequent serious complication of disseminated varicella infection (86).
   2. **Epidemiology.** Although varicella is one of the most common transmittable diseases, adult disease accounts for only 2% of the estimated three to four million cases annually in the United States. Of fatalities, 25% occur in the adult population (87). The virus is acquired by direct contact with varicella or zoster lesions or by inhalation of infectious respiratory secretions. Patients are considered to be contagious from 2 days before onset of rash until all lesions have crusted. In the general population, clinical pneumonia develops in 0.3% to 1.8% of adults with primary varicella (86); radiologic changes occur more frequently (up to 15%) (53). Acute varicella can occur throughout the year, but the peak incidence is in the spring in temperate climates. Pregnant women, patients with chronic obstructive pulmonary disease or immunosuppression, and cigarette smokers appear to develop more severe pulmonary complications (87).
   3. **Clinical manifestations.** Symptoms of varicella pneumonia in normal adults

are usually apparent 1–6 days after the onset of the rash. Symptoms include cough, dyspnea, pleuritic chest pain, and hemoptysis. Respiratory failure with cyanosis may ensue. Physical findings other than fever and tachypnea are often minimal. The intensity of the rash does not necessarily correlate with the severity of pneumonia. However, the development of pneumonia in the absence of fever and after the cessation of new lesion formation is exceedingly rare (87). The characteristic radiographic pattern is that of diffuse nodular (1–10 mm) infiltrates (11,12). With progressive disease, the nodules enlarge and coalesce to form extensive infiltrates (87). In mild cases, the infiltrates may resolve in 3–5 days; however, in widespread severe disease, the radiographic abnormalities may persist for several weeks. Hilar adenopathy, pleural effusions, and peribronchial infiltrates are frequently present. Healed nodules frequently calcify, resulting in diffuse, punctate calcifications.

4. **Diagnosis.** The diagnosis of chickenpox is usually made clinically. Multinucleate giant cells can be demonstrated in a Tzanck smear from the base of a vesicular lesion in varicella, zoster, or herpes simplex infection. Differentiating these viruses requires either direct inoculation of vesicular fluid in cultured cells or detection by direct immunofluorescence staining for antigen, which is the most sensitive and rapid laboratory test (11,12). Serologic tests confirm the diagnosis in 2–3 weeks but are more useful for determining susceptibility to varicella.

5. **Treatment.** Early initiation of intravenous acyclovir appears efficacious in varicella pneumonia in previously healthy adults. The recommended dose for adults with normal renal function is 10 mg/kg every 8 hours (86). Acyclovir therapy must be initiated as early as possible in the course of VZV pneumonia. If treatment is instituted after significant deterioration in pulmonary function has occurred, acyclovir is much less likely to have an effect on the disease process (86). Some argue that patients at high risk for pulmonary complications from primary varicella should be considered for treatment with oral acyclovir (800 mg five times daily) before the development of symptomatic pneumonia (88). Varicella-zoster immune globulin given within 4 days of exposure can reduce the incidence of clinical varicella by 50% in susceptible persons and is indicated for adults with any immunocompromising condition or during pregnancy (89). Pregnant women, especially those in the third trimester, should be referred to an infectious disease specialist for evaluation and therapy.

6. **Complications.** Without treatment, varicella pneumonia is fatal in approximately 11% of otherwise healthy adults and in approximately 35% of pregnant women (86). Bacterial infections due to superinfection of the lung or skin can be expected in about 25% of patients with VZV pneumonia (87). Gram-positive cocci are the leading cause of these infections. Mild diffusion defects and exercise intolerance have been found in some patients from several months to 2 years following the infection. Persistent pulmonary granulomas have been described after recovery from VZV pneumonia (88).

7. **Prevention.** Varicella vaccine is recommended for seronegative adults. While studies demonstrate the cost effectiveness of immunizing children, such studies in adults are lacking. The vaccine appears to be safe and is able to generate acceptable titers in adults.

F. **Cytomegalovirus**
1. **Epidemiology.** CMV is one of the most frequently isolated pathogens in immunosuppressed patients. The availability of treatment options makes this diagnosis important in immunocompromised individuals with pneumonias that do not appear to be bacterial.
2. **Pathogenesis.** Because CMV may depress T- and NK-lymphocyte function, other concurrent infections may be prominent. CMV is contracted from other infected individuals, who are often asymptomatic. Viral shedding may persist for years. Reactivation of latent disease is thought to account for the common occurrence of this disease in patients on immunosuppressive drugs. CMV is itself immunosuppressive.
3. **Clinical manifestations.** Clinical features include fever, nonproductive cough, and dyspnea. Disease may be sudden and rapidly fatal or insidious in onset

over days to weeks. Rales may be heard on examination. Chest radiographs show bilateral diffuse infiltrates in mid- and lower-lung fields (25). A perihilar infiltrate may be confused with pulmonary edema. Diffuse infiltrates, interstitial pneumonitis, and parenchymal opacifications with coexistent nodules <5 mm may be seen (29).

4. **Diagnosis.** CMV pneumonia is hard to diagnose by noninvasive methods. Actual CMV infection is difficult to distinguish from colonization. The presence of virus in blood or urine does not necessarily imply that a pulmonary infiltrate is due to CMV pneumonia. Microscopic examination of stained lung tissue can detect the nuclear and cytoplasmic inclusions of CMV, but lack of these findings does not rule out the diagnosis. The diagnosis may also be confounded by the presence of other opportunistic pathogens. Polymerase chain reaction (PCR) may be useful as a rapid screening technique (90) to exclude the diagnosis (high sensitivity and high negative predictive value); however, a positive PCR result cannot be used to confirm the diagnosis of CMV because of the lower specificity and lower positive predictive value. The combination of positive PCR and positive immunostaining improves sensitivity, specificity, and positive predictive value up to 100% (90).

5. **Treatment.** Ganciclovir for pneumonia is effective in non-AIDS patients and should be used in a dose of 5 mg/kg every 12 hours for 14 days and then at the same dose every day for 30 days or more. CMV immunoglobulin may be used: 400 mg/kg on days 1, 2, and 7 and then 200 mg/kg on days 14 and 21. Untreated cases have a mortality of 85%, which can be reduced to <50% with treatment (91). Acyclovir is active against HSV and VZV, but not against CMV. The adjunctive role of interferon-α in treatment or prophylaxis of viral pneumonia is unclear.

6. **Prevention.** Certain transplantation patients are candidates for ganciclovir prophylaxis. Blood products should be screened. No vaccine is currently available.

G. **Herpes simplex virus**
1. **Epidemiology.** Unlike CMV, other viruses are only rarely isolated from lungs of the immunocompromised patient. HSV and VZV dissemination are more likely in individuals with BMT, cancer, solid organ transplantation, radiation, cytotoxic therapy, malnutrition, and severe burns (53). While cutaneous HSV infection is common, dissemination to the lungs is rare and often fatal.

2. **Pathogenesis.** Suppression of the cellular immune system by immunosuppressive drugs or malignancy can reactivate latent HSV infection. Two mechanisms of pneumonia may occur: extension from the tracheobronchial tree or hematogenous spread.

3. **Clinical manifestations.** While VZV pneumonia is usually found in the presence of skin lesions, HSV may not have concurrent skin or mucocutaneous lesions. Chest x-ray appearance depends on the mode of transmission, with focal or diffuse infiltrates that may be unilateral or bilateral.

4. **Diagnosis.** HSV pneumonitis is rarely diagnosed premortem. While probably more common in intensive care units than previously thought, HSV is not a common cause of CAP. Definitive diagnosis requires obtaining adequate lung biopsy samples for antigen testing and culture. HSV may contaminate the upper airway or cause a tracheobronchitis. If HSV is the only pathogen recovered from lung tissue, initiation of treatment is reasonable in the appropriate clinical setting.

5. **Treatment.** Intravenous acyclovir 5 mg/kg every 8 hours for 7–10 days. Mortality from HSV pneumonitis in immunosuppressed or cancer patients is 10% to 25%.

6. **Prevention.** No vaccine is currently available for HSV.

References

1. Campbell D: Overview of community-acquired pneumonia: prognosis and clinical features. *Med Clin North Am* 1994;78:1035–1048.
2. Niederman MS, Bass JB, Campbell GD, et al.: Guidelines for the initial management of adults with community-acquired pneumonia: diagnosis, assessment of severity, and initial antimicrobial therapy. *Am Rev Respir Dis* 1993;148:1418–1426.

3. Garibaldi R: Epidemiology of community-acquired respiratory tract infection in adults: incidence, etiology, and impact. *Am J Med* 1985;78:32–37.
4. Marston B, Plouffe J, Breiman R, et al.: Preliminary findings in a community-based pneumonia incidence study. In: Barbaree JM, Breiman RF, Dufour AP, eds. *Legionqella: current status in emerging perspectives.* Washington, DC: American Society for Microbiology, 1993:36–37.
5. Mandell L: Community-acquired pneumonia, etiology, epidemiology, and treatment. *Chest* 1995; 108:355–425.
6. Marrie TJ, Durant H, Yates L: Community-acquired pneumonia requiring hospitalization: a 5-year prospective study. *Rev Infect Dis* 1989;11:586–599.
7. Woodhead MA, MacFarlane JT: Comparative clinical laboratory features on Legionella with pneumococcal and mycoplasma pneumonias. *Br J Dis Chest* 1987;81:133–139.
8. Farr BM, Kaiser DL, Harrison BDW, Connolly CK: Prediction of microbial aetiology at admission to hospital for pneumonia from the presenting clinical features. *Thorax* 1989;44:1031–1035.
9. Venkatesan P, Gladman J, MacFarlane JT, et al.: A hospital study of community-acquired pneumonia in the elderly. *Thorax* 1990;45:254–258.
10. Case records of the Massachusetts General Hospital—Case 13. *N Engl J Med* 1996;334:1116–1123.
11. Jansen H, Sachs A, Van Alphen L: Predisposing conditions to bacterial infections in COPD. *Am J Respir Crit Care Med* 1995;151:2073–2080.
12. De Lassence A, Fleury-Feith J, Escudier E, et al.: Alveolar hemorrhage, diagnostic criteria and results in 194 immunocompromised hosts. *Am J Respir Crit Care Med* 1995;151:157–163.
13. Rein MF, Gwaltney JM Jr, O'Brien WM, et al.: Accuracy of Gram's stain in identifying pneumococci in sputum. *JAMA* 1978;239:2671–2673.
14. Boerner DF, Zwadyk P: The value of the sputum Gram's stain in community-acquired pneumonia. *JAMA* 1982;247:642–645.
15. Bartlett J, Mundy L: Community-acquired pneumonia. *N Engl J Med* 1995;333:1618–1624.
16. Caputo GM, Appelbaum PC, Liu HH: Infections due to penicillin-resistant pneumococcus: clinical, epidemiologic, and microbiologic features. *Arch Intern Med* 1993;13:1301.
17. Hofmann J, Cetron M, Farley M, et al.: The prevalence of drug-resistant *Streptococcus pneumoniae* in Atlanta. *N Engl J Med* 1995;333:481–486.
18. Pallares R, Linares J, Vadillo M, et al.: Resistance to penicillin and cephalosporin and mortality from severe pneumococcal pneumonia in Barcelona, Spain. *N Engl J Med* 1995;333:474–480.
19. Schlossberg D: Azithromycin and clarithromycin. *Med Clin North Am* 1995;79:803–815.
20. The Medical Clinics of North America: *Pneumonia: pathogenesis, diagnosis, and management.* Niederman MS, guest editor, Volume 78, No. 5. Philadelphia: WB Saunders Company, 1994.
21. Infectious Disease Clinics of North America: Koziel H, Koziel MJ. *Infections in diabetes mellitus.* March 1995, Vol 9, pp 65–96.
22. Infectious Disease Clinics of North America. *Lower respiratory tract infections,* Sept 1991, Vol 5, No. 3. Wallace R, guest editor, pp 452–615. Clinics in Chest Medicine September 1987: *Respiratory Infections,* Vol. 8 No. 3. Niederman M, guest editor, p 423; Table 2.
23. *Frasier and Pare synopsis of the diseases of the chest.* Chapter 6 page 260, Philadelphia: WB Saunders, 1983.
24. Orens JB, Sitrin RG, Lynch JP. The approach to nonresolving pneumonia. *Med Clinics of N Amer* 1994;78:1143–1168.
25. Murray J, Nadel J: Pyogenic bacterial pneumonia, lung abscess and emphyema. Johnson C, Finegold S, eds. *Textbook of respiratory medicine, 2nd ed.* Philadelphia: W.B. Saunders; 1994, pp 1036–1093.
26. Skerret SJ, Neiderman MS, Fein AM. Respiratory infections and acute lung injury in systemic illness. *Clin Chest Med* 1989;10:469.
27. Infectious Disease Clinics of North America: *Infection in Transplantation.* Rubin RH, guest editor. December 1995; Volume 9, No. 4, pp 965–985.
28. Schimpff S: Empiric antibiotic therapy for granulocytopenic cancer patients. *Am J Med* 1986;80:13–20.
29. Logan P, Primack S, Staples C, Miller R, Muller N: Acute lung disease in the immunocompromised host. *Chest* 1995;108:1283–1287.
30. Fang GD, Fine M, Orloff J, et al: New and emerging etiologies for community-acquired pneumonia with implications for therapy. A prospective multicenter study of 359 cases. *Medicine* 1990; 69:307–316.

31. Light G, Matthay M, Matthay R: Chest medicine. Essentials of pulmonary and critical care medicine, 3rd edition. Niederman M, Sarosi G, eds. *Respiratory tract infections.* Williams and Wilkins, 1995;pp 423–447.
32. Kremsdorf A: Pneumococcal pneumonia. Bordow R, Moser K, eds. *Manual of clinical problems in pulmonary medicine,* 3rd ed. Boston: Little, Brown and Company. 1991; pp. 110–112.
33. Marfin A, Sporrer J, Moore PS, et al: Risk factors for adverse outcomes in persons with Pneumococcal pneumonia. *Chest* 1995;107:457–462.
34. Musher D: Pneumococcal pneumonia including diagnosis and therapy of infections caused by penicillin resistent strains. *Inf Dis Clinics of North Am* 1991;5:509–521.
35. Barret-Connor E: The non-value of sputum culture in the diagnosis of Pneumococcal pneumonia. *Am Rev Respir Dis* 1971;103:845–848.
36. Miller J, Sande M, Hendley J, Gwaltney M: Diagnosis of Pneumococcal pneumonia by antigen detection in sputum. *J Clin Microb* 1978;7:459–462.
37. Recommendations of the Immunization Practice Advisory Committee Pneumococcal Polysaccharide Vaccine. *MMWR* 1989;38:64–76.
38. Landesman SH, Schiffman G: Assessment of the antibody response to pneumococcal vaccine in high~ risk populations. *Rev Inf Dis* 1981;3:S184–S196.
39. Schwartz JS: Pneumococcal vaccine: clinical efficacy and effectiveness. *Ann Int Med* 1982;96:208–220.
40. Lazarus HM, Lederman M, Lubin A, et al: Pneumococcal vaccine response of patients with multiple myeloma. *Am J Med* 1980;69:419–423.
41. Shapiro ED, Berg AT, Austrain R, et al: The protective efficacy of polyvalent pneumococcal polysaccharide vaccine. *N Engl J Med* 1991;325:1453–1460.
42. Ortiz C, LaForce M: Prevention of community-acquired pneumonia. *Med Clin N Am* 1994; 78:1173–1183.
43. Norden C: Haemophilus Influenza infections in adults. *Med Clinics North Am* 1978;62:1037~.
44. Bornstein DL: Pneumonia caused by Haemophilus Influenza type B. *J Resp Dis* 1980;1 :23–41.
45. Murphy T, Apicella M: Nontypable Haemophilus Influenzae: A review of clinical aspects, surface antigen, and the human immune response to infection. *Rev of Inf Dis* 1987;9 1–15.
46. Verghese A, Berk S: Moraxella (Branhamella) catarrhalis. *Inf Dis Clinics North Am* 1991; 5:523–538.
47. Louie MH, Gabay EL, Mathisen GE, et al: Branhamella catarrhalis pneumonia. *West J Med* 1983; 38:47–49.
48. Srinivasan G, Raff M, Templeton WC, et al: Branhamella catarrhalis pneumonia. Report of two cases and review of the literature. *Am Rev Respir Dis* 1981;123:553–555.
49. Bentley DW: Staphylococcus aeurus pneunomia: Coping with a medical emergency. *J Resp Dis* 1980;1:23–41.
50. Mushar DM, Lamm N, Darouiche AO, et al.: The currect spectrum of staphaureus infection in a tertiary care hospital. *Medicine* 1994;73:186–208.
51. Haley RW, Hightower AW, Khabbaz, et al: The emergence of methicillin-resistent Staph aureus infections in U.S. hospitals. *Ann Internal Med* 1982;97:297–308.
52. Woodhead MA, Radvin J, Macfarlane JT: Adult community acquired staphlococcal pneumona in the antibiotic era: a review of 61 cases. *Quarterly J Med* 1987;64:783–790.
53. Huxley E, Viroslav J, Gray W, Pierce A: Pharyngeal aspiration of normal adults and patients with depressed consciousness. *Am J Med* 1978;64:564–568.
54. Johanson W, Harris G: Aspiration pneumonia, anaerobic infections, and lung abscess. *Med Clinics North Am* 1980;64:385–394.
55. Levison ME, Mangura CT, Lorber B, et al: Clindamycin compared with penicillin for the treatment of anaerobic lung abscess. *Ann Int Med* 1983;98:466–471.
56. Moine P, Vercken JB, Chevret S, et al: Severe community-acquired pneumonia: etiology, epidemiology, and prognostic factors. *Chest* 1999; 105:1487–1495.
57. Pachon J, Prados MD, Capote F, et al: Severe community-acquired pneumonia: etiology, prognosis, and treatment. *Am Rev Respir Dis* 1990; 142:369–373.
58. Gilbert K, Fine MJ: Assessing prognosis and predicting patient outcomes in community-acquired pneumonia. *Sem Resp Infect* 1994;9:140–152.
59. Rosenthal S, Tager I: Prevalence of gram-negative rods in the normal pharyngeal flora. *Ann Int Med* 1975;83:355–357.
60. The Medical Clinics of North America: *Antimicrobial Therapy I, Vol 1.* Cunha BA, guest editor. May 1995, No. 3, p 588.

61. Clyde W: Clinical Overview of Typical Mycoplasma Pneumoniae Infections. *Clin Infec Dis* 1993;17(Suppl. l):S32–S36.
62. Kohler RB: ntigen detection for the rapid diagnosis of Mycoplasma and Legionella pneumonia. *Diagn Microb Infec Dis* 1986;4:475—495.
63. Birrer RB, Birrer CD: Mycoplasma pneumonia: a review. *Milit Med* 1908;145:422–424.
64. Pacheco A, Gonzalez-Sainz J, Arocena C, et al: Community-acquired pneumonia caused by Chlamydia pneumoniae Strain TWAR in chronic cardiopulmonary disease in the elderly. *Respiration* 1991;58:316–320.
65. Grayston T: Chlamydia pneumoniae, strain TWAR pneumonia. *Ann Rev Med* 1992;43:317–323.
66. Grayston T, Aldous M, Easton A, et al: Evidence that chlamydia pneumoniae causes pneumonia and bronchitis. *J Inf Dis* 1993;168:1231–1235.
67. Roig J, Domingo C, Norera J: Legionnaires' disease. *Chest* 1994;105:1817–1825.
68. Aguero-Rosenfeld ME, Edelstein PH. Retrospective evaluation of the Du Pont RAI kit for detection of Legionella pneumophilia serogroup I antigenuria in humans. *J Clin Microbiology* 1988; 26:1755–1778.
69. Edelstein PH, Meyer RD, Finegold SM: Laboratory diagnosis of Legionnaires' disease. *Am Rev Respir Dis* 1980;121:317.
70. Pasculle AW, Veto GE, Krystofiak S, McKehey K, Vrsalovic K: Laboratory and clinical evalution of a commercial DNA probe for detection of Legionella. *J Clin Microbiology* 1989;27:2350–2358.
71. Clinics in Chest Medicine: Niederman M, guest editor. *Respiratory infections*, Vol 8; No.3. 1987; pp 423. Table 2.
72. Greenberg S: *Viral pneumonia. Inf Dis Clinics of North Am* 1991; 5:603–621.
73. Ruben FL, Cate TR: Influenza pneumonia. *Semin Respt Infect* 1987;2:222.
74. Glezen WP: Serious morbidity and mortality associated with influenza epidemics. *Epidemiol Rev* 1982;4:25–44.
75. Palese P, Young JF: Variations of Influenza A, B, and C viruses. *Science* 1982;215:1468.
76. Betts RF, Douglas RG, Jr: Influenza virus. In: Mandell GL, Douglas RG, Bennett JE, eds. *Principles and practice of infect disease*, 3rd ed. New York: Churchill Livingstone, 1990.
77. Kimball AM, Foy HM, Cooney MK, et al. Isolation of RSV and influenza virus from the sputum of patients hospitalized with pneumonia. *J Inf Dis* 1983;147:181–184.
78. Advisory Committee on Immunization Practices. Prevention and control of influenza. *MMWR* 1990;39:(RR-7):1–15.
79. Ortiz C, Laforce M: Prevention of community-acquired pneumonia. *Med Clinics of North Am* 1994;78:1173–1183.
80. Recommendations of the Advisory Committee on Immunization: prevention and control of influenza part 1, vaccines. *MMWR* 1993;42:1–14.
81. Nichol K, Lind A, Margolis K, et al: The effectiveness of vaccination against influenza in healthy, working adults. *N Engl J Med* 1995;333:889–893.
82. Anderson L, Partiarca R, Hierblzer J, et al: Viral respiratory illnesses. *Med Clinics of North Am* 1983;67:1009–1020.
83. Wenzel R, McCormick D, Beam W, et al: Parainfluenza pneumonia in adults. *JAMA* 1972; 221:294–295.
84. Hierholzer JC. Adenoviruses in the immunocompromised host. *Clin Microb Rev* 1992;5:262–274.
85. Retalis P, Strange C, Harley R: The spectrum of adult adenovirus pneumonia. *Chest* 1996;109: 1656–1657.
86. Haake DA, Zakowski P, Haake DL, et al: Early treatment with acyclovir for Varicella pneumonia in otherwise healthy adults: retrospective controlled study and review. *Rev Infect Dis* 1990;12: 788–798.
87. Feldman S: Varicella-Zoster Virus Pneumonitis. *Chest* 1994;106:22S–26S.
88. Gogos C, Bassaris H, Vagenakis A, et al: Varicella pneumonia in adults. A review of pulmonary manifestations, risk factors, and treatment. *Respiration* 1992;59:339–343.
89. Recommendations of the Immunization Practices Advisory Committee. Varicella-Zoster immune globulin for the prevention of chickenpox. *Ann Int Med* 1984;100:859–865.
90. Schluger N, Rom W: The PCR in the diagnosis and evaluation of pulmonary infections. *Am J Resp Crit Care Med* 1995;152:11–16.
91. Ho M. Advances in understanding CMV infection after transplant. *Transplant Proc* 1994;25(5): Suppl 4:15–21.

7 Lung Cancer

Christine C. Reardon and
Arthur C. Theodore

Lung cancer is the leading cause of cancer death in the United States for both men and women, with 153,000 deaths attributed to the disease in 1994 (1). The age-adjusted incidence rate for lung cancer in American men peaked in 1988 and decreased slightly in 1989 and 1990. The age-adjusted death rate during the past three decades has increased 121%, from 33.4 per 100,000 in 1956–1958 to 75.6 per 100,000 in 1990. In women, the incidence rate of lung cancer continues to climb, and the death rate has risen a dramatic 425% from 5.4 per 100,000 in 1956–1958 to 31.7 per 100,000 in 1990 (2,3). The overall survival rate for all stages from the time of diagnosis of lung cancer is only 13% and has not changed significantly in recent years, highlighting the fact that lung cancer continues to remain a major problem in the United States.

I. **Predisposing factors**

 A. **Tobacco.** The most common cause of lung cancer (85% to 87%) is the inhalation of carcinogenic chemicals, such as the nitrosamines, in tobacco smoke by active cigarette smokers (4). The risk of lung cancer increases with the duration and quantity of cigarettes smoked, as well as the age when an individual began to smoke (5), and decreases as the interval of smoking cessation increases. Nonsmokers exposed to second hand smoke also have increased rates of lung cancer compared to unexposed nonsmokers (6).

 B. **Oncogene lesions.** Lung cancers resulting from either exposure to cigarette smoke or viral transformation have been associated with mutations of *ras*, *myc* and *HER2/Neu* families of oncogenes, as well as the tumor suppressor genes Rb and p53. Mutations of the p53 gene are the most common genetic alterations in both non–small cell lung carcinoma (NSCLC) and small cell lung cancer (SCLC). *Ras* and *myc* gene mutations correlate with aggressive disease and shortened survival (7).

 C. **Environmental and occupational exposures.** Proven occupational carcinogens for lung cancer include asbestos, arsenic, bis(chloromethyl) ether, chromium, mustard gas, nickel, polycyclic aromatic hydrocarbons, and ionizing radiation. Radon gas, originating as a result of the decay of uranium, can accumulate to levels sufficient to cause lung cancer, especially when combined with cigarette smoke.

 D. **Genetic.** Studies controlling for age, sex, occupation, cigarette smoking, and race have shown an increased relative risk for lung cancer in first-degree relatives of lung cancer patients. Whether this is secondary to true hereditary or other familial factors is unclear, although susceptibility or resistance to carcinogens appears to be involved (8,9).

 E. **Dietary.** Smokers who eat a diet low in vitamin A have an increased risk of developing lung cancer, although this risk is likely related to the quantity of beta-carotene or other compounds in fruits and vegetables (10,11) rather than to vitamin A itself. The anticarcinogenic effects of vitamins E and C have not been conclusively demonstrated to protect against lung cancer.

 F. **Host factors.** The metabolism of carcinogens such as debrisoquin by cytochrome P-450 enzymes has been implicated in the risk of lung cancer development. Abnormal immunosurveillance from drug- or viral-induced defective cell-mediated immunity may be a factor in the development and aggressiveness of many neoplasms including lung cancer.

129

II. **Classification.** The histologic classification of lung cancer is divided into two broad categories based on biological behavior. NSCLC represent 80% of tumors and include squamous cell carcinoma, adenocarcinoma, large cell carcinoma, adenosquamous or other mixed carcinomas, and bronchoalveolar carcinoma. SCLC account for 20% of tumors and require different staging and treatment protocols. Squamous cell and adenocarcinomas may be further classified as moderately or poorly differentiated, correlating with the aggressiveness of the tumor and prognosis.

    A. **Non–small cell lung carcinomas**

        1. **Squamous cell carcinoma or epidermoid carcinoma (EC).** Accounting for 40% of lung cancers, EC arises from bronchial epithelium and tends to be found as central masses that spread intraluminally and invade the bronchial wall. A hilar or perihilar mass is the most common radiographic presentation of these tumors. EC spreads centrally and invades blood vessels and lymphatics, causing involvement of the regional lymph nodes and metastases to distant sites. Squamous tumors arising peripherally are less frequent, have a tendency to cavitate, and may invade the chest wall, diaphragm, or pleura. Histologically, EC is characterized by stratified layers of malignant cells with frequent mitotic figures and conglomerates of keratin called epithelial pearls.

        2. **Adenocarcinoma (AC).** AC represents about 20% of lung cancers and usually presents as peripheral nodules or masses on chest roentgenograms. Early invasion of blood vessels is characteristic of these tumors, and the first symptoms of AC are often due to metastatic lesions or invasion of the chest wall, diaphragm, and/or pleura by the primary tumor. AC tends to form glandular structures of mucin-producing cuboidal or columnar cells.

        3. **Large cell carcinoma (LCC).** Accounting for 10% to 15% of lung cancers, LCC is defined by the absence of pathologic characteristics, such as gland formation or keratin, that might classify it as another cell type. LCC is a fast-growing tumor that tends to arise peripherally, with early invasion of lymphatics and blood vessels leading to nodal and distant metastases. As with AC, the characteristic radiographic presentation is a peripheral mass, but often much larger than AC. Histologically, the cells are large and undifferentiated with abundant cytoplasm.

        4. **Bronchoalveolar cell carcinoma (BAC).** This tumor has a characteristic histologic appearance consisting of well differentiated columnar cells arising from the terminal bronchus and alveoli, leading some authors to consider BAC a type of well differentiated AC. BAC may be slow-growing and present as a peripheral nodule with an air bronchogram or may appear as diffuse infiltrates of one lobe, one lung, or both lungs associated with bronchorrhea. Although rare, BAC is increasing in frequency.

    B. **Small cell (or oat cell) lung carcinomas.** Most often arising in the major bronchi, SCLC account for 15% to 20% of lung cancers and spread by infiltration along the bronchial wall. Early invasion of lymphatics and blood vessels is characteristic, and metastases have often occurred by the time of presentation. While a central hilar or perihilar mass and associated obstructive pneumonitis are the typical presentation, SCLC can also present as a single parenchymal mass. The histologic diagnosis of SCLC precludes surgical intervention except in rare cases when it presents as a small peripheral nodule without demonstrable metastasis. The tumor cells are characterized by small size, abundant mitotic figures, and a paucity of cytoplasm.

    C. **Mixed histologic types.** Many tumors are found to contain two or more cell types when enough specimen is available for examination. Adenosquamous tumors are the most common of these, but virtually all combinations have been reported. The clinical characteristics of mixed tumors reflect the features of the contributing cell types and often pose problems in determining proper treatment.

III. **Signs and symptoms.** Symptoms from lung cancer are often related to the anatomic location of the tumor. Central tumors of the main and lobar bronchi represent 15% of cases and commonly present with cough and hemoptysis. When large enough to cause airway obstruction, atelectasis and pneumonia result. Tumors located in segmental bronchi account for 40% of cases and more often present with bronchial obstruction with atelectasis and/or pneumonia but may also produce cough and hemoptysis. Forty percent of lung cancers are asymptomatic peripheral tumors that are found on an incidental x-ray or after distant metastasis has occurred. Even the most common presenting symptoms, however, may not be apparent until late in the natural history of the disease, when treatment is less likely to be effective.

A. **Thoracic signs and symptoms** (Table 7-1) usually result from invasion of structures from the primary tumor or a postobstructive infection. Cough or change in a chronic cough, shortness of breath, hemoptysis, fever, and wheezing suggest the presence of an airway lesion. The wheezing may be unilateral and often has a monophonic quality. Chest or shoulder pain indicates chest wall and/or pleural involvement with tumor or inflammation. Hoarseness suggests recurrent laryngeal nerve paralysis due to invasion of the aortopulmonary window lymph nodes. Chest tightness, facial swelling, dyspnea, and flushing may indicate obstruction of the superior vena cava. Rarely, tumors can involve the pericardium, producing an effusion and tamponade with tachycardia, hypotension, and neck vein distention. Involvement of the esophagus can cause dysphagia.

B. **Nonspecific signs and symptoms** of lung cancer include weakness, anorexia, cachexia, and weight loss.

C. **Signs and symptoms can be caused by direct metastases** to the skin, central nervous system, lymph nodes, bone, and bone marrow. Although metastases to the liver and adrenal glands are common, symptoms or end-organ failure are unusual.

D. **Paraneoplastic syndromes.** In the absence of bronchopulmonary symptoms, patients may manifest signs and symptoms of disease that are not related to direct metastasis by the lung cancer itself. These paraneoplastic syndromes may precede the discovery of the primary malignancy.

   1. **Endocrinopathies**

   a. **Cushing's syndrome** is most commonly associated with SCLC and results from the ectopic synthesis of ACTH (corticotropin) or its precursors. Patients are likely to present with weakness, fatigue, hyperglycemia, and hypokalemic metabolic alkalosis.

   b. **Hypercalcemia** is present in about 10% of patients with lung cancer, 10% to 15% of whom have no evidence of bony metastases. Squamous cell carcinoma is the tumor most commonly associated with hypercalcemia. The most common signs and symptoms of hypercalcemia are weakness, nausea, vomiting, constipation, change in mental status, polyuria, nocturia, kidney stones, and abdominal pain. The mechanisms of hypercalcemia in pulmonary malignancies appears to be increased osteolysis secondary to:

   i. Direct bony metastasis.

Table 7-1. Initial symptoms of lung cancer

Cough

Hemoptysis

Chest pain

Dyspnea

Extrathoracic pain

Weight loss

Extrathoracic mass

Fatigue

Superior vena cava syndrome

Hoarseness

Central nervous system symptoms

Shoulder pain

Clubbing

    ii. Hormonal influences such as parathyroid hormone-like factors, prostaglandins, and osteoclast-activating factor.

  c. The **syndrome of inappropriate antidiuretic hormone secretion** (SIADH) is most commonly associated with SCLC but may also be seen with adenocarcinoma and bronchoalveolar cell carcinoma. The symptom complex of weakness, lethargy, confusion, headache, coma, seizures, and death is directly related to water intoxication and hypotonicity. Parameters for the clinical diagnosis of SIADH include:

    i. Hyponatremia with extracellular hypo-osmolarity.
    ii. Renal wasting of sodium.
    iii. Absence of volume depletion.
    iv. Inappropriately concentrated urine osmolarity.
    v. Normal kidney and adrenal function.

  2. **Skin and bone** paraneoplastic syndromes.

    a. **Hypertrichosis lanuginosa:** hair growth of extremely fine, silky, lightly pigmented hairs, most apparent on the face and ears but visible on the trunk and extremities.

    b. **Leser-Trélat sign:** abrupt development of seborrheic keratosis.

    c. **Acanthosis nigricans:** bilateral, symmetric hyperpigmentation and hyperkeratosis of intertriginous and flexural regions.

    d. **Dermatomyositis.**

    e. **Hypertrophic pulmonary osteoarthropathy** is most commonly seen with squamous cell carcinoma of the lung. Patients complain of burning pain in the distal aspects of arms and legs, and x-rays demonstrate new periosteal bone formation in the corresponding areas.

    f. **Erythema gyratum repens:** the rare finding of erythematous bands forming parts of circles.

    g. **Clubbing.**

  3. **Neuromuscular manifestations** are most often caused by SCLC.

    a. **Myasthenic and polymyositic myopathies.** The **Eaton-Lambert syndrome** is a myasthenic syndrome characterized by the gradual onset of weakness without pain of the proximal muscles, particularly the hip and lower limbs, with sparing of the ocular and bulbar musculature. Characteristically, the muscles are weak at the beginning of contractions but reach normal strength with sustained effort. An autoimmune etiology has been demonstrated with the finding of IgG Anti-Hu antibodies against calcium channels at the neuromuscular junction. With **polymyositis,** muscle biopsy shows necrosis, inflammation, and fibrosis of individual muscle fibers.

    b. **Polymyopathy and neuromyopathy** are the most common neuromuscular syndromes specifically associated with lung cancer. **Peripheral neuropathy** generally involves both motor and sensory pathways. The presenting symptoms of pain and paresthesias are usually followed by sensory loss and muscle weakness. Rarely, motor neuropathies and neuromyotonia may be seen in the absence of sensory findings.

    c. **Other central nervous system syndromes** include central pontine myelinosis, necrotizing myelopathy, limbic encephalitis, and opsoclonus. **Subacute cerebellar degeneration** is caused by antibodies to cerebellar Purkinje's cells and consists of progressive ataxia, dysarthria, and loss of coordination.

  4. **Other systemic manifestations**

    a. **Membranous glomerulopathy** with nephrotic range proteinuria.

    b. **Hematologic syndromes** are common and include thrombophlebitis, which may be migratory, disseminated intravascular coagulation, thrombocytosis, lymphopenia, granulocytosis or granulocytopenia, and nonbacterial thrombotic endocarditis. Anemia is the most common hematologic derangement in lung cancer.

IV. **Radiographic findings.** Although the radiologic findings in lung cancer are varied and nonspecific, both routine chest films and chest computed tomography (CT) scans are indispensable in the management of lung cancer.

A. The various common patterns of lung cancer observed on **routine chest films** are listed in Table 7-2, but two frequently encountered situations require special discussion.

1. **Solitary pulmonary nodules**, or coin lesions, represent one of the most challenging radiologic abnormalities. The most reliable indicator of malignancy with coin lesions is a demonstrable change in size. Nodules that do not grow or change over a 2-year period are likely to be benign. However, some slow-growing adenocarcinomas and bronchial adenomas with low-grade malignant potential will rarely appear unchanged over a 2-year period. Concentric calcifications or a central nidus of calcium are fairly reliable radiologic signs indicating a benign lesion. Size and shapes of lesions are not reliable indicators of malignancy, although lesions >4 cm in diameter are more likely to be malignant (12).

2. **A slowly resolving pneumonia, recurrent pneumonia** in the same lobe or segment, **segmental atelectasis or lobar collapse**, or **obstructive emphysema** of a lobe or lung may often be the presenting sign of an underlying **neoplasm**.

B. **CT scans of the chest** are extremely useful in discerning the presence of small nodules not visualized on chest x-rays (many of which are benign granulomas) and in determining invasion of the chest wall and mediastinum by the tumor. CT scans provide better resolution for delineating patterns of calcification in coin lesions; in some institutions, the density of the lesion as defined by Hounsfield units has been correlated to the malignant potential of the lesion (13).

V. **Staging.** The American Joint Committee on Cancer and the Union Internationale Contre le Cancer have devised an international staging system for lung cancer (14). The initial T and N stages can usually be determined by diagnostic evaluations with bronchoscopy and chest CT scan. Determination of the final M stage usually requires analysis of any pleural fluid, examination of pleural or lymph node tissue obtained by biopsy procedures, and/or findings at thoracotomy.

A. **The staging classifications for NSCLC** are listed below and described in in detail in Table 7-3. The staging classifications for SCLC will be detailed in a later section.

1. **T status** describes the size, location, and extent of the primary tumor: T1–T4.
2. **N status** delineates lymph node involvement: N0–N2.
3. **M status** represents distant metastases: M0, M1.

B. **Accurate and uniform staging** of lung cancer is essential for the following reasons:

Table 7-2. Radiographic patterns of lung cancer

Solitary lung nodule or "coin" lesion

Parenchymal lung mass

Multiple parenchymal nodules

Unilateral hilar mass

Atelectasis

Lobar collapse

Pleural effusion

Mediastinal mass

Apical or superior sulcus mass

Lobar consolidation

Bilateral alveolar infiltrate

Rib destruction

Elevation of a hemidiaphragm

Table 7-3. Staging for non–small cell lung carcinoma

Primary tumor (T)

TX   Primary tumor cannot be assessed, or tumor proven by presence of malignant cells in sputum or bronchial washings but not visualized by imaging or bronchoscopy

T0   No evidence of primary tumor

Tis   Carcinoma *in situ*

T1   Tumor 3 cm or less in greatest dimension, surrounded by lung or visceral pleura, without bronchoscopic evidence of invasion more proximal than the lobar bronchus* (ie, not in either main bronchus)

T2   Tumor with any of the following features of size or extent: more than 3 cm in greatest dimension; involves main bronchus, 2 cm or more distal to the carina; invades the visceral pleura; or associated with atelectasis or obstructive pneumonitis that extends to the hilar region but does not involve the entire lung

T3   Tumor of any size that directly invades any of the following: chest wall (including superior sulcus tumors), diaphragm, mediastinal pleura, parietal pericardium; or tumor in the main bronchus less than 2 cm distal to the carina* but without involvement of the carina; or associated atelectasis or obstructive pneumonitis of the entire lung

T4   Tumor of any size that directly invades any of the following: mediastinum, heart, great vessels, trachea, esophagus, vertebral body, carina, or tumor with a malignant pleural effusion**

Regional lymph nodes (N)

The regional lymph nodes are the intrathoracic, scalene, and supraclavicular nodes

NX   Regional lymph nodes cannot be assessed

N0   No regional lymph node metastasis

N1   Metastasis in ipsilateral peribronchial and/or ipsilateral hilar lymph nodes, including direct extension

N2   Metastasis in ipsilateral mediastinal and/or subcarinal lymph node(s)

N3   Metastasis in contralateral mediastinal, contralateral hilar, ipsilateral, or contralateral scalene or supraclavicular lymph node(s)

Distant metastases (M)

MX   Presence of distant metastasis cannot be assessed

M0   No distant metastasis

M1   Distant metastasis.

---

*The uncommon superficial tumor of any size that has its invasive component limited to the bronchial wall and may extend proximal to the main bronchus is also classified T1.

**Most pleural effusions associated with lung cancer are due to tumor. However, there are a few patients in whom multiple cytopathologic examinations of pleural fluid are negative for tumor. In these cases, fluid is nonbloody and is not an exudate. When these elements and clinical judgment dictate that the effusion is not related to the tumor, the effusion should be excluded as a staging element and the patient should be staged T1, T2, or T3.

    1. Appropriate treatment selection.
    2. Determination of candidacy for surgical resection.
    3. Assessment of the need for adjuvant or neoadjuvant therapy.
    4. Determination of prognosis.
    5. Comparison of outcomes of different treatment protocols based on stage of disease.
  C. **Upon completion** of the staging process, the patient will have a TNM classification that can then be utilized to assess **stage grouping**: Stage I, II, IIIA, IIIB, or IV (Table 7-4). The TNM and staging systems help assess prognosis, with each successive stage carrying a poorer prognosis.

Table 7-4. AJCC/UICC stage grouping

Occult carcinoma	TX	N0	M0
Stage 0	Tis	N0	M0
Stage I	T1	N0	M0
	T2	N0	M0
Stage II	T1	N1	M0
	T2	N1	M0
Stage IIIA	T1	N2	M0
	T2	N2	M0
	T3	N0	M0
	T3	N1	M0
	T3	N2	M0
Stage IIIB	Any T	N3	M0
	T4	Any N	M0
Stage IV	Any T	Any N	M1

AJCC =American Joint Committee on Cancer; UICC =Union Internationale Contre le Cancer.

VI. Evaluation and diagnosis. Evaluation and diagnosis of potential or suspected lung neoplasms require the determination of the cell type and stage. Since the stage of a lung neoplasm will often be determined in the process of obtaining the cell type, the methods of diagnosis and staging will be considered together.

   A. Screening for lung cancer in high-risk individuals by cytologic examination of serial samples of expectorated sputum (15) has not been found to be useful. Yearly chest x-rays may be justified in individuals with long smoking histories.

   B. Patients with normal chest x-rays require airway surveillance and closer examination of lung parenchyma by bronchoscopy and chest CT scanning when the following conditions are met:

      1. Hemoptysis in an individual over age 40 years with more than a 20-pack-year smoking history.

      2. Malignant cells found on sputum cytology.

   C. Specific diagnostic examinations

      1. Sputum cytology. Examination of three serial early-morning sputum specimens by an expert cytopathologist will often provide a diagnosis of malignancy. Central bronchogenic lesions are more likely to have a positive cytology on sputum analysis than are peripheral lesions, 80% versus 50%, respectively (16). A specific cell type can be diagnosed 85% to 95% of the time if malignant cells are seen in the samples (17).

      2. Flexible fiberoptic bronchoscopy

         a. Diagnosis. Bronchoscopy is a well tolerated technique that visualizes the tracheobronchial tree and permits brushings, washings, and biopsies from any suspicious lesions. Bronchoscopy done with fluoroscopic guidance permits biopsies of more peripheral lesions not directly visualized. The **diagnostic yield** of flexible bronchoscopy with biopsy of endobronchially visible carcinomas is >90% when the optimum number of 6–10 biopsies is obtained. In nonvisualized lesions, the combination of biopsy and brushings yields the diagnosis 60% of the time (18).

         b. Staging. The airways of all patients considered surgical candidates must be examined prior to resection. Bronchoscopy allows exclusion of contralateral endobronchial lesions (M status) and defines the proximal extent of the endobronchial lesion in relation to the main bronchi and trachea (T status). Transtracheal and transbronchial thin-needle aspirations can be used to help define involvement of paratracheal, precarinal, and subcarinal nodes (N status).

3. **Pleural fluid and tissue analysis.** A patient with suspected or documented lung cancer and a pleural effusion requires analysis of the fluid, and possibly a pleural biopsy as well, either to make the initial diagnosis or to define the stage by detecting the presence of malignant cells in the pleural space or pleural tissue.

   a. The **accuracy of cytology in the diagnosis** of malignant pleural effusion varies from 40% to 87% depending on the tumor cell type. Diagnostic accuracy can be maximized from 60% after examination of one pleural specimen to 80% after examination of three independently obtained pleural fluid specimens. Cytopathologic analysis of both cell blocks and smears should be performed (19,20). Pleural biopsy, indicated whenever the cytology of an exudative pleural effusion is nondiagnostic, will be positive for malignancy 39% to 75% of the time (21). In general, pleural fluid analysis provides the diagnosis of malignancy more often than pleural biopsy.

   b. **Staging.** Mandatory examination of the pleura and associated fluid is necessary because malignant effusions automatically stage the patient as having an unresectable T4 lesion. Not all effusions are secondary to pleural involvement with tumor. If repeated fluid and tissue analysis is nondiagnostic and the fluid is exudative, thoracoscopic examination of the pleural surface should be strongly considered prior to resection. The presence of a transudative, nonbloody effusion should not be considered in the determination of stage grouping if the cytopathologic examination is negative.

4. **Transthoracic needle aspiration (TTNA).** TTNA is usually done under CT or fluoroscopic guidance in order to directly visualize needle (18–22 gauge) placement and aspiration within the lesion. The most common complications are pneumothorax (25% to 35%) and minor hemoptysis (1% to 10%). Symptomatic pneumothorax requiring treatment occurs in 5% to 10% of procedures. Less common complications include major bleeding, air embolism, and malignant seeding of the needle tract. The lesions amenable to diagnosis by TTNA as recommended by the American Thoracic Society are summarized in Table 7-5 (22). The **diagnostic sensitivity** of TTNA in lung cancer is 85%. False-negative results are caused by sampling of necrotic tissue or inadequate sampling of the lesion. The false-positive rate of TTNA is 0.1% to 0.5% and is most commonly due to fibrosis or to an inflammatory process such as pneumonia, abscess, or active tuberculosis. TTNA is most useful for determining the cell type in patients who are not candidates for surgery or for staging purposes when either up or down staging would influence management. **TTNA is not indicated for patients who are surgical candidates for resection because the finding of malignant cells adds nothing to the management and TTNA is not a reliable test for diagnosing benign lesions.**

5. **Prethoracotomy assessment of the mediastinum**

   a. The use of **CT scans** in the evaluation of hilar or mediastinal lymphadenopathy is controversial. The sensitivity of CT scanning for nodes >1.0 cm ranges from 64% to 79%, with a specificity of 62% to 66% (23–25). Fifty percent of patients with resected N2 lung cancer may have negative chest CT scans preoperatively (26,27), with adenocarcinomas having the highest rate of false negatives (26). Extension of a chest CT scan to include examination of the liver, adrenals, kidneys, and upper abdominal lymph

Table 7-5. Indications for transthoracic needle aspiration by American Thoracic Society

1. Solitary lung nodules and masses
2. Mediastinal and hilar masses
3. Metastatic disease from extrathoracic malignancy
4. Chest wall invasion in lung carcinoma
5. Pulmonary infections in pulmonary nodules or areas of airspace consolidation

nodes is the most effective tool in delineating metastatic disease to these sites.

b. **Mediastinoscopy** and **anterior mediastinotomy** (Chamberlain procedure) are the most accurate methods for assessing the mediastinum and identifying patients with unresectable disease: contralateral node involvement, extranodal extension of cancer, high paratracheal involvement, or cell type (SCLC) not amenable to surgery. Many centers use CT scanning as a screening tool in the assessment of the mediastinum. Lymph nodes >1.0 cm in the short axis are considered abnormal and require sampling by mediastinoscopy. Patients **with an abnormal mediastinum on chest CT scan should undergo mediastinoscopy or anterior mediastinotomy to obtain tissue to document the presence of malignancy prior to definitive surgical resection.** Cervical mediastinoscopy permits direct imaging and sampling of paratracheal, tracheobronchial, and anterior subcarinal lymph nodes. Anterior mediastinotomy and extended cervical mediastinoscopy allow assessment of the aortopulmonary window and anterior mediastinal nodes. Mediastinoscopy will exclude 30% to 40% of patients initially thought to be surgically resectable from thoracotomy. Indications for mediastinoscopy are summarized in Table 7-6.

6. **Lymph node biopsy.** Patients with palpable cervical or scalene lymph nodes in the setting of suspected lung cancer should be considered for surgical excision of those nodes for histologic evaluation of tissue. This procedure is safe, and evidence of metastasis will usually preclude thoracotomy. In patients with documented lung cancer and palpable scalene nodes, biopsy has been positive in 83% of cases; only 20% of nonpalpable nodes were positive for malignancy after biopsy (28).

7. **Thoracotomy.** Surgical exploration of the chest determines the final T and N status of the cancer and permits decision making regarding the surgical procedure required. Most centers proceed to thoracotomy in any patient with a normal mediastinum on CT scan and sample the mediastinum intraoperatively as long as no other distant site of disease has been detected. All lymph node stations not sampled during mediastinoscopy are assessed at thoracotomy regardless of appearance on CT scan. Samples of nodes from the superior mediastinum, subcarinal, subaortic, peribronchial, and intrapulmonary nodes adjacent to the planned site of bronchial resection are submitted for evaluation. N status often can only be determined at this time.

D. Lung cancer has a propensity to **metastasize** to distant sites, especially bone, brain, liver, adrenals, contralateral lung, extrathoracic lymph nodes, and kidneys. Routine screening for metastases utilizing bone, brain, and liver scans is neither cost effective nor accurate because of the low incidence of true positives and high incidence of false positives (29). The history, physical examination, and biochemical profile of the patient will determine the need for extensive scanning to rule out distant disease. Further diagnostic procedures such as biopsy of adrenal, renal, hepatic, central nervous system, and bone lesions are often required after obtaining the scans looking for distant metastases. It should be remembered that while some radiologic patterns are pathognomonic for metastatic disease, other abnormalities, such as adrenal masses, need to be confirmed by examining tissue samples because of the high incidence of benign adrenal adenomas. Indications for obtaining nuclear

Table 7-6. Indications for mediastinoscopy

1. Presence of enlarged lymph nodes on chest CT scan (>1.5 cm)
2. Primary lung lesion is T2 or T3
3. Cell type is adenocarcinoma or large cell histology
4. Small cell cytology and potentially resectable lesion
5. Left upper lobe lesion with vocal cord paralysis

bone scan, head magnetic resonance (MR) imaging, or contrast-enhanced thoracic CT **and** abdominal CT scans include the following:

1. **Signs and symptoms** suggesting metastatic disease at any site.
   a. **Neurologic complaints:** headache, visual changes, motor or sensory deficits, seizures, confusion.
   b. **Bone pain:** long bones, vertebrae, ribs.
   c. **Abdominal pain:** liver, adrenals, kidneys.
   d. **Abnormal routine laboratory tests,** even if the patient is asymptomatic.
      i. Elevation of serum **calcium.**
      ii. Elevation of serum **alkaline phosphatase.**
      iii. Elevation of **liver function tests.**
2. Histologic diagnosis of **SCLC,** which has a high propensity for early distant metastasis.
3. **Previous history** of cancer.
4. **Likely candidate for surgical resection** of tumor.

VII. **Differential diagnosis.** The differential diagnosis of the signs and symptoms, as well as the radiologic patterns described, includes malignant, metastatic, and benign lesions (Table 7-7) and other etiologies that are discussed elsewhere.

VIII. **Complications of lung cancer**

A. **Malignant pleural effusions** are always exudative and usually bloody. Cytologic examination of the fluid reveals malignant cells 70% to 80% of the time. The presence of a malignant effusion is a poor prognostic sign, with a mean survival of only 3–6 months and a negligible 5-year survival.

1. **Pathogenesis**
   a. **Obstruction of lymphatic channels** by tumor occlusion of stomata of parietal pleura.
   b. **Mediastinal lymph node invasion** by tumor resulting in lymphatic backup.
   c. **Direct involvement** of the pleura by malignancy.
2. **Presentation**
   a. Patients may be completely **asymptomatic,** with the effusion found incidentally on physical examination or radiographic study.
   b. Commonly, patients will complain of increasing dyspnea, initially only with exertion but then at rest.
3. **Management**
   a. If the patient is **asymptomatic, treatment may be deferred** until symptoms develop.
   b. The effusion may be **removed by thoracentesis** and monitored for recurrence. In cases of SCLC, removing the effusion and then instituting chemotherapy will result in definitive management of the effusion.
   c. NSCLC is less likely to respond to chemotherapy, and further interventions are required to manage the effusion.
      i. Placement of a **chest tube** to allow complete drainage of the effusion, followed by instillation of a sclerosing agent such as bleomycin or doxycycline to permit pleurodesis.
      ii. **Thoracoscopy** with talc poudrage will also provide effective pleurodesis.
   d. **Experimental** management techniques
      i. Intracavitary chemotherapy.
      ii. Pleuroperitoneal shunting of refractory pleural fluid.
      iii. Intrapleural *C. parvum.*

B. **Superior vena cava (SVC) syndrome.** Eighty percent of cases of SVC syndrome are secondary to lung cancer, with SCLC being the most common cell type involved. The median survival is 46 weeks following the diagnosis of SVC syndrome caused by SCLC.

1. **Presentation.** Acute or subacute onset of facial fullness, flushing, headache, dyspnea, cough, and edema of the upper extremities are the most common presenting signs and symptoms. Symptoms may worsen while leaning forward.

Table 7-7. Differential diagnosis of malignant and benign pulmonary neoplasms

Malignant
Bronchogenic carcinoma
Squamous cell carcinoma
Small cell carcinoma
Adenocarcinoma
Large cell carcinoma
Mixed adenosquamous cell carcinoma
Bronchoalveolar cell carcinoma
Bronchial adenomas (low-grade malignant potential)
    Carcinoid
    Bronchial gland
    Papillary
Lymphoma
    Hodgkin's
    Non-Hodgkin's
Sarcoma (primary)
Malignant teratoma
Mixed carcinosarcoma
Mesothelioma
Melanoma
Metastatic from distant site
    Solitary
    Multiple
Multiple myeloma
Plasmacytoma
Pulmonary blastoma

Benign
Bronchial adenoma
Benign mesothelioma
Granular cell myoblastoma
Hamartoma
Hemangioma
Papilloma
Leiomyoma
Fibroma
Lipoma
Chondroma
Pericytoma
Neurogenic tumor
Plasma cell granuloma
Pseudolymphoma
Teratoma

     2. Physical examination reveals a prominent venous pattern of the face and upper trunk, papilledema, and facial plethora.

     3. Pathogenesis. The SVC syndrome results from extrinsic compression of the thin-walled superior vena cava by the primary tumor or associated adenopathy within the mediastinum. Secondary intraluminal thrombosis is often present.

     4. Management. Although SVC syndrome is considered an oncologic emergency, a tissue diagnosis should be made prior to radiotherapy or chemotherapy. The signs and symptoms of the SVC syndrome usually respond to initial therapy.

  C. Bronchial obstruction by malignant tumors will often lead to pneumonitis, atelectasis, total lung collapse, or emphysematous hyperinflation. If surgical resection is not possible, tumor size may be reduced by radiotherapy or chemotherapy.

     1. Other palliative techniques to relieve endobronchial obstruction refractory to standard measures include (30):

        a. Neodymium:yttrium-aluminum-garnet (Nd:YAG) laser delivers radiation in the neon infrared region and provides both thermal necrosis of the lesion and photocoagulation to control bleeding.

           i. Indications for use of the Nd:YAG laser include airway obstruction unresponsive to other treatment, protrusion of the lesion into the bronchial lumen, tumor extent <4 cm, and the presence of viable and functional lung distal to the obstruction.

           ii. Complications of Nd:YAG laser include development of bronchopleural fistula and hemorrhage from tumor necrosis or from perforation of a large blood vessel.

        b. Endobronchial prosthetic devices. Bronchial obstruction may be secondary to extrinsic compression by tumor or lymph nodes rather than an intraluminal process. If the patient is not a candidate for surgery or radiotherapy, a bronchial stent may be placed to relieve the obstruction.

           i. Placement of an intraluminal stent made of either metal or silicone may relieve symptoms of obstruction.

           ii. Complications of intraluminal stents include migration of the stent or continued tumor growth and development of granulation tissue with occlusion of the airway, particularly when metal stents are used.

  D. Brain metastases are the site of recurrence in one-third of patients with NSCLC, with the majority of cases due to adenocarcinoma. The median survival in patients with symptomatic brain metastases is 1 month. A solitary brain metastasis has a better prognosis if the primary tumor and the brain metastasis can both be completely resected. Surgical resection of both lesions, followed by radiotherapy to the brain, can prolong median survival to 9.2 months compared with 3.4 months for palliation alone (31).

IX. Treatment of non–small cell lung carcinoma. The overall 5-year survival for patients with NSCLC is a dismal 14% (32). Pulmonary resection is the best available treatment and provides the only potential cure. Radiation alone has a <5% to 10% cure rate but is a reasonable alternative therapy for inoperable patients. Chemotherapy alone has shown poor results in curing NSCLC. Survival statistics based on stage are outlined in Table 7-8. Management options include the following:

     1. Surgical resection for cure.

     2. Chemotherapy to alleviate symptoms.

     3. Radiotherapy to relieve pain related to bony metastases or neurologic symptoms related to brain metastases.

     4. No treatment if asymptomatic.

     5. Experimental protocols.

  A. Stage I. Complete surgical resection is the treatment of choice for operable lesions and is associated with a 5-year survival rate of 75% in T1 disease. In general, tumors involving a main bronchus or a lobar orifice within 2 cm of the proximal orifice require a complete pneumonectomy for optimal control. **Adjuvant chemother-**

Table 7-8. Postoperative 5-year survival in non–small cell lung carcinoma

TNM subset	Stage (International 1986)	5-Year survival (%)	
		Mountain (14)	Naruke (14a)
T1 N0 M0	I	68.5	76.4
T2 N0 M0		59.0	56.9
T1 N1 M0	II	54.1	43.6
T2 N1 M0		40.0	37.6
T3 N0 M0	IIIa	17.6	33.7
Any T N2 M0		28.8	13.7
Any T N3 M0			0.0
T4 Any N M0	IIIb	3.9	8.4
Malignant effusion			
Any T, Any N M1	IV	1.3	6.8

apy has no role in the treatment of stage I lesions. Clinical trials have failed to show any added benefit in survival rates with postoperative chemotherapy (33).

B. **Stage II.** The treatment of choice is **surgical resection followed by adjuvant radiotherapy.** By definition, stage II cancer has hilar or peribronchial nodal involvement with tumor cells (N1). **Adjuvant radiotherapy is utilized** to sterilize remaining nodal disease and potentially decrease the local recurrence of the tumor within the chest, but it does not improve overall survival (34).

C. **Stage IIIA**
1. **Standard surgery and radiotherapy.** Although this stage is considered advanced disease, the median survival of potentially resectable patients with T3N0 or T3N1 tumors is 12 months, with a 5-year survival rate of 15%. The median survival of inoperable stage IIIA disease treated with standard radiotherapy is 10 months, with a 5-year survival rate of 5%. The overall survival of stage III patients remains quite poor.
2. **Surgery and neoadjuvant chemoradiotherapy.** Because of the poor survival outcomes of this stage, investigative clinical trials have been conducted using **neoadjuvant chemoradiotherapy** to downstage the primary tumor and convert patients into more favorable surgical candidates. Initial protocols with this approach have increased the percentage of disease-free patients, but the median survival is only slightly improved and the toxicity of treatment is extremely high (35). The criteria for enrolling stage III patients into an experimental clinical protocol include:
   a. Good surgical candidate (T3N0 or T3N1 status).
   b. Good performance status based on ability to participate in activities of daily living, ability to work, and care for oneself.
   c. Ability to tolerate chemoradiotherapy.
3. **Palliative therapy.** Since asymptomatic patients have no improvement in survival with radiotherapy, this treatment should be **used for the relief of symptoms** related to the disease. If the patient is not a surgical candidate, has a poor performance status, or is unwilling to be placed on a protocol, radiotherapy can be utilized to improve symptoms (bone pain, hemoptysis, neurologic deficits) related to the tumor. If the patient is asymptomatic, therapy should be withheld until the development of symptomatic disease.

D. **Stage IIIB.** Patients with stage IIIB disease are **categorically unresectable.** The median survival is 8 months, with a 5-year survival rate of <5%. Radiotherapy alone is ineffective. Treatment combining cisplatin-based chemotherapy with radiotherapy may increase survival by 3 months.

E.   **Stage IV.** With the exception of solitary brain nodules, patients with metastases to the brain, liver and adrenal glands, skin, bones, kidneys, or lung have **tumors that are unresectable**. The 5-year survival of stage IV disease is negligible. **Cisplatin-based chemotherapy may help improve symptoms** related to metastatic disease. Responders to chemotherapy may survive 2–4 months.

F.   **Pancoast tumors** arise in the **superior sulcus of the lung** and often extend to involve the lower roots of the brachial plexus, intercostal nerves, sympathetic chain, stellate ganglion, and adjacent ribs and vertebrae (36). Squamous cell neoplasms account for half of Pancoast tumors, with the remaining half equally distributed between adenocarcinoma and large cell cancers. These tumors deserve special consideration because of their **response to radiation and their improved survival** when compared to other NSCLC lesions of similar stage.

1.   **Signs and symptoms.** Pulmonary symptoms are seldom present. **Pain** is the most common presenting symptom (90%) and is localized to the shoulder or the ulnar distribution of the hand and arm. **Muscle-wasting** of the hand and associated **Horner's syndrome** (ptosis, miosis, and hemifacial anhidrosis) are present in 62% of cases and are caused by extension of the tumor through the chest wall.

2.   **Diagnosis and staging.** The characteristic NSCLC cell types, radiologic appearance, and symptom complex are often sufficient to eliminate the need for a specific tissue diagnosis prior to the initiation of therapy. Many centers will begin radiation in the absence of a tissue diagnosis. If histologic diagnosis is required, **TTNA** usually produces the greatest yield. **Bronchoscopy** should be performed prior to surgery in all cases in order to rule out extension of the tumor to the mainstem bronchus or contralateral airway. Staging is best determined by CT scan to define the extent of bony and mediastinal involvement. MR imaging is particularly useful in visualizing tumor involvement of the brachial plexus and vertebrae.

3.   **Treatment and survival.** T3N0–2 Pancoast tumors **may be resectable**, although N2 disease has a negligible survival at 2 years. Since true Pancoast lesions extend through the visceral and parietal pleura to the chest wall, surgical treatment involves resection of the lung, the lower trunk of the brachial plexus, and en-bloc resection of the chest wall. **Preoperative radiotherapy** of 3000–5000 Gy is given to the tumor 2–4 weeks prior to the en-bloc resection to decrease the size of the primary tumor, as well as sterilize any tumor located in proximate lymphatics. The survival of patients with T3N0M0 Pancoast lesions treated with surgery and chemotherapy is 34% at 5 years and 29% at 10 years. Pancoast tumors are not resectable if the tumor extensively involves the brachial plexus, extends to nodes outside the mediastinum, or invades the vertebrae, transverse processes, or subclavian artery. Single modality radiation for unresectable lesions offers palliation and is associated with long-term survival rates of 6% at 5 years. Cord compression is a feared complication and portends a poor prognosis.

G.   **Poor prognostic factors for relapse**
1.   Pretreatment **weight loss.**
2.   **Advanced** disease **stage.**
3.   Identified **vascular invasion.**
4.   **Oncogenic abnormalities**, particularly K-*ras* point mutations.

X.   **Preoperative assessment of patients undergoing pulmonary resection.** All patients with surgically resectable lung cancer require assessment of the ability to tolerate thoracotomy and removal of lung parenchyma.

A.   A complete **history and physical examination** are essential to assess comorbid medical conditions that increase the risk of major surgery, such as coronary artery disease, hypertension, diabetes, cerebrovascular disease, or underlying lung disease. Age alone is not a contraindication for thoracotomy.

B.   **Spirometry** alone has not been clearly established as a definitive test for identifying patients at high risk for mortality or perioperative complications (37). However, a preoperative forced expiratory volume in 1 second (FEV_1) of <800 mL renders patients inoperative. Prediction of a postoperative FEV_1 of <800 mL is sufficient to allow a wedge resection, but patients may be dyspneic at rest after surgery (38). Sex and height are important considerations for predicting postoperative FEV_1, since an FEV_1 of <800 mL may be perfectly adequate in a small female patient.

C. **Arterial blood gases.** Anecdotal reports suggest that preoperatve **hypoxemia** with Pao_2 <50 and **hypercarbia** with $Paco_2$ >45 are associated with an **increased risk of morbidity and mortality**.

D. **Perfusion scanning** prior to surgery is indicated for patients with severe obstructive pulmonary disease to help **predict the postoperative lung function** (39). The percentage of perfusion distributed to the remaining lobes multiplied by the preoperative FEV_1 is a good predictor of postoperative FEV_1.

E. **Pulmonary exercise testing.** Patients with a maximum oxygen consumption ($\dot{V}o_2$) of **<10 mL/kg/min are at increased risk** for postoperative morbidity and mortality. Exercise testing may be useful in assessing risk for thoracotomy when other studies have been inconclusive (40,41).

F. **Preoperative interventions** that optimize pulmonary status prior to thoracotomy should be performed in all patients.
   1. **Smoking cessation** for at least 2 weeks prior to surgery.
   2. Aggressive **pulmonary toilet** with bronchodilator therapy and antibiotics to reduce sputum production.
   3. **Education** regarding the use of incentive spirometry, deep-breathing exercises, and coughing techniques.
   4. Participation in a **pulmonary rehabilitation** program to improve baseline level of function prior to surgery.
   5. Scheduling of patients with chronic sputum production as **late-morning or afternoon cases** to allow for sputum clearance.

XI. **Small cell lung carcinoma.** SCLC represents 20% of all cases of lung cancer (42) and has the strongest association with cigarette smoking. A neuroendocrine stem-cell origin is suggested by the presence of neurosecretory granules in the cytoplasm, along with expression of neuromembrane antigens on the cell surface (43). SCLC is the cell type most commonly associated with the Eaton-Lambert syndrome and ectopic production of antidiuretic hormone and ACTH. The disease is almost always metastatic at the time of diagnosis; only 10% of patients present without apparent metastases at the time of diagnosis.

A. **Signs and symptoms.** The thoracic signs and symptoms are similar to those in NSCLC. Patients with SCLC are more likely than those with NSCLC to **present with symptoms and signs related to metastatic disease** to the brain, liver, bone marrow, and adrenals or related to complications associated with a paraneoplastic syndrome.

B. **Chest radiograph** usually reveals a **central lung mass with bulky hilar and mediastinal adenopathy**. On occasion, SCLC will present as a solitary pulmonary nodule that is asymptomatic.

C. **Evaluation.** Once a diagnosis of SCLC has been made, a careful staging evaluation must be completed to look for metastatic disease.
   1. **CT scan** of chest, liver, and adrenals.
   2. **Mediastinoscopy** to stage mediastinal involvement.
   3. **Head CT scan** with contrast or MR imaging to look for occult brain metastases.
   4. **Bone scan** to assess for bony metastases.
   5. Bilateral **bone marrow aspirates and biopsies** if the patient has an abnormal hematologic panel.

D. **Staging.** Of the two staging systems applied in SCLC, the **Veterans Administration staging system** (limited and extensive disease) has more utility than the TNM staging system (44).
   1. **Limited stage.** The tumor is restricted to one hemithorax and mediastinum with or without supraclavicular lymph node involvement.
   2. **Extensive disease.** The tumor has spread beyond the limits defined by limited stage. All distant metastatic involvement is deemed extensive disease. At the time of diagnosis, 50% to 66% of patients have extensive disease.

E. **Treatment.** The major difficulties in treating SCLC are the presence of distant metastases at presentation and the rapid acquisition of resistance to chemotherapeutic agents. **Chemotherapy is intrinsic to all treatment protocols** for SCLC, as it provides systemic coverage for distant metastatic foci.

1. **Limited stage.** SCLC patients with a solitary pulmonary nodule may benefit from surgical resection and chemotherapy. Limited-stage disease is associated with 5-year survival rates of 25% to 35% (45). For other limited-stage patients, combination **chemotherapy** with cisplatin, etoposide, cyclophosphamide, doxorubicin, and vinca alkaloids is used. Response rates are 80% to 90%, with 40% to 60% of patients having a complete response. Median survival is 12–18 months, with a 2-year survival rate of 20% (42).

   a. Combined modality with the use of concurrent radiotherapy and chemotherapy has been attempted in randomized trials. The addition of radiotherapy appears to improve local control and may increase median survival (46).

   b. Maintenance chemotherapy does not prolong survival and is not a part of most treatment protocols.

2. **Extensive stage. Combination chemotherapy** is the treatment of choice. Response rates to chemotherapy are 60% to 80%, with 20% to 40% having a complete clinical remission. The 2-year survival rate is 10% to 20% (42).

3. **Prophylactic cranial irradiation (PCI).** Chemotherapy does not appear to decrease the rate of brain metastases in SCLC. This may be related to the poor penetration of the chemotherapeutic agents through the blood–brain barrier. PCI has been shown to **decrease the rate of central nervous system relapse**; however, it has not shown to increase survival (47).

   a. **Toxicity** may be exacerbated by concurrent chemotherapy and includes memory disturbances, gait abnormalities, urinary incontinence, and dementia.

   b. **Indications.** PCI should be reserved for patients with limited disease who have had a complete response to chemotherapy. PCI should be used in patients with extensive disease only for palliation of symptoms.

4. **Investigational** treatment options

   a. **Autologous bone marrow transplantation** increases disease-free survival.

   b. **Immunotoxin therapy** with monoclonal antibodies linked to potent toxins that recognize cancer cell surface antigens results in cell destruction.

F. **Prognostic factors** in SCLC (48)

   1. **Performance** status.
   2. Disease **stage.**
   3. **Sex:** women have a better response and survival than men.
   4. **Age:** older ages tend to have a worse prognosis.
   5. Presence of **supraclavicular nodes** worsens prognosis in patients with limited disease.

XII. **Future directions in lung cancer treatment**

A. **Neoadjuvant chemotherapy** and chemoradiotherapy trials are underway with the goals of controlling local recurrence and eliminating distant metastases.

B. **Protocols** using alternative methods of radiotherapy to maximize tumor killing and minimize toxicity are in progress. Techniques being assessed include hyperfractionation of radiation and continuous hyperfractionated accelerated radiotherapy.

C. **In immunotoxin therapy** with monoclonal antibodies delivering cytotoxic agents to tumor cells, a monoclonal antibody, designed to recognize a surface antigen on the lung cancer cells, is linked to a cytotoxin. Tumor binding is followed by internalization of the toxin and cell death. Studies using a toxic monoclonal antibody, N901-blocked ricin, have shown improved response rates in relapsed SCLC (49).

D. The utilization of **newer chemotherapeutic agents** including navelbine, CPT-11, taxol, and edatrexate. Colony-stimulating factors are being used to improve hematologic status, allowing for a reduction in the intervals between chemotherapy cycles.

E. **Chemoprevention** is the systemic use of natural or synthetic chemicals to reverse or suppress the progression of a premalignant lesion to avoid the development of invasive cancer. Agents being tested include the retinoids, which are thought to control differentiation through effects on peptide growth factor and oncogene expression (50).

References

1. Boring CC, Squires TS, Tong T, Montgomery S: Cancer statistics. *CA Cancer J Clin* 1994;44:7–26.
2. Boring CC, Squires TS, Health CW Jr: Cancer statistics. *CA Cancer J Clin* 1992;42:19–38.
3. Boring CC, Squires TS, Tong T: Cancer statistics. *CA Cancer J Clin* 1993;43:7–26.
4. U.S. Surgeon General: *Smoking and health.* Washington, DC: U.S. Department of Health, Education, and Welfare, 1964; publication 1103.
5. Doll R, Peto R: Cigarette smoking and bronchial carcinoma: dose and time relationships among regular smokers and lifelong nonsmokers. *J Epidemiol Community Health* 1978;32:303–313.
6. Department of Health and Human Services, Centers for Disease Control: *Health consequences of involuntary smoking: a report of the* Surgeon General. Washington, DC: U.S. Government Printing Olfice, 1986; publication CDC 87-8398.
7. Slebos R, Kibbelaar R, Dalesio O, et al.: K-ras oncogene activation as a prognostic marker in adenocarcinoma of the lung. *N Engl J Med* 1990:323;561–565.
8. Tokuhata GK: Familial factors in human lung cancer and smoking. *Am J Public Health* 1964; 54:24–32.
9. Ooi WL, et al.: Increased familial risk for lung cancer. *J Natl Cancer Inst* 1986;76:217–222.
10. Mettlin G, et al.: Vitamin A and lung Cancer. *J Natl Cancer Inst* 1979;62:1435–1438.
11. Kvale G, Bjelke E, Gart JJ: Dietary habits and lung cancer risk. *Int J Cancer* 1983;31:397–405.
12. Cummings SR, Lillington GA, Richard RJ: Estimating the probability of malignancy in solitary pulmonary nodules. *Am Rev Respir Dis* 1986;134:449.
13. Siegelman SS, Zerhouni EA, Leo FP, et al.: CT of the solitary pulmonary nodule. *AJR* 1980; 135:1–13.
14. Mountain CF: A new international staging system for lung cancer. *Chest* 1986;89:225s–33s.
14a. Naruke T. Prognosis and survival based on the new staging system. *J Thorac Cardiovasc Surg* 1988;96:440.
15. Strauss GM, Gleason RE, Sugarbaker DJ: Screening for lung cancer re-examined: a reinterpretation of the Mayo lung project randomized trial on lung cancer screening. *Chest* 1993;103: 337s–341s.
16. Carr DT, Cortese DA: The value of cytologic examination in the management of lung cancer. *Curr Probl Cancer* 1980;5:20–34.
17. Hess FG, et al.: Pulmonary cytology: current status of cytologic typing of respiratory tract tumors. *Am J Pathol* 1981;103:323–333.
18. Popovich J Jr, Kvale PA, Eichenhorn MS, et al.: Diagnostic accuracy of multiple biopsies from flexible bronchoscopy: a comparison of central versus peripheral carcinoma. *Am Rev Respir Dis* 1982;125:521–523.
19. Light R: *Pleural diseases,* 2nd ed. Philadelphia: Lea and Febiger, 1990.
20. Light RW, et al.: Cells in pleural fluid: their value in differential diagnosis. *Arch Intern Med* 1973;132:854–860.
21. Von Hoff DD, Livolsi V: Diagnostic reliability of needle biopsy of the parietal pleura. *Am J Clin Pathol* 1975;64:200–203.
22. Sanders C: Transthoracic needle aspiration. *Clin Chest Med* 1992;13:11–16.
23. Libshitz HI, McKenna RJ jr, Haynie TP, McMutrey MJ, Mountain CT: Mediastinal evaluation in lung cancer. *Radiology* 1984;151:295–299.
24. Staples CA, Muller NL, Miller RR, Evans KG, Nelems B: Mediastinal nodes in bronchogenic carcinoma: comparison between CT and mediastinoscopy. *Radiology* 1988;167:367–372.
25. McCloud TC, et al.: Bronchogenic carcinoma: analysis of staging in the mediastinum with CT by correlative lymph node mapping and sampling. *Radiology* 1992;182:319–322.
26. Cybulsky IJ, Lanza LA, Ryan MB, et al.: Prognostic significance of computed tomography in resected N2 lung cancer. *Ann Thorac Surg* 1992;54:533–537.
27. Shields TW: The use of mediastinoscopy in lung cancer: the dilemma of mediastinal lymph nodes. In: Kittle CF, ed. *Current controversies in thoracic surgery.* Philadelphia: WB Saunders, 1986: 145–161.

28. Brantigan JW, Brantigan CO, Brantigan OC: Biopsy of nonpalpable scalene lymph nodes in carcinoma of the lung. *Am Rev Respir Dis* 1973;107:962–974.
29. Ramsdell JW, Peters RM, Taylor AT Jr, Alazraki NP, Tisi GM: Multiorgan scans for staging lung cancer: correlation with clinical evaluation. *J Thorac Cardiovasc Surg* 1977;73:653–659.
30. Edell ES, Cortese DA, McDougall JC: Ancillary therapies in the management of lung cancer: photodynamic therapy, laser therapy, and endobronchial prosthetic devices. *Mayo Clin Proc* 1993; 68:685–690.
31. Patchell RA, Tibbs PA, Walsh JW: A randomized trial of surgery in the treatment of single metastases to the brain. *N Engl J Med* 1990;322:494–500.
32. Humphrey EW, Smart CR, Winchester DP: National survey of the pattern of care for carcinoma of the lung. *J Thorac Cardiovasc Surg* 1990;100:837–843.
33. Feld R, Rubinstein l, Thomas PA: Adjuvant chemotherapy with cyclophosphamide, doxorubicin, and cisplatin in patients with completely resected stage I non-small cell lung cancer. *J Natl Cancer Inst* 1993;85:299–306.
34. Weisenberger TH, Gail MH: Effects of postoperative mediastinal radiation on completely resected stage II and III epidermoid cancer of the lung. *N Engl J Med* 1986;315:1377–1381.
35. Strauss GM, Herndon JE, Sherman DD: Neoadjuvant chemotherapy and radiotherapy followed by surgery in stage IIIa non-small cell carcinoma of the lung: report of a cancer and leukemia group b phase II study. *J Clin Oncol* 1992;10:1237–1244.
36. Pancoast HK: Superior pulmonary sulcus tumor: tumor characterized by pain, Horner's syndrome, destruction of bone and atrophy of hand muscles. *JAMA* 1932;99:1391.
37. Zibrak JD, O'Donnell CR, Marton K: Indications for pulmonary function testing. *Ann Intern Med* 1990;112:763–771.
38. Gaensler EA et al: The role of pulmonary insufficiency in mortality and invalidism following surgery for pulmonary tuberculosis. *J Thorac Surg* 1955;29:163–187.
39. Corris PA, Odom NJ, Jackson NJ, McGregor CG: Use of radionuclide scanning in the preoperative estimation of pulmonary function after pneumonectomy. *Thorax* 1987;42:285–291.
40. Bechard D, Weinstein L: Assessment of exercise oxygen consumption as preoperative criteria for lung resection. *Ann Thorac Surg* 1987;44:344–349.
41. Smith TP, Kinasewitz GT, Tucker WY, Spillers WP, George RB: Exercise capacity as a predictor of post-thoracotomy morbidity. *Am Rev Respir Dis* 1984;129:730–734.
42. Inde DC: Current status of therapy for small cell carcinoma of the lung. *Cancer* 1984;54;2722–2728.
43. Sheppard MN: Neuroendocrine differentiation in lung tumors. *Thorax* 1991;46:843–850.
44. Hyde L, et al.: Cell type and the natural history of lung cancer. *JAMA* 1965;193:52–57.
45. Prasad US, Naylor AR, Walker WS, et al.: Long-term survival after pulmonary resection for small cell carcinoma of the lung. *Thorax* 1989;44:784–787.
46. Turrisi AJ: Incorporation of radiotherapy fractionation in the combined-modality treatment of limited small-cell lung cancer. *Chest* 1993;103:418s–422s.
47. Abner A: Prophylactic cranial irradiation in the treatment of small-cell carcinoma of the lung. *Chest* 1993;103:445s–448s.
48. Spiegelman D, Maurer LH, Ware JH, et al.: Prognostic factors in small-cell carcinoma of the lung; an analysis of 1521 patients. *J Clin Oncol* 1989;7:344–354.
49. Lynch TJ: Immunotoxin therapy of relapsed small-cell lung cancer. *Chest* 1993;103:436s–439s.
50. Shepherd FA: Future directions in the treatment of non-small cell lung cancer. *Semin Oncol* 1994;21(3)4:48–62.

8 Tuberculosis

Bernadette R. Gochuico and
John Bernardo

I. Overview

A. Tuberculosis (TB) is an infectious disease caused by the pathogenic organism, *Mycobacterium tuberculosis*. This organism infects an estimated one-third of the world's population, and today TB remains the leading cause of death from infectious disease in the world. In the United States, the introduction of antituberculosis medications in the 1940s and 1950s, combined with extended public health efforts to combat the disease, resulted in a decline in the incidence of TB. Unfortunately, the 1980s witnessed a recrudescence of the disease in this country. Several factors have been cited, including a waning interest in and familiarity with TB by public health officials and health care practitioners, a consequent lack of recognition of the medical and public health issues related to the diagnosis and treatment of TB, and an increasing incidence of disease in vulnerable populations, especially among foreign-born persons and people with human immunodeficiency virus (HIV) infection.

B. Recent declines in disease incidence in the United States in the 1990s have come at considerable expense and yet leave many unresolved issues for public health programs regarding the human and fiscal costs of disease management and control. Timely diagnosis and proper treatment of tuberculous disease, as well as preventive treatment of tuberculous infection in high-risk populations, remain the cornerstones of TB control that must be supported in the future if TB is to be eliminated as a threat to the public health.

II. Pathogenesis and epidemiology (1,2)

A. *M. tuberculosis* is transmitted via infected droplet nuclei (generally, particles 1–5 μm in diameter).

    1. An infectious source with pulmonary TB commonly aerosolizes these organisms by coughing, although other methods of transmission have been described.

    2. Infection occurs by inhalation of the droplets, which impact the epithelium of the lower respiratory tract and induce an inflammatory response. This response often goes unrecognized clinically, and asymptomatic lymphohematogenous spread from the primary focus follows, because organisms survive within alveolar macrophages that are cleared from the lung.

    3. In immunocompetent persons, a host response usually develops and successfully contains the infection within granulomas (collections of lymphocytes and monocytes) in the lung and in remote sites accessed by the lymphohematogenous spread of the ingested organisms, such as the adrenal glands, the kidneys, the central nervous system, or lymph nodes.

        a. Organisms remain viable but minimally active metabolically within granulomas.

        b. These organsims constitute a potential source of reactivation TB.

B. **Primary TB** is a disease that actively progresses following the initial tuberculous infection and occurs in a minority of normal hosts (<5%) and in HIV-infected persons. Primary TB is most commonly seen in young children (especially younger than 4 years), as well as in immunocompromised persons.

   C. Most persons infected with *M. tuberculosis* never develop disease, but a few will develop **reactivation TB** after a variable period of containment.

     1. Reactivation TB (also called adult-type TB) results from breakdown of host defenses at sites of previous containment (ie, infected granulomas) and proliferation of organisms at these locations.

     2. Reactivation TB most commonly occurs within the lungs (75% to 85% of cases in nonimmunocompromised persons), usually in the apical and/or posterior segments of the upper lobes or the superior segments of the lower lobes. In a minority of cases, reactivation occurs at any site where granulomas had formed following the initial infection, such as the kidneys, adrenal glands, lymph nodes, or within the central nervous system.

     3. The risk of non-HIV-infected adults developing TB is greatest in the 2 years following infection (roughly 2% to 4% per year for the first 2 years); overall, approximately 10% of persons with tuberculous infection will develop active disease during their lifetimes.

       a. As noted previously, HIV-infected persons have a greater chance of developing active primary TB following the initial infection than noncompromised persons.

       b. In addition, the HIV-infected who also are infected with *M. tuberculosis* **have up to 7% to 10%** *annual* **risk of developing active TB. In this latter group, reactivation occurs with increased frequency (up to 50%) at** *extrapulmonary* **sites.**

III. Risk factors and screening for tuberculosis (3,4)

   A. Identification of TB-infected persons and provision of preventive services where indicated are necessary in order to eliminate the infected reservoir that will become the future cases of TB (see below). However, "routine" screening of low-risk persons (eg, school children) is generally not effective in this regard, and screening programs should be targeted at certain high-risk groups (Table 8-1). Screening of additional selected populations or groups also may be warranted, based on epidemiologic data within specific communities provided by ongoing TB surveillance activities by health departments.

Table 8-1. Risk factors for tuberculosis (TB)

Close contacts of known TB cases (especially if the index case has identifiable organisms on
    smears)

Persons infected with HIV

Persons born in countries with high TB prevalence
    Represent 35% of cases in the U.S. in 1995 reported to the CDC
    Majority of cases present within 5 years of entry into the U.S.

Persons whose chest radiographs suggest old TB (if previously untreated)

Homeless persons

Prison inmates

Nursing home residents

Health care workers

Substance abusers (alcoholics and intravenous drug users)

Various medical conditions:
    Silicosis
    Postgastrectomy
    Post–jejunoileal bypass
    Diabetes mellitus
    Hemodialysis (especially extrapulmonary disease)
    Post–organ transplantation (especially extrapulmonary disease)
    Selected malignancies
    Weight less than 90% of ideal body weight
    Prolonged high-dose corticosteroid therapy

IV. **Clinical features**
  A. **Site of infection** (5,6)
       1. The **clinical presentation of TB is variable and depends on the site of disease, as well as the host's underlying immune status.**
            a. Pulmonary TB is the most common site of disease; in non-HIV-infected adults, approximately 75% to 85% of TB occurs in the lungs and encompasses both primary and reactivation disease.
            b. In HIV-infected persons, isolated pulmonary TB develops in 50% to 75% of cases; the remainder of HIV-infected patients develop concomitant pulmonary and extrapulmonary TB.
       2. In 1995, the Centers for Disease Control (CDC) reported the extent and nature of TB in the United States. Of 22,860 reported cases of TB, 77% were pulmonary, 18% extrapulmonary, and 5% both pulmonary and extrapulmonary. The most common extrapulmonary sites were lymph nodes, the pleura, bones and/or joints, the genitourinary tract, the central nervous system (meninges), and the peritoneum.
  B. **Classic symptoms of active TB** include fever, cough (with or without hemoptysis), dyspnea, night sweats, and weight loss. Persons with extrapulmonary disease also may have symptoms localized to the site of involvement. TB in immunocompromised hosts, especially HIV-infected persons, may present with unusual manifestations. Clinicians should maintain a high index of suspicion for TB in such patients.
  C. The **diagnosis of TB** can be established using modalities that are readily available to the clinician. Tuberculin skin testing, chest radiographs, and various microbiologic studies are commonly used in combination to diagnose tuberculous infection and disease.
       1. **Tuberculin skin testing** is a simple method used to screen for TB infection in *high-risk* populations and in suspected TB cases (4,7). Routine screening of low-risk persons is generally not indicated; the decision to screen and the frequency of skin test screening depend on the risk of TB within a given population.
            a. Administration and interpretation of the skin test using the **Mantoux technique** is a highly standardized procedure; these tasks should be undertaken *only* by persons who have been trained in their performance. Purified protein derivative (PPD) tuberculin solution (0.1 mL), containing 5 tuberculin units (5 TU) of tuberculin and stabilized using Tween-80 detergent, is injected intracutaneously. The injection is administered on the palmar surface of a forearm, although it may be given elsewhere, and must result in a noticeable bleb for the test to be accurate.
            b. By convention, the **diameter of the area of induration (*not* erythema) is measured after 48–72 hours *across the forearm* (rather than lengthwise). Patients or other untrained persons never should be relied on to interpret skin tests. Since induration is a result of a delayed-type hypersensitivity (DTH) reaction, the criterion for a significant (positive) skin test is dependent on an individual's ability to develop an adequate cellular immune response (Table 8-2).

Table 8-2. Interpretation of PPD reaction

Measured induration	Persons considered infected
≥5 mm	Persons infected with HIV, contacts of infectious TB cases, persons with fibrotic lesions on chest radiograph (old TB)
≥10 mm	Other at-risk adults and children (see Table 8-1 for risk factors for TB)
≥15 mm	No identifiable risk factors

PPD =purified protein derivative.

    c. **Positive reactions** usually indicate prior tuberculous infection; negative reactions usually indicate either that there is no tuberculous infection or that the subject is unable to develop a DTH skin-test response (termed skin-test anergy). The tuberculin skin test may also be negative in recently acquired tuberculous infection (the capacity to mount a skin test response to tuberculin may take up to 12 weeks following infection) or in active TB disease.

    d. Since many persons with active TB (up to 30% in some studies) may not express a reaction to PPD tuberculin, **a negative skin test should never dissuade clinicians from beginning anti-TB therapy in a suspected case if treatment is indicated**. Such a patient should receive empiric anti-TB therapy and undergo repeat tuberculin skin testing 12 weeks following the negative test, if indicated.

    e. The tine test is not standardized and should not be used to screen persons for TB infection.

2. **The interpretation of PPD tuberculin reactions in persons who have received previous bacille Calmette-Guérin (BCG) vaccine** is sometimes difficult.

    a. Prepared from live, attenuated strains of *M. bovis*, BCG vaccine for TB is administered in many parts of the world by injection. However, the preparations of BCG vaccine available, the number of doses administered to an individual, and the schedules for administration have never been standardized.

    b. The ability of BCG vaccine to cause the PPD tuberculin skin test to become positive (ie, to convert a negative skin test) is variable; when the skin test is converted by BCG vaccine, the reaction size tends to be small (ie, <15 mm induration) and wanes with time.

    c. For these reasons, and since BCG vaccine is usually used in places where TB is endemic, **a history of BCG vaccination *should not* influence the interpretation of a positive PPD tuberculin reaction in adults; a significant reaction to a tuberculin skin test in a BCG-vaccinated person should be interpreted as indicating previous tuberculous infection.**

3. **Chest radiographs** in pulmonary TB may reveal various findings that depend on the stage of disease and a patient's underlying immune status.

    a. **Primary pulmonary TB presents as a bronchopneumonia**, usually involving a lower lobe or the right middle lobe or lingula. Hilar lymphadenopathy may be associated, although adenopathy may be the sole finding.

    b. **The classic chest radiographic findings of *reactivation* TB include upper lobe (apical or posterior segments) or lower lobe (superior segment) infiltration with or without cavitation.**

    c. Although these typical radiographic findings are common in patients with intact immune systems, unusual radiographic presentations have been described, especially in immunocompromised persons. In these cases, findings include infiltrates in atypical locations, lung nodules, miliary infiltrates, pleural effusion, and/or lymphadenopathy.

    d. Rarely, some individuals with active pulmonary TB may have a normal chest radiograph.

4. **Examination of appropriately stained and cultured specimens** can confirm a diagnosis of TB in suspected cases (1,8,9). Suitable specimens for analysis include **sputum; bronchoalveolar lavage fluid; transbronchial, pleural, and other biopsy specimens; pleural fluid; lymph node and other tissue aspirates; synovial fluid; urine** (note: acid-fast bacilli [AFB] stains of urine or gastric aspirates should not be performed because of high false-positive rates); **peritoneal fluid; and cerebrospinal fluid**. Since the yield of stains and cultures from these specimens can be variable, multiple specimens should be obtained and analyzed, if possible.

    a. AFB **stains** can aid a clinician in making a rapid diagnosis of TB and in identifying a case as infectious **(approximately 10^4 organisms/mm^3 of specimen are needed to reliably produce a positive smear).**

   i. In addition to the Ziehl-Neelsen stain, fluorochromes (auramine and rhodamine) are available in some clinical laboratories. False-positive results may be obtained with fluorochromes; positive fluorochrome specimens should be confirmed by traditional AFB stains.

   ii. AFB stains cannot discriminate between mycobacterial species or provide antibiotic resistance information; all specimens positive by stain should be confirmed by culture.

   b. **Cultures for *M. tuberculosis* are more specific than AFB stains,** and growth of *M. tuberculosis* from a body fluid or a tissue specimen establishes a diagnosis with certainty. Cultures can also provide information regarding drug susceptibility of the isolate, and susceptibility testing should always be performed on positive cultures.

   i. The main disadvantage of routine cultures is delay of up to 8 weeks before identification of *M. tuberculosis* is confirmed.

   ii. **Newer, rapid culture systems are available in many clinical laboratories and allow for identification of *M. tuberculosis* within 1–3 weeks.**

   iii. Nucleic acid amplification tests recently approved by the FDA for use in specific situations are presently being evaluated by the CDC for clinical applications.

5. Other diagnostic techniques are available in some research laboratories, including immunoassays for mycobacterial antigens and antimycobacterial antibodies, and gas and liquid chromatography.

6. Other characteristic findings that may be used to support the diagnosis of TB include:

   a. Reduced glucose levels (<60 mg/dL), reduced pH (<7.2), and elevated protein levels in pleural, peritoneal, cerebrospinal, and synovial fluid.

   b. Pleural, peritoneal, and cerebrospinal lymphocytosis (synovial fluid tends to exhibit a predominance of polymorphonuclear leukocytes).

   c. <2% mesothelial cells in pleural fluid.

   d. Urinalysis may reveal microscopic hematuria or white blood cells in the absence of bacteria (sterile pyuria).

   e. Peritoneal fluid may have elevated activity of adenosine deaminase (this assay is not commonly available).

   f. Biopsy specimens may reveal characteristic caseating granulomas.

V. **Classification of tuberculosis** (10). Information derived from the history, physical examination, PPD tuberculin skin test result, chest radiograph, and microbiologic studies is used to classify TB cases. The classification scheme used by the American Thoracic Society and the CDC is provided in Table 8-3. Classification of a given case allows stratification that aids in the monitoring of treatment and the development of epidemiologic profiles by public health officials.

VI. **Treatment**

Table 8-3. Classification of tuberculosis

Class 0	No exposure; no infection
Class 1	Exposure; no infection
Class 2	Infection; no disease (ie, positive PPD reaction but no evidence of active TB)
Class 3	Disease, clinically active
Class 4	Disease, not clinically active (ie, evidence of previous TB or following therapy for tuberculous disease)
Class 5	Suspected disease, diagnosis pending

A. **General principles** (1,11,12)
   1. Although TB is generally a treatable disease, **the use of multiple antibiotic agents and prolonged durations of treatment are necessary to assure eradication of the organism and prevent relapse.** The main goal of treatment is to provide the most effective and safe regimen in the shortest period of time and in a manner that optimizes the likelihood of adherence to therapy. Many possible treatment regimens and conditions for administration of anti-TB therapy are presently available.
   2. The treatment of TB must be addressed within the framework of the individual's culture and society; if the patient does not receive proper treatment, the disease will not be cured. This often extends the treatment for TB far beyond the prescribing of medications for a given patient.
      a. Physicians must consider the method of administration of medications in addition to the best choice of drug combinations, which depends on individual case information and local epidemiologic data
      b. Treatment regimens must be tailored to meet community, program, and individual patient needs.
   3. Many TB programs have successfully employed **case-management strategies** centered around patient self-treatment. However, treatment policies based on universal self-administered therapy frequently generate uncertainties about adherence.
      a. More restrictive management requirements may be implemented, such as **voluntary directly observed therapy (DOT), mandatory DOT (used for *all* persons with active disease in some locales), or involuntary incarceration for those who demonstrate persistent nonadherence and pose a threat to the public health of the community.**
B. **Rationale for combination chemotherapy**
   1. Most persons with active TB harbor a large number of viable organisms. Since *spontaneous* **resistance to anti-TB medications may occur among a population of organisms within an individual** (risk for spontaneous resistance to ethambutol alone is 1 in 10^4 organisms, to isoniazid or streptomycin 1 in 10^6, and to rifampin 1 in 10^8), and since such resistance usually occurs in a given organism to a single drug and not to others, multiple drugs are required for the treatment of active TB to minimize the possibility of selecting for drug-resistant organisms.
      a. For example, if a person with a total of 10^9 organisms is treated with isoniazid alone, 10^3 spontaneously isoniazid-resistant organisms will survive isoniazid treatment and be free to continue to proliferate.
      b. Since spontaneous resistance in any single organism is unique to a single drug, the risk of resistance to both isoniazid and rifampin is 1 in 10^{14} (1 in 10^6 for isoniazid and 1 in 10^8 for rifampin). Since this person is harboring only 10^9 organisms, the risk of any one of his organisms being resistant to the combination of isoniazid and rifampin is 1 in 10^5. Therefore, treatment with isoniazid and rifampin is likely to eradicate all organisms.
   2. Combination therapy is also useful because different agents act on various subpopulations of *M. tuberculosis*.
      a. Isoniazid is effective against intracellular and extracellular organisms.
      b. Rifampin, similar to isoniazid, is effective against intracellular and extracellular organisms but is also effective against slowly metabolizing organisms.
      c. Pyrazinamide is active in environments with an acidic pH; thus, it is particularly effective against intracellular organisms.
C. **Antituberculosis medications**
   1. **First-line medications** (11,12,13) include those anti-TB drugs with the highest antimycobacterial activity and an acceptable incidence of toxicity. They may be used as single agents for preventive therapy (most commonly isoniazid or rifampin; see H. Pregnancy and tuberculosis below) or in combination for either preventive therapy or treatment of active disease. First-line medications are listed in Table 8-4.

Table 8-4. First-line antituberculosis medications: daily dosing

Drug	Daily dose	Side effects
Isoniazid	5–20 mg/kg (max 300 mg)	Hepatitis (especially with alcohol use or age >35 years), peripheral neuropathy (administer pyridoxine, especially in persons with diabetes mellitus, alcoholism, renal insufficiency, malnutrition, pregnancy, and seizure disorder to reduce risk), CNS, rash
Rifampin	10–20 mg/kg (max 600 mg)	Discolored body fluids, GI, hepatitis, rash, fever, flu-like symptoms, thrombocytopenia
Pyrazinamide	15–30 mg/kg (max 2000 mg)	Hepatitis, hyperuricemia, rash, GI, difficult to control diabetes mellitus
Ethambutol	15–25 mg/kg (max 2500 mg)	Retrobulbar neuritis (especially with underlying renal insufficiency; dose related)
Streptomycin/ kanamycin	15–20 mg/kg (max 1000 mg)	Ototoxicity and nephrotoxicity (cumulative dose related)

2. **Second-line medications** generally are less effective against *M. tuberculosis* than first-line drugs and/or have more substantial toxicity. These drugs include capreomycin, ethionamide, para-aminosalicylic acid, and cycloserine (12,13). Usually reserved for use in relatively complex situations, these medications should be administered only with consultation from a TB specialist.

3. Other potentially effective medications include other aminoglycosides (eg, gentamicin and amikacin), quinolones, ansamycin, clofazimine, and combinations of β-lactam antibiotics and β-lactamase inhibitors (12).

   a. The effectiveness of these classes of medications in the treatment of TB has not been conclusively demonstrated. As with second-line medications, they should be used only upon the recommendation of a TB specialist, who should also monitor their use.

D. **Combination therapy** (1,8,11,12,13,14)

1. **Successful treatment regimens include at least two agents to which the patient's organism is susceptible.** Assurance of patient adherence to therapy is key to achieving a cure and in preventing spread of disease to others.

2. Chemotherapeutic agents administered regularly for a prolonged period of **6–12 months are generally required for adequate treatment for pulmonary and extrapulmonary TB.**

3. The CDC and the American Thoracic Society in collaboration with the American Academy of Pediatrics have recently published treatment guidelines for the management of tuberculous infection and disease in adults and children.

   a. In most cases, **initial therapy for adults with active TB should include four drugs: isoniazid, rifampin, pyrazinamide, and either ethambutol or streptomycin. In communities where the rate of drug resistance is <4%, initial therapy with isoniazid, rifampin, and pyrazinamide is acceptable.** Vitamin B_6 (pyridoxine at 50 mg/d PO) usually is administered with isoniazid to prevent isoniazid-associated peripheral neuropathy.

   b. This initial intensive-treatment phase targets rapidly dividing organisms; medications are usually **administered daily for at least 8 weeks.**

4. If cultures and drug susceptibility studies indicate that the organism is sensitive to the drugs before 8 weeks of therapy have been completed, either ethambutol or streptomycin may be stopped.

5. After 8 weeks of three-drug therapy, pyrazinamide may be discontinued, and isoniazid and rifampin should be administered for at least 4 additional months (6 months total therapy).

6. Alternatively, if pyrazinamide is administered for <8 weeks or if it was omitted from the initial treatment regimen, isoniazid and rifampin should be administered for a total of at least 9 months. **These recommended lengths of therapy assume a good clinical response to treatment, supported by negative cultures for the final 3 months and 6 months, respectively, where culture material is easily obtainable** (eg, sputum).

7. Immunocompromised and HIV-infected persons require more prolonged therapy, and treatment should be individualized. In addition, **all cases of miliary or bone/joint TB should be treated for at least 12 months.** Similarly, tuberculous meningitis in children should be treated for at least 12 months.

8. **If cultures and drug susceptibility studies yield a drug-resistant organism, administration of at least two agents to which there is known susceptibility is essential. Consultation with a TB expert should be sought for all cases of multiple drug resistance.**

9. If cultures of adequate specimens remain without growth at 8 weeks in a person with active TB who has responded to treatment, isoniazid and rifampin should be administered to complete a total of 4 months of therapy. Other agents may be stopped after 8 weeks if all cultures are negative.

E. **Evaluation during treatment** (12)

1. **Routine follow-up** for persons receiving chemotherapy for TB is essential to assess adequate response to therapy, to monitor for potential side effects, and to assure adherence to medications.

   a. **Response to therapy** is monitored by symptomatic response, serial microbacteriologic studies, physical examinations, and chest radiographs.

      i. For persons with smear- or culture-positive specimens, **smears and cultures should be repeated at least monthly** until cultures become negative. The sputum will convert to negative within the first 2 months of therapy for 85% of patients receiving isoniazid and rifampin. If conversion occurs, a final specimen should be examined at the completion of therapy, if one can be obtained.

      ii. If conversion does not occur within 2 months, repeat cultures with drug susceptibility testing should be performed at least monthly, **and directly observed therapy should be started to insure that drugs are taken.**

      iii. **If conversion does not occur within 3–6 months of therapy, the person should be regarded as a treatment failure and should be referred to a TB specialist.** Repeat susceptibility testing should be performed, and the addition of three drugs not given previously should be considered until results of repeat testing are available.

      iv. For persons with smear- and culture-negative sputum specimens, clinical and radiographic responses should be monitored.

   b. Abnormal chest radiographs should be monitored serially during therapy for TB to assess response to therapy. A chest radiograph should also be obtained routinely in all patients following completion of therapy for possible future comparison.

   c. Regular monitoring for **potential adverse reactions to medications** should be performed. Patients should be educated about potential medication side effects at the initiation of therapy, and this education must be repeatedly reinforced throughout treatment.

      i. Baseline measurements of serum transaminases (AST and ALT) should be obtained in all persons receiving hepatotoxic drugs.

      ii. Visual acuity and red-green color perception should be documented prior to therapy with ethambutol. Adequate assessment of visual function may be difficult in young children; thus, alternative medications (eg, streptomycin or kanamycin) should be considered for these patients.

      iii. Monthly evaluations by a health care provider must be performed in every patient receiving anti-TB medication. These examinations should include screening for symptoms and physical findings suggestive of adverse drug reactions, follow-up laboratory studies in high-risk individuals or if otherwise indicated, and suspension of treatment if a serious adverse reaction is suspected. Similarly, patients should be instructed to contact their health care provider immediately and, in some cases, to hold therapy if they suspect they are experiencing an adverse reaction to a medication.

2. **Directly observed therapy (DOT) should be instituted at the outset of treatment in potentially noncompliant patients.** This may be accompanied by enablers or incentives (eg, bus passes, taxi vouchers, etc) to improve the likelihood of adherence. Generally, three options exist for the administration of DOT (Table 8-5).

   a. Both symptomatic response and conversion to negative smears and cultures are expected after 3 months of any DOT regimen.

   b. If the patient remains symptomatic or if smears and cultures do not convert after 3 months of DOT, the patient should be referred to a TB specialist. Dosage adjustments for adults receiving twice or thrice weekly regimens are given in Table 8-6.

F. **Drug resistance and multidrug resistance** (11,12,15–19)

   1. **Resistance of *M. tuberculosis* to anti-TB medication may be due to either initial infection with a drug-resistant organism, termed primary resistance (ie, from an index case with resistant TB), or secondarily by development of drug-resistant disease due to incorrect administration of anti-TB medications.** Mechanisms responsible for selection of drug-resistant organisms by administration of inadequate therapy have been addressed earlier. Incorrect prescription of a treatment regimen by a health care provider or irregular, intermittent ingestion of medications by the patient may also induce secondary drug resistance. Measures that have been used to minimize treatment variables that select for secondary resistance include drug administration regimens that encourage adherence (eg, DOT, incarceration) and the use of fixed drug-combination medications, such as capsules containing isoniazid

Table 8-5. Regimen options for directly observed therapy (12)

Option 1	Isoniazid, rifampin, and pyrazinamide daily for 8 wk followed by isoniazid and rifampin daily or twice/thrice weekly for 16 wk (in areas where drug resistance rate is <4%); add ethambutol or streptomycin to initial daily regimen until susceptibility to isoniazid and rifampin is confirmed (in areas where drug resistance rate is >4%)
Option 2	Isoniazid, rifampin, pyrazinamide, and ethambutol or streptomycin daily for 2 wk followed by the same four drugs twice weekly for 6 wk; then isoniazid and rifampin twice weekly for 16 wk
Option 3	Isoniazid, rifampin, pyrazinamide, and ethambutol or streptomycin thrice weekly for 6 mo

For all regimens, consult TB expert if patient remains symptomatic or is smear or culture positive after 3 months of treatment.

Table 8-6. Dosage adjustments for twice or thrice weekly regimen options in adults (12)

Drug	Twice weekly regimen	Thrice weekly regimen
Isoniazid	15 mg/kg (max 900 mg)	15 mg/kg (max 900 mg)
Rifampin	10 mg/kg (max 600 mg)	10 mg/kg (max 600 mg)
Pyrazinamide	50–70 mg/kg (max 4000 mg)	50–70 mg/kg (max 3000 mg)
Ethambutol	50 mg/kg	25–30 mg/kg
Streptomycin/kanamycin	25–30 mg/kg (max 1500 mg)	25–30 mg/kg (max 1500 mg)

150 mg + rifampin 300 mg (Rifamate) and tablets containing isoniazid 50 mg + rifampin 120 mg + pyrazinamide 300 mg (Rifater), to assure that patients will not selectively take or exclude individual drugs. (Note: Fixed combinations of Rifater make it unsuitable for intermittant 2 or 3 times a week therapy.)

2. **Multidrug-resistant *M. tuberculosis* is defined by resistance to both isoniazid and rifampin.**

   a. Populations at highest risk for multidrug resistance include HIV-infected persons, institutionalized persons, and homeless individuals. Since the cure rate decreases (and mortality increases) for persons with multidrug-resistant TB, adequate control of this disease is essential. Local TB control programs and TB specialists should be involved in all cases.

G. **HIV infection and tuberculosis (4,12)**

   1. **A clear association exists between HIV infection and TB.**

      a. Persons coinfected with HIV and TB are at great risk of developing reactivation disease, and HIV-infected persons appear to be very susceptible to new infection that may become rapidly progressive.

      b. Those at greatest risk include HIV-infected injecting drug users and the foreign born. Data from San Francisco indicate that 29% of non-Asian TB patients 18–65 years of age are infected with HIV. In addition, a review of registries of acquired immunodeficiency syndrome (AIDS) cases and TB cases in several states reveals that 4% of cases appear in both registries.

   2. Several clinical features are notable regarding TB in HIV-infected persons. **Unusual clinical presentations of TB are common among HIV-infected persons with active TB, presenting diagnostic challenges to the clinician.**

      a. Extrapulmonary TB may be present in 40% to 70% of these patients and often occurs concomitantly with pulmonary TB.

      b. Skin test reactions may be falsely negative due to immunosuppression; thus, tuberculin skin test reactions of ≥5 mm induration suggest tuberculous infection.

   3. Concomitant infection with HIV and *M. tuberculosis* will prolong the duration of therapy for both tuberculous infection and active disease.

      a. Preventive treatment for HIV-infected persons also infected with TB requires 12 months of isoniazid.

      b. Multidrug therapy for active TB must be administered for at least 12 months, and more prolonged therapy may be necessary depending on individual clinical response.

H. **Pregnancy and tuberculosis** (12,20)

   1. Drug therapy for pregnant patients must be carefully prescribed and monitored. Fortunately, adequate multidrug therapy for active TB in pregnant women is associated with an excellent prognosis.

      a. Isoniazid, rifampin, and ethambutol have not been shown to be teratogenic and can be used at standard doses. Pyridoxine should be administered along with isoniazid to pregnant patients. Pyrazinamide is not recommended during pregnancy due to inadequate data regarding potential teratogenic effects.

      b. Streptomycin has been demonstrated to affect development of the ear and may cause congenital deafness. Since kanamycin and capreomycin may have teratogenic effects similar to those of streptomycin, these three agents should be avoided in pregnant patients.

   2. Preventive therapy for TB (see section H) should be delayed until after delivery in most pregnant patients. However, recently infected pregnant women who have high-risk medical conditions such as HIV infection should receive preventive therapy with isoniazid without delay.

VII. **Tuberculosis prophylaxis** (6,8,12,21)

   A. In 1990, the CDC estimated that 10–15 million persons in the United States were infected with *M. tuberculosis*. Since >90% of TB cases develop after a period of containment following initial infection, preventive therapy administered before the development of disease has been shown to reduce the progression to active TB. Effective TB control requires public health screening programs of high-risk persons to identify those for whom preventive therapy is indicated. Adequate resources must be available to provide preventive services to high-risk persons: clinical evaluations of skin test reactors, low-cost or free medications, and monthly medical follow-up for those receiving treatment.

B. The decision to institute TB prophylaxis should be based on an individual's potential benefits of treatment weighed against the risk of adverse drug reactions (especially hepatotoxicity).

  1. The lifetime risk of progression from tuberculous infection to disease among the general, tuberculous-infected population is estimated to be approximately 10%; however, this risk is substantially higher in selected groups with comorbid conditions **(HIV infection, diabetes, end-stage renal disease, corticosteroid or other immunosuppressive therapy, recent significant rapid weight loss and chronic malnutrition, hematologic or reticuloendothelial diseases)**.

  2. Risk of progression appears to be highest in TB/HIV-coinfected persons (estimated at 7% to 10% per year) and recently infected persons (2% to 4% per year for 2 years following new infection). The risk of hepatotoxicity is highest in persons older than 35 years, daily alcohol users, and pregnant or postpartum women.

C. Conditions meeting requirements for preventive therapy, regardless of the age of the patient (if not previously treated), are listed in Table 8-7. Conditions meeting requirements for preventive therapy in patients younger than 35 years are listed in Table 8-8.

  1. Other populations that may be considered for preventive therapy include health care workers, staff of facilities housing institutionalized persons, and school staff.

  2. Other persons younger than 35 years without risk factors for TB and a PPD tuberculin reaction ≥15 mm induration also may be considered for preventive therapy, based on individual and/or programmatic considerations.

D. **Since adherence to prolonged treatment regimens (generally 6–12 months) is necessary for preventive therapy to be effective, clinicians should begin preventive therapy only in patients who are likely to complete treatment.**

  1. **Preventive therapy consists of daily administration of isoniazid at 10–15 mg/kg (maximum, 300 mg) for a minimum of 6 months.** Children should receive treatment for 9 months. Persons with HIV infection or fibrotic lesions

Table 8-7. Candidates for preventive therapy regardless of age

HIV-infected persons with PPD ≥5 mm induration

Close contacts of infectious TB cases with PPD ≥5 mm induration

Children and adolescents who are close contacts of infectious TB cases with PPD <5 mm induration, until a repeat skin test is performed in 3 mo

Persons with fibrotic lesions on chest radiographs suggestive of old TB with PPD ≥5 mm induration

Skin test converters (conversion within a 2-year period: if <35 years of age, ≥10 mm increase in induration over previous test; if ≥35 years of age, ≥15 mm increase)

Injecting drug users with PPD ≥10 mm induration

Persons with a high-risk medical condition (see Table 8-1) with PPD ≥10 mm induration

PPD =purified protein derivative test.

Table 8-8. Candidates for preventive therapy (age ≤35 years)

Foreign-born persons with high-prevalence countries with PPD ≥10 mm induration

High-risk, medically underserved populations with PPD ≥10 mm induration

Institutionalized persons with PPD ≥10 mm induration

on their chest radiograph consistent with old, untreated TB should be treated for 12 months. Alternatively, persons with fibrotic lesions may be treated with a combination of daily isoniazid (10–15 mg/kg; maximum, 300 mg) and rifampin (10–20 mg/kg; maximum, 600 mg) for 4 months.

2. **Persons infected with isoniazid-resistant, rifampin-sensitive TB or persons who cannot tolerate isoniazid may be treated with a 6–12-month course of rifampin (600 mg/d) (12,24); those infected with multidrug-resistant (ie, isoniazid- and rifampin-resistant) TB should be referred to a TB specialist.**

E. Persons receiving preventive therapy must be monitored monthly for hepatotoxicity and other possible drug toxicities.

   1. Baseline AST and ALT levels should be measured before treatment is initiated; if active hepatitis is discovered, preventive therapy should be deferred in most cases until these issues are resolved.

   2. For persons younger than 35 years, a monthly clinical examination is adequate; periodic examination of serum transaminases is not necessary in low-risk persons. Patients should be instructed to seek prompt medical evaluation if any signs or symptoms of an adverse reaction develop. These include anorexia, nausea, emesis, icterus, dark urine, abdominal pain, fever, rash, or paresthesias. Repeat AST and ALT determinations should be made if adverse hepatic reactions are suspected. If these enzymes are elevated to >3–5 times normal, discontinuation of isoniazid preventive therapy should be considered.

   3. **For persons 35 years and older, monthly AST and ALT measurements should be routinely obtained.**

   4. **In addition, other persons at increased risk for hepatotoxicity (ie, daily alcohol users, injecting drug users, persons with chronic liver disease, pregnant or postpartum women, and postpubertal black and Hispanic women) should be considered for routine liver function test measurements.**

VIII. **Tuberculosis and the public health.** The treatment of a case of TB extends far beyond the prescription of a course of medication (22,23). State and local health departments must be concerned with issues related to patient adherence and safe completion of appropriate therapy, contact investigation, education of the patient, family, and coworkers, and provision of preventive services.

A. **TB is a reportable disease in the United States; all TB cases and suspects must be reported to local and/or state departments of public health.** Data compiled by health departments and supplied to the CDC are analyzed to identify trends and help direct resources as required for more effective TB control.

B. Health departments should be expected to provide resources and expertise to providers who manage active TB cases and patients suspected of having TB, such as provision of expert consultation and/or direct clinical services (diagnostic and subsequent management), free medications, provider education, and culturally appropriate assistance in managing cases and contacts.

C. The treatment of TB will be most successful if medical management is considered within the social context of the patient. A multidisciplinary case-management approach coordinated by direct care providers in collaboration with health departments assures that appropriate aspects of TB control are addressed to achieve a cure in the index case and minimize the spread of infection within the community.

References

1. Glassroth J: Tuberculosis. In: Niederman, Sarosi, Glassroth, eds. *Respiratory infections.* Philadelphia: WB Saunders, 1994:449–458.
2. Hopewell PC, Bloom BR: Tuberculosis and other mycobacterial diseases. In: Murray, Nadel, eds. *Textbook of respiratory medicine.* Philadelphia: WB Saunders, 1994:1094–1160.
3. Recommendations of the Advisory Council for the Elimination of Tuberculosis: Tuberculosis among foreign-born persons entering the United States. *MMWR* 1990;39(18):1–16.

4. Recommendations of the Advisory Council for the Elimination of Tuberculosis: Screening for tuberculosis and tuberculous infection in high-risk populations. *MMWR* 1990;39(8):1–12.
5. Centers for Disease Control and Prevention: Reported tuberculosis in the United States, 1993. October 1994, 10–11.
6. Recommendations of the Advisory Council for the Elimination of Tuberculosis: Tuberculosis and human immunodeficiency virus infection. *MMWR* 1989;38(14):236–250.
7. Use of BCG vaccines in the control of tuberculosis: a joint statement by the ACIP and the Advisory Council for the Elimination of Tuberculosis. *MMWR* 1988;37(43):663–675.
8. Barnes PF, Barrows SA: Tuberculosis in the 1990s. *Ann Intern Med* 1993;119:400–410.
9. Voigt MD, Kalvaria I, Trey C: Diagnostic value of ascites adenosine deaminase in tuberculous peritonitis. *Lancet* 1989;1:751–4.
10. Diagnostic standards and classification of tuberculosis: joint statement of the American Thoracic Society and the Centers for Disease Control. *Am Rev Respir Dis* 1990;142:725.
11. Recommendations of the Advisory Council for the Elimination of Tuberculosis: Initial therapy for tuberculosis in the era of multidrug resistance. *MMWR* 1993;42(7):1 –8.
12. Treatment of tuberculosis and tuberculous infection in adults and children: joint statement of the American Thoracic Society and the Centers for Disease Control. *Am J Respir Crit Care Med* 1993;149:1359–1374.
13. Drugs for tuberculosis. *Med Lett* 37(954):67–70.
14. Combs DL, O Brien RJ, Geiter LJ: USPHS tuberculosis short-course chemotherapy trial 21: effectiveness, toxicity, and acceptability. A report of final results. *Ann Intern Med* 1990;112:397–406.
15. Pearson ML, Jereb JA, Frieden TR: Nosocomial transmission of multidrug resistant *Mycobacterium tuberculosis*. *Ann Intern Med* 1992;117:191–196.
16. Dooley SW, Jarvis WR, Martone WJ, Snider DE Jr: Multidrug-resistant tuberculosis (editorial). *Ann Intern Med* 1992;117:257–258.
17. Iseman MD: Treatment of multidrug-resistant tuberculosis. *N Engl J Med* 1993;329:784–791.
18. Meeting the challenge of multidrug-resistant tuberculosis: summary of a conference. *MMWR* 1992; 41(11):51–57.
19. Centers for Disease Control. Management of persons exposed to multidrug-resistant tuberculosis. *MMWR* 1992;41(11):61–71.
20. Snider D: Pregnancy and tuberculosis. *Chest* 86S(3):10S–13S.
21. Recommendations of the Advisory Council for the Elimination of Tuberculosis: The use of preventive therapy of tuberculous infection in the United States. *MMWR* 1990;39(8):9–12.
22. Bloom BR, Murray CJL: Tuberculosis: commentary on a reemergent killer. *Science* 1992;257: 1055–1064.
23. Reichman LB: The U-shaped curve of concern. *Am Rev Respir Dis* 1991;144:741–742.
24. Polesky A, Farber HW, Gottlieb DJ, et al. Rifampin preventive therapy for tuberculosis in Boston's homeless. *Amer J Respir Crit Care Med* 1996;154:1473–1477.

9 Fungal Infections

Hardy Kornfeld

I. Introduction

A. More than 100,000 species of fungi are found in nature; several hundred have been associated with human disease, but only a handful are usually encountered in clinical practice. The widespread use of immunosuppressive drugs and the global epidemic of acquired immunodeficiency syndrome (AIDS) have greatly increased the frequency of pulmonary and systemic fungal infections.

B. In contrast to bacteria, fungi possess a true nucleus. Their cell wall and lack of chlorophyll differentiate them from other eukaryotic cells of plants or animals. Fungi may produce spores (a common vehicle for infection by inhalation) and may organize into filamentous structures, a property shared by certain bacteria that will also be covered in this chapter. Fungi are widely disseminated in the environment, and most pulmonary mycoses are caused by organisms that grow in soil.

C. Morphologically, fungi may be characterized as molds or yeasts. **Molds** are colonies of fungal cells **(hyphae)** that form networks called **mycelia**. Growth occurs at the hyphal tip with periodic branching of the filaments. In contrast, **yeast** exist as individual cells that reproduce by budding or fission. Certain fungi are dimorphic, growing as molds in soil or in culture at room temperature but converting to yeast-like forms at body temperature and *in vivo*.

D. Pulmonary mycoses covered in this chapter include aspergillosis, histoplasmosis, coccidioidomycosis, cryptococcosis, paracoccidioidomycosis, mucormycosis, and pneumonia due to *Candida* species. There are several recent sources for more comprehensive information (1,2). The bacterial infections actinomycosis and nocardiosis that clinically and morphologically bear a closer resemblance to fungal infections than to typical bacterial pneumonia are also covered in this chapter.

II. Aspergillosis

A. The spectrum of host responses to pulmonary challenge with *Aspergillus* species ranges from hypersensitivity reactions to colonization of airways with conidia, through noninvasive infection of parenchymal cavities, to fulminant invasive pulmonary and systemic infection (usually in the setting of impaired host defenses) with high mortality. Further complicating this picture is the fact that crossover between these various manifestations may occur. Aspergillosis is seen more frequently as a result of the increasing use of immunosuppressive medical therapies and broad-spectrum antibiotics, as well as the AIDS epidemic.

B. Aspergillus lung disease may present as four distinct forms:
1. Allergic bronchopulmonary aspergillosis (hypersensitivity reaction).
2. Chronic mycetoma (noninvasive infection).
3. Suppurative bronchitis and chronic necrotizing pneumonia (minimally invasive disease).
4. Acute necrotizing pneumonia (invasive parenchymal infection).

C. Allergic bronchopulmonary aspergillosis (ABPA) is characterized by asthma and proximal bronchiectasis. Its true prevalence is uncertain, but ABPA is probably underdiagnosed, since it affected a sizable fraction of steroid-dependent asthmatic patients in some series (3).
1. **Presenting signs and symptoms** include episodic wheezing, sputum production with expectoration of blood or brown plugs, fever, chest pain, and

malaise. Chest x-ray abnormalities reflect intermittent airway obstruction by impacted secretions, as well as chronic bronchial changes (wall thickening and dilatation). Transient patchy infiltrates are frequent, and lobar consolidation and collapse may be observed. Mucoid impaction of bronchi may be reflected by hilar tubular or branched gloved-finger opacities.

  2. **Pathogenesis.** ABPA is caused by hypersensitivity to *Aspergillus fumigatus;* a similar syndrome may be evoked by other fungal species (see chapter 4). The disease may progress from an acute to a chronic phase; prolonged inflammation characterized by steroid-dependent asthma may lead to bronchiectasis and airway fibrosis.
  3. **Diagnosis.** Typical patients with ABPA have preexisting asthma, cystic fibrosis, or some other chronic lung disease. In the absence of a pathognomonic feature or single diagnostic laboratory test, the diagnosis of ABPA is usually established by a pattern of several characteristics (5) (Table 9-1).
  4. **Management.** Corticosteroids are the therapy of choice for ABPA. A typical regimen is prednisone 0.5 mg/kg/d for 2 weeks, then every other day for 3 months, followed by a taper of 5 mg every 2 weeks, although higher doses and longer durations may be required. Response to treatment may be monitored by improvement of radiographic changes and reductions in total IgE antibody. Itraconazole (200 mg PO BID) may be a beneficial adjunct to steroids in refractory cases (6).
D. **Chronic mycetoma.** Preexisting pulmonary cavities are subject to saprophytic colonization by fungi resulting in a mass of mycelia (fungus ball) filling the space. In this setting, parenchymal invasion is minimal or absent, although life-threatening hemoptysis may occur.
  1. **Presenting signs and symptoms.** Mycetomas may be asymptomatic, but the majority will ultimately give rise to symptoms, which most commonly include cough and hemoptysis. Weight loss and fever are less frequently encountered. Hemoptysis is often recurrent and may be massive.
  2. **Etiology and pathogenesis.** The vast majority of mycetomas are due to aspergilli **(aspergilloma)**; *Mucor* species can also produce mycetomas. Predisposing conditions include any cavitary lung disease, with most occurring in the setting of healed tuberculosis or histoplasmosis, sarcoidosis, or bronchiectasis. The natural history of mycetomas is variable. Spontaneous resolution occurs in about 10% of cases. The majority of patients will have at least one episode of hemoptysis. Massive hemoptysis may occur in up to 20% of cases; the risk for this increases with the duration of disease.
  3. **Diagnosis.** The chest x-ray typically reveals a thick-walled upper lobe cavity containing a round mass that changes its position with changes in the position of the patient. An **air crescent sign** may also be present and is pathognomonic for mycetoma. Chest computed tomography (CT) scan permits the identification of mycetomas even in cases in which the intracavitary air space is obliterated and the fungus ball is immobile (7).
      a. Nearly all patients with aspergilloma will have positive serum precipitins for *A. fumigatus*, while a negative result suggests mucormycosis or a di-

---

Table 9-1. Diagnostic criteria of allergic bronchopulmonary aspergillosis

Episodic bronchial obstruction

Eosinophilia

Immediate cutaneous reactivity to *A. fumigatus* (sensitive, not specific)

Precipitating antibodies to *A. fumigatus*

Elevated total IgE (sensitive, not specific; useful to follow response to treatment)

Elevated specific IgE and IgG to *A. fumigatus* (supportive)

Proximal bronchiectasis

agnosis other than mycetoma. A positive skin test and positive sputum cultures for aspergillus are nonspecific and do not rule out mycetoma due to other fungi.

    b. Because of the characteristic x-ray features, bronchoscopy or percutaneous needle biopsy are usually not required for diagnosis. The differential diagnosis includes entities that may produce filled cavities, including hematomas, lung cancer, bacterial lung abscess, and hydatid cyst.

  4. Management. Intravenous antifungal therapy is ineffective for mycetoma. Asymptomatic mycetomas require no treatment but should be followed clinically for progression (enlargement). Minor episodes of hemoptysis may be managed conservatively by postural drainage and empiric antibiotic treatment for associated bacterial infection. Intracavitary instillation of amphotericin B may be attempted for persistent or recurrent symptoms (8). Long-term itraconazole treatment may provide an alternative to invasive therapy (9), but experience is limited. Massive hemoptysis can be controlled by bronchial artery embolization, but recurrence is common. Surgical resection provides a definitive cure for mycetoma and should be considered when potentially life-threatening hemoptysis occurs. The decision to proceed with surgery is often complicated by the nature of the patient's underlying lung disease and correspondingly poor pulmonary function. Early consultation with pulmonary and thoracic surgery specialists is recommended for persistently symptomatic patients with mycetoma.

E. Chronic necrotizing pulmonary aspergillosis and **aspergillus tracheobronchitis.** Minimally invasive aspergillosis syndromes are characterized by minimal-to-moderate invasion of parenchymal tissue by fungus without symptoms or signs of classical invasive pulmonary aspergillosis. These less invasive infections typically occur in the context of mild-to-moderate immune deficiency and lie midway between saprophytic colonization and severe acute pneumonia and disseminated infection.

  1. Presenting signs and symptoms of both chronic necrotizing aspergillosis and aspergillus tracheobronchitis include cough and fever. Hemoptysis is more commonly seen with necrotizing infection. Chest x-ray findings include slowly evolving patchy infiltrates, sometimes seen in association with a mycetoma or with another chronic lung disease. Aspergillus tracheobronchitis is frequently associated with AIDS and may produce atelectasis due to inflammatory mucous plugs.

  2. Pathogenesis. Minimally invasive aspergillus lung disease nearly always occurs in the context of associated predisposing conditions. Necrotizing infection may start from the wall of a preexisting mycetoma; other typical settings include those of chronic obstructive or cavitary lung disease. The infection is slowly progressive.

    a. Aspergillus tracheobronchitis **(pseudomembranous necrotizing bronchial aspergillosis)** has been identified as a comorbid condition in the human immunodeficiency virus (HIV)-infected host (10). This process features true invasive infection of the airway mucosa without penetration to deep parenchymal structures of the lung.

    b. Minimally invasive aspergillosis may also occasionally be seen in HIV-seronegative hosts associated with chronic bronchitis or bronchiectasis, where the suppurative process is exacerbated. Pathologically, circumferential bronchial infection occurs with pseudomembrane formation. As part of the spectrum of aspergillus lung disease, these semi-invasive conditions may progress to more acute invasive pulmonary and systemic aspergillosis.

  3. Diagnosis. The diagnosis of chronic necrotizing aspergillosis is usually made on the basis of circumstantial evidence. Sputum culture for *Aspergillus* is frequently positive but does not differentiate invasive disease from colonization. In contrast to acute aspergillus pneumonia, serum precipitins are frequently positive in chronic disease. Chest CT scan can be helpful in defining semi-invasive infection (11). Tracheobronchitis should be suspected in an

HIV-seropositive individual presenting with persistent cough and chest x-ray signs of atelectasis, especially if sputum cultures grow the fungus. Mucous plugs containing fungal hyphae may be expectorated, and bronchoscopic examination of the airways reveals pseudomembranous inflammation. Diagnosis may be confirmed by biopsy and culture.

4. **Treatment.** By virtue of their subacute presentation and minimal tissue penetration, the minimally invasive aspergillosis syndromes may usually be treated with itraconazole (200 mg PO BID). A good response to itraconazole may be anticipated in patients with tracheobronchitis, while the response of chronic necrotizing aspergillosis may be complicated by the morbidity of the underlying lung disease. Definitive treatment with amphotericin B should be reserved for symptomatic cases unresponsive to itraconazole.

F. **Invasive aspergillosis.** Acute aspergillus pneumonia and disseminated, systemic aspergillar infection are life-threatening conditions that usually occur in immunocompromised patients, often following prolonged treatment with broad-spectrum antibiotics.

1. **Presenting signs and symptoms** of invasive aspergillosis can mimic acute bacterial pneumonia with fever, cough, and pleuritic chest pain. A syndrome indistinguishable from gram-negative septic shock may be seen.

2. **Pathogenesis.** Invasive pulmonary aspergillosis is nearly always associated with defective neutrophil number or function, as occurs during organ transplantation or induction chemotherapy for acute leukemia. Less common predisposing factors include prolonged corticosteroid therapy, alcoholism, diabetes mellitus, and chronic renal failure. Phagocytic defenses are relatively preserved in HIV-1 infection, and invasive aspergillosis is among the less frequent mycotic complications in the HIV-infected host. An occurrence in this setting is usually associated with end-stage AIDS and neutropenia. It may also rarely occur in apparently normal hosts.

   a. The pathologic spectrum of aspergillus lung disease includes acute bronchopneumonia, angioinvasive disease with tissue necrosis, miliary infection, chronic necrotizing pneumonitis, tracheobronchitis, and pleural involvement. Acute mycetomas may arise in the course of disease when necrotic cavities become filled with hyphae.

3. **Diagnosis.** Chest x-ray findings include virtually any pattern, with multifocal infiltrates being the most common. Patterns indicating pulmonary infarction are frequent and suggest the possibility of invasive aspergillosis in a compatible clinical setting. Acute infiltrates may cavitate and progress to mycetomas.

   a. Although the culture yield from bronchoalveolar lavage (BAL) is approximately 50%, definitive diagnosis of invasive pulmonary aspergillosis requires tissue obtained by transbronchial or open lung biopsy, since aspergilli can be airway saprophytes. However, positive fungal culture of sputum or BAL fluid from an immunosuppressed patient in a compatible clinical setting is suggestive of invasive disease and may be a sufficient basis for initiating treatment.

   b. Empiric treatment is often initiated in the absence of any culture data in febrile neutropenic patients unresponsive to antibiotic therapy. Serologic tests are not helpful for the diagnosis of acute invasive aspergillosis, and a test for *Aspergillus* antigens is not yet widely available.

4. **Treatment.** Amphotericin B remains the drug of choice for life-threatening invasive aspergillosis; prompt initiation of therapy is crucial for rapidly progressive disease. Itraconazole may be used in less critical situations.

   a. Administration of amphotericin B for aspergillosis follows guidelines that are generally applicable to the treatment of other pulmonary mycoses. Amphotericin B should be started with a test dose of 1 mg IV, followed by the full therapeutic dose in 2–4 hours if the test dose is tolerated. In a critically ill patient, the test dose may be skipped. A daily dose of 1.0–1.5 mg/kg given over 2–4 hours should be administered until a cumulative dose of 1–4 g is achieved, generally over 1–4 months. Lower daily doses of 0.3–0.6 mg/kg may be used for indolent infection.

b. Premedication with acetaminophen and meperidol with every dose is recommended to minimize the fevers, chills, and myalgias that can occur during amphotericin B infusion. The risk of thrombophlebitis may be reduced by alternating venous access sites if peripheral veins are used for infusion.

c. Amphotericin B treatment may be accompanied by significant toxicity, including renal dysfunction with azotemia, renal tubular acidosis, hypokalemia, and hypomagnesemia. When the serum creatinine level exceeds 3 mg/dL during amphotericin B treatment, the drug should be held for several days and reinstituted at a lower dose or on alternate days. The duration of treatment depends on the clinical response and the underlying condition of the patient. Decisions regarding the duration of treatment should be made in consultation with a pulmonary or infectious disease specialist.

d. A liposomal preparation of amphotericin B with reduced potential for renal toxicity has recently become available. It has been initially approved for salvage therapy in patients whose infections are not responding to conventional administration or who are having unacceptable toxicity. The indications for using the liposomal preparation are likely to expand in the coming years. It may become the first-line treatment for patients with coexisting renal failure. Consultation with an infectious diseases specialist regarding its use is advised.

e. The addition of flucytosine or rifampin to conventional amphotericin B therapy for possible synergy has not been demonstrated to be beneficial in acute invasive or systemic aspergillosis. Itraconazole (200 mg PO BID) may be used to treat invasive pulmonary aspergillosis in less acutely ill patients, particularly those with AIDS. Itraconazole may also be used for secondary prophylaxis (200 mg/d PO) in patients with chronic immunodeficiency. It may also prove beneficial for secondary prophylaxis during induction chemotherapy in patients previously treated for invasive aspergillosis or undergoing a second round of intensive chemotherapy.

    i. Food enhances the absorption of itraconazole, while drugs that decrease gastric acidity reduce absorption. Rifampin, phenobarbital, phenytoin, cisapride, and carbamazepine, among others, decrease serum itraconazole levels, while itraconazole increases serum concentrations of cyclosporine, digoxin, terfenadine, and astemizole. The latter two have been associated with cardiac arrhythmias including torsades de pointes (12).

    ii. Common adverse effects of itraconazole include nausea and abdominal discomfort. Edema and hypokalemia may occur with high doses, and hepatitis has been reported. No dosage adjustment is required for renal or hepatic failure

III. Histoplasmosis. *Histoplasma capsulatum* is present in temperate areas around the world and is one of the most widely disseminated pathogenic fungi in the United States (13). Over 20% of the United States population are estimated to be histoplasmin skin test reactors, while in endemic areas, the valleys of the Ohio and Mississippi Rivers, >80% of residents are positive. Fortunately, acute and chronic disease caused by infection with *H. capsulatum* is relatively infrequent, compared with the degree of exposure.

A. Presenting signs and symptoms of histoplasmosis depend on host factors, including immune function, previous infection with the fungus, and the presence of chronic lung disease. Acute pulmonary histoplasmosis is usually an unrecognized asymptomatic event in normal hosts, although it may present as a typical flu-like illness with fever, chills, headache, arthralgia, myalgia, and cough. The disease is usually self-limited and resolves within 2 weeks. Occasionally, more severe or complicated illness may occur in apparently normal hosts. This may include arthritis, erythema nodosum, pleural or pericardial effusion, or bronchial obstruction due to enlarged mediastinal lymph nodes. Although rare, severe acute pneumonia and respiratory failure in normal hosts can occur following heavy exposure to infectious microconidia. Inactive infection in normal individuals is often identified by coin lesions on chest x-ray that must be differentiated from neoplasms.

1. **The presentation of histoplasmosis in abnormal hosts** depends on the specific underlying host defect. Patients with impaired cell-mediated immunity can develop progressive disseminated histoplasmosis with subacute onset of fevers, fatigue, malaise, and weight loss. More acute presentations include life-threatening pneumonitis, respiratory failure, and septic shock. Alternatively, patients with underlying chronic lung disease may develop chronic pulmonary histoplasmosis with clinical features resembling tuberculosis. These patients experience waxing and waning symptoms of cough, fever, and weight loss.

B. **Etiology and pathogenesis.** *H. capsulatum* is a dimorphic fungus found in mycelial form in soil and in yeast form at body temperature in the infected host. Infection follows exposure to microconidia released in dust from soil during mycelial growth. Disturbance of soil containing bird droppings or decaying organic matter during construction or demolition activities can result in heavy exposure to spores. Following inhalation, microconidia germinate into yeasts within several days. An early neutrophil response is effective against the microconidia, but not against yeast. The yeast are partially contained by alveolar macrophages, leading to subclinical dissemination and the induction of cell-mediated immunity and an effective granulomatous response. The outcome of infection is determined by the intensity of the initial exposure and the adequacy of the host response.

1. **Normal hosts** may have no clinically apparent disease or self-limited **acute pulmonary histoplasmosis** (Table 9-2) that progresses in a subacute fashion with mild systemic symptoms, anemia, and liver function test abnormalities. Chest involvement is marked by diffuse and progressive infiltrates.

   a. A less frequent presentation of symptomatic disease following *H. capsulatum* infection is **chronic pulmonary histoplasmosis**. This typically occurs in patients with chronic obstructive lung disease and shares many clinical features with tuberculosis, although it is less severe. Chest involvement is marked by fibrocalcific changes in the lung apices, cavity formation, and pleural reaction. Repeated bouts of exacerbated pneumonitis are followed by scarring and cavity formation with progressive loss of functioning parenchyma.

   b. With **fibrosing mediastinitis**, chest disease may progress even in the absence of active infection. In this condition, morbidity arises not from proliferation of the fungus but from an excessive inflammatory and fibrotic reaction to previous infection. Compression of pulmonary or systemic arteries and veins, airways, or the esophagus can occur. Fibrosing mediastinitis due to histoplasmosis is associated with characteristic radiologic features (eggshell calcifications of mediastinal and hilar nodes) that distinguish it from other causes of this disorder (14). The response to therapy is poor, and death from respiratory failure, cor pulmonale, superior vena cava syndrome, or other complications occurs in as many as 20% of such cases.

2. **In patients with impaired cellular immune function, progressive disseminated histoplasmosis** may occur following primary exposure to the organism or by reactivation of latent infection. Multiple organs in addition to the lung are involved, including the central nervous system, bone and joints, heart valves, liver, spleen, lymph nodes, bone marrow, and adrenal glands. A more

Table 9-2. Clinical presentation of histoplasmosis

Acute pulmonary histoplasmosis (often a mild self-limited illness)

Chronic pulmonary histoplasmosis (shares clinical features with tuberculosis)

Progressive disseminated histoplasmosis (associated with defective cell-mediated immunity)

rapid course may be seen particularly in AIDS patients, with a clinical picture of septic shock and acute respiratory failure (15).

C. Diagnosis

1. The **histoplasmin skin test is not useful** for diagnosis because of the high incidence of positive reactions in the general population, the lack of correlation with disease activity, and the possibility of reversion from positive to negative reactions over time. The histoplasmin skin test may also cause a rise in serum antibodies to *H. capsulatum* and *Coccidioides immitis* in patients previously exposed to those fungi.

2. **Complement fixation** is the most useful diagnostic serologic test. Serum titers >1:32 suggest acute disease, while cerebrospinal fluid (CSF) titers >1:8 are evidence of meningeal involvement.

3. The **immunodiffusion test** is more specific than complement fixation and may be useful when the complement fixation result is borderline. Antigen detection tests for blood, urine, and spinal fluid are becoming more generally available and are particularly useful for monitoring the response to therapy. A majority of patients with disseminated histoplasmosis will have antigen detected in the serum or urine, while positive results are less frequently seen in mild disease.

4. A definitive diagnosis is established by culture, and the yield is influenced by the manner of disease presentation. Sputum culture is infrequently positive in acute pulmonary histoplasmosis, but sputum and particularly BAL fluid are frequently positive in disseminated or chronic pulmonary forms of the disease. In disseminated histoplasmosis, other sources with a high yield of positive cultures include bone marrow, blood, urine, and spinal fluid. Overall, >90% of disseminated cases will have a positive culture from at least one site.

D. Treatment is not required for most cases of acute pulmonary histoplasmosis in normal hosts but should be considered when symptoms continue for >2 weeks. A 2-week course of itraconazole (200 mg PO BID) or intravenous amphotericin B totaling 500 mg is probably sufficient. More aggressive treatment is indicated for cases of severe exposure, chronic pulmonary disease, or disseminated histoplasmosis. Amphotericin B in a total dose of up to 3 g is recommended for progressive disseminated histoplasmosis. Alternatively, patients who stabilize rapidly after receiving at least 500 mg of amphotericin B may be switched to itraconazole (200 mg PO BID) for at least 6 months.

1. **AIDS patients** treated for histoplasmosis have a high rate of relapse, and amphotericin B therapy in these patients should be followed by lifelong suppression with itraconazole (200–400 mg/d PO). Serum concentrations of itraconazole should be measured periodically because of erratic absorption and multiple drug interactions.

2. Amphotericin B is also effective in **chronic pulmonary histoplasmosis**, although itraconazole is an effective alternative therapy. Itraconazole should be given orally for 12 months or 6 months beyond achieving sputum conversion. Ketoconazole (400–800 mg/d PO) is a less expensive option but has significant side effects, including suppression of plasma testosterone with gynecomastia and decreased libido in men and menstrual irregularities in women. Mild hepatic toxicity is common and the drug must be discontinued if jaundice or symptomatic hepatitis occurs.

3. Hemoptysis occurring as a complication of chronic airways disease may require surgical intervention.

IV. Coccidioidomycosis. *C. immitis* is a dimorphic fungus endemic in the southwestern United States. Infection is acquired by inhalation of spores, with outdoor activities, excavation work, and exposure to windstorms the most common risks. The disease has myriad presentations (16).

A. Presenting signs and symptoms of coccidioidomycosis (as with histoplasmosis) depend on the infecting dose and the immune status of the host (Table 9-3).

1. **Primary pulmonary coccidioidomycosis** commonly presents with cough, fever, and headache. A skin rash is present in 50% of cases, and erythema no-

Table 9-3. Clinical presentation of coccidioidomycosis

Primary pulmonary coccidioidomycosis (valley fever)
Persistent primary coccidioidomycosis
Chronic pulmonary coccidioidomycosis
    Cavitary disease
    Fibrocalcific disease
    Chronic progressive pulmonary coccidioidomycosis
Disseminated coccidioidomycosis
Coccidioides meningitis

---

dosum or erythema multiforme is present in >10%. Most cases present with minor, transient symptoms and do not require medical attention.

2. **Persistent primary coccidioidomycosis** is characterized by continuous symptoms for longer than 1 month, often with a very productive cough and chest pain. Stable pulmonary infiltrates are seen on chest x-ray, and the symptoms neither progress nor resolve.

3. **Coccidioidal pneumonia** may be encountered in otherwise normal hosts following heavy exposure or in patients with moderate defects in antifungal defenses. The clinical presentation ranges from fatigue and cough to an acute septic condition with extensive pneumonia, pleural effusion, cavitation, and respiratory failure. Roentgenographic features of primary coccidioidal pneumonia include patchy subsegmental infiltrates, often with hilar lymphadenopathy. Severe cases will progress to lobar consolidation; necrosis is common, with cavity formation leading to hemoptysis or hydropneumothorax. When miliary disease, respiratory failure, or the adult respiratory distress syndrome occurs, mortality is high.

4. **Disseminated coccidioidomycosis** occurs when the host fails to contain the initial coccidioidal lung infection. Despite the systemic nature of the infection, the clinical presentation may range from mild to severe. Patients typically present with fever, sweats, dyspnea, and a miliary pattern on chest x-ray.

   a. Single or multiple nodular skin lesions from disseminated infection may be seen after the chest x-ray has cleared and may be the only identifiable site of extrapulmonary disease. Alternatively, extensive skin lesions may develop during the early presentation of disseminated disease in more severe cases.

   b. Dissemination to the meninges (coccidioidal meningitis) may be mild initially, with an ordinary headache as the only presenting symptom. More advanced cases will demonstrate meningismus and abnormalities of gait and mental status.

   c. Local symptoms may also arise from bone or joint infection. Soft tissue abscesses may arise in virtually any organ and produce symptoms related to a mass effect without the pain and tenderness associated with pyogenic infection.

B. **Pathogenesis.** Following inhalation, arthroconidia shift from a saprobic to a parasitic growth cycle with the generation of spherules that multiply as a result of the formation of endospores. Infection is rarely acquired by percutaneous inoculation. The initial dose of arthroconidia inhaled along with a variety of host factors determines the outcome. Clinical evidence suggests that disseminated disease affects men more often than women, and the risks are higher for African-Americans and Asians than for European-Americans, and for infants and the elderly than for other age groups. The infected host responds to the fungal spherule via multiple cellular (neutrophils, macrophages, T lymphocytes, NK cells) pathways.

   1. The importance of **T-lymphocyte function** in defense against coccidioidomycosis is underscored by the impact of coinfection with HIV-1 on the outcome

of disease. Coccidioidomycosis in patients with AIDS may be primary or result from reactivation of latent infection. Extensive and severe pulmonary infiltration and extrapulmonary dissemination with a high mortality are more likely in AIDS, although milder presentations have been recognized (17).

2. **Patients receiving chemotherapy**, immunosuppression for organ transplantation, and high-dose corticosteroid therapy are all at greater risk for severe coccidioidal lung infection and dissemination.

3. **Chronic sequelae** of coccidioidal lung infection include cavities that may become secondarily infected with bacteria or mycetomas that result in cough and hemoptysis. Fibrocalcific scarring may occur, similar to that in histoplasmosis and tuberculosis. These lesions are typically stable, but a chronic progressive symptomatic fibrocavitary disease may occur in some individuals. Previous coccidioidomycosis can leave patients with solitary or multiple pulmonary nodules that may raise the suspicion of malignancy in certain settings.

C. **Diagnosis.** A definitive diagnosis of coccidioidomycosis is established by the identification of *C. immitis* in clinical specimens. While person-to-person spread of the organism does not occur, growth of the fungus in the laboratory and spread to hospital personnel easily occurs; *C. immitis* should be considered an extreme biohazard. The organism can be isolated from BAL fluid, transbronchial biopsy specimens, skin biopsies, and body fluids including blood, urine, CSF, and pleural fluid. When pleural disease is present, pleural biopsy provides a better diagnostic yield than simple thoracentesis. In cases of disseminated disease, bone scan should be performed to identify subclinical lesions that may progress during antifungal treatment and may require surgical debridement.

1. **Serologic tests** for coccidioidomycosis can be useful adjuncts when biopsy or culture data are lacking. Mild-to-moderate lung infection is usually associated with IgG complement fixation titers $\geq 1:8$, and the titer typically declines within 6 months following clinical resolution. A rising titer $\geq 1:32$ is an early indication of dissemination; the overall disease activity correlates well with the level of complement-fixing antibody. Very high antibody levels suggest a poor outcome.

2. **Skin testing** is of limited value because acute disease cannot be distinguished from remote infection, the response may be suppressed during active disease, and the frequency of cross-reactions is high.

D. **Treatment.** While self-limited cases of valley fever require no treatment, the type and duration of treatment for intermediate cases may sometimes be less clear. Treatment is usually offered to patients with pulmonary coccidioidomycosis at risk for dissemination, with mild but prolonged symptomatic lung disease, and with extensive pulmonary involvement. These cases may be treated with itraconazole (200 mg PO BID), fluconazole (400–600 mg/d PO), or ketoconazole (400 mg/d PO). The drug of first choice has not been established, but relapse rates, toxicity, and drug interactions appear to be less frequent with itraconazole than with fluconazole or ketoconazole.

1. All cases of **disseminated disease** must be treated with systemic amphotericin B up to 3 g total dose. In stable cases, a minimum of 1 g amphotericin B may be followed by an azole for 1 year. Severe refractory cases may require as much as 6 g. Patients with significant toxic symptoms may be given 50 mg/d of amphotericin B until symptoms are controlled, followed by a taper from alternate day to twice-weekly administration over 3–6 months.

2. Patients with **AIDS** and coccidioidomycosis do not respond as well to initial treatment and must be placed on indefinite suppressive therapy with an azole or amphotericin B.

3. Because of **poor penetration to the central nervous system,** intrathecal amphotericin B should be given to patients with coccidioidal meningitis by repeated lumbar puncture or by reservoir under the direction of infectious disease and neurosurgical specialists. High-dose fluconazole (800–1600 mg/d) is an effective alternative to amphotericin B in the treatment of coccidioidal meningitis, but lifelong administration of the drug may be required.

V. **Cryptococcosis.** *Cryptococcus neoformans* is a yeast found worldwide, associated with bird droppings. In the infected host, the yeast produces a characteristic thick capsule that is a virulence factor and also serves as the basis for a sensitive diagnostic antigen test. The exposure rate for humans is unknown in the absence of a diagnostic skin test, but presumably it is quite high, given the ubiquitous distribution of the fungus. Cryptococcosis is rare in immunocompetent hosts but is the most common life-threatening mycotic infection in AIDS. Up to 10% of persons infected with HIV-1 develop cryptococcosis during the course of their disease (18).

A. **Presenting signs and symptoms** of pulmonary infection with *C. neoformans* vary greatly, depending on the immune status of the host.

   1. **Normal host.** Although the lung is the portal of entry, pulmonary infection is asymptomatic in the majority of immunocompetent individuals. Pneumonia in an immunocompetent host is characterized by low-grade fever and cough with a single or multiple nodules on chest x-ray. *C. neoformans* has a strong predilection for the central nervous system and often presents as meningitis in the absence of identifiable lung involvement.

   2. **Immunodeficient host.** Individuals with immunodeficiencies due to malignancy, immunosuppressive therapies, or HIV-1 infection may present with severe cryptococcal pneumonia. Findings range from diffuse nodular interstitial infiltrates with respiratory failure in the most profoundly immunosuppressed AIDS patients, to single or multiple nodules with or without cavitation and associated hilar lymphadenopathy in those with less severe decrements in immune status. No single clinical feature readily distinguishes cryptococcal infection from other pulmonary mycoses, inflammatory lung diseases, or metastatic malignancies.

B. **Pathogenesis.** Following inhalation, yeast that reach the alveolar compartment may be eliminated by primary phagocytic defenses or through cell-mediated immune responses. If not contained, the organism disseminates and has a predilection for the central nervous system, skin, and prostate. There may be minimal inflammation, or an exuberant granulomatous response may develop. Since *C. neoformans* elaborates no toxins, no tissue necrosis, hemorrhage, or fibrocalcific scarring occurs, in contrast to other mycoses. Even with clinically apparent cryptococcal lung infection, dissemination in normal hosts is rare, and spontaneous resolution is frequent. The single most important risk factor for disseminated cryptococcosis is a defect in cell-mediated immunity; no increased risk is associated with either neutropenia or an isolated impairment of humoral immunity.

C. **Timely diagnosis** of cryptococcosis often depends on a high index of clinical suspicion. The frequent occurrence of cryptococcal meningitis and of skin involvement (characterized by multiple nodules or circumscribed ulcers) in disseminated cryptococcosis provides important clues to early diagnosis.

   1. **Cryptococcal pneumonia** may be readily diagnosed by bronchoscopy (BAL or transbronchial biopsy) or CT-guided fine-needle aspiration.

   2. **Lumbar puncture** is the diagnostic procedure of first choice if neurologic symptoms are present.

   3. **Serology.** While no clinically useful antibody test exists for cryptococcosis, cryptococcal antigen may be detected in the blood, urine, or CSF. Antigen is nearly always present in the serum with disseminated disease but may be absent in cases of isolated lung infection.

   4. **Invasive testing.** A positive culture, a positive cryptococcal antigen test, or a positive India ink capsule stain of CSF obviates the need for more invasive tests in cases with compatible chest x-ray findings and appropriate clinical settings. Examination of swabs and biopsies of skin lesions can provide a rapid diagnosis of disseminated disease. Detection of the antigen in serum mandates lumbar puncture even in the absence of neurologic symptoms or signs. Yeast may be cultured from blood, CSF, BAL fluid, and urine and can be detected in cytologic specimens or biopsies by mucicarmine or silver stains.

D. **Treatment** of isolated pulmonary cryptococcosis with amphotericin B is usually not necessary in the immunocompetent host, if disseminated infection is excluded by testing serum and CSF for cryptococcal antigen, as well as by culturing blood, CSF, and urine (following prostate massage). However, with the availability and safety of the newer azoles, many physicians would elect to treat most patients with pulmonary cryptococcosis for several weeks until clinical improvement is apparent. The majority of immunosuppressed patients with cryptococcal pneumonia will progress to disseminated disease if not treated.

   1. **All cases of cryptococcal meningitis or any form of disseminated disease** should be treated with amphotericin B alone (0.5–0.8 mg/kg/d IV) or in combination with flucytosine (75–150 mg/kg/d in four divided doses). Flucytosine treatment is often limited by potentially lethal bone marrow toxicity and enterocolitis. Its metabolite, fluorouracil, accumulates in renal failure. The dose of flucytosine should be adjusted to provide peak serum levels of 60–80 µg/mL and trough levels of 20–40 µg/mL. Treatment should be continued for 4–6 weeks in immunocompetent individuals and in those with transient immunosuppression.

   2. **AIDS patients and possibly organ transplant recipients** with disseminated cryptococcal infection should receive suppressive treatment with fluconazole (200 mg/d PO) indefinitely. Fluconazole or itraconazole is a suitable alternative to amphotericin B in stable patients who cannot tolerate amphotericin B.

VI. **Blastomycosis.** *Blastomyces dermatitidis* is a dimorphic fungus present in soil. Originally thought to be localized to North America, it appears to be more widespread (19). Human disease occurs primarily in rural areas and is associated with outdoor activities. Clinically apparent blastomycosis is a rare disease. The number of identified cases is probably only a fraction of the incidence of minimally symptomatic or asymptomatic cases.

   A. **Presenting signs and symptoms** of blastomycosis vary from asymptomatic infection to acute disseminated disease. The lung is the portal of entry and site of primary infection. Disease is characterized by the acute onset of fever, chills, arthralgia and myalgia. A productive cough is often seen, and the clinical picture may resemble acute bacterial pneumonia. Chest x-ray findings are quite variable, with nodules, large round infiltrates, lobar consolidation, and acute lung injury patterns reported. The clinical course is unpredictable; the infection is self-limited in about one-third of cases, while others may progress rapidly to fulminant pneumonia. Relapse may occur locally or at distant sites years after resolution of an initial infection. Disseminated disease may present with meningeal signs or cutaneous nodules or ulcers. A predilection for the prostate has been noted in patients with disseminated disease. Erythema nodosum has been reported.

   B. **Pathogenesis.** Inhaled arthrospores reaching the alveolar compartment convert to the parasitic yeast form. A primary neutrophilic pneumonitis is followed by a granulomatous response that may contain the infection with a moderate degree of residual fibrosis and limited calcification, compared with histoplasmosis or coccidioidomycosis. Lung and mediastinal infections may involve vertebral and chest wall structures and lead to fistula formation similar to that in actinomycosis. In the absence of an effective cell-mediated response, dissemination occurs with involvement of skin, bone, meninges, prostate, or adrenal glands. Disseminated infection is therefore more common in patients with defects in T-lymphocyte number or function and is virtually always associated with progressive disease.

   C. **Diagnosis.** *B. dermatitidis* is readily isolated from sputum, pus, or other clinical specimens. The organism is slow-growing and may require up to 3 weeks to be identified. Potassium hydroxide preparations of sputum are simple and rapid and have a relatively high yield. The large yeasts (8–15 µm) have a characteristic broad-based bud. Transbronchial biopsies or biopsies of other affected tissues should be stained with silver for the best yield. No clinically useful serologic test is available.

   D. **Treatment** may not be needed for cases of mild isolated pulmonary disease in immunocompetent hosts. Treatment is mandated whenever the infection does not resolve, the pneumonitis is severe, dissemination has occurred, or the host is immunodeficient.

      1. Fulminant infection should be treated with amphotericin B to a total dose of at least 2 g. Patients stabilized on amphotericin B may be switched to itraconazole (100–200 mg PO BID) or ketoconazole (400–800 mg/d PO) for a minimum 6-month course.

2. Less critically ill patients should be treated initially with itraconazole. Fluconazole in doses of 400 mg/d or less has been associated with higher failure and relapse rates than itraconazole.

VII. Paracoccidioidomycosis. The dimorphic fungus *Paracoccidioides brasiliensis* is endemic in subtropical Latin and South America (particularly Brazil), but sporadic cases are imported to the United States and may be encountered more frequently because of rising immigration.

   A. Presenting signs and symptoms depend on the patient's age and preexisting state of health. The infection is asymptomatic and subclinical in many cases. In children, and patients of any age with defective cell-mediated immunity, the disease may present with fever, weight loss, leukocytosis, eosinophilia, lymphadenopathy, hepatosplenomegaly, or ulcerated skin lesions (20). In this setting, pulmonary involvement is uncommon. Immunocompetent adults present with a more chronic illness limited to the lung and characterized by cough, fever, and sputum production. Mucocutaneous lesions or lymph node involvement may be present, with the latter resembling scrofula. Unifocal or multifocal infiltrates on chest x-ray can progress to bilateral perihilar infiltration with hilar lymph node enlargement. Resolution is associated with scarring and cavity formation. Reactivation of latent foci may occur.

   B. Pathogenesis. Infection is acquired by inhalation of conidia and may be limited to the lung or may hematogenously disseminate. The course of disease is typically chronic and progressive, with both granulomatous and suppurative lesions seen histopathologically. The relative infrequency of apical involvement, pleural effusion, or calcification helps discriminate paracoccidioidomycosis from tuberculosis and histoplasmosis.

   C. Diagnosis is based on the demonstration of the fungus in clinical specimens. Sputum, BAL fluid, purulent drainage from involved lymph nodes, or tissue biopsies may reveal spherical yeasts with double refractile walls and one or more thin-necked buds on silver-stained preparations. The organism can be easily cultured; serologic tests are clinically useful, as most patients will generate a humoral response. Changes in antibody titer over time provide useful information for prognosis and monitoring the response to treatment. Paracoccidioidomycosis can mimic tuberculosis, other mycoses, and Wegener's granulomatosis.

   D. Treatment for severe disease may be initiated with amphotericin B to a total dose of at least 1.5 g, followed by a 6-month course of itraconazole (200 mg PO BID). In less severe cases, itraconazole or fluconazole (200–400 mg/d PO) alone is sufficient. Ketoconazole (200–400 mg/d PO) and sulfadiazine (4–6 g/d) are alternatives.

VIII. Pulmonary mucormycosis. Pulmonary mucormycoses are rare but often fatal infections caused by one of several related fungi. Within the class Zygomycetes are the orders Murcorales and Entomophthorales. The former includes *Rhizopus* and *Mucor* species, as well as *Absidia corymbifera*, all of which have varying degrees of pathogenic potential. In contrast, organisms of the order Entomophthorales are generally not pulmonary pathogens. These thermotolerant fungi are commonly found in decaying organic matter and cause disease in compromised hosts.

   A. Presenting signs and symptoms of pulmonary mucormycosis include fever and pulmonary infiltrates resistant to empiric antibiotic therapy, in the setting of neutrophil deficiency. These fulminant infections resemble invasive aspergillosis with progressive vascular invasion leading to pulmonary infarction and hemoptysis with late dissemination. Chest x-ray findings include pneumonic infiltrates and consolidation, cavitation, and acute mycetoma. On chest CT scan, upper lobe nodules or wedge-shaped consolidation are the most frequent findings (21).

   B. Pathogenesis. Three typical patterns of mucormycosis are recognized: pulmonary infection (associated with neutropenia or high-dose corticosteroid therapy), rhinocerebral infection (associated with diabetes mellitus), and disseminated infection. Pulmonary disease is acquired by inhalation of asexual sporangiospores that germinate and develop hyphae unless cleared by alveolar macrophages. A locally invasive bronchopneumonia ensues, marked by hyphal invasion of blood vessels with infarction and hemorrhage. Rarely, a more subacute infection may be seen.

   C. Diagnosis of pulmonary mucormycosis requires a biopsy of affected tissue for culture and histologic examination. The infection may be suggested by the rapid progression of pneumonia and infarction in the typical host. Sputum examination is often negative, while a positive result in a compromised host with fever and pulmonary infiltrates should not be dismissed. Skin or mucocutaneous lesions should always be biopsied. No useful serologic test is available.

D.   Treatment. Amphotericin B is the drug of choice for pulmonary mucormycosis and is given to a total dose of 2–4 g. In severe cases, high-dose treatment of 1–1.5 mg/kg/d may be needed. There is no proven synergy with flucytosine, azoles, or other drugs. Surgical debridement, often required for rhinocerebral disease, may be beneficial in selected cases of lung infection (22).

IX.   Sporotrichosis. The dimorphic fungus *Sporothrix schenckii* is a very rare cause of lung disease. Infection with this saprophytic organism with worldwide distribution usually occurs following cutaneous infection through exposure to rose thorns, timber, or sphagnum moss.

A.   Presenting signs and symptoms. Symptomatic pulmonary sporotrichosis is an indolent disease characterized by cough and low-grade systemic symptoms. Chest x-ray reveals fibronodular upper lobe infiltrates, often with cavity formation, that may be mistaken for tuberculosis.

B.   Pathogenesis. Lung disease is acquired by inhalation of spores and may often escape detection. In addition to subacute lung infection, hematogenous dissemination may occur. Alcoholism and chronic obstructive pulmonary disease have been recognized as risk factors for pulmonary disease (23). In the setting of AIDS, the infection may be disseminated and respond poorly to treatment (24).

C.   Diagnosis may be made from an examination of sputum or lung biopsy specimens but cannot be established by morphology alone. Definitive diagnosis requires fungal culture or a positive direct fluorescent antibody test. Serum agglutinins may be useful, but a negative result does not exclude the diagnosis.

D.   Treatment consists of amphotericin B given to a total dose of 2 g in most cases. Surgery may also be curative when disease is limited. Iodides used for cutaneous infection are of no benefit for lung disease. Experience with azoles is limited, but itraconazole, which is very useful for the more common lymphocutaneous manifestation of sporotrichosis, may also be effective for treating pulmonary sporotrichosis.

X.   *Candidal* pneumonia. While various infections due to *Candida* species are among the most frequent clinical mycoses, lung infection is very rare. *Candida albicans* and *C. tropicalis* are the most common pathogens. Ubiquitous throughout the world, they are normal residents of human skin, the gastrointestinal tract, and the female genital tract.

A.   Presenting signs and symptoms of candidal pneumonia are nonspecific but typically include sustained fever and pneumonitis unresponsive to antibiotic therapy in a compromised host. Chest x-ray findings include patchy pneumonic or diffuse infiltrates. Cavitation is distinctly rare. Advanced disease may present with septic shock.

B.   Pathogenesis. Candidal pneumonia in adults probably most often results from hematogenous dissemination. Predisposing factors include disruption of the skin or mucosal barriers, intensive broad-spectrum antibiotic therapy (typically for febrile neutropenia), and total parenteral nutrition.

C.   Diagnosis requires documentation of lung invasion, since *Candida* is frequently found in sputum or BAL fluid in the absence of infection (25). Transbronchial or open lung biopsy are high yield procedures, but patients are often too medically compromised to undergo these procedures. Treatment is often initiated empirically. Endophthalmitis or skin lesions from disseminated infection may aid in the diagnosis when present.

D.   Treatment. Amphotericin B (0.5–1.0 mg/kg IV) has been considered the drug of choice for candidal pneumonia, with total doses of 1.5–3 g typically given. Flucytosine (100–150 mg/kg/d PO) provides effective synergy and can be added as tolerated for documented infection. Fluconazole may also be used for this indication in selected patients. Experience with itraconazole is more limited.

XI.   Actinomycosis. Actinomycosis is an indolent infection caused by *Actinomyces israelii* or related species *(A. naeslundii, A. viscosus, A. myeri,* and *Arachnia propionica).*

These anaerobic bacteria are normal commensals of the oral cavity but may cause serious pulmonary, cervicofacial, or abdominal infections.

A. **Presenting signs and symptoms** of pulmonary actinomycosis include the insidious onset of productive cough, fever, and weight loss. Chest x-ray findings include dense or mass-like infiltrates, cavitation, and pleural effusion. Complete blood cell counts typically show a neutrophilic leukocytosis and anemia. Characteristic dense yellow colonies of bacteria called **sulfur granules** may be discharged from draining fistulas in the chest wall (or other sites of infection).

B. **Pathogenesis.** *Actinomyces* species cannot invade normal mucosa, but periodontal disease predisposes to cervicofacial infection and lung infection by aspiration. Pulmonary infection can also occur by hematogenous or lymphatic spread from oral lesions. The infection does not respect anatomic boundaries (26), passing through interlobar fissures and frequently forming abscesses and fistulas through the chest wall or vertebrae (but without spread to the disc space). An intense neutrophilic inflammatory response is incited with production of white odorless pus.

C. **Diagnosis** may be complicated by the fact that these organisms are normal upper respiratory tract flora. The diagnosis is suggested by finding sulfur granules (which do not contain sulfur, despite their coloration) in sputum or fistula drainage. Potassium hydroxide preparations reveal typical branching mycelia that are not readily distinguished from *Nocardia*. The organism may be cultured anaerobically from BAL fluid or biopsies, fine-needle aspirates, blood, or abscesses. No serologic test is available for the diagnosis of actinomycosis.

D. **Treatment.** Penicillin is the drug of choice for actinomycosis and should be given in doses of 10–20 million U/d for severe infection. Treatment with parenteral followed by oral penicillin should be continued for 6–12 months. Tetracycline or clindamycin are effective alternative agents.

XII. **Nocardiosis.** Nocardiosis is an indolent infection caused by *Nocardia asteroides* and related species. These aerobic, gram-positive bacteria grow in branching filaments and are found throughout the world. They are not a part of the normal human commensal flora.

A. **Presenting signs and symptoms** of nocardiosis include the subacute onset of pneumonia and/or lung abscess over weeks to months with fever, weight loss, and malaise. Remissions and exacerbations are common, and the infection may develop at a more rapid pace in immunosuppressed patients. Chest x-ray findings include infiltrates, nodules, cavitation, and empyema (27).

B. **Pathogenesis.** Pulmonary infection is most likely acquired by inhalation of airborne organisms. A neutrophilic inflammatory response leading to abscess formation is common, and the infection may spread to adjacent pericardium or mediastinum, but local spread is less common than in actinomycosis. Half of patients with pulmonary nocardiosis will experience dissemination to brain, sinuses, or skin. Nocardiosis typically occurs in compromised hosts, including patients with lymphoreticular neoplasms, a variety of chronic lung diseases (notably alveolar proteinosis), and AIDS.

C. **Diagnosis** may be suggested by finding gram-positive branching filamentous organisms in sputum. *Nocardia* organisms grow slowly in culture, so that blood cultures should be maintained for 30 days and urine and CSF should be concentrated to obtain the highest yields. For these reasons, notifying the bacteriology laboratory that nocardiosis is suspected is critical for proper handling of clinical specimens. Head CT scans should be obtained if neurologic symptoms are identified or if dissemination is suspected. No clinically useful serologic test is yet available.

D. **Treatment.** Sulfonamides are the drugs of choice for nocardiosis. Sulfisoxazole (4–12 g/d in four divided doses) or trimethoprim/sulfamethoxazole (8–20 mg/kg/d trimethoprim in four divided doses) should be given for 6–12 months, with longer courses when central nervous system infection is present. In patients unable to tolerate sulfonamides, minocycline, chloramphenicol, ampicillin, and amikacin have been used. Many strains of *Nocardia* are also susceptible to third-generation cephalosporins and other β-lactam antibiotics, as well as imipenem. Some patients with brain abscesses may require surgical intervention.

References

1. Sarosi GA, Davies SF, eds: *Fungal diseases of the lung*, 2nd ed. New York: Raven Press, 1993.
2. Kibbler CC, Mackenzie DWR, eds. *Principles and practice of clinical mycology.* Chichester, UK: Wiley, 1996.
3. Schwartz HJ, Greenberger PA: The prevalence of allergic bronchopulmonary aspergillosis in patients with asthma, determined by serologic and radiologic criteria in patients at risk. *J Lab Clin Med* 1991;117:138.
4. Kauffman HF, Tomee JF, van der Werf TS, et al.: Review of fungus-induced asthmatic reactions. *Am J Respir Crit Care Med* 1995;151:2109. (An up-to-date discussion of pathogenesis.)
5. Vaughan LM: Allergic bronchopulmonary aspergillosis. *Clin Pharm* 1993;12:24. (Reviews diagnostic criteria, clinical stages, and treatment.)
6. Denning DW, Van Wye JE, Lewiston NJ, Stevens DA: Adjunctive therapy of allergic bronchopulmonary aspergillosis with itraconazole. *Chest* 1991;100:813.
7. Roberts CM, Citron KM, Strickland B: Intrathoracic aspergilloma: role of CT in diagnosis and treatment. *Radiology* 1987;165:123.
8. Hargis J, Bone R, Stewart J, Rector N: Intracavitary amphotericin B in the treatment of symptomatic pulmonary aspergilloma. *Am J Med* 1980;68:389.
9. Jennings TS, Hardin TC: Treatment or aspergillosis with itraconazole. *Ann Pharmacother* 1993; 27:1206.
10. Kemper CA, Hostetler JS, Follansbee SE, et al.: Ulcerative and plaque-like tracheobronchitis due to infection with *Aspergillus* in patients with AIDS. *Clin Infect Dis* 1993;17:344.
11. Aquino SL, Kee ST, Warnock ML, Gamsu G: Pulmonary aspergillosis: image findings with pathologic correlation. *AJR* 1994;163:811.
12. *Med Lett* 1994;36:16. (A review of antifungal therapies.)
13. Goodwin RA Jr, Des Prez RM: Histoplasmosis: state of the art. *Am Rev Respir Dis* 1978:117:929.
14. Sherrick AD et al: The radiologic findings of fibrosing mediastinitis. *Chest* 1994;106:484.
15. Wheat J: Histoplasmosis and coccidioidomycosis in individuals with AIDS: a clinical review. *Infect Dis Clin North Am* 1994;8:467.
16. Stevens DA: Coccidioidomycosis. *N Engl J Med* 1995;332:1077.
17. Fish DG et al: Coccidioidomycosis during human immunodeficiency virus infection. *Medicine* 1990;69:384.
18. Eng RHK et al: Cryptococcal infections in patients with acquired immunodeficiency syndrome. *Am J Med* 1986;81:19.
19. Bradsher RW: A clinician's view of blastomycosis. *Curr Top Med Mycol* 1993;5:181.
20. Brummer E, Casteneda E, Restrepo A: Paracoccidioidomycosis: an update. *Clin Microbiol Rev* 1993;6:89.
21. Jamadar DA et al: Pulmonary zygomycosis: CT appearance. *J Comput Assist Tomogr* 1995;19:733.
22. Tedder M et al: Pulmonary mucormycosis: results of medical and surgical therapy. *Ann Thorac Surg* 1994;57:1044.
23. England DM, Hochholzer L: Sporothrix infection of the lung without cutaneous disease: primary pulmonary sporotrichosis. *Arch Pathol Lab Med* 1987;111:298.
24. Heller HM, Fuhrer J: Disseminated sporotrichosis in patients with AIDS: case report and review of the literature. *AIDS* 1991;5:1243.
25. Haron E et al: Primary *Candida* pneumonia: experience at a large cancer center and review of the literature. *Medicine* 1993;72:137.
26. Conant EF, Wechsler RJ: Actinomycosis and norcardiosis of the lung. *J Thorac Imaging* 1992; 7:75.
27. Buckley JA, Padhani AR, Kuhlman JE. CT features of pulmonary nocardiosis. *J Comput Assist Tomogr* 1995;19:726.

I. Introduction. Sarcoidosis is a **multisystemic disease of unknown etiology**. Noncaseating granulomas are characteristically found in involved organs. Sarcoidosis affects the lungs and thoracic lymph nodes but may involve any organ, especially the eyes, skin, liver, central nervous system (CNS), kidneys, and heart. Several organs systems may be involved simultaneously, or disease may become apparent after variable periods of time, even after pulmonary abnormalities have regressed. The diagnosis is established with clinical, radiologic, and histologic evidence. The course of sarcoidosis varies, and the prognosis depends on the clinical presentation and the organs involved. Many patients are asymptomatic despite organ involvement. The disease may undergo spontaneous resolution or may progress to pulmonary fibrosis and multiple organ system dysfunction. Corticosteroids are the therapy of choice.

II. Epidemiology and pathogenesis (1)

   A. The worldwide estimated prevalence of sarcoidosis is 10 cases per 100,000 population, based on radiologic patterns consistent with the diagnosis. In the United States, the prevalence is estimated at 10–40 per 100,000.

   1. Sarcoidosis is reported to be more common in some ethnic populations (eg, 40/100,000 in African-Americans, 36/100,000 in mainland Puerto Ricans). However, the prevalence data may be unreliable because there are variations in the clinic populations studied and the disease is often asymptomatic (2). While sarcoidosis has no sex predilection, some manifestations of the disease are more common in women (2). The disease generally begins in the third or fourth decade and tends to be rare in children and the elderly (3).

   B. The etiology of sarcoidosis remains unknown. Studies investigating the potential role of infectious, genetic, autoimmune/immunologic, or environmental factors have been unrevealing (4). The propensity to develop sarcoidosis may depend on genetic or environmental factors, with clusters of cases reported in identical twins and in certain families (5).

   C. Sarcoidosis is characterized by a compartmentalization of activated immune cells. This immunologic dysregulation is initially seen as a CD4-lymphocytic alveolitis, with subsequent formation of granulomas and occasionally fibrosis. Despite evidence of cellular activation at sites of granulomatous reactions, there is a paradoxical systemic anergy (6)

   1. Bronchoalveolar lavage (BAL) from patients with sarcoidosis shows a marked CD4+ lymphocytic alveolitis (7). This interstitial pneumonitis may be more prominent than granulomas. The CD4/CD8 ratio is increased by a factor of 6–10 (6). Numerous cytokines have been identified in the BAL fluid from patients with sarcoidosis: interleukin-1 (IL-1), IL-2; tumor necrosis factor-α (TNF-α), and interferon-γ (IFN-γ) (8). Recruitment, activation, and proliferation of T lymphocytes and blood monocytic cells by these and other cytokines may play an important role in the formation of granulomas (7).

   2. The hallmark of sarcoidosis is the noncaseating granuloma. The sarcoid granuloma consists of a central area of macrophages, epithelial cells, and Langhans' giant cells (fused epithelioid cells), surrounded by CD4 lymphocytes, monocytes, and fibroblasts (9). Granulomas probably represent a localized immune reaction to an as yet unidentified antigen and may occur in any organ. Once established, the granuloma may regress without scar formation, or subsequent fibroblast infiltration may result in hyalinizing fibrosis (10).

3. The pathogenesis of the **interstitial fibrosis** of sarcoidosis is not understood. Many cytokines identified with sarcoidosis, particularly IL-1, insulin-like growth factor 1 (IGF-1), and TNF-α, may play important roles. However, none of these is either predictive or universally associated with the fibrotic state (10).

4. **Cutaneous delayed-type hypersensitivity reactions** to skin test antigens, such as purified protein derivative (PPD) tuberculin, *Candida*, mumps, and streptokinase/streptodornase, are depressed (11). As many as two-thirds of patients with sarcoidosis will be anergic to PPD tuberculin (12). Despite this anergy, the distribution of memory T cells in the blood is normal, humoral immune responses are normal to hyperreactive, and opportunistic infections are rare (13). The mechanism of this anergic reaction in sarcoidosis is not understood.

III. **Clinical features**
A. **The signs and symptoms** will vary depending on the organs involved and the severity of involvement (12). **One of the hallmarks of this disease is the clinically silent nature of organ involvement.** Almost half of patients with sarcoidosis are asymptomatic, with incidental chest X-rays showing bilateral hilar adenopathy with or without parenchymal lung disease (14,15). Approximately 20% to 40% of the symptomatic patients have respiratory symptoms, and 10% to 40% have eye pain, rashes, arthralgias, or other symptoms (Table 10-1). Systemic symptoms such as fever, weight loss, or fatigue may be present in 20% to 30% of patients (15).

B. **Staging of disease** is assessed by chest x-ray appearance (12).

Stage
0: Normal chest x-ray.
I: Normal parenchyma with adenopathy.
II: Parenchymal changes and adenopathy.
III: Diffuse parenchymal changes without adenopathy.
IV: Advanced fibrosis.

C. Some patients with sarcoidosis present with distinct constellations of findings.
1. **Löfgren's syndrome** is characterized by the acute onset of erythema nodosum and/or migratory arthritis, uveitis, and hilar adenopathy (seen in 10% of patients).
2. **Heerfordt's syndrome** is characterized by fever, parotid enlargement, anterior uveitis, and facial nerve palsy (12).

D. **Subacute sarcoidosis**, sarcoidosis of <2 years' duration, usually occurs in younger patients and often undergoes spontaneous remission. **Chronic sarcoidosis**, with a duration >2 years, is characterized by a more insidious onset with constitutional symptoms. Chronic sarcoidosis often leads to fibrosis in the affected organs, including pulmonary fibrosis, retinal fibrosis, and nephrocalcinosis (15).

E. **Intrathoracic manifestations**
1. The common **pulmonary symptoms** include dry cough, dyspnea, and chest pain. Wheezing may occur when endobronchial involvement is present. Hemoptysis is infrequent and is usually associated with later stages of the disease (3,14,16).
2. **Thoracic adenopathy** may be totally asymptomatic, or impingement of the bronchi by enlarged lymph nodes may cause wheezing. The nodes are enlarged bilaterally and are nontender and mobile (12).

F. **Extrathoracic manifestations**
1. **Ocular manifestations** occur in approximately 25% of patients of sarcoidosis, most commonly manifested as uveitis, conjunctivitis, or lacrimal gland involvement. However, any part of the eye may be involved including the retina (15,17). Ocular involvement may be asymptomatic, and a thorough ophthalmologic examination (slit-lamp examination) is necessary in every patient with a suspected diagnosis of sarcoidosis. Ocular involvement may lead to visual loss in some patients.

Table 10-1. Sarcoidosis: organ involvement and clinical picture

	Organ involvement (%)	Clinically evident (%)	Symptoms	Physical exam
Lungs	90	30–50	Dyspnea, cough, wheezing	Wheezing
Intrathoracic lymph nodes	90	see text	Wheezing	Wheezing
Extrathoracic lymph nodes	40	30		Adenopathy
Skin	25	25	Nodules, plaques	
Eyes	33	20	Pain, tearing, photophobia	Conjunctivitis
Kidney	15	see text	Renal colic	Decreased mental status due to hypercalcemia
Nervous system	5–15	10	Headache, seizures, hearing loss, confusion, paresthesias	cranial nerve palsy, decreased mental status, abnormal sensory exam
Salivary glands	20	5	Dry mouth	
Liver	50–75	20		Hepatomegaly
Spleen	50	15		Splenomegaly
Musculoskeletal system	10–30	10	Arthritis, painful muscles	Abnormal joint exam
Heart	25	5	Syncope, dyspnea	Congestive heart failure

Not a complete listing. Data from Mayock R, Bertrand P, Morrison C. Manifestations of sarcoidosis. *Am J Med* 1963;35:67; Sharma O. Sarcoidosis. *Disease-a-Month* Sept:469, 1990; and Katz S. Clinical presentation and natural history of sarcoidosis. In: Fanburg B, ed. *Sarcoidosis and other granulomatous diseases of the lung*. New York: Marcel Dekker, 1983:3.

2. About 25% of patients will have **dermatologic manifestations**. The most common is erythema nodosum, present in up to one-third of patients (3,12). Typical lesions are shiny, erythematous, tender, and symmetrical and are usually found along the anterior aspect of the lower legs. **Lupus pernio**, a chronic violaceous induration on the face, nose, ears, and lips, may be associated with progressive pulmonary fibrosis, chronic uveitis, and bone cysts. Other skin lesions include plaques and maculopapular eruptions (12).

3. About 25% of patients with sarcoidosis will manifest **arthritis** involving the knees, ankles, elbows, and wrist. The arthritis may be transient, relapsing, or chronic. **Bone involvement**, usually asymptomatic and most commonly affecting the middle and distal phalanges of the fingers and toes, has been associated with skin lesions, particularly lupus pernio (12).

4. Sarcoidosis commonly affects the **liver**, and hepatic granulomas are found in 60% to 90% of patients (12,18). Hepatomegaly is appreciated in only 20%, and fever may be a prominent symptom in 50% of patients with liver involvement. Only 50% of liver granulomas found on liver biopsy can be attributed to sarcoidosis; other causes include infections (eg, tuberculosis, schistosomiasis) and other liver diseases (eg, primary biliary cirrhosis) (18).

5. About 15% of patients will have **renal involvement**, manifested as hypercalciuria (30% to 50%) and/or hypercalcemia (10% to 20%) that may result in nephrolithiasis (10%) or nephrocalcinosis (5%). Abnormal calcium metabolism results from increased levels of calcitriol produced by activated pulmonary sarcoid macrophages. Fewer than 5% of patients will develop nephrocalcinosis, but these account for 50% of sarcoidosis patients with renal insufficiency. Granulomatous infiltration of the kidney or renal arteries (leading to renal artery stenosis) may occur (19).

6. Asymptomatic **involvement of the spleen** occurs in about 50% of patients, but splenomegaly is seen in only about 15%. Hypersplenism (thrombocytopenia, anemia) and spontaneous rupture of the spleen may rarely occur once splenomegaly is present (12).

7. **Cardiac involvement** is present in approximately 20% of patients with sarcoidosis, although only 5% are recognized clinically (20). The most common cardiac manifestations are arrhythmias, conduction disturbances, chest pain, congestive heart failure, valvular dysfunction, and sudden death. This emphasizes the necessity of performing a full cardiac evaluation in all patients with sarcoid (20).

8. **Neurologic abnormalities** are clinically recognized in 5%, although careful neurologic evaluation can detect involvement in approximately 20% of patients (21). Symptoms are present in half of patients with neurosarcoidosis. Associated systemic manifestations of sarcoidosis are present in 50%, with thoracic manifestations being the most common. CNS manifestations include cranial nerve palsies (most commonly, facial nerve palsy), meningitis, space-occupying lesions, spinal cord abnormalities, hypothalamic and pituitary dysfunction leading to diabetes insipidus or endocrine failure, and peripheral neuropathies. These manifestations may result from granulomatous infiltration, hemorrhagic infarction, or demyelination (21).

9. **Peripheral lymphadenopathy,** particularly involving the cervical, axillary, epitrochlear, and inguinal nodes, is seen in 75% of patients.

10. Involvement of **other organ systems** is much less common, but sarcoidosis has been described in almost every organ (15).

G. **Physiology**
   1. **Pulmonary function tests**
      a. **Lung volumes** are preserved in stages 0 and I, including vital capacity (VC) and total lung capacity (TLC). Moderate-to-severe decreases in VC and TLC are present in two-thirds of stage II and III patients (22). However, advanced disease may be associated with cyst formation and subsequent increases in TLC.
      b. Most patients with pulmonary involvement will have a **decreased diffusing capacity** (D_LCO) (22). Because the D_LCO is so sensitive, a de-

crease may be found in patients with early stage I disease, but it will not be as severe as in the other stages (22).

c. An **obstructive physiologic pattern** seen in some patients is usually caused by granulomatous infiltration of the bronchial mucosa, enlarged hilar nodes compressing bronchi, or narrowing and distortion of peripheral airways by parenchymal fibrosis (22,23).

d. **Increases in the alveolar-arterial oxygen difference (A-a)Do$_2$** may occur in all stages of the disease. Approximately 50% of patients with stage II or stage III disease will have abnormal gas exchange (22). Resting hypoxemia is usually observed only in patients with advanced fibrotic disease. Exercise testing may help detect abnormal gas exchange in patients with normal arterial blood gases (24).

IV. **Differential diagnosis and approach**
   A. The differential diagnosis of pulmonary sarcoidosis is extensive and best approached by radiographic stage of disease.
      1. Tuberculosis and fungal infections are included in the differential diagnosis at all stages, stressing the importance of obtaining microbiologic data as part of the diagnostic approach. Other disease processes should be considered depending on the stage of disease (Table 10-2).
      2. Beryllium exposure induces a systemic granulomatous disease similar to sarcoidosis. Hypersensitivity pneumonitis is induced by exposure to specific antigens, with pathologic findings restricted to the lung. The specific precipitating antigen can often be identified, and the disease resolves after removal of the offending antigen. In contrast to sarcoidosis, the granulomas are less well defined and associated with a more diffuse mononuclear infiltrate (12).
   B. The diagnosis of sarcoidosis is made on the basis of compatible clinical, radiologic, and pathologic data. Microbiologic culture and special stains should be done to exclude tuberculous and fungal infection (15). Given the extensive differential diagnosis of sarcoidosis, the diagnostic criteria listed in Table 10-2 must be met in order to confidently make the diagnosis. Biochemical data may help detect extrapulmonary involvement and monitor disease activity.

Table 10-2. Differential diagnosis by stages of sarcoidosis

Stage	Infection	Cancer	Miscellaneous

I Adenopathy only	Tuberculosis
	Histoplasmosis
	Coccidioidomycosis
	Brucellosis
		Lymphoma
		Bronchogenic
		  carcinoma
		Metastasis
			Drugs: methotrexate,
			  phenytoin

II Infiltrates and
  adenopathy
	Tuberculosis
	Histoplasmosis
	Coccidioidomycosis
		Lymphoma
		Lymphangitic
		  carcinomatosis
			Pneumoconiosis: silicosis,
			  berylliosis

III Infiltrates only	Tuberculosis
	Fungal infections
		Lymphangitic
		  carcinomatosis
			Collagen vascular diseases
			Hypersensitivity pneumonitis
			Eosinophilic granulomatosis
			Idiopathic pulmonary fibrosis
			  (IPF)
			Alveolar proteinosis
			Drugs: chemotherapeutic
			  agents, nitrofurantoin

IV Fibrosis	Tuberculosis Fungal infections		Pneumoconiosis Bronchiectasis IPF

Not a complete listing.

1. The systemic nature of this illness emphasizes the importance of a **complete history and physical examination**. Once symptoms or physical findings are identified, possible sites for tissue biopsy should be considered. A patient with erythema nodosum, uveitis, and bilateral hilar adenopathy may not need tissue taken for confirmation of the diagnosis of sarcoidosis, but many patients will not have this classic presentation (2).

2. In most cases, **definitive diagnosis will require biopsy of the most accessible abnormal tissue**. Although the clinical appearance may be highly suggestive of sarcoidosis (bilateral hilar adenopathy and parenchymal infiltrates), available therapies are not benign and should not be administered without pathologic confirmation. With the exception of erythema nodosum, which has a poor diagnostic yield, biopsy of skin lesions and palpable lymph nodes often shows noncaseating granulomas and can make the diagnosis. Conjunctival biopsy should be performed if there is an obvious abnormality of the conjunctiva. A portion of the specimen should be sent for culture to exclude tuberculosis.

3. **In the absence of an easily accessible biopsy site, transbronchial biopsy through a flexible fiberoptic bronchoscope is the procedure of choice.** The overall diagnostic yield approximates 85%; even with a normal chest radiograph, the yield is over 60% (25). If a diagnosis is not obtained by transbronchial biopsy, mediastinoscopy and biopsy of enlarged intrathoracic lymph nodes will likely be diagnostic. Open lung biopsy is rarely needed to establish the diagnosis (25).

4. **Other potential biopsy sites** include the liver, skeletal muscle, lacrimal gland, nasal mucosa, minor salivary gland, endomyocardium, or spleen, if local symptoms or abnormalities are present (26). However, detection of granulomas should be interpreted cautiously in some tissues such as liver. Biopsy of another tissue, such as the lung, may be necessary in certain situations to clarify the diagnosis.

5. **Radiology**
   a. **Chest x-ray.** The chest x-ray may be normal or reveal parenchymal and/or lymph node abnormalities. Serial chest x-rays are used to follow the course of disease.
      i. **Hilar adenopathy and paratracheal adenopathy** are classically bilateral but maybe asymmetric. **Mediastinal adenopathy** is less frequent. Unilateral hilar adenopathy and calcification of the nodes are rare but can occur.
      ii. **Parenchymal abnormalities** are usually bilateral and reticulonodular in nature. Acinar (alveolar) sarcoid infiltrates (fluffy opacities with irregular borders), as well as nodular and miliary infiltrates may occur as well (8). Unilateral infiltrates are rare. Macronodular disease with nodules >1 cm in diameter is uncommon. Nodules rarely cavitate. Other uncommon radiologic appearances of sarcoid include: pleural effusion, pneumothorax, and lobar atelectasis. Hilar retraction, bullous changes, and honeycombing are usually associated with advanced fibrotic disease (8).
   b. **Computed tomography** (CT) and high-resolution CT (HRCT) scans are helpful when the parenchyma appears normal on chest X-ray. CT is superior to standard chest x-ray in showing nodules and infiltrates. HRCT allows the detection of micronodules, peribronchial cuffing, thickened septa and pleura, small cystic air spaces, bronchiectasis, pleural thickening, and ground-glass attenuation (27).
   c. **Magnetic resonance (MR) imaging and contrast-enhanced CT are both useful in the detection of CNS involvement.** The leptomeningeal predilection of neurosarcoidosis, especially the basal cistern, and the meninges are optimally evaluated by gadolinium-enhanced MR imaging (28).
   d. **Gallium scans** lack specificity and should not be used alone for the diag-

nosis of sarcoidosis. The "lambda-panda" pattern (uptake of gallium in the intrathoracic lymph nodes and in the salivary and tear glands, respectively) was shown to be highly sensitive and specific for sarcoidosis when chest radiographs show typical bilateral adenopathy and/or bilateral diffuse parenchymal involvement in the appropriate clinical context (29). Making a diagnosis of sarcoidosis based solely on these findings is not recommended.

6. **Biochemistry**
   a. **Assessment of calcium metabolism** is important to detect the presence of hypercalciuria and hypercalcemia (19).
      i. Hypercalciuria is seen in 30% to 50% of patients and is twice as common as hypercalcemia. A 24-hour urine calcium determination is indicated when hypercalcemia is present.
      ii. Hypercalcemia is present in 10% to 20% of sarcoidosis patients.
   b. **Angiotensin-converting enzyme** (ACE) is produced by epithelioid cells in granulomas. ACE levels are increased in about 60% of patients with sarcoidosis but have limited diagnostic value (12). Elevated ACE levels are nonspecific and seen in several disease processes, including pneumoconiosis, hypersensitivity pneumonitis, lymphoma, and miliary tuberculosis (12). **While ACE levels should not be used alone to follow disease activity, elevations occurring during therapy may help predict relapse and identify patients who require closer follow-up** (30).
   c. **Kveim-Siltzbach intradermal test** involves the intracutaneous injection of a meticulously processed and tested suspension of human sarcoid spleen. If positive, biopsy of the nodule that forms at the site of injection 2–6 weeks later shows the characteristic noncaseating granulomatous reaction (31). While very sensitive and specific, the test is only available at a few selected centers and therefore not widely used.
   d. Other tests. **PPD with controls shows anergy** in most patients. Examination of the cerebrospinal fluid in neurosarcoidosis shows increased protein and immunoglobulin levels. Leukopenia is frequent.

V. **Management**
   A. **General principles**
      1. **Many patients will undergo remission without specific treatment.** Three-quarters of patients will experience resolution of the disease within 2 years, while the others experience a progressive course highlighted by periods of exacerbations. Mortality is 5% to 10%, with death resulting from end-organ damage, usually pulmonary fibrosis (32). The likelihood of spontaneous resolution is inversely correlated with the length and severity of disease: 90% of patients with Löfgren's syndrome, 65% with stage I disease, 46% with stage II disease, and 20% with stage III disease (32).
      2. Therapy for sarcoidosis depends on the symptoms and organs involved and includes nonsteroidal anti-inflammatory drugs (NSAIDs), systemic corticosteroids, topical agents, and occasionally immunosuppressive agents. **Absolute indications for therapy include ocular, cardiac, and CNS involvement and hypercalcemia** (2).
   B. **Intrathoracic involvement**
      1. Management decisions are based on an assessment of disease activity that requires data on symptom progression, measurements of pulmonary function and diffusing capacity, evaluation of chest radiographic findings, and measurements of other indicators of disease activity such as ACE levels and sedimentation rates. No treatment is necessary for asymptomatic stage 0, I, or II disease in the absence of objective signs of pulmonary impairment. If pulmonary or extrathoracic symptoms arise or pulmonary function tests worsen during this observation period, therapy may need to be instituted.
      2. The precise treatment protocols for pulmonary sarcoidosis vary among institutions and individual physicians. Generally, patients with stage II disease and

abnormal pulmonary function studies and those with symptoms of cough or dyspnea should be started on corticosteroids. Most patients in stage III will demonstrate pulmonary function impairment and will require therapy. Asymptomatic stage III patients with progressive lung function impairment may respond to therapy, as active granuloma formation is a likely component of the disease process. The same applies to patients presenting with fibrosis (2,31).

3. **Sarcoidosis will generally respond to low-to-moderate doses of steroids.** The usual starting dose can be 40 mg prednisone or 0.5 mg/kg/d, although some clinicians start with lower doses. Alternate-day therapy can be instituted initially or after a clinical response has been obtained; this schedule has been associated with fewer side effects than daily steroids (2,33). The duration of therapy is individually based. Most patients will require minimal-effective-dose steroid therapy for several months, followed by slow tapering to a maintenance dose of 10–15 mg/d over a course of 6 months, for a total length of therapy of approximately 12 months (2,34,33). Some patients may require long-term therapy or increased doses because of frequent relapses during steroid taper (2). Some of these patients may require alternative therapy as discussed below. The benefit of inhaled corticosteroids as monotherapy or as a systemic steroid-sparing adjunct has been supported by a few studies, although no large controlled trials have been completed to date (35,36).

C. **Extrathoracic involvement**
   1. **Corticosteroid therapy is absolutely indicated for ocular, CNS, and cardiac involvement, as well as the presence of hypercalciuria and hypercalcemia.**
      a. All forms of **ocular sarcoidosis** should be treated with corticosteroids. For anterior uveitis, topical corticosteroids can be used initially, with systemic corticosteroids utilized if symptoms worsen or there is no improvement. Loss of vision, cataracts, glaucoma, or choreoretinal fibrosis may occur as a result of ocular sarcoid (17).
      b. **Cardiac involvement** may require a combination of systemic corticosteroids and antiarrhythmic drugs. Pacemakers or defibrillators may be necessary to treat life-threatening arrhythmias and conduction abnormalities. Cardiac sarcoidosis is associated with a 10-fold increase in mortality as compared to sarcoidosis of other organs (20,37).
      c. Systemic corticosteroids and high-dose pulsed steroids may be required to control **neurosarcoidosis**. Antiseizure medications or ventriculoperitoneal shunts may be required. CNS sarcoid is associated with a 10-fold increase in mortality compared to other organ involvement. Irradiation may be considered if steroids fail to stem the progression of the disease (21,37).
      d. **Hypercalcemia** is responsive to systemic corticosteroids. Calcium chelation may be necessary for persistent hypercalciuria (37). If untreated, hypercalcemia results in nephrolithiasis and nephrocalcinosis and can lead to renal failure (19).
      e. **Skin manifestations** can be treated with topical steroids, methotrexate, or chloroquine; in the case of erythema nodosum, NSAIDs or a brief course of low-dose systemic steroids may be used (12,37). The dermatologic manifestations of sarcoidosis are particularly sensitive to methotrexate and chloroquine.
      f. If **hypersplenism** is present clinically, corticosteroids may control thrombocytopenia and anemia. Splenectomy may occasionally be necessary (12).
      g. **Hepatic involvement** may require long-term steroid therapy when associated with prolonged high fevers and persistent fatigue or with a rapid deterioration in liver function (38).

D. **Other therapy**
   1. **The use of cytotoxic and immunosuppressive drugs is controversial.** These agents are generally used when corticosteroid treatment is contraindicated or ineffective, or as a steroid-sparing measures. Chlorambucil, metho-

trexate, chloroquine, cyclophosphamide, azathioprine, and cyclosporine have all been used with variable success in sarcoidosis (39–44).

2. **Irradiation** has occasionally been used in rapidly progressive neurologic and systemic sarcoidosis when systemic therapy has failed (45).

3. **Transplantation** can be an option in patients with end-stage pulmonary fibrosis and other end-organ fibrosis (kidney, heart, liver). However, recurrence of sarcoidosis has been reported in transplanted lungs and liver (9,37).

E. **Dosage**

1. **Therapy and dosing will vary depending on symptoms and organ involvement.** The dose of NSAID necessary to achieve optimal effect varies by the particular agent chosen for therapy. Corticosteroid doses vary according to the indication for treatment, from low doses taken orally to pulsed high doses given intravenously for indications such as neurologic deterioration. Topical corticosteroids are often sufficient for the treatment of anterior uveitis (Table 10-3).

2. **Immunosuppressive agents** are rarely used and are reserved for special situations. Common doses as suggested by various reports in the literature are as follows: methotrexate (10 mg/wk for 3 months), cyclophosphamide (50 mg/d for 3 months), azathioprine (50 mg TID for 3 months, with possible repetition), and chlorambucil (5 mg/d for 3 months) (38,40–44).

F. **Disease activity. No one single test can or should be used to follow the progression or improvement of sarcoidosis.** Furthermore, one organ system may improve while others worsen during therapy or observation, making the elucidation of a true marker of disease activity difficult. The "activity" of the disease is idiosyncratic and best measured by comprehensive clinical, radiographic, biochemical, and pulmonary function evaluations on an individual basis (46,47).

Table 10-3. Treatment of extrapulmonary sarcoidosis*

Ocular
  Topical corticosteroids (only for anterior uveitis): triamcinolone acetonide 1% (8)
  Systemic corticosteroids (if no improvement or other ocular manifestations): prednisone 40–80 mg (4,36)
Dermatologic
  Erythema nodosum
    Nonsteroidal anti-inflammatory drugs: indomethacin 25 mg po TID (2)
    Corticosteroids: prednisone 20 mg po QOD (2)
  Lupus pernio, plaques
    Corticosteroids (39)
    Chloroquine 250 mg QOD 9 mo (40)
    Methotrexate 10 mg once weekly (39)
Neurologic
  Systemic corticosteroids: prednisone 60–80 mg po QD or equivalent IV (33)
Cardiac
  Systemic corticosteroids: prednisone 60–80 mg po QD or equivalent IV (11,33)
  Pacemaker or defibrillator may be indicated
Hepatic, if progressive deterioration (33)
  Systemic corticosteroids
Renal (hypercalcemia)
  Prednisone (10,39)

*For duration, see text, references. Not a complete listing.

G. Problems and complications of therapy

1. The usual side effects of **steroid therapy** may be observed: new or worsening diabetes, cushingoid syndrome, cataracts, avascular necrosis of the hip, and peptic ulcer disease. Alternate-day dosing of steroids should be instituted whenever possible to avoid suppression of the hypothalamic-pituitary-adrenal axis. Steroids should be taken with food, antacids, or acid-suppressing agents whenever possible.

2. A **PPD tuberculin test and anergy panel** must be placed in patients without a previously documented positive PPD prior to the initiation of long-term steroid therapy. A positive PPD in patients with sarcoidosis whose clinical picture is also consistent with tuberculosis requires evaluation for isoniazid prophylaxis or full treatment of tuberculosis while cultures are pending from sputum or biopsy specimens.

3. **Cyclophosphamide** and **azathioprine** are associated with hematologic complications. The hepatic fibrosis associated with **methotrexate** is not seen with weekly low doses suggested for the treatment of sarcoidosis (39). Routine eye examinations are necessary to assess potential **chloroquine** ocular toxicity (12).

4. The **fibrotic lung** in sarcoidosis is similar to other forms of chronic pulmonary fibrosis. Severe lung fibrosis leads to pulmonary hypertension and cor pulmonale (15). Assessment may require echocardiography and right heart catheterization. Such patients may require supplemental oxygen therapy and other vasodilator therapies.

5. Upper lobe cavitations that result from fibrosis can become colonized with **fungus,** most commonly *Aspergillus,* as determined by repeated sputum cultures, leading to the development of a mycetoma. The development of invasive aspergillosis requires treatment with antifungal medications. Hemoptysis may also result from bronchiectasis but may respond to antibiotic treatment. Patients with severe hemoptysis due to either bronchiectasis or mycetoma should be evaluated for surgical resection of the affected area (16).

VI. Referrals to specialists. The diagnosis of sarcoidosis may require evaluation and consultation by a variety of specialists. Sarcoidosis can involve almost any organ, and hence the referrals necessary for diagnosis and management will vary from patient to patient. The importance of these evaluations is underscored by the silent involvement of certain organs that can be life-threatening and require aggressive therapy.

A. Pulmonologists can perform endobronchial evaluation/ biopsy and transbronchial biopsy with bronchoscopy.

B. Ophthalmologic evaluation is of utmost importance, since a diagnosis can be made without further invasive procedures.

C. Cardiothoracic surgeons may provide the diagnosis with mediastinoscopy and/or lung biopsy.

D. Cardiologic evaluation may be necessary for echocardiography or more invasive testing such as myocardial biopsy, as well as for therapy (pacemaker placement).

E. Dermatologists may provide the diagnosis with skin biopsy whenever skin involvement is present.

F. Gastroenterologists may perform a liver biopsy to search for granulomas. Hepatic granulomas should be interpreted with caution and only in combination with microbiologic cultures and special stains.

VII. Pregnancy. The course of sarcoidosis appears to be improved during pregnancy and has been attributed to higher endogenous corticosteroid levels during pregnancy. A normal pregnancy and delivery are to be expected. Chest x-rays should be avoided, and the disease should be monitored with ACE levels or other parameters. After delivery, sarcoidosis will usually return to the level of activity prior to pregnancy, although occasionally the disease can progress or worsen (12,48).

VIII. Necrotizing sarcoid granulomatosis. Necrotizing sarcoid granulomatosis is considered by some to be a variant of sarcoidosis. As in sarcoidosis, noncaseating granulomas are present and the clinical course may be benign, with or without therapy. Confluent granulomas are found on histologic examination, associated with a minimal granulomatous vasculitis involving the pulmonary arteries and veins. Unlike sarcoidosis, adenopathy is generally not found (49).

References

1. Teirstein A, Lesser M: Worldwide distribution and epidemiology of sarcoidosis. In: Fanburg B, ed. *Sarcoidosis and other granulomatous diseases of the lung.* New York: Marcel Dekker, 1983: 101.
2. DeRemee R: Sarcoidosis. *Mayo Clin Proc* 1995;70:177.
3. Mayock R, Bertrand P, Morrison C: Manifestations of sarcoidosis. *Am J Med* 1963;35:67.
4. Joyce-Brady M: "Tastes great, less filling:" the debate about mycobacteria and sarcoidosis. *Am Rev Respir Dis* 1992;145:986.
5. Nowack D, Goebel K: Genetic aspects of sarcoidosis. *Arch Intern Med* 1987;147:481.
6. Thomas P, Hunninhake G: Current concepts of the pathogenesis of sarcoidosis. *Am Rev Respir Dis* 1987;135:747.
7. Hunninghake G, Crystal R: Pulmonary sarcoidosis: a disorder mediated by excess helper T-lymphocyte activity at sites of disease activity. *N Engl J Med* 1981;1981:429.
8. Kirks D, McCormick V, Greenspan R: Pulmonary sarcoidosis: roentgenologic analysis of 150 patients. *AJR* 1973;117:777.
9. Turner-Warwick M, McAllister W, Lawrence R, et al.: Corticosteroid treatment in pulmonary sarcoidosis: do serial lavage lymphocyte counts, serum angiotensin converting enzyme measurements, and gallium-67 scans help management? *Thorax* 1986;41:903.
10. Semenzato G, Agostini C: Immunology of sarcoidosis. In: King T et al, ed. *Infiltrative lung diseases.* 1993.
11. Daniele R, Dauber J, Rossman M: Immunologic abnormalities in sarcoidosis. *Ann Intern Med* 1980;92:406.
12. Sharma O: Sarcoidosis. *Disease-a-Month* 1990;Sept:469.
13. Hudspith BN, Flint K, James DG, et al.: Lack of immune deficiency in sarcoidosis: compartmentalisation of the immune response. *Thorax* 1987;42:250.
14. Siltzbach L, James D, Neville E, et al.: Course and prognosis of sarcoidosis around the world. *Am J Med* 1974;57:847.
15. Katz S: Clinical presentation and natural history of sarcoidosis. In: Fanburg B, ed. *Sarcoidosis and other granulomatous diseases of the lung.* New York: Marcel Dekker, 1983:3.
16. Israel H, Lenchner G, Atkinson G: Sarcoidosis and aspergilloma: the role of surgery. *Chest* 1982; 82:430.
17. Karma A, Huhti E, Poukkula A: Course and outcome of ocular sarcoidosis. *Am J Ophthalmol* 1988; 106:467.
18. Klatskin G: Hepatic granulomata: problems in interpretation. *Ann N Y Acad Sci* 1976;278:427.
19. Muther R, McCarron D, Bennett W: Renal manifestations of sarcoidosis. *Arch Intern Med* 1981; 141:643.
20. Sharma O, Maheshwari A, Thaker K: Myocardial sarcoidosis. *Chest* 1993;103:253.
21. Scott T: Neurosarcoidosis: progress and clinical aspects. *Neurology* 1993;43:8.
22. Winterbauer R, Hutchinson J: Clinical significance of pulmonary function test: use of pulmonary function tests in the management of sarcoidosis. *Chest* 1980;78:640.
23. Dines D, Stubbs S, McDougall J: Obstructive disease of the airways associated with stage I sarcoidosis. *Mayo Clin Proc* 1978;53:788.
24. Matthews J, Hooper R: Exercise testing in pulmonary sarcoidosis. *Chest* 1983;83:75
25. Gilman M, Wang K: Transbronchial lung biopsy in sarcoidosis: an approach to determine the optimal number of biopsies. *Am Rev Respir Dis* 1980;122:721.
26. Israel H, Sones M: Selection of biopsy procedures for sarcoidosis diagnosis. *Arch Intern Med* 1964;113:147.
27. Remy-Jardin M, Remy J, Deffontaines C, et al.: Assessment of diffuse infiltrative lung disease: comparison of conventional CT and high-resolution CT. *Radiology* 1991;181:157.
28. Sherman J, Stern B: Sarcoidosis of the CNS: Comparison of unenhanced and enhanced MR images. *AJR* 1990;155:1293.
29. Sulavik S, Spencer R, Palestro C, et al.: Specificity and sensitivity of distinctive chest radiographic and/or ^{67}Ga images in the noninvasive diagnosis of sarcoidosis. *Chest* 1993;103:403.
30. Allen R: A review of angiotensin converting enzyme in health and disease. *Sarcoidosis* 1991;8:95.
31. Siltzbach L: The Kveim test in sarcoidosis. *JAMA* 1961;178:476.
32. Siltzbach L: Sarcoidosis. In: Fishman A, ed. *Pulmonary diseases and disorders.* New York: McGraw-Hill, 1980.

33. Sharma O: Pulmonary sarcoidosis and corticosteroids. *Am Rev Respir Dis* 1993;147:1598.
34. DeRemee R, Offrod K: The treatment of pulmonary sarcoidosis: the house revisited. *Sarcoidosis* 1992;9:17.
35. Spiteri M: Inhaled corticosteroids in pulmonary sarcoidosis. *Postgrad Med J* 1991;67:327.
36. Selroos O: Inhaled corticosteroids and pulmonary sarcoidosis. *Sarcoidosis* 1988;5:104.
37. Geraint James D. Treatment. In: Geraint James D, ed. *Sarcoidosis and other granulomatous disorders*. New York: Marcel Dekker, 1994:607.
38. Israel H, Margolis M, Rose L: Hepatic granulomatosis and sarcoidosis: further observations. *Dig Dis Sci* 1984;29:353.
39. Israel H, McComb B: Chlorambucil treatment of sarcoidosis. *Sarcoidosis* 1991;8:35.
40. Lower E, Baughman R: The use of low-dose methotrexate in refractory sarcoidosis. *Am J Med Sci* 1990;299:153.
41. Morse S, Cohn Z, Hirsch J, Schaedler: The treatment of sarcoidosis with chloroquine. *Am J Med* 1961; 779.
42. Demeter S: Myocardial sarcoidosis unresponsive to steroids— treatment with cyclophosphamide. *Chest* 1988;94:202.
43. Pacheco Y, Marechal C, Marechal F, et al.: Azathioprine treatment of chronic pulmonary sarcoidosis. *Sarcoidosis* 1985;2:107.
44. York E, Kovithavongs T, Man S, et al.: Cyclosporine and chronic sarcoidosis. *Chest* 1990;98:1026.
45. Ahmad K, Kim Y, Spitzer A, et al.: Total nodal irradiation in progressive sarcoidosis. *Am J Clin Oncol* 1992;15:311.
46. Baudouin S, du Bois R: Disease activity. In: Geraint James D, ed. *Sarcoidosis and other granulomatous disorders*. New York: Marcel Dekker, 1994:573.
47. Oni A, Hershberger R, Norman D, et al.: Recurrence of sarcoidosis in a cardiac allograft: control with corticosteroids. *J Heart Lung Transplant* 1992;11:367.
48. Selroos O: Sarcoidosis and pregnancy: a review with results of a retrospective survey. *J Intern Med* 1990;227:221.
49. Churg A, Carrington C, Gupta R: Necrotizing sarcoid granulomatosis. *Chest* 1979;76:406.

11 — Hypersensitivity Lung Disease

Frank S. Becker and Jeffrey Glassroth

Hypersensitivity pneumonitis (HP), or extrinsic allergic alveolitis, is an immunologically mediated disease of the lungs that results from the inhalation of a multitude of different organic antigens, from the ingestion of certain drugs, and, rarely, from exposure to relatively simple inorganic chemicals. Although the antigens differ widely, the clinical syndromes that result are very similar. HP may present in an acute and/or a chronic form.

I. Acute hypersensitivity pneumonitis

A. Presenting signs and symptoms (1–8)

1. The acute disease presents as a febrile illness with an onset usually 4–6 hours after the exposure. Patients complain of fever, chills, myalgias, and a nonproductive cough. Physical examination reveals a tachypneic and tachycardic patient with diffuse mid- to late-inspiratory rales. Wheezing is usually not present but can be found in particularly severe cases. Cyanosis may be present in severe cases, and the level of hypoxemia may appear to be out of proportion to the level of toxicity of the patient. The presentation is frequently mistaken for mycoplasmal or viral pneumonia. The duration of symptoms varies but typically lasts several hours. Minor symptoms may persist for 24–48 hours.

2. In occupational exposures, there can be a cyclical nature to the symptoms due to repetitive exposure to, then removal from, the particular antigen. The term *Monday-morning fever* describes the acute exacerbation often seen upon return to the workplace after a weekend or longer away from exposure.

B. Etiology and pathogenesis

1. The etiology of most of the hypersensitivity syndromes is the inhalation of an antigen that triggers a common immune response. Reactions of both type III (immune-complex deposition) and type IV (cellular immune reactions) have been implicated (9). The antigen may be derived from animal (feces, urine, fur, feathers), insect (wheat weevils), or plant material. Reactions to plant products may be due to the plant itself or, more commonly, to a fungal or bacterial antigen that grows on the plant (thermophilic *Actinomyces, Aspergillus,* and *Penicillium* species).

2. Other hypersensitivity syndromes can be seen as a result of exposure to certain chemicals (toluene diisocyanate, trimellitic anhydride, diphenylmethane diisocyanate). These chemicals act as haptens interacting with the patient's own proteins to create antigens that can result in a HP-like syndrome.

C. Relevant physiology

1. Pulmonary function tests usually demonstrate a restrictive pattern with decreased vital capacity and lung volumes. Forced expiratory volume in 1 second (FEV_1) is usually reduced in proportion to the vital capacity. Obstruction is not typical, unless there is superimposed reactive airways disease; however, obstruction may be seen in severe cases. The diffusing capacity for carbon monoxide (D_LCO) is usually decreased. Arterial hypoxemia is common and, if not present at rest, may be elicited with exercise.

2. In the acute form of the disease, the pulmonary function tests return to normal

between episodes. In the chronic form, a restrictive ventilatory defect generally remains.

D. Differential diagnostic possibilities

1. **Infections** (10). The presenting symptoms of acute HP are similar to a flu-like illness with an associated pneumonitis. As patients with HP are reexposed to the offending antigen, recurring symptoms result.

2. **Drugs.** Many drugs can cause a syndrome similar to HP (see chapter 27).

3. **Allergic bronchopulmonary aspergillosis (ABPA)** shares a number of characteristics with acute HP. However, ABPA typically occurs in the setting of asthma, is not associated with extrinsic exposures, and has a stereotypical immune pattern with skin test reactivity to aspergillin and the presence of antibodies specific for *Aspergillus*. Serum IgE immunoglobulin is also elevated in active cases.

E. Diagnostic approach

1. **History.** Symptoms characteristically occur in a temporal relation to an environmental exposure. A history of recurrent pulmonary symptoms or "infections" should prompt questions about possible exposures to agents that could cause HP. Patients should be asked about recent exposure to hay, especially damp hay (Farmer's lung), or to birds including pigeons, chickens, turkeys, and pet birds (parrots, parakeets, finches). Those employed in laboratories should be asked about exposure to animals (rats, rabbits, dogs) and to certain chemicals (Pauli's reagent).

2. **Radiologic studies**

   a. **The chest x-ray** findings are nonspecific. Generally, bilateral nodular infiltrates are seen. Diffuse interstitial infiltrates can be seen with and without Kerley's B lines. Patchy, linear, streaky opacities can be seen in the lung periphery. The picture can mimic acute pulmonary edema, with interstitial and alveolar infiltrates with hilar prominence. In mild cases, the chest x-ray may be totally normal.

   b. **High-resolution computed tomography** (HRCT) is more sensitive than chest radiography but is also nonspecific. Generally, reticular and nodular infiltrates are seen using both modalities (11,12).

   c. **Magnetic resonance (MR) imaging** is less sensitive than CT and plays no role in the diagnosis of HP (13).

3. Precipitating antibodies may be found in the majority of cases. However, the presence of precipitating antibodies is more useful as a marker of exposure than as an indicator of disease. For instance, many farmers exposed to moldy hay will have precipitating antibodies to actinomycetes without having clinical evidence of disease. However, those with disease will generally have higher antibody titers than healthy subjects. Nevertheless, the history of exposure to an antigen and the presence of precipitating antibodies in a clinical setting consistent with HP are generally enough to confirm the diagnosis.

   a. The conventional **Ouchterlony double-diffusion test** is generally sufficient to make the diagnosis. More sensitive tests are available, such as the enzyme-linked immunosorbent assay, radioimmunoassay, and radioallergosorbent test. Hypersensitivity screening panels containing the most common antigens are widely available commercially. If an unusual exposure is suspected, a referral to an allergy center may be useful. The antigen could be extracted from the source and the patient's serum tested for antibodies.

4. **Bronchoscopy and lung biopsy** generally have no role in the diagnosis of HP but can be useful to exclude other diseases.

   a. Bronchoalveolar lavage (BAL) usually demonstrates abnormally large numbers of lymphocytes. Decreases in the CD4+/CD8+ (T-helper/T-suppressor cell) ratio of alveolar lymphocytes have been reported, which is the inverse of what is seen in sarcoidosis (14). Others have disputed these findings. Overall, BAL can be a useful research tool but does not aid in diagnosis (15).

   b. Examination of **lung biopsy specimens** reveals nonspecific changes. In the acute form, alveolar and interstitial inflammation is seen, along with hyaline membranes and edema. Lymphocytic infiltration may be present. An increased number of alveolar macrophages with foamy cytoplasm has been described. The presence of bronchiolar inflammation and non-caseating granulomas may suggest HP (16).

5. **Routine laboratory tests** are generally normal. Mild leukocytosis may occur, but eosinophilia is rare. Serum IgE is not elevated. Skin tests with the offending antigen may show reactivity, but this is a nonspecific finding.

F. **Management**
   1. **Avoidance of the offending antigen** is crucial in the management of HP and in many cases is all that is required. In acute HP, improvement will be rapid. In the chronic forms of the disease, improvement will generally occur over several days to weeks. In situations where avoidance is impossible, **mask respirators** have been shown to be effective in limiting exposure. However, compliance with respirators is difficult, especially if they are to be worn during heavy labor.
   2. **Corticosteroids** decrease the length of the illness. However, after the medication is discontinued, reexposure to an antigen will provoke another acute episode. Symptomatic patients should be started on prednisone 0.5–1.0 mg/kg/d. This dose should be continued until the patient is asymptomatic and the pulmonary function tests have normalized. This can often take 1–2 weeks to occur. Prednisone should then be tapered and discontinued over a period of 2–4 weeks. In chronic exposure, there is some evidence that low-dose prednisone may prevent fibrosis.

G. **Problems and complications of therapy**
   1. Complications of therapy are essentially those of short- or long-term use of corticosteroids, which can increase susceptibility to bacterial, viral, and fungal infections. Other complications include glucose intolerance, gastrointestinal irritation, fluid retention, osteoporosis, agitation, myopathies, and accelerated cataract formation.
   2. The risk of steroid complications needs to be considered on an individual basis. Mild cases of HP should be treated with antigen avoidance alone.

H. **Specialist referrals**
   1. **Acute HP** can be diagnosed on clinical grounds based on a history of environmental exposure and the characteristic symptomatologies. If the exposure is clear and avoidance achievable (eg, an acute self-limited illness following work around pigeon droppings, and future exposure is not anticipated), then generally further evaluation by a specialist is not warranted.
   2. In some situations, the etiology of the syndrome must be definitively established. This is especially true in medicolegal cases or if avoidance of the antigen would require a major change in profession or lifestyle (eg, in farmer's lung or where a pet is concerned). Although precipitating antibodies lend credibility to the diagnosis, they can be found in individuals without clinical disease. Inhalational challenges can be performed by specialists in allergy to confirm the diagnosis. These can be done either "in the field" (with the patient returning to the place of exposure, followed by close monitoring of pulmonary functions and clinical signs and symptoms) or as an inhalational challenge in the hospital laboratory. A laboratory challenge requires hospitalization, as 24 hours or more of monitoring may be required. Because these challenges involve exposure to pure extracts of the antigen, they can result in severe cases of bronchospasm and/or pneumonitis. As such, they should only be performed in specialized laboratories familiar with the procedure.

II. **Chronic hypersensitivity pneumonitis.** Chronic HP often mimics other chronic pulmonary conditions such as sarcoidosis, interstitial lung disease, miliary tuberculosis, alveolar cell carcinoma, and alveolar proteinosis. As the diagnosis frequently requires tissue confirmation, referral to a pulmonologist is generally indicated.

A. **Etiology and pathogenesis.** This condition presents with the insidious onset of malaise, cough, dyspnea, weight loss, and weakness. Less commonly, fever may be seen. Patients may pass from acute to chronic disease as their level of exposure to the inciting antigen changes.

B. Differential diagnosis

1. Chronic HP can resemble any of the chronic interstitial lung diseases on chest imaging studies and can present with symptoms and radiologic studies that mimic miliary tuberculosis. As such, it is crucially important to rule out tuberculosis before initiating steroids.

2. Diagnostic consideration should be given to all of the following: sarcoidosis, talc granuloma, usual interstitial pneumonitis (UIP), desquamative interstitial pneumonitis (DIP), and alveolar cell carcinoma. Alveolar proteinosis can have a similar radiologic pattern but is more insidious in onset and is not associated with fever. Sarcoidosis may have a similar clinical and radiologic presentation. Discriminating features favoring sarcoidosis are the presence of extrapulmonary symptoms and prominent hilar adenopathy. The histologic appearance may be helpful in separating HP from sarcoidosis, as determined by a study of 60 patients with farmer's lung (17). In sarcoidosis, there is minimal alveolitis, whereas in HP alveolitis is the predominant lesion. Although noncaseating granulomas occur in both diseases, they are not always present in HP. When identified in HP, the granulomas are centrilobular in location, whereas in sarcoidosis granulomas tend to locate along the lymphatics. Fibrosis is present in the end-stage of both sarcoidosis and chronic HP.

3. Chronic HP is associated with decreased lung volumes and bilateral interstitial infiltrates resembling pulmonary fibrosis on chest x-ray. As the disease becomes chronic, fibrotic changes in the upper lobes are seen on HRCT scanning.

C. Relevant physiology. Pulmonary function tests are consistent with a restrictive lung disease as evidenced by reductions in all capacities and volumes. The FEV_1 is usually reduced in proportion to the vital capacity. Again, obstruction will not be found unless there is superimposed reactive airways disease. The D_LCO will be reduced. Arterial hypoxemia at rest or exercise is common. These findings will persist with time in patients with chronic disease.

D. Diagnostic approach

1. As in acute HP, a detailed history offers the best hope for establishing a diagnosis. Because the symptoms are more insidious in nature, it may be more difficult to establish which antigen may be causative. Serologies may be helpful in establishing the exposure but are not pathognomonic for disease.

2. **Bronchoscopy and lung biopsy** are useful in the exclusion of other diseases. The diagnoses of many diseases in the differential of HP, such as alveolar cell carcinoma, lymphangitic spread of carcinoma, and alveolar proteinosis, can readily be made by bronchoscopy. BAL and lung biopsy can be helpful in ruling out tuberculosis. However, in miliary tuberculosis bronchoscopy may be negative. If there is a high index of suspicion for miliary tuberculosis, a bone marrow or liver biopsy should be considered to exclude mycobacterial infection. Granulomas may be seen in both sarcoidosis and chronic HP.

3. Open lung biopsy may be considered if the roentgenographic pattern of disease suggests the possibility of UIP or DIP.

E. Treatment

1. **Avoidance of the offending antigen** is of critical importance. In some occupational exposures, consideration should be given to a change in job. However, many occupational exposures can be avoided by reassigning the employee to an area where the exposure is unlikely.

2. **Prednisone** is generally begun at 0.5–1.0 mg/kg/d and continued until symptoms resolve. This generally requires several weeks to months. The dose of prednisone is then tapered over the following 8–12 weeks until the lowest dose that maintains the response is achieved. In situations where avoidance of the antigen is impossible, low-dose prednisone may be continued indefinitely.

III. Specific forms of hypersensitivity pneumonitis

A. Farmer's lung (humidifier lung) is the most common and best described of the hypersensitivity syndromes. The etiology is usually thermophilic actinomycetes, but it can be due to other organisms. A similar syndrome can occur when these organisms infect free-standing water in humidifiers (humidifier lung) or in saunas (sauna-taker's lung).

1. **Etiology and pathogenesis.** Farmer's lung was originally described in the 1930s. It was originally thought to be a fungal infection of the lung. The acute syndrome consists of typical HP that occurs 4–8 hours after the hay is raked or turned. It may also present as a slowly progressive pulmonary fibrosis. **The organisms responsible are generally thermophilic actinomycetes *(Micropolyspora faeni, Thermoactinomyces vulgaris)* or *Aspergillus* species.** Hay stored in damp conditions generates heat that is conducive to the growth of these organisms. Raking the hay releases large amounts of aerosolized antigen that is then inhaled. The illness may also occur in cattle. When originally described, the illness was more common in the summer months. Currently, there appears to be a winter predominance, which may be due to changes in storage practices.

2. **Differential diagnostic possibilities**
    a. The presentation of farmer's lung is usually straightforward. However, consideration should be given to other sources of antigen that may be present on a farm. These include avian products (feathers, feces) and animal urine and dander. Furthermore, the source of the exposure to the thermophilic actinomycetes may not be the hay directly but may be due to an inadequate ventilation system or other sources of humidity.
    b. **Inhalation of nitrogen dioxide (silo filler's disease)** can present in a manner similar to HP. Nitrogen dioxide is formed in silos due to the fermentation of grain. Peak levels of nitrogen dioxide occur a few weeks after filling of the silo. Inhalation of the gas causes lung injury. Two phases have been described. Acute silo filler's disease generally occurs within hours of being exposed to a silo and presents with cough and upper airway irritation, followed by increasing dyspnea, cyanosis, and pulmonary edema. Generally, patients are much more toxic than with HP. After the patient recovers from the acute phase, a second, sometimes more severe phase can occur. The severity of the initial phase appears to be a poor predictor of the occurrence or severity of the second phase. In farm workers, HP from other environmental exposures could coexist with lung injury due to nitrogen dioxide.

3. **Management**
    a. As in all forms of HP, avoidance is crucial. However, this is usually not possible for most farmers. If feasible, the job of raking hay should be given to someone less sensitive. The farmer should be instructed to contact the local agricultural agency for instructions on storing hay. Proper drying and storage of hay can dramatically reduce the amount of spore formation and may significantly decrease the severity of attacks. Respirators should be worn when the hay is disturbed.
    b. Even with these precautions, the sensitive individual is at risk for developing chronic HP. Individuals in the farming industry should be questioned about respiratory symptoms temporally related to working around hay. The pulmonary examination should be monitored for the presence of inspiratory rales.
    c. Individuals with chronic HP who cannot avoid exposure and have instituted the above measures should be treated with steroids. Prednisone should be started at 0.5–1.0 mg/kg/d and continued until pulmonary function tests have normalized or have stopped improving. The dose is then tapered over the following weeks to months to the lowest dose that maintains the response. Frequent measurement of vital capacity is indicated. The advent of low-cost home spirometers has made daily monitoring of vital capacity feasible; such monitoring should be instituted in highly sensitive individuals.

B. **Hypersensitivity pneumonitis due to exposure to birds.** Several syndromes of HP are caused by exposure to bird-derived antigens. The most common are **pigeon-breeder's lung and bird fancier's lung.**

1. **Presenting signs and symptoms.** The presentation is similar to other forms of HP. The clinical course is often similar to chronic HP with frequent acute and subacute exacerbations. The disease is probably the most common cause of HP in children.
2. **Etiology and pathogenesis.** Any one of a number of sources of antigen can cause a picture consistent with HP. Individuals who are sensitive to birds frequently will demonstrate serum precipitins to bird serum, droppings, or feathers.
3. **Differential diagnostic possibilities.** The diagnosis can be more difficult than in other forms of HP because hypersensitivity to any one of a number of antigens may be present. There is considerable heterogeneity in these antigens among species, although some cross-reactivity may occur. Because of the large number of species that can cause HP, along with the numerous sources of antigen in each species, serum tests can often be falsely negative. If routine screening tests for precipitins are negative, referral can be made to a specialty laboratory. A history of exposure and a clinical picture consistent with HP may be the only evidence to support the diagnosis.
   a. **Psittacosis** should be considered in any patient who presents with respiratory complaints with a history of exposure to birds. Usually, patients present with high spiking fevers, headaches, arthralgias, and a severe hacking cough. The infection is due to *Chlamydia psittaci*, an obligate intracellular parasite. The organism can be cultured on selective media; however, this can present a hazard to laboratory personnel, and should only be performed in laboratories that are familiar with the handling of this organism. The diagnosis can also be confirmed with a fourfold increase in antibody titers or with a single titer of 1:16 or greater. The infection responds to tetracycline, but recovery is slow.
4. **Management.** As in other forms of HP, avoidance is crucial. Simply removing the bird from the environment may not be sufficient. Studies have shown that bird droppings and feathers can permeate an enclosed area even months after the pet is removed and can cause clinical disease (18). Exposed surfaces must be thoroughly cleaned after the pet is removed, and consideration should be given to replacing carpeting and furniture.
C. **Chemical-induced hypersensitivity pneumonitis.** Workers employed in chemical manufacturing can develop an HP-like syndrome. It appears that a smaller chemical reacts with proteins found within the susceptible individual, resulting in either an alteration of the protein or a hapten reaction. Although these syndromes are not a consequence of inhaling an organic dust, the clinical, laboratory, and x-ray findings are similar to those in other forms of HP and are usually regarded as a subset of HP.
   1. **Presenting signs and symptoms.** Chemical-induced HP is most commonly seen in industry, and the most common form of chemical HP is due to isocyanate exposure. Generally, the presentation is similar to that of other forms of HP. Because isocyanates are also known to cause asthma, the presentation is often that of HP in the setting of a preexisting case of asthma. The asthmatic symptoms appear to predominate, and therefore the prevalence of HP due to isocyanates may be underestimated (19). Isocyanates are used in the plastic-manufacturing industry, and this form of hypersensitivity is most commonly seen in workers within that industry. They are also used in polyurethane-based paints and furniture finishes; and spray painters and woodworkers can have high exposures. Because the use of plastic products and polyurethane is ubiquitous in industry, any person presenting with an HP-like syndrome should be questioned about work exposures to heated plastic products,
   2. **Etiology and pathogenesis.** Chemical HP has been best described with isocyanates. Other chemicals implicated in HP include toluene diisocyanate, hexamethylene diisocyanate, diphenylmethane diisocyanate, Pauli's reagent (sodium diazobenzenesulfonate), and phthalic anhydrides (used in epoxy resin).
   3. **Management.** As in other forms of HP, avoidance is crucial. Corticosteroids are of benefit and should be instituted. Because repeated exposure to isocyanates can also cause progressive asthma, avoidance of these chemicals is of even greater importance than in other causes of HP.

D. **Drug-related hypersensitivity pneumonitis.** Many drugs have been associated with HP. These include gold, methotrexate, and amiodarone. These will be discussed in chapter 25.

E. **Japanese summer-type hypersensitivity disease** is an unusual form of HP that appears to be of clinical significance only in Japan. It is caused by *Trichosporon cutaneum*. The disease occurs in the summer months, with peak incidence in July. It is most common in female homemakers and is associated with homes with poor sanitation, dampness, and poor ventilation (20).

IV. **Organic dust toxic syndrome** (ODTS) (21–23). ODTS has many similarities to HP but is currently regarded as being a separate entity due to its different clinical presentation, laboratory findings, and treatment.

A. **Presenting signs and symptoms.** ODTS presents as an acute respiratory illness consisting of fever, chills, cough, and dyspnea. Headache, myalgia, and generalized malaise are common. The presentation occurs shortly after an exposure to organic dust. Unlike HP, frequent exposures do not seem to be required to cause illness, and the full spectrum of the disease can occur after only one heavy exposure.

B. **Etiology and pathogenesis.** ODTS generally occurs 1–8 hours after exposure to a large amount of organic dust. Sources can include grain, wood chips, or other plant products. It appears that damp, moldy conditions increase the likelihood of a reaction. For this reason, fungal antigens were initially suspected. However, the antigens involved have not been definitively identified, and the area is one of active investigation.

C. **Relevant physiology.** Pulmonary function abnormalities are distinctly unusual, in contrast to HP. Some have described mild obstructive or restrictive pulmonary function tests; however, a normal study is the rule. Hypoxemia is also distinctly unusual and is transient, if present. Chest x-ray abnormalities are not seen. BAL will reveal the presence of a neutrophilic alveolitis, and not the lymphocyte-predominant alveolitis with inverted T-helper/T-suppressor cell ratios characteristic of HP.

D. **Differential diagnosis** of ODTS includes HP and asthma. Silo filler's disease should also be considered. Generally, those with silo filler's disease will be much more toxic, have physical findings demonstrating crackles, and are much more likely to have chest x-ray abnormalities, abnormal pulmonary function tests, and hypoxemia.

E. **Management.** Unlike HP, treatment with steroids is not indicated. With avoidance, spontaneous recovery is the rule, and long-term sequelae have not been described.

References

1. Gurney J: Hypersensitivity pneumonitis. *Radiol Clin North Am* 1992;30:1219–1230.
2. Kaltreider H: Hypersensitivity pneumonitis. *West J Med* 1993;159:570–578.
3. Levy M, Fink J: Hypersensitivity pneumonitis. *Ann Allergy* 1985;54:167–171.
4. Fink J: Epidemiologic aspects of hypersensitivity pneumonitis. *Monogr Allergy* 1987;21:59–69.
5. Fink J: Hypersensitivity pneumonitis. *Clin Chest Med* 1992;13:303–309.
6. Lopez M, Salvaggio J: Epidemiology of hypersensitivity pneumonitis/allergic alveolitis. *Monogr Allergy* 1987;21:70–86.
7. Sharma O: Hypersensitivity pneumonitis. *Disease-A-Month* 1991;37:409–471.
8. Walker C, Grammer L: Hypersensitivity pneumonitis. *Allergy Proc* 1993;14:167.
9. Costabel U: The alveoloitis of hypersensitivity pneumonitis. *Eur Respir J* 1988;1):5–9.
10. Marinelli W, Davies S: Granulomatous diseases of the lung that mimic respiratory infections. *Semin Respir Infect* 1988;3:181–202.
11. Buschman D, Gamsu G, Waldron J, et al.: Chronic hypersensitivity pneumonitis: use of CT in diagnosis. *AJR* 1992;159:957–960.
12. Lynch D, Rose C, Way D, King T: Hypersensitivity pneumonitis: sensitivity of high-resolution CT in a population-based study. *AJR* 1992;159:469–472.
13. Muller N, Mayo J, Zwirewich C: Value of MR imaging in the evaluation of chronic infiltrative lung diseases: comparison with CT. *AJR* 1992;158:1205–1209.
14. Semenzato G, Ambello R, Trentin L, Agostini C: Cellular immunity in sarcoidosis and hypersensitivity pneumonitis: recent advances. *Chest* 1993;103:139S–143S.

15. Daniele R, Elias J, Epstein P, Rossman M: Bronchoalveolar lavage: role in the pathogenesis, diagnosis and management of interstitial lung disease. *Ann Intern Med* 1985;102:93–108.
16. Hensley G, Garancis J, Cherayil G, Fink J: Lung biopsies of pigeon breeder's disease. *Arch Pathol* 1969;87:572.
17. Reyes CN, Wenzel FJ, Lawton BR, Emanuel DA. The pulmonary pathology of farmer's lung disease. *Chest* 1982;81:142–146.
18. Craig T, Hershey J, Engler R, et al.: Bird antigen persistence in the home environment after removal of the bird. *Ann Allergy* 1992;69:510–512.
19. Vandenplas O, Malo J, Dugas M, et al.: Hypersensitivity pneumonitis-like reaction among workers exposed to diphenylmethane diisocyanate (MDI). *Am Rev Respir Dis* 1993;147:338–346.
20. Ando M, Arima K, Yoneda R, Tamura M: Japanese summer-type hypersensitivity pneumonitis: geographic distribution, home environment, and clinical characteristics of 621 cases. *Am Rev Respir Dis* 1991;144:765–769.
21. von Essen S, Robbins R, Thopson A, Rennard S: Organic dust toxic syndrome: an acute febrile reaction to organic dust exposure distinct from hypersensitivity pneumonitis. *J Toxicol* 1990;28:389–420.
22. Weber S, Kullman G, Petsonk E, et al.: Organic dust exposures from compost handling: case presentation and respiratory exposure assessment. *Am J Ind Med* 1993;24:365–374.
23. do Pico G: Hazardous exposure and lung disease among farm workers. *Clin Chest Med* 1992;13:311–328.

12

Pleural Effusions

Leslie H. Zimmerman

I. **Overview**
  A. The pleural space between the visceral and parietal pleurae normally contains a very thin layer of fluid. The primary function of this fluid and the serous pleural membranes is the mechanical coupling of the movement of the lung and the chest wall in a low-resistance manner. Pleural fluid arises from systemic vessels supplying the visceral and parietal pleurae and exits the pleural space by bulk flow (not diffusion) via parietal pleural stomas and pleural lymphatics. **Pleural fluid accumulates due to either an increased rate of fluid formation, a decreased rate of removal, or both.**
  B. The initial step in establishing the etiology of a pleural effusion is to determine whether the fluid is a transudate or an exudate. Defining an effusion as a transudate limits the differential diagnosis to a small number of disorders and also limits the need for further work-up in most cases. The classic definition described by Light and colleagues (1) remains the best way to distinguish transudates from exudates and remains superior to more recent reports using the serum to pleural fluid albumin gradient, the pleural fluid cholesterol concentration, or the pleural fluid/serum bilirubin ratio (2). Measurments of the pleural fluid/serum lactate dehydrogenase (LDH) and protein ratios should be obtained, as should full cell counts and differentials. Cultures should be obtained as the clinical situation warrants (Table 12-1).

II. **Transudates**
  A. **Presenting signs and symptoms**
    1. Small transudative effusions are usually asymptomatic and often discovered incidentally on a chest radiograph. Larger effusions may cause dyspnea, especially in the presence of underlying cardiac or pulmonary disease. Cough may occur, probably secondary to distortion of the lung parenchyma.
    2. Physical examination reveals absent breath sounds, decreased vocal and tactile fremitus, and dullness to percussion over the effusion. An accentuation of breath sounds and increased egophony may be noted over the area of compressed lung above large effusions.
    3. Hypoxemia is unusual with small-to-moderate effusions, probably because of similar decreases in both ventilation and perfusion, but it may occur in patients with very large effusions.
  B. **Etiology and pathogenesis.** Transudative pleural effusions are an ultrafiltrate of plasma. The finding of a transudative effusion generally implies that the pleural membranes are not diseased and the fluid accumulation is caused by systemic (nonlung, nonpleural) factors affecting the formation and absorption of pleural fluid. **The most common cause of a transudative effusion, as well as the most common cause of all effusions, is congestive heart failure (CHF).**
  C. **Differential diagnostic possibilities.** Atelectasis, pneumonia, pleural mass, or pleural thickening may cause absent breath sounds, dullness to percussion, and opacification on chest radiographs. Transudative effusions are typically free-flowing on lateral decubitus films and thereby easily distinguishable radiographically from these other processes. Fluid can occasionally collect in the major or minor fissures and appear to be a mass, usually in the setting of heart failure. Resolution of these "pseudotumors" with diuresis distinguishes them from true lung masses.

Table 12-1. Exudative effusions (one or more criteria)

Pleural fluid to serum protein ratio >0.5
Pleural fluid to serum LDH ratio >0.6
Pleural fluid LDH value >2/3 upper normal limit for serum LDH

LDH =lactate dehydrogenase.
Adapted from Light RW, MacGregor MI, Luchsinger PC, Ball WC. Pleural effusions: the diagnostic separation of transudates and exudates. *Ann Intern Med* 1972;77:507–513.

D. Specific approach

1. Free-flowing pleural fluid gravitates to the most dependent part of the thoracic cavity; when upright, this is the posterior costophrenic sulcus. More than 150 mL of fluid is required to blunt the costophrenic angle on a lateral chest radiograph. If the costophrenic angle appears blunted, bilateral decubitus films should be ordered to determine whether the fluid is free-flowing (nonloculated). If the effusion is free-flowing, the decubitus film with the abnormal side "down" permits estimation of the size of the pleural effusion; the decubitus film with the abnormal side "up" permits examination of the underlying, previously obscured lung parenchyma.

2. If the distance between the fluid inside the thoracic cage and the outside of the lung is <10 mm on lateral decubitus films, the pleural effusion will be difficult to obtain by thoracentesis and not likely to be clinically significant.

3. Because transudative and exudative pleural effusions can have similar radiographic appearances, a diagnostic thoracentesis (removal of 50–100 mL) should be considered in nearly all patients with free-flowing pleural fluid >10 mm thick on lateral decubitus films. Thoracentesis should be performed one interspace below the upper border of a moderate free-flowing effusion, identified by dullness to percussion and the loss of tactile and vocal fremitus, about 5–10 cm lateral to the spine. The needle should be introduced into the intercostal space just above the upper margin of the rib to avoid inadvertent laceration of the intercostal artery or nerve.

4. Observation of small effusions in patients with clinical heart failure or recent uncomplicated thoracic or abdominal surgery is appropriate. However, the presence of a large or loculated effusion, fever, or pleuritic chest pain raises the possibility of an exudative process and should prompt a thoracentesis.

E. Causes of transudative effusions are listed below. CHF, pulmonary embolism, and cirrhosis account for >90% of transudative effusions (Table 12-2).

F. Management. Management of transudative effusions is directed at treatment of the underlying problem (CHF, renal failure, cirrhosis). Diuresis can change a transudative effusion into an exudative effusion (3), although this is an unusual occurrence (4). Of note, pulmonary emboli may be associated with a transudative effusion in 25% of patients (5).

G. Problems and complications of thoracentesis

1. **Relative contraindications** to thoracentesis include very small pleural effusions, anticoagulation therapy, or other bleeding diatheses. The risks of thoracentesis include local pain and bleeding, hemothorax, pneumothorax, infection (rare), puncture of intra-abdominal organs including spleen and liver, and reexpansion pulmonary edema (6–8).

2. The risk of pneumothorax varies from 3 to 18% (8,9); risk is minimized when thoracentesis is performed under ultrasonographic guidance (8). Ultrasonographic guidance is especially useful in small or loculated effusions or in patients on positive-pressure mechanical ventilation in whom accidental lung puncture could cause a tension pneumothorax. Other factors that increase the risk of pneumothorax include large-volume thoracentesis and use of needles >20 gauge.

3. Reexpansion pulmonary edema may occur when large volumes of pleural fluid are removed (usually >1 L), especially in the setting of a long-standing pleural

Table 12-2. Causes of transudative effusions

Congestive heart failure
Pulmonary embolism
Cirrhosis
Nephrotic syndrome
Peritoneal dialysis
Myxedema
Urinothorax
Atelectasis
Constrictive pericarditis
Superior vena cava obstruction

effusion or the generation of high negative pressures during fluid removal (10). We therefore recommend that no more than 1 L be removed during an individual procedure.

H. **Specialist referrals.** Moderate-to-large transudative effusions may cause significant symptoms in patients with poor cardiopulmonary reserve. If response to treatment of the underlying disease is poor, pleurodesis should be considered in individuals who have experienced symptomatic relief of dyspnea after repeated therapeutic thoracenteses (11).

III. **Exudates**
A. **Presenting signs and symptoms**
  1. Moderate-to-large exudative effusions may also cause dyspnea (especially in the presence of underlying cardiac or pulmonary disease) and cough. Even small exudative effusions may be associated with pleuritic chest pain (from parietal pleural inflammation via intercostal nerves) or ipsilateral referred shoulder pain (from diaphragmatic parietal pleural inflammation via the phrenic nerve).
  2. The physical examination is identical to that found with transudates, with absent breath sounds, decreased fremitus, and dullness to percussion over the area of effusion; however, the presence of a pleural friction rub with an effusion strongly suggests an exudative process.
B. **Etiology and pathogenesis.** Exudates typically arise from leakage of fluid across an injured capillary bed in the pleura itself or in the adjacent lung. The injured capillaries permit fluid with a high protein content to leak across a disrupted endothelial barrier. Less commonly, an exudative pleural effusion can originate from an infected or inflammatory fluid collection in the mediastinum, retroperitoneum, or peritoneum and can track into the low-pressure-potential space of the pleural cavity.
C. **Differential diagnostic possibilities**
  1. Pneumonia, malignancy, and pulmonary embolism account for the majority of exudative effusions. Exudative effusions may be confused with atelectasis, pneumonia, pleural mass, or pleural thickening on physical examination and by chest radiograph. Again, free-flowing, small-to-moderate effusions can be distinguished from these other processes by lateral decubitus films.
  2. Loculated exudative effusions do not shift on decubitus films and may be difficult to distinguish from pulmonary parenchymal processes or pleural masses. Ultrasonography can differentiate these processes and identify the optimal site for pleural-fluid sampling of a loculated fluid collection. Decubitus films are not useful when the entire hemithorax is opacified. The differential diagnosis for an opacified hemithorax includes massive effusion, complete lung atelectasis, or tumor with or without associated effusion.
  3. Computed tomography (CT) scan may be used to distinguish peripheral lung abscesses from empyemas with air–fluid levels and to identify pleural masses

such as mesotheliomas in patients with undiagnosed exudative effusions. Magnetic resonance (MR) imaging does not appear to be as useful as ultrasonography or CT scan in the work-up or management of pleural effusions, mass, and lung collapse. Mediastinal shift toward the opacified side suggests atelectasis; shift away from the opacified side suggests an effusion. However, ultrasonography or CT may be necessary to distinguish these different processes.

D. Specific approach

    1. The first step is to diagnose the effusion as exudative. An effusion is considered to be an exudative if it meets any of the criteria listed above (1). After obtaining appropriate imaging studies including CT scan to evaluate the underlying lung parenchyma and pleural surface for masses, a thoracentesis should be performed to obtain fluid. Because exudative effusions have many possible etiologies (Table 12-3), a stepwise approach to making the diagnosis is useful.

    2. Step 1—check appearance of pleural fluid.

        a. Frank pus is diagnostic of an empyema; immediate tube thoracostomy placement should be considered.

        b. Hemothorax (pleural fluid hematocrit >50% of peripheral blood hematocrit) may also require tube thoracostomy depending on the volume of the effusion and the clinical situation. Since effusions may appear sanguineous with >10,000 red blood cells (RBCs) per milliliter of fluid, a spun hematocrit should be ordered on bloody-appearing effusions.

        c. Milky or opalescent-appearing fluid suggests a chylothorax.

    3. Step 2—obtain chemistries, cell counts, cultures, and cytologies. Once the diagnosis of exudate is confirmed by protein or LDH ratios and the fluid does not appear to be pus, blood, or chyle, the following additional pleural fluid studies should be ordered: RBC count, white blood cell count and differential, glucose, amylase, Gram's stain and cultures, and cytology.

    4. Step 3—obtain other studies in selected individuals. Pleural fluid pH should be obtained if the diagnosis of empyema remains in doubt. Pleural fluid antinuclear antibody, complement levels, rheumatoid factor, and lipid analysis should be obtained to rule out vasculitic and connective tissue disease as causes of exudates (Table 12-4).

    5. Step 4—perform percutaneous pleural biopsy in selected individuals. Although a specific diagnosis can be made in up to 75% of patients with exudative pleural effusions by the studies listed above, percutaneous pleural biopsy may be required in the remaining cases (12).

Table 12-3. Causes of exudative effusions

Parapneumonic
Malignancy
Pulmonary embolism
Tuberculosis
Gastrointestinal diseases
Connective tissue diseases
Trauma
Asbestos-related effusion
Dressler's syndrome
Uremia
Meig's syndrome
Drug reaction
Radiation therapy
Sarcoidosis
Yellow nail syndrome

Table 12-4. Assessment of pleural fluid

Test	Comment
RBC per mm³ >100,000	Trauma, malignancy, pulmonary embolism
Hct >50% of peripheral blood	Hemothorax
WBC per mm³	
>50,000–100,000	Grossly visible pus, otherwise total WBC less useful than WBC differential
>50% neutrophils	Acute inflammation or infection
>50% lymphocytes	Tuberculosis, malignancy
>10% eosinophils	Most common: hemothorax, pneumothorax; also benign
>5% mesothelial cells	Asbestos effusions, drug reaction, paragonimiasis; tuberculosis *less likely*
Glucose <60 mg/dL	Infection, malignancy, tuberculosis, rheumatoid pleuritis
Amylase >200 units/dL	Esophageal perforation, pancreatic disease, malignancy, ruptured ectopic pregnancy
	Isoenzyme profile: salivary—esophageal disease, malignancy (esp. lung)
	Isoenzyme profile: pancreatic—pancreatic disease
pH <7.2	Infection (complicated parapneumonic effusion and empyema), malignancy, esophageal rupture, rheumatoid or lupus pleuritis, tuberculosis, systemic acidosis, urinothorax
Triglyceride >110 mg/dL	Chylothorax
Microbiological studies	Etiology of infection
Cytology	Diagnostic of malignancy

Hct =hematocrit; RBC =red blood cell; WBC =white blood cell.
Adapted from Sahn SA. State of the art: the pleura. *Am Rev Respir Dis* 1988;138:184–234.

    a. Percutaneous pleural biopsy should be performed to evaluate undiagnosed exudative effusions in which tuberculosis or malignancy is suspected. The diagnostic yield of percutaneous pleural biopsy for tuberculosis is approximately 80% (13). Because of the non-uniform nature of pleural metastases, the pleural biopsy yield for malignancy is approximately 45% to 55% (12–14).

    b. Contraindications to percutaneous pleural biopsy include an obliterated pleural space, concurrent anticoagulation therapy or other bleeding diatheses, and renal insufficiency because of platelet effects (12).

    c. Of the remaining "idiopathic" effusions, a definitive diagnosis can be made in the vast majority (with malignancy the most common finding) by direct thoracoscopic examination and directed biopsy of the pleura (15–17).

  5. In the absence of associated hemoptysis or radiographic abnormalities such as a mass lesion or atelectasis, bronchoscopy rarely adds to the diagnostic yield of an unexplained pleural effusion (18).

 E. **Management.** The specific management of an exudative effusion depends on the underlying diagnosis.

IV. **Specific types of pulmonary effusions**

 A. **Parapneumonic effusions** are those associated with a pneumonia, lung abscess, or occasionally bronchiectasis. Pneumonias from aerobic organisms such as *Streptococcus pneumoniae*, *Staphylococcus aureus*, and various gram-negative rods typically present with an acute febrile illness. The frequency of an infected pleural space in the setting of a pneumonia varies with the infectious agent. For example, pleural effusions are quite common with pneumococcal pneumonia, being found in 50% of patients, but the effusion is culture positive for the organism in <5% of patients (19). Effusions are less common in *S. aureus* pneumonia, but pleural fluid cultures are positive in approximately 20% of cases. The majority of effusions associated with gram-negative pneumonias are culture negative (19).

1. Anaerobic and mixed anaerobic/aerobic infections account for the majority of culture-positive parapneumonic effusions. Anaerobic pneumonias and associated effusions more typically present with a subacute illness, and most patients have some predisposing risk factor for aspiration.
2. Parapneumonic effusions can range from sterile exudates with slightly abnormal pleural fluid characteristics that resolve with prompt antibiotic treatment of the pneumonia to grossly infected pus requiring prompt tube thoracostomy drainage, antibiotic therapy, and occasionally surgical debridement. Recommendations for tube thoracostomy drainage in parapneumonic effusions have been debated for years (19–22), although some basic recommendations remain the same. "Uncomplicated" sterile parapneumonic effusions, with normal glucose and pH values, typically resolve spontaneously with antibiotic therapy alone.
3. **Empyema, as defined by gross pus or a positive Gram's stain, or a "complicated" parapneumonic effusion with a glucose <40 mg/dL or pH <7.1 require prompt tube thoracostomy drainage in addition to antibiotics for adequate resolution of the infection.** Between these two extremes, the challenge is to differentiate those effusions that will resolve spontaneously with antibiotics from those that behave like empyemas and require tube drainage. The standard approach is to use pleural fluid chemistries to guide the need for tube thoracostomy placement.
    a. Those patients with intermediate chemistries, that is, pleural fluid pH between 7.1 and 7.3 and glucose between 40 and 60 mg/dL, may either be managed with chest tube drainage or serial thoracenteses. Younger, healthier patients and those with pneumococcal pneumonia are more likely to clear the associated effusion with antibiotics alone. A falling pH or glucose suggests that the infection is not controlled with antibiotics alone. Although the absolute level of pleural fluid LDH is less useful for determining need for tube thoracostomy, a rising pleural fluid LDH level over serial thoracenteses indicates poor control of infection, and tube drainage should be considered. Lastly, worsening clinical status, persistent or recurrent fever, or an increasing pleural fluid volume suggests the need for drainage.
    b. Once a decision is made to drain an infected or potentially infected effusion, prompt drainage is critical since the infection can spread rapidly over the pleural surface. A pleural infection induces fibrin deposition that can compartmentalize the effusion into loculated pockets, making adequate drainage much more problematic. Once a chest tube is placed, most patients should defervesce within several days.
    c. 20% to 30% of patients with empyemas fail to improve after chest tube placement; this is usually due to undrained fluid in one or more locules. Additional chest tube placement with or without intracavitary fibrinolysis (23), minithoracotomy, or full thoracotomy for debridement may be required.
B. **Malignant effusions.** Effusions due to metastatic disease are the second most common cause of exudative effusions. More than half of "idiopathic" exudative effusions, that is, those that remain without apparent cause despite thoracentesis, are due to malignancy (15). Metastatic lung, breast, gastric, or ovarian cancer or lymphoma account for the vast majority of malignant effusions (12,14). Ninety percent of malignant effusions are exudative and approximately one-third are bloody (12, 14). Seventy percent of massive effusions that opacify an entire hemithorax on presentation are due to malignancy (24).
    1. Pleural fluid cytology is positive in up to 60% of malignant effusions on the first thoracentesis; diagnostic yield increases with the volume of fluid analyzed. A second or third thoracentesis improves the yield to 70% to 80% (14). Percutaneous pleural biopsy (more likely to be positive with extensive pleural tumor burden) or thoracoscopic visualization of the pleura and biopsy of abnormal areas will provide a diagnosis, respectively, in 45% to 55% and 90% of cases of malignant pleural effusion (12,14,16).

2. Immunocytometry and gene-rearrangement analysis can increase diagnostic yield and help differentiate tumor cells from a polyclonal inflammatory reaction in patients with lymphoma.

3. Patients with malignant effusions are not curable by any modalities currently in use; such patients have a mean life expectancy of 6 months to 1 year. Such individuals may be candidates for palliative measures. Patients with malignant effusions who experience symptomatic improvement in their dyspnea with repeated thoracentesis should be considered for tube thoracostomy with chemical pleurodesis in order to maximize comfort and time out of the hospital. This can be accomplished by instillation of doxycycline, minocycline, bleomycin, or talc through a chest tube at a time when most of the malignant effusion has been drained. This procedure should not be performed if the patient has atelectatic lung, which is not reexpandable by suction. Of note, pleural fluid with lower pH statuses correlates with a higher tumor burden, shorter survival, and less successful pleurodesis (25).

4. Paramalignant effusions are not caused by direct pleural metastases and may be due to lymphatic obstruction from mediastinal lymph node involvement, endobronchial tumor with airway obstruction, atelectasis, or obstruction of the thoracic duct with development of a chylothorax (14).

C. **Pulmonary embolism.** Pleural effusions occur in up to 50% of patients with pulmonary emboli (26), although the clinical presentation is similar in those with or without effusions. The effusion may be caused by parenchymal and pleural ischemia, changes in local hydrostatic pressure, and/or increased capillary permeability (12). Pleural fluid characteristics are highly variable and not diagnostic. Effusions can be transudative (20%), exudative, and even bloody (27). While not diagnostic, bloody effusions are more common secondary to a pulmonary infarction. Therapy is directed at the underlying thromboembolic disease, and **the presence of a bloody effusion is not a contraindication to anticoagulation.**

D. **Tuberculous effusions.** Tuberculous pleuritis classically accompanies primary tuberculosis (28). Effusions tend to be unilateral and small to moderate in size, most commonly occurring 3–6 months after the initial infection. Radiographically apparent associated parenchymal disease occurs in only one-third to one-half of cases (29).

1. **Primary tuberculous pleuritis** typically occurs in younger patients and presents either as an acute febrile illness with nonproductive cough and pleuritic chest pain or a subacute illness with anorexia, weight loss, and low-grade fever. Up to one-third will have a negative purified protein derivative (PPD) tuberculin test on presentation, although most will convert in the next 1–2 months (12). Thoracentesis reveals a serous or serosanguineous exudate with a lymphocytic predominance (neutrophils may predominate very early in the course of the effusion [30]). **The presence of >5% mesothelial cells on the differential cell count makes the diagnosis of tuberculous pleuritis less likely.** Primary tuberculous pleuritis probably represents a hypersensitivity reaction to a small subpleural focus of infection.

   a. The pleuritis is a granulomatous reaction with a very low mycobacterial load; acid-fast bacillus stain and culture of pleural fluid from primary tuberculous pleuritis are positive in only about 15% of patients (13). Percutaneous pleural biopsy improves the diagnostic yield to 80% (13); finding caseating granuloma in the biopsy specimen provides a presumptive diagnosis in patients with lymphocytic exudative effusions (12).

   b. Accurate diagnosis and therapy with regimens used for active pulmonary tuberculosis are important because untreated patients are at high risk for subsequent pulmonary reactivation despite the fact that the effusion is self-limited (29).

2. **Pleural effusions as a manifestation of reactivation tuberculosis** are typically associated with radiographic evidence of upper lung-field parenchymal disease. Patients tend to be older than those with primary tuberculosis, with a higher frequency of positive PPD tuberculin reactions and a greater likelihood of having sputum and pleural fluid cultures positive for tuberculosis (31).

Tube thoracostomy drainage is unnecessary in these effusions, unless a true tuberculous empyema with thick purulent exudate is present.

    a. Primary and reactivation tuberculous-associated effusions are associated with high levels of adenosine deaminase (ADA) activity; ADA isoenzymes may help to separate tuberculous pleuritis from parapneumonic pleuritis, although the clinical utility of this test is still uncertain (32).

E. **Effusions due to pancreatic diseases.** Any intra-abdominal inflammatory or infectious process may cause a sympathetic pleural effusion. Pancreatitis and pancreatic pseudocysts are remarkable for causing exudative effusions with an elevated pleural fluid amylase (33). Pleural effusions are present in 15% of patients with acute pancreatitis, are usually small to moderate in size, and are left-sided in 60% of patients (12).

    1. The diagnosis is confirmed by an **elevated pleural fluid amylase** (greater than serum amylase). Patients present with abdominal symptoms consistent with acute pancreatitis; the effusion resolves as the pancreatitis subsides, and usually no specific therapy for the effusion is required (other than diagnostic thoracentesis). If the effusion does not resolve in 2–3 weeks, a pancreatic abscess or pseudocyst may be present.

    2. Chronic pancreatitis may be accompanied by massive recurrent exudative pleural effusions, and patients usually have symptoms of dyspnea or cough related to the effusion. While most patients have a history of alcoholism, only one-half have a previous history of pancreatitis.

    3. The etiology of these effusions in most patients is a pancreatic pseudocyst that has decompressed into the pleural space via a sinus tract. Although serum amylase may not be elevated, pleural fluid amylase is typically very high. CT scan will usually confirm the presence of a pancreatic pseudocyst (34).

    4. Conservative therapy with bowel rest, hyperalimentation, therapeutic pleural drainage (as needed for dyspnea), and possibly a regimen of somatostatin or analogs is successful in 40% of cases; surgery may be required for those who fail to respond (34). A pancreatic abscess may also form as a consequence of acute or chronic pancreatitis and cause a sympathetic effusion. The treatment is drainage of the underlying abscess.

F. **Mesothelioma.** Malignant mesothelioma is a primary pleural tumor. The risk of developing mesothelioma is generally related to the duration and intensity of exposure to asbestos (35), although minimal exposure has also been associated with this tumor. Mesothelioma is seen more commonly in men as a consequence of workplace exposure. Because of the long latency period after asbestos exposure (>30 years) (12), the incidence appears to be rising and will likely continue to rise through the next decade (35). Most patients present with nonpleuritic chest pain and dyspnea, although fever, weight loss, and easy fatigabilty are also seen. More than half of patients will have a large pleural effusion at the time of presentation. The tumor grows and invades locally, eventually encasing the ipsilateral lung. Chest radiographs reveal effusions, and one-third of patients have coincident pleural plaques in the opposite lung (36). The effusion may initially cause a mediastinal shift away from the affected side, but as the tumor gradually encases and traps the lung, the mediastinum shifts toward the affected side.

    1. **Chest CT scans are very useful in diagnosis, revealing a characteristically thickened, nodular pleural surface** (36). Thoracentesis can reveal serous, serosanguineous, or bloody exudative fluid. Cytologic distinction between benign and malignant mesothelial cells and between malignant mesothelioma and metastatic adenocarcinoma may be difficult.

    2. Although diagnosis by needle biopsy is possible, the specimen size obtained by this procedure is usually not sufficient for accurate histopathology. **Thoracoscopy is currently the best method for diagnosis, with a sensitivity of approximately 90%** (12,15–17).

G. **Hemothorax** (37,38). A hemothorax is a bloody pleural effusion with a hematocrit >50%. Trauma is the most common cause of hemothorax: either blunt trauma with rib fracture or penetrating trauma, including procedural complications. Most large or expanding traumatic hemothoraces should be managed with tube thoracostomy.

Chest tube placement allows quantification of blood loss and may slow the bleeding through apposition of the pleural surfaces. Whenever the chest tube drainage is >200 mL/h, thoracotomy should be considered. Bloody effusions not due to trauma are most likely due to malignancy.

H. Chylothorax (12,39). Ingested fat enters the blood stream through the thoracic duct in the form of triglycerides and lipoprotein-rich chylomicrons. A chylothorax results from disruption of the thoracic duct or, less commonly, from tracking of chylous ascites from the peritoneum. Thoracentesis usually reveals a sterile, opalescent or milky fluid with a triglyceride level between 50–110 mg/dL.

  1. Malignancy, typically lymphoma with intrathoracic lymphatic obstruction, is the most common cause of a chylous effusion. Other causes include injury to the thoracic duct during thoracic surgery, complications of central line placement or other procedures, blunt chest trauma, and rare diseases such as lymphangiomyomatosis.

  2. Patients typically present with dyspnea, as chylous effusions can be quite large. Active pleuritis is not a feature. Patients without a history of trauma or surgery should have a chest CT scan to evaluate the mediastinum for lymphoma or other malignancies.

  3. Management of a chylothorax includes initial drainage of the effusion, if needed for symptomatic relief of dyspnea, and then dietary interventions to minimize oral intake of fat, including the use of hyperalimentation for nutrition. The decrease in chyle formation may allow spontaneous healing of a ruptured thoracic duct. In addition, radiation therapy for lymphoma, surgical repair of a traumatically injured thoracic duct, and pleurodesis for patients with poorly responsive malignancies may be required for management. Repeated thoracenteses or chronic chest tube drainage lead to malnutrition and immunologic incompetence and should be avoided.

  4. Long-standing effusions from any cause may contain large amounts of cholesterol crystals and give a milky appearance to pleural fluid. These "pseudochylous" effusions are not related to problems with the thoracic duct and can be differentiated from true chylous effusions by lipoprotein analysis, which reveals elevated cholesterol and low triglyceride levels.

V. Referrals to specialists. Exudative pleural effusions of unclear etiology require consultation with a pulmonary specialist. Percutaneous pleural biopsy, thoracoscopic pleural biopsy, or pleurodesis requires referral to a specialist.

VI. Problems and complications of therapy. The risks and relative contraindications to thoracentesis are the same for transudates and exudates. For percutaneous pleural biopsy, risks are primarily pneumothorax, bleeding from intercostal artery laceration, and (rarely) puncture of intra-abdominal organs. Pneumothorax occurs in 10% of cases, although only 1% will require placement of a chest tube (13). The risks associated with thoracoscopic pleural biopsy include bleeding, local infection, air leak from inadvertent lung puncture, and the risks of local or general anesthesia. Death or major complications are rare, while minor complications are reported in 5% to 19% of cases (15–17). It is very important to remember that malignant seeding can occur along the biopsy tract of patients found to have malignant mesothelioma by needle biopsy or thoracoscopic biopsy. Local radiotherapy at the biopsy site may minimize local tumor spread (40).

References

1. Light RW, MacGregor MI, Luchsinger PC, Ball WC: Pleural effusions: the diagnostic separation of transudates and exudates. *Ann Intern Med* 1972;77:507–513.
2. Burgess LJ, Maritz FJ, Taljaard JJF: Comparative analysis of the biochemical parameters used to distinguish between pleural transudates and exudates. *Chest* 1995;107:1604–1609.
3. Chakko S: Pleural effusion in congestive heart failure. *Chest* 1990;98:521–522.
4. Shinto RA, Light RW: Effects of diuresis on the characteristics of pleural fluid in patients with congestive heart failure. *Am J Med* 1990;88:230–234.

5. Light RW: Pleural diseases. *Disease-a-Month* 1992;38:261–331.
6. Grogan DR, Irwin RS, Channick R, et al.: Complications associated with thoracentesis: a prospective, randomized study comparing three different methods. *Arch Intern Med* 1990;150:873–877.
7. Grogan DR, Irwin RS: Risk of thoracentesis. *Ann Intern Med* 1991;114:431.
8. Raptopoulos V, Davis LM, Lee G, et al.: Factors affecting the development of pneumothorax associated with thoracentesis. *AJR* 1991;156:917–920.
9. Bartter T, Mayo PD, Pratter MR, et al.: Lower risk and higher yield for thoracentesis when performed by experienced operators. *Chest* 1993;103:1873–1876.
10. Mahfood S, Hix WR, Aaron BL, et al.: Re-expansion pulmonary edema. *Ann Thorac Surg* 1988;45:340–345.
11. Sudduth DC, Sahn SA: Pleurodesis for nonmalignant pleural effusions: recommendations. *Chest* 1992;102:1855–1860.
12. Sahn SA: State of the art: the pleura. *Am Rev Respir Dis* 1988;138:184–234.
13. Bueno CE, Clemente G, Castro BC, et al.: Cytologic and bacteriologic analysis of fluid and pleural fluid biopsy specimens with Cope's needle. *Arch Intern Med* 1990;150:1190–1194.
14. Fenton KN, Richardson JD: Diagnosis and management of malignant pleural effusions. *Am J Surg* 1995;170:69–74.
15. Harris RJ, Kavuru MS, Mehta AC, et al.: The impact of thoracoscopy on the management of pleural diseases. *Chest* 1995;107:845–852.
16. LoCicero J: Thoracoscopic management of malignant pleural effusion. *Ann Thorac Surg* 1993;56:641–643.
17. Menzies R, Charbonneau M: Thoracoscopy for the diagnosis of pleural disease. *Ann Intern Med* 1991;114:271–276.
18. Feinsilver SH, Barrows AA, Braman SS: Fiberoptic bronchoscopy and pleural effusion of unknown origin. *Chest* 1986;90:518–519.
19. Light RW, Girard WM, Jenkinson SG, George RB: Parapneumonic effusions. *Am J Med* 1980;69:507–512.
20. Berger HA, Morganroth ML: Immediate drainage is not required for all patients with complicated parapneumonic effusions. *Chest* 1990;97:731–735.
21. Poe RH, Marin MG, Israel RH, Kallay MC: Utility of pleural fluid analysis in predicting tube thoracostomy/decortication in parapneumonic effusions. *Chest* 1991;100:963–967.
22. Sahn SA: Management of complicated parapneumonic effusions. *Am Rev Respir Dis* 1993;148:813–817.
23. Moulton JS, Benkert RE, Weisiger KH, Chambers JA: Treatment of complicated pleural fluid collections with image-guided drainage and intracavitary urokinase. *Chest* 1995;108:1252–1259.
24. Maher GG, Berger HW: Massive pleural effusion: malignant and nonmalignant causes in 46 patients. *Am Rev Respir Dis* 1972;105:458–460.
25. Sahn SA, Good JT: Pleural fluid pH in malignant effusions. *Ann Intern Med* 1988;108:345–349.
26. Stein PD, Saltzman HA, Weg JG: Clinical characteristics of patients with acute pulmonary embolism. *Am J Cardiol* 1991;68:1723–1724.
27. Bynum LJ, Wilson JE: Characteristics of pleural effusions associated with pulmonary embolism. *Arch Intern Med* 1976;136:159–162.
28. Seibert AF, Haynes J, Middleton R, Bass JB: Tuberculous pleural effusion: twenty-year experience. *Chest* 1991;99:883–886.
29. McAdams HP, Erasmus J, Winter JA: Radiologic manifestations of pulmonary tuberculosis. *Radiol Clin North Am* 1995;33:655–678.
30. Antony VB, Repine JE, Harada RN, et al.: Inflammatory responses in experimental tuberculous pleurisy. *Acta Cytol* 1983;27:355–361.
31. Antoniskis D, Amin K, Barnes PF: Pleuritis as a manifestation of reactivation tuberculosis. *Am J Med* 1990;89:447–450.
32. Ungerer JP, Oosthuizen HM, Retief JH, Bisbbort SH: Significance of adenosine deaminase activity and its isoenzymes in tuberculous effusions. *Chest* 1994;106:33–37.
33. Joseph J, Viney S, Beck P, et al.: A prospective study of amylase-rich pleural effusions with special reference to amylase isoenzyme analysis. *Chest* 1992;102:1455–1459.
34. Rockey DC, Cello JP: Pancreaticopleural fistula: report of 7 patients and review of the literature. *Medicine* 1990;69:332–344.
35. Antman KH: Natural history and epidemiology of malignant mesothelioma. *Chest* 1993;103:373S–376S.

36. Aisner J: Current approach to malignant mesothelioma of the pleura. *Chest* 1995;107:332S–344S.
37. Light RW: Hemothorax. In: Light RW, ed. *Pleural diseases*. Philadelphia: Lea Febiger, 1990:263–268.
38. Martinez FJ, Villanueva AG, Pickering R, et al.: Spontaneous hemothorax. Report of 6 cases and review of the literature. *Medicine* 1992;71:354–368.
39. Marts BC, Naunheim KS, Pennington DG: Conservative versus surgical management of chylothorax. *Am J Surg* 1992;164:532–534.
40. Boutin C, Rey F, Viallat JR: Prevention of malignant seeding after invasive diagnostic procedures in patients with pleural mesothelioma: a randomized trial of local radiotherapy. *Chest* 1995; 108:754–758.

13 Pneumothorax

John L. Berk

I. **Definitions. Pneumothorax** is defined as the presence of air in the pleural space.
   A. **Spontaneous pneumothorax** is defined as a pneumothorax occurring in the absence of trauma to the chest.
      1. **Primary spontaneous pneumothorax** occurs in an otherwise healthy individual without identifiable lung disease.
      2. **Secondary spontaneous pneumothorax** occurs in a person with preexisting lung disease.
   B. **Traumatic pneumothorax** is defined as a pneumothorax caused by chest trauma that injures the pleural surface or disrupts the wall of a bronchus, an alveolus, or the esophagus.
      1. **Iatrogenic pneumothorax** is caused by the intentional or accidental entry of air into the pleural space during an invasive medical procedure.
   C. **Tension pneumothorax** occurs when persistent displacement of air into the pleural cavity causes the intrapleural pressures to exceed ambient barometric pressure. The respiratory and cardiovascular consequences of positive pressure in the pleural space constitute a medical emergency.

II. **Pathophysiology.** During spontaneous respiration, two opposing forces generate negative pleural pressures: the outward recoil of the chest wall and the inward tendency of the lung to collapse (elastic recoil). Sudden communication of the pleural space with alveolar or external air results in gas entry, until either the pressure gradient dissipates or the pleural defect is repaired. The air in the pleural space causes the ipsilateral lung to collapse, decreasing the vital capacity and lowering arterial oxygen levels. The cause of the hypoxemia is multifactorial. In addition to preventing full expansion of the ipsilateral lung, the pneumothorax induces ventilation–perfusion (V/Q) mismatching, pulmonary shunting, and regional alveolar hypoventilation (1,2). An increase in anatomic shunting occurs only when the pneumothorax occupies >25% of the hemithorax.

III. **Quantitation of pneumothorax size.** The volume of the hemithorax occupied by pleural air may be estimated by the following equation: Percentage pneumothorax = $[1 - (\text{lung diameter})^3/(\text{hemithorax diameter})^3] \times 100]$. Lung diameter may be estimated on a plane chest radiograph as the average distance from the hilum to the edge of the pneumothorax. For example, if the average diameter of the hemithorax is 12 cm and the average diameter of the collapsed lung is 10 cm, then the percentage of hemithorax occupied by the pneumothorax = $[1 - (10^3/12^3)] \times 100 = 42\%$. Since air in the pleural space is spontaneously resorbed at a rate of 1.25% of the hemithorax volume per day, it would take approximately 33 days (42/1.25) for a pneumothorax of this size to resolve.

IV. **Primary spontaneous pneumothorax**
   A. **Incidence.** The age-adjusted annual rate of primary spontaneous pneumothorax is about 7.4 events per 100,000 men and 1.2 events per 100,000 women (3). The male-to-female predominance varies internationally; the ratio is approximately 6:1 in the United States, versus 15:1 in Singapore (4). The peak incidence for primary spontaneous pneumothorax is in the third and fourth decades of life, and tall thin men are predisposed (5,6).
   B. **Etiology.** By definition, primary spontaneous pneumothorax occurs in people without clinically evident lung disease or disease present on a chest radiograph. How-

ever, chest computed tomography (CT) scans usually reveal subpleural blebs and bullae at the lung apices (7,8).

1. The cause of these emphysematous changes is unclear, although several theories exist. Apical pleural bleb formation may be related to alveolar distending pressures, which increase with the height of the thorax. The overrepresentation of tall young men with increased thoracic height supports this hypothesis. Alternatively, abnormal collagen deposition and bleb formation may explain the increased prevalence of spontaneous pneumothorax in patients with Marfan's syndrome or mitral valve prolapse (9). A familial predisposition to spontaneous pneumothorax has been rarely reported (10,11).

2. **Most important, smoking predisposes to spontaneous pneumothorax in a dose-related fashion** (12). In women, smoking 1–12 cigarettes per day increases the relative risk of pneumothorax fourfold over nonsmokers; 13–22 cigarettes daily increase the relative risk 14-fold, and >22 cigarettes per day increases the risk 68-fold. The relative risk of pneumothorax is 50% higher among men than women at each level of daily cigarette consumption.

C. **Presentation**

1. **Dyspnea** or **acute chest pain** localized to the affected lung are reported in 90% of cases, with both symptoms present in approximately two-thirds of cases (13). Rarely, Horner's syndrome (ptosis, miosis, and anhidrosis) may result from traction on the sympathetic ganglion (14). Among patients with normal lung function, dyspnea may resolve within 24 hours of initial lung collapse despite the persistence of the pneumothorax. Up to 18% of patients delay medical evaluation for >7 days (15).

2. **Primary spontaneous pneumothorax typically occurs at rest**, with <10% of cases occurring during exercise (16). Activities associated with marked swings in atmospheric pressure (eg, rapid altitude changes or underwater ascents) may induce the rupture of apical pleural blebs or intraparenchymal bullae.

D. **Physical findings**

1. **Moderate tachycardia may be the only abnormal vital sign.** Breath sounds are usually decreased over the affected hemithorax, while percussion resonance is increased. Hamman's sign, extra sounds heard throughout the cardiac cycle due to the juxtaposition of pleural air and the heart, occurs with left-sided pneumothorax. Tracheal shift away from the pneumothorax indicates a large collection of air in the pleural space. **Heart rates >140/min in the presence or absence of pulseless electrical activity, peripheral cyanosis, or hypotension suggest tension pneumothorax.**

E. **Diagnosis**

1. The identification of a pleural line on a **chest x-ray** is diagnostic. Expiratory or lateral chest films may accentuate the presence of pleural air. Associated pleural effusions are noted in 9% to 26% of cases (15). Two-thirds of these effusions are serous, while one-third are bloody. Spontaneous hemopneumothorax is extremely rare, however.

2. **Electrocardiographic (ECG) findings** are limited and nonspecific. Left-sided pneumothoraces may result in diminished QRS forces in the limb leads, decreased R-wave magnitudes precordially, and inverted T waves (17).

3. **Arterial blood gases** reveal an increased alveolar-arterial oxygen gradient, reflecting a decreased vital capacity, increased V/Q mismatching, and anatomic shunting in the collapsed lung.

F. **Recurrence rate**

1. All patients are at risk for recurrence of spontaneous pneumothorax, although the exact rate of repeated pneumothorax is debated. **Spontaneous pneumothorax recurs in 26% to 52% of patients within 5 years of the first event.** Recurrence rates in patients with **primary spontaneous pneumothorax** (31.8%) are lower than in patients with **secondary spontaneous events** due to underlying lung disease (43%) (18).

2. **Recurrent spontaneous pneumothorax** occurs most frequently within 2 years of the first event. A Department of Veterans Affairs Cooperative Study

demonstrated that 66% of the first year recurrences among patients with secondary spontaneous pneumothorax were within 1 month of the first event, and 89% occurred within 3 months of the first event (18). The incidence of recurrent spontaneous pneumothorax increases with each repeated event (62% after one recurrence and 83% after two recurrences). Contralateral recurrence occurs in <10% of patients (19).

  3. **Smoking cessation** after a first primary spontaneous pneumothorax has little impact on recurrence rates. This lack of effect probably reflects the short time interval between the first and second pneumothoraces relative to the prolonged effects of smoking on airway inflammation and bleb formation.

V. **Secondary spontaneous pneumothorax**

  A. **Incidence.** The age-adjusted incidence of secondary spontaneous pneumothorax is about 6.3/100,000 per year for men and 2.0/100,000 per year for women (3.2:1 male:female ratio) (3). The incidence of secondary spontaneous pneumothorax increases with age regardless of sex.

  B. **Etiology** (Table 13-1). Secondary spontaneous pneumothorax most frequently occurs (55% to 67%) in patients with chronic obstructive pulmonary disease (COPD) (3,18). The incidence of spontaneous pneumothorax among patients with COPD increases with the severity of airway obstruction (18). The rupture of intrapulmonary bullae, often found with secondary spontaneous pneumothoraces, causes lung collapse. Unlike apical pleural bleb formation in patients with primary spontaneous pneumothorax, these subpleural air spaces result from either enzymatic destruction of lung tissue (emphysema) or abnormal elastic recoil properties (fibrosis). Thoracic cavity length does not affect the incidence of secondary spontaneous pneumothorax. Necrotizing processes (infections, vasculitides, parenchymal infarction) also predispose to pleural rupture.

Table 13-1. Causes of secondary spontaneous pneumothorax

Infection	Pulmonary diseases
Necrotizing bacterial pneumonias	Cystic fibrosis
Infective endocarditis	Chronic obstructive airways disease
Mycobacterium tuberculosis	Asthma
Pneumocystis carinii	Idiopathic pulmonary hemosiderosis
Echinococcosis	Idiopathic pulmonary fibrosis
Paragonimiasis	Pulmonary infarction
	Berylliosis
Gastrointestinal disease	Pulmonary alveolar proteinosis
	Lymphangioleiomyomatosis
Colo- and gastropleural fistulas	Interstitial pneumonitis
Biliary cirrhosis	Desquamative interstitial pneumonitis
	Usual interstitial pneumonitis
Cardiac disease	
Mitral valve prolapse	
Systemic disease	**Cancer**
Eosinophilic granuloma/histiocytosis X	Primary lung carcinomas
Sarcoidosis	Pleural metastases
Wegener's granulomatosis	Sarcoma
Rheumatoid arthritis	Germ cell tumors
Catamenia	Adenocarcinomas
Scleroderma	Wilms' tumors
Neurofibromatosis	Radiation-related lung injury
Tuberous sclerosis	
Xanthomatosis	
Ankylosing spondylitis	
Marfan's syndrome	

C. **Presentation.** Patients with secondary spontaneous pneumothorax are more symptomatic than those with primary spontaneous pneumothorax. The dyspnea is typically disproportionate to the size of the pneumothorax, reflecting the severity of underlying lung disease, the degree of lung dysfunction induced by lung collapse, and the lack of pulmonary functional reserve. All patients with COPD experience shortness of breath, and 75% complain of unilateral pleuritic chest pain (20). Recognizing the classically asymmetric auscultatory and percussion findings may be difficult in patients with severe underlying lung disease.

D. **Diagnosis**

1. Identifying the visceral pleural line on **chest x-ray** is diagnostic. Concomitant lung disease may complicate radiographic recognition of the pleural air collection.

2. **Particular care must be taken to distinguish large subpleural air collections, such as bullae, from pneumothorax.** Chest tube placement into a **bulla** risks creation of bronchopleurocutaneous fistulas. **Chest CT** studies can differentiate air in the pleural space from large intraparenchymal bullae.

3. **Arterial blood gases** may reveal profound hypoxemia (mean $PaO_2 = 48$ Torr) and hypercapnia in patients with COPD. Lobar collapse in the setting of pneumothorax may represent bronchial obstruction, particularly if no air bronchograms are detected in the atelectatic lung. **If a large segment of lung does not fully reinflate following chest tube placement, bronchoscopy should be performed to rule out an endobronchial lesion.**

E. **Mortality.** Mortality due to pneumothorax has been thought to be approximately 15% to 20% in patients with COPD. However, a recent study reported only 1% mortality directly due to pneumothorax over a 5-year follow-up, but 36% of the study population died from unrelated causes within 5 years (18). Thus, spontaneous pneumothorax in COPD patients is an indicator of poor prognosis.

F. **Recurrence rate. Secondary spontaneous pneumothorax recurs more frequently than primary spontaneous events**. During 5-year follow-up periods, recurrences occurred in approximately 46% of patients with underlying COPD versus 33% of patients with apparently normal lungs (18,21). Nearly 50% of children with cystic fibrosis will experience a second pneumothorax unless pleurodesis is performed (22). A repeat pneumothorax typically occurs in the same hemithorax, but contralateral recurrence is noted in about 5% of patients (18).

VI. **Therapeutic approaches to spontaneous pneumothorax**

A. **Observation.** Conservative management is recommended only for patients with otherwise normal lungs, a small pneumothorax (<15%), and no shortness of breath or hemodynamic instability. As air is resorbed from the pleural space at 1.25% per day (23), small pneumothoraces should resolve in less than 12 days (15%/1.25% per day.) These patients do not need to be hospitalized.

B. **Oxygen administration.** Supplemental oxygen accelerates the rate of pneumothorax resorption fourfold over untreated controls (24). Exogenous oxygen dilutes the nitrogen gas concentration in the capillaries of the alveoli and the pleura, establishing a gradient of nitrogen gas between the pleural air and the vessels of the lung. All patients hospitalized with a pneumothorax should receive high-level oxygen supplementation.

C. **Simple needle aspiration**

1. **A first time primary spontaneous pneumothorax of >15% may be treated with simple needle aspiration.** This low-risk procedure can be performed on an outpatient basis. Cumulative experience with needle aspiration indicates successful treatment of primary spontaneous pneumothorax in >70% of reported cases. In contrast, needle aspiration is successful in only 31% of patients with secondary spontaneous pneumothorax. Therefore, **needle aspiration is not recommended for secondary spontaneous pneumothorax or patients with recurrent primary spontaneous events.**

2. **Technique.** Following local anesthesia, a 16-gauge needle (attached to a 60-mL syringe by a three-way stopcock) is inserted in the midclavicular line into the second intercostal space. Air is removed by aspiration until resistance is felt, the patient coughs persistently, or the patient complains of pain. The needle is then removed, and a chest x-ray obtained immediately and again several

hours later. If the pneumothorax recurs or the total air aspirated is >4 L, a small-bore thoracostomy and Heimlich valve attachment may be necessary.

D. Chest tube drainage. Patients with primary spontaneous pneumothorax who fail needle aspiration or experience a recurrent spontaneous event, as well as most patients with secondary spontaneous pneumothorax, should have the pleural space evacuated by chest tube. This approach is highly effective in primary spontaneous pneumothorax (96% of cases have complete resolution), and requires only a 4-day hospital stay on average. Chest tube management of patients with secondary spontaneous events is more complex, reflecting the effect of the underlying parenchymal lung disease on closure of the pleural defect. In a third of cases, persistent air leaks in patients with cystic fibrosis or COPD require multiple chest tubes to evacuate the pneumothorax.

   1. Chest tube management
      a. Placement. The tube should be placed in an apical and anterior aspect of the pleural space to facilitate air drainage. The tube should not be placed in a dependent area of the hemithorax.
      b. Suction. Waterseal alone generally resolves the pneumothorax. Placing the chest tube initially to suction risks reexpansion pulmonary edema due to rapid reinflation of atelectatic lung. If the pneumothorax or air leak persists after 12–24 hours, applying 15–20 cm H_2O of suction to the chest tube may facilitate closure of the pleural defect.
      c. Following resolution. Eighteen to 24 hours after complete drainage of the pneumothorax (no air leak, normal chest x-ray), the chest tube should be placed to waterseal, and an expiratory chest x-ray should be repeated in 3–6 hours. If pleural air does not reaccumulate, consider clamping the chest tube for 12–24 hours to assess for slow air leaks. Clamping is controversial, although advocated by a majority of thoracic surgeons. The patient must be closely monitored for the recurrence of a large pneumothorax. If the pneumothorax reappears, return the chest tube to wall suction. If no signs of pleural air are noted on repeat chest x-ray, the chest tube may be removed. **Removal of the chest tube immediately after resolution of the pneumothorax results in recurrence in 25% of cases.**

E. Pleurodesis (Table 13-2). Pleurodesis is usually required in the setting of recurrent primary spontaneous pneumothorax or secondary spontaneous events accompanied by respiratory compromise. **Before pleurodesis is undertaken in patients with severe underlying lung disease, the impact of the procedure on future lung transplantation must be considered.**
   1. Sclerosing strategies

Table 13-2. Costs of pleurodesis for spontaneous pneumothorax

Sclerosing agent	Dosing	Cases	Failures (%)	Cost
Thoracotomy/pleurectomy		>750	<6	$3,500
Tetracycline HCl	500 mg to 30 mg/kg	173	20	<$50
Minocycline HCl	300 mg	7	14	$80
Doxycycline HCl	500 mg	5*	0	$125
Bleomycin	15–240 U	1	0	$15/U
Talc poudrage via thoracoscopy	2–10 g	702	9	$2,253
Video-assisted thoracoscopy/pleurectomy		76	15	$2,900

*Successful pleural symphysis often requires multiple administrations of the drug.
Adapted from Berger R. Pleurodesis for spontaneous pneumothorax: will the procedure of choice please stand up? *Chest* 1994;106:992–994.

a. **Open thoracotomy.** This is the traditional approach. Typically, sizable blebs or bullae are resected, and pleurodesis is induced by partial pleurectomy, physical abrasion of the pleural surfaces, or the instillation of chemicals into the pleural cavity. Retrospective reviews indicate a low rate of recurrence (<10%) over an average follow-up of 9.1 years. Complications include postoperative fever (10%), wound infection (6.7%), air leak for >5 days (6.7%), and pneumonia (2.4%) (25). This therapy is expensive (operative and costs of hospitalization) and has the associated risks of general anesthesia.

b. **Chest tube–guided chemical sclerotherapy.** The instillation of chemicals into the pleural space via chest tubes is inexpensive and easily administered. Pain and fever are the primary complications, although drug-specific events have been reported. After the lung has reexpanded, sclerosants are administered through the chest tube (18).

   i. Patients should be pretreated with 150 mg lidocaine (15 mL of a 1% solution, epinephrine free) injected into the chest tube.

   ii. Reconstituted sclerosant (50 mL) is then injected into the chest tube.

   iii. Clamp the chest tube for 1–2 hours, periodically repositioning the patient to distribute the drug throughout the pleural space. (Although sclerosing agents are well distributed without position change in patients with pleural effusion, no data exist for patients with pneumothorax.)

   iv. Return the chest tube to wall suction for at least 24 hours.

c. **Sclerotherapeutic agents.** Agents used to induce pleurodesis in the setting of pneumothorax include bleomycin, tetracycline (no longer manufactured, but still available), minocycline, doxycycline, and asbestos-free talc.

   i. **Tetracycline hydrochloride** 500 mg (up to 30 mg/kg) is diluted in 50 mL of sterile saline and injected through the chest tube. Cumulative experience indicates a 20% recurrence rate at >12 months follow-up in spontaneous pneumothorax. In a 5-year prospective Veterans Affairs cooperative study, tetracycline pleurodesis decreased pneumothorax recurrence rates from 43% (untreated controls) to 28% among patients with obstructive airways disease (18). Among patients without underlying lung disease (primary spontaneous pneumothorax), tetracycline treatment decreased recurrent pneumothorax rates from 32% (untreated group) to 11% (treated group). Notably, the recurrence rate was greater in patients pretreated with lidocaine instillation (28%) versus those not receiving lidocaine (9%). Complications of tetracycline and its derivatives are minor (fever and pain). Acute renal failure has been reported following sclerosis of a patient's pleural space. However, tetracycline is no longer manufactured.

   ii. **Minocycline hydrochloride** 300 mg is diluted in 50 mL of sterile saline. Experience with minocycline is small, limited to malignant effusions, and inadequate to determine accurate rates of either successful pleurodesis (no reaccumulation of pleural fluid) or 1-year recurrences.

   iii. **Doxycycline hydrochloride** 500 mg is diluted in 30–50 mL of sterile saline. Experience with doxycycline sclerotherapy is also largely limited to malignant effusions (>87 cases). Only 5 cases of spontaneous pneumothorax in patients with the acquired immunodeficiency syndrome (AIDS) have been treated with doxycycline. Persistent air leaks and pneumothorax were successfully treated in four of these cases; follow-up data could not be obtained due to the short survival of the study population (26). Malignant effusions recur in >25% of treated cases at 1-year follow-up.

    iv. **Bleomycin** 60 mg is reconstituted in 100 mL of sterile saline. The published experience is limited to one patient with *Pneumocystis carinii* pneumonia (PCP) complicated by pneumothorax refractory to tetracycline pleurodesis. Bleomycin obliterated the pleural space, preventing recurrence over the 7-month follow-up. Bleomycin is not recommended in patients with pneumothorax and normal pleural surfaces.

    v. **Talc** poudrage (aerosolized) involves instilling 2–10 g of the powder, asbestos and heavy metal free, through a thoracoscope into the pleural space. Particles range from 10–50 μm in diameter. The talc must be sterilized, generally by dry-heat treatment. If blebs or bullae are noted, oversewing or excision is performed by thoracotomy or video-assisted thoracoscopy (VATS). Talc slurry can be instilled via a chest tube, although poudrage is the most frequently used technique. Talc successfully treats pneumothorax in 91% of cases, regardless of the talc preparation used (27). **Early complications include** fever in 16% to 69% of cases, usually 4–12 hours after administration and lasting <3 days, and NOTE: empyema in <3% of cases; anecdotal reports have noted acute pneumonitis, respiratory failure, adult respiratory distress syndrome (ARDS), pneumonia, and death. **Late complications include** only minor restrictive lung disease (decreased total lung capacity without changes in forced expiratory volume in 1 second).

  2. **Video-assisted thoracoscopy and pleurodesis**
    a. Operative intervention is recommended for patients with an air leak that persists for >7 days, failure to respond to chemical pleurodesis, recurrent pneumothorax with identified bullae, and selected patients who perform high-risk activities (eg, deep-water diving, aviators). Direct visualization of the pleural surface allows:
      i. Identification and removal of subpleural blebs and bullae.
      ii. Lysis of adhesions that limit lung reexpansion and the proper distribution of the sclerosant.
      iii. Directed delivery of aerosolized talc (poudrage).
    b. The anticipated advantages of thoracoscopy over thoracotomy include limited anesthesia (costal nerve block vs. general anesthesia), lesser effects on lung function postoperatively, minimal wound-related pain, and possibly shortened hospital stays. Properly controlled studies involving patients with secondary spontaneous pneumothorax indicate that although VATS requires less anesthesia both during and after the procedure, it is associated with longer operative time, more prolonged hospitalizations, and a greater incidence of treatment failures (16%) than standard thoracotomy (7%). In contrast, VATS compares favorably with thoracotomy in patients with complicated primary spontaneous pneumothorax: shorter chest tube drainage times (2.4 days vs. 6.3 days) and postoperative hospitalizations (4.2 days vs. 9 days) (28,29). **VATS therefore appears to be the surgical procedure of choice in patients with secondary spontaneous pneumothorax in whom general anesthesia represents an unacceptable risk and in patients with complicated primary spontaneous pneumothorax.**

VII. **Pneumothorax in AIDS.** The incidence of spontaneous pneumothorax in AIDS is 2% to 4% (30,31), nearly 1000 times the rate of secondary spontaneous pneumothorax in an immunocompetent population.
  A. **Etiology. *P. carinii* lung infections account for the majority of cases (89% to 95%) of nontraumatic AIDS-related pneumothorax.** Surgical specimens from AIDS patients with pneumothorax reveal subpleural tissue necrosis or pneumatocele formation, and methenamine silver staining demonstrates *Pneumocystis* trophozoites. The degree of parenchymal lung destruction impairs maneuvers to seal the pleural defect, leading to protracted treatment and multiple pneumothoraces. The prevalence of PCP and the frequency of complicating pneumothorax (6%

to 9% of all PCP cases) readily explain the high rate of spontaneous pneumothorax in AIDS patients (30,32).

B. Presentation

1. **Risk factors for AIDS-related pneumothorax include active PCP, prior treatment with aerosolized pentamidine, and repeated episodes of PCP.** Nearly 5% of patients receiving aerosolized pentamidine prophylaxis suffer pneumothorax. Positive-pressure ventilation and transbronchial biopsy are also associated with pneumothorax in this population.

2. AIDS patients with pneumothorax have low CD4-lymphocyte counts (<100/ mm³) and high mortality rates. Persistent air leaks, prolonged hospitalizations, and high recurrence rates (36% to 65%) typify these pneumothoraces. Half of all recurrences occur in the contralateral lung.

C. Treatment

1. **All AIDS patients with spontaneous pneumothorax should be treated empirically for active PCP**, given the high prevalence of the infection in surgical specimens. **Chest tube drainage** is effective in only 26% of these cases, with patients often requiring placement of multiple tubes for prolonged periods. In one series, the median time of chest tube drainage was 20 days. Over half of the study population underwent pleurodesis, and 25% required surgical management (30). **Sclerotherapy** with doxycycline (500 mg) is effective, although the published experience is limited and repeated administrations may be necessary. **Video-assisted talc poudrage** has been successful in >60% of cases refractory to nonsurgical management and may shorten the length of hospitalization when used early in treatment (33).

2. Notably, certain PCP treatments (steroids and dapsone) diminish the inflammatory response to tetracycline-induced pleurodesis.

3. AIDS patients with persistent or recurrent pneumothoraces may be treated with chronic chest tube drainage outside the hospital as an alternative to prolonged hospitalization or surgical intervention. The Heimlich valve, a one-way flow device, permits continuous tube drainage of air from the pleural space. If chronic drainage of the pleural space fails to resolve the pneumothorax, surgical intervention is recommended.

VIII. Catamenial pneumothorax

A. Etiology. Recurrent pneumothorax temporally related to menstrual periods represents 5% to 6% of secondary pneumothorax in woman (34). Fewer than 100 cases have been reported to date. The pathogenesis is unknown. The passage of air from the peritoneal cavity to the pleural space can occur via surgically identified fenestrations in the diaphragm leaflets in 19% to 33% of cases reported. Ectopic endometrial tissue lining the pleural space or a bronchial wall has been found in women with menses-related pneumothorax, yet its role in generation of pneumothorax is unclear.

B. Presentation. Recurrent pneumothorax at the time of menstrual flow must occur before the diagnosis can be considered. Typically, women will have five pneumothoraces before the diagnosis is entertained. Catamenial pneumothorax occurs within 1–3 days of the onset of menses, with **first episodes most frequently in women >30 years old**. Right-sided pneumothorax is characteristic (87.5% cases), with left-sided and bilateral events occurring in 5% to 6% of all cases (35).

C. Treatment. A woman must ovulate to generate catamenial pneumothorax. Therefore, **inducing an anovulatory state prevents repeated pneumothorax**. Favored drugs include danazol, medroxyprogesterone, or gonadotropin-releasing hormone analogues. Surgical repair of diaphragmatic defects, physical pleurodesis, and/or hysterectomy with bilateral oophorectomy should be considered if drug therapy cannot be tolerated.

IX. Iatrogenic pneumothorax

A. Etiology. Pneumothorax is a complication of many procedures (Table 13-3), and the incidence of iatrogenic pneumothorax exceeds that of all spontaneous events (36). The settings most frequently associated with pneumothorax include transthoracic fine-needle aspiration, thoracentesis, closed pleural biopsy, transbronchial biopsy, and mechanical ventilation of acutely injured lungs.

Table 13-3. Frequent causes and incidence of iatrogenic pneumothorax

Transthoracic needle aspiration		33%
Thoracentesis		10%
Closed pleural biopsy		8%
Transbronchial lung biopsy		<5%
Mechanical ventilation		4%
Aspiration pneumonia	37%	
Positive end-expiratory pressure	15%	
Main-stem intubation	13%	
Transbronchial needle aspiration (Wang needle)		2%

Adapted from Light RW. Pneumothorax. In: Murray JF, Nadel JA (eds). *Textbook of respiratory medicine.* Philadelphia: WB Saunders, 1988:1752–1753.

B. Procedures

1. In patients undergoing transbronchial biopsies, fluoroscopy is often used to guide biopsy forceps to solitary parenchymal lesions and to avoid disruption of the visceral pleura. In patients with diffuse lung processes, however, fluoroscopic guidance does not alter the rate of iatrogenic pneumothorax (37,38), and chest x-ray adds little to the detection rate. Rarely, a pneumothorax will be identified by chest x-ray 4 or more hours after transbronchoscopic biopsies.

2. Transbronchial needle aspiration (Wang needle) has been associated with a much lower rate of pneumothorax (0.5%).

3. Transthoracic needle biopsy (TTNB) with fluoroscopic guidance is complicated by a high rate of pneumothorax in most series (5% to 61%; mean, 27%). Notably, CT-guided TTNB has an even higher pneumothorax complication rate than the fluoroscopy-directed approach (mean, 37%). Evidently, the improved visualization of solitary lesions by CT allows TTNB of smaller, less accessible lesions, increasing the complication rates. As many as 15% of patients with TTNB-associated pneumothorax require chest tube placement.

   a. The risk of pneumothorax from TTNB increases significantly when performed in patients with COPD. The pneumothorax rate was noted to be 46% in COPD patients versus 7% in patients with normal lung function (39). Moreover, the COPD population was much more likely to require chest tube drainage than patients with normal pulmonary spirometric function (19% vs. none, respectively).

   b. Other factors that increase the risk of TTNB-associated pneumothorax include (a) repeated pleural passes, (b) long distance of the lesion from the chest wall, and (c) older patients.

   c. Maneuvers that may decrease the rate and size of TTNB-related pneumothorax are unproven but include (a) roll-over technique (positioning the patient on the instrumented hemithorax), (b) strict bedrest for 3 hours postinstrumentation, and (c) autologous blood patching. Although the blood-patch technique (injecting blood clot into the needle tract) is advocated by some, randomized studies have failed to demonstrate an effect on the rates of pneumothorax (40).

C. Risk factors for pneumothorax in mechanically ventilated patients include acutely injured lung (necrotizing pneumonia, the fibroproliferative phase of ARDS, status asthmaticus, COPD, and aspiration pneumonia), high levels of positive end-expiratory pressure (PEEP) (>15 cm H_2O), large tidal volumes (Vt >12 mL/kg), and high peak (or mean) airway pressures (41).

1. **Presentation.** Patients who are mechanically ventilated and develop a pneumothorax associated with thoracentesis may complain of chest or shoulder pain (diaphragmatic irritation) or shortness of breath if on assist-control mode. However, symptoms may be delayed for 1–2 days after the event. Lung

compliance will decrease (increased peak and plateau airway pressures), Pao_2 will decrease, and hemodynamic instability (tachycardia and hypotension) may ensue.

2. **Intubated patients are at risk for pneumothorax due to the misplacement of oro- or nasogastric tubes (Salem sump) into the pleural space.** The endotracheal balloon imperfectly seals the trachea, occasionally allowing oro- or nasogastric tubes to enter the trachea. Obtunded, intubated patients may not respond to placement of a feeding tube into the trachea or to accidental rupture of the visceral pleura. Moreover, localizing the position of the tube by the auscultation of insufflated air is unreliable; suctioning gastric contents is a more reliable indicator of correct placement. **The position of an oro- or nasogastric tube must be determined by chest x-ray prior to administration of medications or nutritional products through the tube. Following accidental placement of a feeding tube into the tracheobronchial tree, subsequent efforts at tube positioning should proceed under direct visualization of the hypopharynx.**

3. **Diagnosis**
    a. Recognition of pneumothorax may be difficult in the mechanically ventilated patient. **Pleural air always collects in the most superior aspect of the chest, the location of which varies with body positioning.** Thus, views of mechanically ventilated patients generally depict a semirecumbent or fully recumbent thorax. **Consequently, pneumothorax is most frequently seen in the anterior medial or subpulmonic areas of the pleural space in mechanically ventilated individuals.** A hyperlucent costophrenic sulcus that extends caudally is classically labeled the *deep sulcus sign.* Erect or decubitus x-ray films may accentuate the pneumothorax. Chest CT is the most sensitive test but is often not a practical approach.
    b. The majority of TTNB-related pneumothoraces (89%) can be detected by chest x-ray within 15 minutes of the procedure (42). However, about 10% of pneumothoraces first appear 1 hour after the biopsy, so that later films (approximately 4 hours postprocedure) should be obtained. All large pneumothoraces will be clinically evident within 1 hour of the biopsy.
    c. Pneumothorax occurring during fluoroscopically directed transbronchial lung biopsy will be readily identified by fluoroscopy. Transbronchial biopsies performed without fluoroscopic guidance require a postprocedure chest x-ray within 4 hours.

4. **Treatment.** The management of iatrogenic pneumothorax depends on its size, the presence of underlying lung disease, and the degree of respiratory compromise. Pneumothoraces due to thoracentesis, TTNB, or pleural biopsy are usually small and not physiologically significant. Consequently, several treatment options are available.
    a. **Small pneumothoraces in patients with normal lungs.** When the postprocedure chest x-ray demonstrates a small pneumothorax (<15%) and the patient remains asymptomatic, repeat chest films every 2 hours are recommended to determine whether the pneumothorax size is increasing. If the pneumothorax is unchanged and the patient is symptom free, the patient may be discharged to home with instructions to return if symptoms occur.
    b. **Pneumothoraces that are large, increasing in size, or associated with respiratory compromise.** Large or growing pneumothoraces in patients with normal lung function, as well as respiratory compromise in any patient, warrant chest tube placement. Generally, as the pleural defect is small and readily sealed upon lung reinflation, a small-bore chest tube (6–9 French) and Heimlich valve suffice. Typically, the chest tube is placed in the second intercostal space in the midclavicular line. Supplemental oxygen should be administered in all patients admitted to hospital to accelerate resorption of air in the pleural space. Complete resolution occurs within 48 hours in most cases. If persistent air leak occurs, chang-

ing the Heimlich valve to a waterseal system may improve lung expansion and eliminate the leak.

c. **Pneumothoraces due to transbronchial biopsy** often occur in the setting of interstitial lung disease. The increased elasticity of the lung often limits its spontaneous reexpansion, resulting in a persistent pneumothorax. Even in the absence of respiratory compromise, many of these patients require chest tube placement to facilitate full resolution of the pneumothorax.

d. **Mechanically ventilated patients developing a pneumothorax should undergo chest tube placement.** The presence of underlying lung disease and continued positive-pressure ventilation risk generation of a large-volume, highly pressurized, collection of air in the pleural space: a tension pneumothorax. Consequently, chest tube drainage must be performed in all patients on positive-pressure mechanical ventilation. To prevent reaccumulation, the chest tube should be left in place for 48 hours after the air leak has resolved.

X. **Bronchopleural fistula.** A bronchopleural fistula (BPF) is a persistent communication between the bronchial tree and the pleural space. BPF is a difficult management problem regardless of whether the patient is mechanically ventilated or breathing spontaneously. Approximately two-thirds of cases occur as a complication of lung resection, while the remaining BPFs are associated with necrotizing pneumonias, empyemas, or pleural space infections (43). Mortality in patients with BPF ranges from 18% to 50%, and the magnitude of airflow through the BPF predicts outcome: Patients with >500 mL per breath flow through the BPF have an extremely poor prognosis (44). Patients with ARDS complicated by BPF frequently die.

A. **Presentation.** The initial manifestations of BPF vary with its postoperative timing, the extent of pleural space infection, and the mobility of the mediastinum. **Early in the postoperative period**, patients with BPF may present with the sudden expectoration of purulent material arising from an infected pleural space. Inability to clear the secretions from the airways (aspiration) may result in acute lung injury and respiratory failure. Tension pneumothorax can complicate the presentation of these patients, as the mediastinum remains freely mobile. **Late postoperative presentations** tend to be more indolent, with prolonged fevers and a modestly productive cough. Pleural-space and mediastinal fibrosis induced by chronic infection impedes mediastinal movement in these patients. Therefore, tension pneumothorax rarely occurs in late-postoperative fistulas.

B. **Evaluation.** Persistent air leak following chest tube placement represents either a dysfunctioning drainage system or a BPF. **Problems with the chest tube system must be ruled out.**

1. **Chest tube positioning.** Improper placement of the chest tube often results in air under pressure dissecting into the soft tissue of the chest wall. The patient should be examined for subcutaneous emphysema. Chest tube anchoring at the skin insertion site should be evaluated for leak. The location of the proximal port of the chest tube must be inside the chest wall (visualized by chest x-ray) to prevent persistent air leak, subcutaneous emphysema, and incomplete drainage of the pleural space. To avoid pleural-space contamination, **improperly positioned chest tubes should be replaced** and never be readvanced through an established tract.

2. **Chest tubing or hose connector failure.** To quickly determine the source of a persistent air leak, clamp the chest tube as it exits the chest. If the air leak stops, the problem is in the chest proximal to the clamp. If bubbling through the waterseal persists, the problem lies between the clamp and the waterseal, in the tubing, the connectors, or the drainage bottles. To define the exact point of leakage, advance the clamp down the tubing toward the drainage bottles. When the leak disappears, the defect lies proximal to the clamp site.

3. **Positioning of the chest tube within the chest.** A **chest CT** scan should be obtained to assess the degree of lung destruction in the area of the pleural defect and the positioning of the chest tube(s). Accidental placement of the chest tube into the lung parenchyma will result in continued air leak.

C. Treatment. Correct chest tube placement is paramount in the treatment of BPF. Other important considerations include appropriate antibiotic coverage of cultured bacteria and careful attention to the nutritional state of the patient to promote tissue healing.

  1. Chest tubes

  a. Proper size. The magnitude of the air leak through chest tubes varies from <1 L/min to 16 L/min (45). To properly drain the pleural space of air, prevent further lung collapse and tension pneumothorax formation, a large-bore tube is needed. Thoracostomy tubes with a 6-mm internal diameter are capable of evacuating 15 L/min at -10 cm H_2O negative pressure. Consequently, a 32 French chest tube (9-mm internal diameter) is recommended. The capacity of chest tube drainage systems varies as well (Table 13-4)(46).

  b. Multiple chest tubes. Persistent pneumothorax or air leak through a properly placed chest tube should prompt placement of additional tubes.

  c. Detrimental effects. Chest tube treatment of BPF in the mechanically ventilated patient may be complicated by (a) decreased Vt returned through the endotracheal tube, (b) decreased oxygenation and carbon dioxide excretion, (c) inappropriate cycling of the ventilator, and (d) persistence of the BPF. In mechanically ventilated patients with ARDS and BPF, nearly 25% of the minute ventilation exits out the chest tube, reducing the "effective" Vt. However, up to 20% of carbon dioxide excretion may occur via this flow through the chest tube (47). Cycling of the ventilator results when sufficiently negative pressure is transmitted from the chest drainage system to the proximal airway to trigger the machine. Paradoxically, chest tube management may sustain the BPF in both spontaneously and mechanically ventilated settings. **Placing a chest tube on high suction rates may induce large flows through the pleural defect, impairing its closure.** If high suction does not promote closure, putting the chest tube to waterseal may sufficiently decrease flows across the defect to promote healing. In the mechanically ventilated patient, the size and stability of the pneumothorax must be monitored closely when the chest tube is placed to waterseal.

  2. Ventilator management. Aggressive evacuation of pleural air using high suction settings may impede BPF healing, while measures to decrease flow across the defect compromise alveolar ventilation and risk large pneumothorax formation. Potential ventilator strategies to decrease airway and alveolar pressures are limited by the oxygen needs of the patient. The higher the $Paco_2$, the lower the alveolar (PAo_2) and the arterial (Pao_2) oxygen tensions. While hypercarbia is well tolerated, hypoxemia is dangerous, so that it is most important to oxygenate the patient regardless of the $Paco_2$ levels. Consequently, patients need close monitoring when the following ventilator strategies are implemented, as the physiologic response of the patient is unpredictable.

  a. Minimize airway pressures

    i. Decrease delivered Vt without significantly limiting $Paco_2$.

    ii. Decrease the respiratory rate.

Table 13-4. Air-flow capacities of chest tube drainage systems

Device	Maximal flow (L/min)
Emerson pump	35.5
Pleur-Evac A4000	34.0
Thora-Klex	19.7
Sentinel seal	2.3

Adapted from Capps JS, Tyler ML, Rusch VW, Pierson DJ. Potential of chest drainage units to evacuate bronch-pleural air leaks. *Chest* 1988;88:57S.

      iii. Decrease the inspiratory time.

      iv. Use the least amount of PEEP possible.

  b. Alternative strategies

      i. Positioning. Placing the lung with BPF in a dependent position may decrease ventilation to the BPF.

      ii. Differential lung ventilation. Selective ventilation of one lung may be helpful in patients with profound, unilateral BPF. One option is to advance a standard endotracheal tube into the mainstem bronchus of the good lung and ventilate only it. The disadvantage of this technique is that the contralateral lung may collapse. Further, if the short right mainstem bronchus must be intubated, care must be taken to avoid occlusion of the right upper lobe orifice by the balloon. Another option is to have an experienced anesthesiologist place a double-lumen (Carlan's) endotracheal tube and differentially ventilate each lung, with reduced ventilation of the lung with the BPF. This is difficult to do, since both ventilators must be synchronized or mediastinal shift will occur. In addition, Vt must be decreased (approximately 4 mL/kg), and the lung compliance (plateau pressures) must be monitored to avoid volutrauma.

  c. Chest tube pressurization. The risk of each of the following chest tube maneuvers is inadequate drainage of the pneumothorax, resulting in a tension pneumothorax. Patients must be carefully monitored at all times when these maneuvers are employed.

      i. Expiratory phase maneuvers. In patients requiring PEEP to sustain acceptable arterial oxygen levels, the chest tube can be pressurized to the level of PEEP during the expiratory phase of respiration. This may sufficiently decrease BPF flows during expiration to allow continued use of PEEP. Inspiratory-phase air leaks will persist, however.

      ii. Inspiratory phase maneuvers. Occluding the chest tube during the inspiratory phase will limit BPF flows during the period of greatest airway pressures.

      iii. Inspiratory and expiratory maneuvers. Clamping of the chest tube during the inspiratory limb may be combined with chest tube pressurization during the expiratory limb of the respiratory cycle.

  d. High-frequency ventilation (HFV). Studies indicate that gas exchange is better maintained by HFV than conventional ventilation modes in animal models of BPF with proximal fistulas (trachea or mainstem bronchial defects) and normal lung parenchyma. Human beings with proximal BPFs seem to respond similarly (48). HFV in patients with ARDS (acute lung injury) does not improve gas exchange or reduce mean chest tube leakage when compared to conventional ventilation management (49).

3. Bronchoscopic management. BPF following lobectomy or pneumonectomy warrants endoscopic visualization of the bronchial stump. Bronchoscopy in nonsurgical patients with diffuse parenchymal disease is used to localize the defect and treat it by obstructing the appropriate bronchiole.

  a. Proximal airway BPF. Visualize disruption of the bronchus and surgically repair.

  b. Distal airway BPF. To localize the fistula, a Fogarty (occluding) balloon must be passed selectively into third or fourth generation bronchi, and the chest tube air leak monitored during inflation of the balloon. Significant decrease or elimination of the air leak indicates that the bronchus leading to the BPF has been identified. The balloon should stay inflated for no longer than 24–48 hours to avoid pressure necrosis. Various materials can be injected through the port distal to the balloon to occlude the fistula more permanently (Table 13-5) (50). Postobstructive pneumonia is a theoretical complication but has not been reported.

4. Surgical management. Patients with air leaks present for 7 days despite appropriate chest tube management should undergo thoracotomy or VATS. Pleu-

Table 13-5. Fistula-occluding agents delivered via bronchoscopy

Agent	Cases	Experience
Blood-tetracycline	1	Success
Gelfoam	1	Success
Silver nitrate	3	Multiple administrations needed
Cyanoacrylate	7	Multiple administrations needed in 50% of cases
Fibrin formulations	8	Complete seal in 75%; multiple administrations needed in 16% of cases

Adapted from Baumann MH, Sahn SA. Medical management and therapy of bronchopleural fistulas in the mechanically ventilated patient. *Chest* 1990;97:721–728.

rodesis of a BPF has been successful in patients without underlying lung disease. Whether patients with significant lung disease and BPF benefit from chemical pleurodesis is unknown. Surgical closure of fistulas in the noninfected patient with or without pleurodesis is the favored approach. BPF complicated by an infected pleural space (empyema) should undergo rib resection and open drainage or an Eloesser flap procedure.

XI. Traumatic pneumothorax. Noniatrogenic injury to the chest wall resulting in lung collapse defines traumatic pneumothorax. This usually occurs in drug-abuse-related chest trauma or blows to the chest wall.

  A. Illicit-drug-related pneumothorax

    1. Intravenous (IV) drug users. In some centers, >21% of pneumothoraces are related to illicit IV drug use (51). Characteristically, the pneumothorax occurs during efforts to inject material into the subclavian or internal jugular veins. Bilateral pneumothoraces have been reported.

    2. Drug inhalation. Pneumothorax due to Valsalva's maneuvers can occur during the inhalation of foreign materials such as cocaine and marijuana (52). The risk of pneumothorax appears greatest with "buddy breathing" and free-basing.

  B. Chest trauma. Three types of pneumothorax occur with trauma to the chest: (a) open pneumothorax, (b) closed pneumothorax, and (c) tension pneumothorax.

    1. Open pneumothorax results from penetrating injury to the chest wall, allowing direct communication of the pleural space with the atmosphere. The degree of respiratory distress reflects the size of the chest wall defect, the pretrauma condition of the lungs, and other associated lung injuries. Usually, the wound is easily identified, often by audible air exchange across the defect. Chest wall defects that exceed the size of the trachea (approximately 3 cm) may induce preferential air movement through the wound, which then impairs gas exchange through the tracheobronchial tree.

    2. Closed pneumothorax from blunt chest trauma results from either laceration of the visceral pleura by a fractured rib or sudden deceleration injury of the airways. After laceration, rapid compression of the chest raises transalveolar pressures, disrupting the alveolar membrane–bronchovascular interface. Alternatively, the tracheobronchial tree may be fractured by a sudden deceleration injury, typically occurring within 2.5 cm of the main carina. Right mainstem bronchial injury is most common, usually sparing the pulmonary vasculature (53). Patients sustaining a pneumothorax from tracheobronchial disruption present with dyspnea, subcutaneous emphysema, and, rarely, hemoptysis (25% of cases).

  C. Diagnosis

    1. Chest x-rays will demonstrate the pneumothorax (with or without pneumomediastinum), as well as **fractures of the first three ribs, sternum, or clavicles** (frequently seen in adults) (54). Several features of chest x-rays in patients with pneumothorax suggest the presence of tracheobronchial injury:

      a. A large, persistent, pneumothorax despite good chest tube drainage.

  b. Combined pneumothorax and pneumomediastinum in the absence of a pleural effusion.

  c. Mediastinal or deep cervical emphysema following chest trauma in a patient not treated with positive-pressure mechanical ventilation (55).

 2. Bronchial obstruction and lung collapse can follow complete displacement of the bronchus. Collapse of the lower lobe toward the chest wall—the **fallen lung sign**—suggests bronchial disruption with loss of the ligamentous attachments supporting the distal lung (56). Notably, **pneumothorax may not be evident in 30% of cases with tracheobronchial disruption.**

 3. Damage to other visceral organs can mimic airway disruption. Traumatic esophageal rupture may produce pneumomediastinum and/or hydropneumothorax. **Esophageal injury does not cause pneumothorax in the absence of pleural effusion.** The consequences of esophageal perforation (acute mediastinitis) warrant rapid radiographic evaluation, antibiotic administration, and surgical consultation.

D. Treatment

 1. Illicit-drug-related pneumothorax. The treatment of pneumothorax from needle use is identical with that of iatrogenic causes. Inhalational-drug-related pneumothoraces are managed as spontaneous events, with the aggressiveness of pneumothorax evacuation reflecting the extent of underlying lung disease and the degree of respiratory compromise.

 2. Open traumatic pneumothorax. Initially, a petroleum-laden gauze pad should be placed over the open chest wound to prevent external air entry into the pleural space during inspiration. Three sides of the pad should be fixed to the chest wall; the free side allows pleural air to escape, preventing tension pneumothorax formation. After placement of a chest tube, the pad can be completely taped in place.

 3. Closed traumatic pneumothorax. Following chest tube placement, physical and radiographic signs of tracheobronchial disruption should be sought. Bronchoscopy should be performed if airway injury is suspected. If tracheobronchial injury occurred, open thoracotomy is recommended. Dysphagia, pneumomediastinum, and hydropneumothorax suggest esophageal rupture. Elevated pleural fluid amylase levels occur within several hours of injury in virtually all patients with esophageal disruption; low pH status is also characteristic. Barium or meglumine diatrizoate (Gastrografin) studies of esophageal integrity should be performed promptly, as mortality is directly related to delayed diagnosis.

XII. Tension pneumothorax. Tension pneumothorax constitutes 2% to 3% of all pneumothoraces and occurs when the pleural pressure is greater than atmospheric pressure throughout the expiratory phase of respiration. Generation of tension pneumothorax in spontaneously breathing patients requires the presence of a one-way valve that allows the movement of air into the pleural cavity during inspiration but prevents its egress during expiration. Tension pneumothorax in mechanically ventilated patients does not require check-valve physiology. The high inspiratory airway pressures during positive-pressure ventilation drive air into the disrupted pleural space. Consequently, pleural pressures may exceed atmospheric pressure throughout the inspiratory and expiratory phases of respiration.

A. Physiology. In spontaneously breathing patients, **hypoxemia and tachycardia, not hypotension, are the earliest physiologic changes**. Atelectasis of the involved lung results in shunting, V/Q mismatching, and hypoxemia. In contrast, $Paco_2$ is maintained, despite smaller Vt, by increasing the respiratory rate and inspiratory effort. Hemodynamically, diminished venous return to the heart does occur due to the transmittance of positive intrapleural pressures to the superior and inferior vena cavae. In the early phase of tension pneumothorax, however, tachycardia compensates for decreases in left ventricular stroke volume, preserving cardiac output. **Hypotension is a late manifestation**, occurring only after metabolic and respiratory acidoses are present.

B. Presentation. Patients may be agitated, restless, even confused or combative. On examination, cyanosis may be evident due to hypoxemia and impedance to venous return from the head and extremities. Neck veins may be distended. Often the trachea shifts toward the contralateral side. The involved hemithorax may appear distended, the rib interspaces increased, and the liver edge displaced inferiorly. A supra-clavicular soft tissue mass representing lung herniation may appear. Typically, there is little movement of the ipsilateral chest wall during expiration.

1. **Chest x-rays** classically reveal ipsilateral lung collapse, caudal movement of the hemidiaphragm, and mediastinal shift away from the pneumothorax. In patients with pleural adhesions, localized tension pneumothorax may occur without lung collapse or changes in mediastinal position.

2. **ECG** manifestations include low voltage, poor R-wave progression due to rotation of the heart, T-wave inversions, electrical alternans, and ventricular tachycardia. All these electrical signs are more often reported with right-sided pneumothoraces. **In patients with a Swan-Ganz catheter,** progressive lung collapse causes distal migration of the catheter tip, producing a permanently "wedged" tracing.

3. **Arterial blood gases** reveal decreased PaO_2 and an increased $P(A-a)O_2$.

4. **The effects of tension pneumothorax on lung mechanics in the mechanically ventilated patient are similar to the findings in patients with simple pneumothorax.** Peak and plateau pressures rise simultaneously, indicating decreasing lung compliance. Auto-PEEP and increased airway resistance may make manual bagging difficult.

C. **Treatment. Tension pneumothorax requires immediate decompression of the pleural space and must not await radiographic confirmation of tension.** Placement of a large-bore needle (14 gauge) into the pleural cavity at the second intercostal space in the midclavicular line is recommended. Several variations are available for the drainage apparatus attached to the needle:

1. No attachments: Listen for a rush of air from the pleural space.

2. 30-mL syringe containing sterile saline: Remove the plunger when the needle has been placed into the pleural space. Bubbling represents escaping air. The water prevents entrance of air into the pleural space in patients mistakenly diagnosed with tension pneumothorax.

3. IV tubing connected directly to the 14-gauge needle, with the free end of the tubing immersed in fluid to create a waterseal: If an air rush or significant bubbling is noted on placement of the needle into the pleural space, the needle must be kept in place until a thoracostomy tube can be inserted.

References

1. Anthonisen NR: Regional function in spontaneous pneumothorax. *Am Rev Respir Dis* 1977;115: 873–876.

2. Norris RM, Jones JG, Bishop JM: Respiratory gas exchange in patients with spontaneous pneumothorax. *Thorax* 1968;23:427–433.

3. Melton LJ III, Hepper NGG, Offord KP: Incidence of spontaneous pneumothorax in Olmsted County, Minnesota: 1950 to 1974. *Am Rev Respir Dis* 1979;120:1379–1382.

4. Chan TB, Tan WC, Tech PC: Spontaneous pneumothorax in medical practice in a general hospital. *Ann Acad Med Singapore* 1985;14:457.

5. Kawakami Y, Irie T, Kamishima K: Stature, lung height, and spontaneous pneumothorax. *Respiration* 1982;43:55.

6. Peters RM, Peters BA, Benirschke SK: Chest dimensions in young adults with spontaneous pneumothorax. *Ann Thorac Surg* 1978;25:193–196.

7. Gobbel WGJ, Rhea WGJ, Nelson IA, Daniel RAJ: Spontaneous pneumothorax. *J Thorac Cardiovasc Surg* 1963;46:331–345.

8. Lesur O, Delorme N, Fromaget JM, et al.: Computed tomography in the etiologic assessment of idiopathic spontaneous pneumothorax. *Chest* 1990;98:341–347.

9. Dwyer EM, Jr, Troncale F: Spontaneous pneumothorax and pulmonary disease in the Marfan syndrome. Report of a case and review of the literature. *Ann Intern Med* 1965;62:1285–1292.

10. Sharpe IK, Ahmad M, Braun W: Familial spontaneous pneumothorax and HLA antigens. *Chest* 1980;78:264–268.

11. Rashid A, Sendi A, Al-Kadhimi A: Concurrent spontaneous pneumothorax in identical twins. *Thorax* 1986;41:971.

12. Bense L, Eklung G, Wiman LG: Smoking and the increased risk of contracting spontaneous pneumothorax. *Chest* 1987;92:1009–1012.
13. Vail WJ, Alway AE, England NJ: Spontaneous pneumothorax. *Chest* 1960;38:512–515.
14. Aston SJ, Rosove M: Horner's syndrome occurring with spontaneous pneumothorax. *N Engl J Med* 1972;287:1098.
15. Seremetis MG: The management of spontaneous pneumothorax. *Chest* 1970;57:65–68.
16. Bense L, Wiman LG, Hedenstierna G: Onset of symptoms in spontaneous pneumothroax: correlations to physical activity. *Eur J Respir Dis* 1987;71:181–186.
17. Walston A, Brewer DL, Kitchens CS, Krook JE: The electrocardiographic manifestations of spontaneous left pneumothorax. *Ann Intern Med* 1974;80:375–379.
18. Light RW, O'Hara VS, Moritz TE, et al.: Intrapleural tetracycline for the prevention of recurrent spontaneous pneumothorax: results of a Department of Veterans Affairs cooperative study. *JAMA* 1990;264:2224–2230.
19. Hickok DG, Ballenger FP: The management of spontaneous pneumothorax due to emphysematous blebs. *Surg Gynecol Obstet* 1965;120:499.
20. Dines DE, Clagett OT, Payne WS: Spontaneous pneumothorax in emphysema. *Mayo Clin Proc* 1970;45:481–487.
21. Videm V, Pillgram-Larsen J, Ellingsen O: Spontaneous pneumothorax in chronic obstructive pulmonary disease: complications, treatment and recurrences. *Eur J Respir Dis* 1987;71:365–371.
22. Luck SR, Raffensperger JG, Sullivan HJ, Gibson LE: Management of pneumothorax in children with chronic pulmonary disease. *J Thorac Cardiovasc Surg* 1977;74:834–839.
23. Kircher J, LT, Swartzel RL: Spontaneous pneumothorax and its treatment. *JAMA* 1954;155:24–29.
24. Northfield TC: Oxygen therapy for spontaneous pneumothorax. *BMJ* 1971;4:86–88.
25. Donahue DM, Wright CD, Viale G, Mathisen DJ: Resection of pulmonary blebs and pleurodesis for spontaneous pneumothorax. *Chest* 1993;104:1767–1769.
26. Read CA, Reddy VD, O'Mara TE, Richardson MSA: Doxycycline pleurodesis for pneumothorax in patients with AIDS. *Chest* 1994;105:823825.
27. Kennedy L, Sahn SA: Talc pleurodesis for the treatment of pneumothorax and pleural effusion. *Chest* 1994;106:1215–1222.
28. Waller DA, Forty J, Soni AK, et al.: Videothoracoscopic operation for secondary spontaneous pneumothorax. *Ann Thorac Surg* 1994;57:1612–1615.
29. Waller DA, Forty J, Morritt GN: Video-assisted thoracoscopic surgery versus thoracotomy for spontaneous pneumothorax. *Ann Thorac Surg* 1994;58:372–377.
30. Sepkowitz KA, Telzak EE, Gold JW, et al.: Pneumothorax in AIDS. *Ann Intern Med* 1991;114: 455–459.
31. Truitt T, Bagheri K, Safirstein BH: Spontaneous pneumothorax in *Pneumocystis carinii* pneumonia. *AJR* 1992;158:916–917.
32. McClellan MD, Miller SB, Parsons PE, Cohn DL: Pneumothorax with *Pneumocystis carinii* pneumonia in AIDS. *Chest* 1991;100:1224–1228.
33. Wait MA, Dal Nogare ARD: Treatment of AIDS-related spontaneous pneumothorax: a decade of experience. *Chest* 1994;106:693–696.
34. Carter EJ, Ettensohn DB: Catamenial pneumothorax. *Chest* 1990;98:713–716.
35. Shiraishi T: Catamenial pneumothorax: report of a case and review of the Japanese and non-Japanese literature. *J Thorac Cardiovasc Surg* 1991;39:304–307.
36. Despars JA, Sassoon CS, Light RW: Incidence and significance of iatrogenic pneumothorax. *Chest* 1990;98:138S.
37. Mulligan SA, Luce JM, Golden J, et al.: Transbronchial biopsy without fluoroscopy in patients with diffuse roentgenographic infiltrates and the acquired immunodeficiency syndrome. *Am Rev Respir Dis* 1988;137:486–488.
38. Anders GT, Johnson JE, Bush BA, Matthews JI: Transbronchial biopsy without fluoroscopy: a seven-year perspective. *Chest* 1988;94:557–560.
39. Fish GD, Stanley JH, Miller KS, et al.: Postbiopsy pneumothorax: estimating the risk by chest radiography and pulmonary function tests. *AJR* 1988;150:71–74.
40. Bourgouin PM, Shepard JA, McLoud TC, et al.: Transthoracic needle aspiration biopsy: evaluation of the blood patch technique. *Radiology* 1988;166:93–95.
41. Jantz MA, Pierson DJ: Pneumothorax and barotrauma. *Clin Chest Med* 1994;15:75–91.
42. Perlmutt LM, Johnston WW, Dunnick NR: Percutaneous transthoracic needle aspiration: a review. *AJR* 1989;152:451–455.
43. Steiger Z, Wilson RF: Management of bronchopleural fistulas. *Surgery* 1984;158:267–271.

44. Pierson DJ, Horton CA, Bates PW: Persistent bronchopleural air leak during mechanical ventilation: a review of 39 cases. *Chest* 1987;90:321–323.
45. Rusch VW, Capps JS, Tyler ML, Pierson DL: The performance of four pleural drainage systems in an animal model of bronchopleural fistula. *Chest* 1988;93:859–863.
46. Capps JS, Tyler ML, Rusch VW, Pierson DJ: Potential of chest drainage units to evacuate bronchopleural air leaks. *Chest* 1988;88:57S.
47. Bishop MJ, Benson MS, Pierson DJ: Carbon dioxide excretion via bronchopleural fistulas in adult respiratory distress syndrome. *Chest* 1987;91:400–402.
48. Carlson GC, Kahn RC, Howland WS, et al.: Clinical experience with high frequency jet ventilation. *Crit Care Med* 1981;9:1–6.
49. Bishop MJ, Benson MS, Sato P, Pierson DJ: Comparison of high-frequency jet ventilation with conventional mechanical ventilation for bronchopleural fistula. *Anesth Analg* 1987;66:833–838.
50. Baumann MH, Sahn SA: Medical management and therapy of bronchopleural fistulas in the mechanically ventilated patient. *Chest* 1990;97:721–728.
51. Douglass RE, Levison MA: Pneumothorax in drug abusers: an urban epidemic. *Am Surg* 1986;52:377–380.
52. Seaman ME: Barotrauma related to inhalational drug abuse. *J Emerg Med* 1990;8:141–149.
53. Collins JP, Ketharanathan V, McConchie I: Rupture of major bronchi resulting from closed chest injuries. *Thorax* 1973;28:371–375.
54. Campbell DB: Trauma to the chest wall, lung, and major airways. *Semin Thorac Cardiovasc Surg* 1992;4:234–240.
55. Fraser RG, Paré JAP, Paré PD, et al.: Diseases of the thorax caused by external physical agents. In: Fraser RG, Paré JAP, Paré PD et al., eds. *Diagnosis of diseases of the chest*, 3rd ed. Philadelphia: WB Saunders, 1991.
56. Unger JM, Schuchmann GG, Grossman JE, Pellett JR: Tears of the trachea and main bronchi caused by blunt trauma: radiologic findings. *AJR* 1989;153:1175–1180.
57. Eijgelaar A, Homan van der Heide JN: A reliable early symptom of bronchial or tracheal rupture. *Thorax* 1970;25:120–125.

14

Emphysema

Joel B. Karlinsky

Emphysema is a commonly encountered pulmonary condition in the smoking population (1).

I. **Definition**
- A. Emphysema has been defined by the **Emphysema Working Group** as a pathologic entity **characterized by abnormal, permanent enlargement of airspaces distal to the terminal bronchiole, accompanied by the destruction of their walls without obvious fibrosis**. Thus, emphysema primarily affects the parenchymal portion of the lung involved in gas exchange and only secondarily makes the conducting airways more collapsible by a reduction of elastic tethering (2,3).
- B. New alveolar units cannot be formed in adults, and thus the functional pulmonary impairment produced by emphysema is irreversible. Therapy of pure emphysema is symptomatic.
  1. Emphysema is usually accompanied by **bronchitic** (mucus hypersecretion) and/or **asthmatic** (wheezing) components; these components often respond to medical therapy.
  2. Thus, the presence of these other components in patients with emphysema must be defined if treatment is to be optimal.
  3. Under certain circumstances, functional improvement may be obtained in moderate to severe emphysema using newly developed surgical interventions (lung reduction surgery).
- C. **Types of emphysema**
  1. **Centrilobular emphysema** is most common in smokers and tends to localize to the upper lung zones.
  2. **Panacinar emphysema** is most frequently found in patients with α_1-protease inhibitor deficiency and tends to be found in the lower lobes.
  3. **Paraseptal emphysema** is also most commonly found in smokers and tends to be located peripherally. This type predisposes to large bullae.

II. **Clinical presentation (4)**
- A. **History.** Middle-aged to elderly patients with emphysema usually have a smoking history and will present with dyspnea on exertion that has been worsening over time. A seasonal or allergic component to the dyspnea is not found. Dyspnea may be accompanied by a productive cough that worsens with recumbency. Weight loss is common with severe disease, as well as complaints of insomnia and sexual dysfunction. Younger patients will also have similar complaints but may not give a significant smoking history; α_1-protease inhibitor deficiency or other genetic abnormalities (eg, Swyer-James-Macleod syndrome marked by a unilateral hyperlucent lung) must be suspected in such individuals.
- B. **Physical examination.** The basal respiratory rate will usually be increased. A normal physical examination may be found. However, most patients with moderate-to-severe emphysema will have a barrel-shaped chest and evidence of hyperinflation on examination. Breath sounds will be decreased, while increased tympanic sounds will be noted on percussion. Soft dry rales may be appreciated on auscultation of the lung bases. Evidence of pulmonary hypertension, including an increased second heart sound, jugular venous distention, and right ventricular heave, may be found. A right-sided S_3 gallop may be heard substernally. Patients may have supraclavicular

wasting and nasal flaring. Cyanosis will not usually be present unless emphysema is far advanced. Patients will not exhibit clubbing.

C. **Diagnostic evaluation** (4,5). A diagnostic work-up must be done to confirm the clinical suspicion of emphysema made by the history and physical examination. This evaluation should include the following components:

1. **Pulmonary function testing** (6). A full set of pulmonary function tests should be obtained, including measurements of airflow, lung volumes, and the single breath diffusing capacity. Measurements of airflow will be reduced, including the forced vital capacity (FVC), the forced expiratory volume in 1 second (FEV_1), and the FEV_1/FVC ratio. In particular, the FEV_1/FVC ratio will be <75% of the predicted value. The vital capacity (VC) may be normal or reduced, but the functional residual capacity (FRC) will be >100% of predicted, mainly due to increases in residual volume (RV). The ratio of RV to total lung capacity (RV/TLC) will also be >100% of the predicted value and is a marker of hyperinflation. The diffusing capacity for carbon monoxide ($D_L CO$) will be reduced, even when corrected for the alveolar volume. Patients with severe emphysema (FEV_1 <0.8 L) will not be able to perform the 10-second breath-hold necessary to obtain a valid $D_L CO$. Arterial blood gas determinations at rest should be obtained in all patients to determine the baseline degree of hypoxemia and hypercapnemia.

2. **Imaging of the lung parenchyma**
   a. Posteroanterior (PA) and lateral view **chest radiographs** should be obtained on every patient suspected of having emphysema. Although a diagnosis of emphysema may not be made with complete certainty using the chest radiograph, certain features are characteristic of the disease. These features include the presence of flattened diaphragms on the lateral film, increased lung volumes with increases in the retrosternal airspace, a narrowed cardiac silhouette, and vascular attenuation peripherally. None of these findings correlates with the extent of pulmonary function abnormality; chest radiographs may be normal in patients with mild degrees of emphysema.
   b. **Computed tomography** (CT) of the thorax is more sensitive than chest radiography in detecting mild degrees of airspace enlargement and should be obtained in individuals with relatively normal pulmonary function tests who have symptoms of dyspnea on exertion and a smoking history (7–11). Mean attenuation numbers obtained via this modality correlate with the degree of emphysema found in lung specimens (7). In addition, these numbers also correlate with common pulmonary function tests, including the FEV_1 and the FEV_1/FVC and $D_L CO/V_A$ ratios. High-resolution CT (HRCT) can be helpful in the evaluation of pulmonary vasculature, especially involving large bullae being evaluated for surgical resection to alleviate symptoms (9). Whether HRCT scans will be useful in identifying lucent areas compatible with small bullae in patients with emphysema being considered for lung reduction surgery remains controversial.

3. **Testing for α_1-protease inhibitor deficiency** (12–14). The diagnosis of α_1-protease inhibitor deficiency should be considered in any young, nonsmoking individual with moderate-to-severe emphysema defined by the criteria listed above (FEV_1 and $D_L CO$ <50% predicted). Serum protein electrophoresis should be done to measure the α_1-protease inhibitor level, which will be <35% of the normal predicted level in individuals with the deficiency. Phenotyping should then be carried out to further evaluate patients. Most patients will be homozygous (Pi ZZ phenotype); heterozygous patients are usually of the Pi SZ or Pi FZ phenotype.

4. **Giant bullous disease** (15)
   a. Bullae are usually found in the upper lung zones, most frequently in the right lung of smokers. The presence of basilar bullae seen in a nonsmoker should raise the possibility of α_1-protease inhibitor deficiency.

Bullae in patients who have little generalized emphysema usually begin in paraseptal foci and enlarge by a check-valve mechanism.

    b. Resection should be considered for a single large bulla or multiple localized bullae that constitute greater than one-third to one-half of a hemithorax in symptomatic patients. The major consideration in deciding whether to do surgery relates to the structure of the underlying compressed lung, which should be relatively free of small bullae or emphysema. This may be assessed by several techniques including HRCT or pulmonary angiography. CT should be performed at full inspiration and full expiration to determine whether the bulla or bullae communicate with the lung and can empty. Angiography is invasive but can yield information about the number and state of the arteries in the underlying lung. If the number is reduced or the arteries are attenuated distally, then there is a high likelihood that the underlying compressed lung contains bullae or emphysematous areas that will enlarge soon after resection. Angiography is far less frequent now that the same information can be obtained by CT.

    c. If the underlying compressed lung is normal by HRCT and/or angiography, then the emphysematous process will continue at a reduced rate after resectional surgery. In all cases, a judgment must be made regarding the benefit to be gained from lung resectional surgery. Pulmonary function testing should be performed prior to surgery, since some patients will exhibit little abnormality. Comparisons between the FRC measured by the helium dilution and the plethysmographic technique can be used to estimate the volume of gas contained within noncommunicating bullae; this may be several liters or more. If the volume of gas is large (>2 L), the diffusing capacity relatively preserved, hypocapnia not present, and the patient young, working, and moderately to severely disabled, then resectional surgery of a single large bulla should be performed, because an improvement in function will almost always occur.

    d. If a bulla is small and the remaining lung not compromised, function will not greatly improve after resectional surgery. All patients with bullae should stop smoking.

III. Medical therapy

A. Smoking cessation (16–20)

    1. Smoking cessation is the cornerstone of therapy for emphysema. About 1–2 mg of nicotine, the addictive substance found in cigarettes, is delivered to the lungs for each cigarette smoked. An addicted or dependent individual is defined as one who smokes more than one pack of cigarettes per day, smokes within 30 minutes of rising in the morning, or smokes in nonsmoking environments. Nicotine is rapidly absorbed, has a half-life of 2 hours, and continuously accumulates in the blood. Metabolism is by the liver, and cotinine, the major metabolite of nicotine, has a longer half-life and is filtered by the kidney. Cotinine levels may be measured in the plasma. Nicotine withdrawal may occur during the first week after stopping smoking and is manifested by anxiety, irritability, anger, fatigue, disordered sleep, and depression.

    2. Patients who smoke should be told directly by the physician to stop, since the increased rate of pulmonary function decline found in smokers will slow once smoking has ceased. However, patients will not stop smoking until they are ready; the physician should ascertain whether patients are indeed at this stage. The time to act is when this stage is reached.

    3. No single cessation technique is effective for every individual who desires to quit smoking (see chapter 31 for further details). Conditions should be optimized to aid patients who desire to quit; this includes encouraging family members to refrain from smoking in the presence of the patient and reducing stress by pharmacologic means. Nicotine replacement via gum or transdermal patch decreases withdrawal symptoms in addicted patients and may decrease recidivism. Nicotine polacrilex is available in gum form (2 mg/piece), and transdermal nicotine patches may be used according to the manufacturer's instruction; this involves starting off with patches containing 21 mg of nicotine for 2–4 weeks and tapering the dosage to 14 mg and then to 7 mg over 2–3 months. Nicotine patches should be used carefully in patients with known coronary disease since angina and infarction can occur if patients continue to smoke while using the patches. Transdermal patches are generally well tolerated; half of patients will develop a mild erythema over the patch site that may be minimized by rotating the patches to different skin sites. The long-term (6-month) success rates are about (22% to 42%) with patches; efficacy may improve when replacement regimens are combined with adjuvant programs (counseling or group therapy). Abstinence during the first 2 weeks of therapy is associated with higher success rates; patch therapy beyond 6–8 weeks is probably not useful. A typical smoking cessation protocol is given in Table 14-1.

   4. **Agents aiding in smoking cessation.** The use of clonidine, an α_2-adrenergic agent, sometimes improves short-term abstinence but does not improve ultimate success rates. The use of buspirone, an anxiolytic, will improve withdrawal symptoms and aid in smoking cessation.

   5. **Acupuncture and hypnosis** have not been proved to be useful.

B. **Pulmonary rehabilitation** (21–26) (Chapter 18). Pulmonary rehabilitation was defined by the American College of Chest Physicians Committee on Pulmonary Rehabilitation at the 1974 annual meeting as that art of medical practice wherein an individually tailored, multidisciplinary program is formulated that, through accurate diagnosis, therapy, emotional support, and education, stabilizes or reverses both the physio- and psychopathology of pulmonary diseases and attempts to return the patient to the highest possible functional capacity allowed by his or her pulmonary handicap and overall life situation.

   1. The **benefits of pulmonary rehabilitation** are listed in Table 14-2. The FEV_1

Table 14-1. Smoking cessation protocol

1. Patient must decide to quit. Physician or other trusted health care worker must explain risks of smoking and benefits of quitting. Physicians must be flexible and decide to work with patients over a long period of time to help with quitting. It is usually helpful to have a formal smoking cessation group available for patients who respond to group support. Patients must understand that once a quit date is agreed on and the patient stops, "falling off the wagon" does not indicate failure. The patient begins again, as often as necessary.

2. Reinforcement. Follow-up in person or by telephone within 1 week. Follow-up every month or on an as-needed/tolerated basis. Can measure carbon monoxide or serum, urine, or saliary cotinine levels, but this implies mistrust of the patient and should not routinely be done. If patients require additional help, can prescribe nicotine replacement in the form of slow-release patches or gum. Elderly patients must agree not to smoke while using exogenous nicotine, as further nicotine derived from cigarettes may result in extremely high blood levels and produce angina or myocardial infarction. Nicotine replacement therapies have a higher success rate when used in conjunction with smoking cessation groups.

3. Success. Success should be verbally rewarded; follow-up should be continued on a monthly basis.

4. Failure. If patients relapse, the program should be reviewed and the use of pharmacologic therapies can be offered. Patients should not be made to feel that one or more failures precludes ultimate success; efforts should be continued as long as necessary to achieve success. There is no evidence that hypnosis or acupuncture influences results; these modalities may be used if patients desire and can afford them.

Table 14-2. Benefits of pulmonary rehabilitation

Decrease in symptoms, primarily dyspnea
Reduced anxiety, depression
Improved exercise tolerance
Possible reduced hospitalizations

for patients with emphysema decreases 40–80 mL/yr, as opposed to 20–30 mL/yr for normal individuals. Pulmonary rehabilitation does not alter this decrease but may improve survival, if smoking is stopped and a comprehensive rehabilitation program with close follow-up is instituted. Several studies have documented the positive effect of rehabilitation programs on exercise tolerance. Patients have reported decreases in dyspnea, cough, and sputum production.

2. **Pulmonary rehabilitation is usually performed on an outpatient basis.** All programs assume a correct pulmonary diagnosis and require a careful assessment of the degree of pulmonary impairment by pulmonary function and exercise testing so that objective measurements of improvement may be made. All concomitant comorbidities, especially cardiovascular and neurologic, should be evaluated prior to designing the individually based rehabilitation program. Patients with significant cardiac dysfunction require a different kind of program. Patients should be committed to the rehabilitation program and should not have any significant underlying psychiatric conditions. Psychiatric consultation may be required in some cases to provide advice on medication use. Realistic functional goals should be clearly stated at the outset; these goals should be based on achieving decreases in perceived dyspnea and on improved exercise tolerance, and not on improvements in FEV_1 or FVC. Families need to be actively involved and fully supportive. Obviously, any patient undergoing pulmonary rehabilitation should not smoke.

3. The **components** of a successful rehabilitation program include: chest physical therapy to aid with clearance of secretions; an exercise conditioning program that closely follows daily activities (walking, cycling) involving the use of large muscle groups;and respiratory therapy, including use of bronchodilators delivered by metered dose inhaler (MDIs) or by updraft nebulizers if patients cannot perform the necessary respiratory maneuvers required by MDIs.

4. In particular, exercise should include **upper extremity training**. Dyspnea is common when using the upper extremities to perform the activities of daily life, possibly because the accessory muscles of breathing are destabilized while using the arms, and these muscles are of prime importance in emphysematous patients. Training can improve the functioning of these accessory muscles, although improvement in overall exercise tolerance may not be realized. Rehabilitation sessions should take place 3–5 days per week. The intensity of exercise varies according to the program used; no standards are available. Rehabilitation should include training in optimal breathing techniques (diaphragmatic and pursed-lip breathing) involving conscious slowing of the ventilatory rate with increases in tidal volumes to improve synchrony of the movement of the abdomen and thoracic cage. Overall mechanical function of the lung is not likely to improve with rehabilitation, but overall exercise tolerance is likely to improve and should be periodically measured with results communicated to the patient and families. A long-term commitment to the patient by the health care team is necessary.

C. **Oxygen** (27–29)
1. **Continuous oxygen administration** via nasal cannula should be offered to all patients with **hypoxemia** (Pa_{O_2} <55 Torr, oxygen saturation [Sa_{O_2}] <88%) to be used under the following conditions: at rest, only with exertion, or during sleep. Virtually all emphysematous patients who are hypoxemic during wakeful rest will be hypoxemic during sleep, since ventilation–perfusion relationships are adversely affected by the recumbent position. Enough oxygen should be supplied to maintain the Pa_{O_2} >60 Torr at all times.

2. Oxygen has been shown to lower the pulmonary artery pressures and reduce mortality in hypoxemic patients. Oxygen will also improve exercise performance and endurance and reduce symptoms of dyspnea. Patients should have at least two baseline arterial blood gas determinations to verify hypoxemia, since oxygen is an expensive treatment modality. These determinations will also identify those patients with carbon dioxide retention, whose oxygen needs must be very carefully titrated against carbon dioxide increases by an

experienced pulmonologist. Flows as low as 1 L/min may be necessary for individuals who retain carbon dioxide and may be delivered via several modalities, including compressed gas oxygen, oxygen concentrators, and liquid oxygen systems.

3. Arterial blood gases should be obtained and flow rates adjusted during chronic obstructive pulmonary disease (COPD) exacerbations and other changes in medical condition. Once instituted, room-air arterial blood gases (or at least SaO_2) should be measured at least twice yearly to demonstrate continued need for oxygen therapy.

D. **Bronchodilator therapy** (30–33)

1. **β_2 Agonist bronchodilators.** Although most patients with emphysema and little bronchitic component will not have an objective response (ie, an acute increase in FEV_1 by >15% to 20%) to inhaled selective β_2-agonist bronchodilators (sympathomimetic compounds), these drugs nonetheless improve symptoms and should be used as a first-line therapy, even though overall mortalty is not altered. Salmeterol, albuterol, pirbuterol, or metaproterenol are examples of relatively pulmonary-selective drugs that are preferred because they are associated with less cardiotoxicity. Initially, 2 puffs TID of a moderately long-acting or 2 puffs QID of a long-acting sympathomimetic preparation should be used. A spacer may be added to increase drug delivery to the lungs; this reduces the necessity of performing a correct inhalational maneuver. The dosing can be gradually increased to 4 puffs 4–6 times/d if the patient is reliable and has no history or evidence of coronary artery disease. Overuse of this medication is common because the rapid onset of action provides immediate symptomatic relief, and these patients must be carefully watched and counseled. Slow-release oral drugs may be used to prevent nighttime wheezing in emphysematous patients. If the patient is unable to perform the inhalational maneuver correctly, then the medication may be delivered by an updraft nebulizer.

2. **Anticholinergics.** Aerosolized anticholinergics may be more effective than aerosolized β_2-agonist compounds in some emphysematous individuals. Ipratropium bromide has a slower onset of action and longer duration than albuterol and should be dosed 2–4 puffs TID–QID. Ipratropium via aerosol may be added to a β_2-agonist regimen. There is no proof that these compounds improve long-term mortality.

3. **Theophylline**

   a. Due to a narrow therapeutic range (serum concentration 10–20 µg/mL) and considerable gastrointestinal, cardiac, and neurologic toxicity, the use of theophylline in the elderly emphysematous population has declined. A long-acting form of theophylline may still be quite useful in the treatment of nocturnal wheezing. The drug is also useful in patients who are noncompliant or unable to use aerosols but willing to take tablets. The nonbronchodilator activities (increased diaphragmatic contractility, stimulation of the respiratory center, improved cardiac output, reduced pulmonary vascular resistance) make theophylline a useful drug in emphysematous patients with cardiac disease or cor pulmonale. A synergistic benefit may be provided when used in conjunction with β-agonists and ipratropium. Theophylline therapy has no effect on the long-term course of emphysema. Table 14-3 gives information on when to check theophylline levels and common drug interactions.

   b. Patients who have the following conditions or are taking one or more of the medications found in Table 14-3 should have a theophylline level checked after five half-lives of the drug have been taken. If the drug is given on a TID basis, this will be after 48 hours; if the drug is given on a BID basis, this will be after 72 hours. The theophylline dosage should be adjusted to give a serum concentration of 10–20 µg/mL under baseline, stable conditions. In the elderly, it is wise to maintain a concentration toward the lower end of this range.

E. **Mucolytics.** The efficacy of mucolytics in emphysema is not proven. These agents (oral acetylcysteine, DNAase) may provide symptomatic benefit in emphysematous

Table 14-3. When to check theophylline level

Theophylline level too low in	Theophylline level too high in
Cigarette smokers	Patients with
Patients taking	Hepatic failure
Phenytoin	Cardiac failure
Rifampin	Cor pulmonale
Isoproterenol IV	Viral pneumonia
Phenobarbital	Patients taking
Carbamazepine	Cimetidine
Aminoglutethimide	Mexiletine
Isoniazid	Qinolone compounds (eg, ciprofloxacin)
Ketoconazole	Allopurinol
	Erythromycin
	Propranolol
	Oral contraceptives
	Tetracycline
	Calcium channel blockers
	Aluminum and magnesium hydroxide

patients with a significant bronchitic component and thick viscid sputum that is difficult to clear because of impaired cough from muscle weakness.

F. Psychoactive drugs. Older emphysematous patients experience depression, anxiety, insomnia, and pain. Benzodiazepines and other psychoactive drugs should be avoided in severe emphysema because they depress the respiratory center, especially during sleep. Safer drugs include sedating antihistamines, chloral hydrate, or the serotonin-reuptake inhibitor class of antidepressants.

G. α1-protease inhibitor replacement (12). Reformulated α_1-protease inhibitor replacement is indicated in the young patient with homozygous disease when blood levels are below the safe range. Therapy should be given every 1–2 weeks, as the half-life of α_1-protease inhibitor is about 7 days.

H. Immunizations. Patients with emphysema should receive the pneumococcal vaccine every 5–10 years and a yearly influenza vaccine as preventive measures.

I. Nutrition (34–37)

1. Patients with advanced emphysema (FEV_1 <750 mL) may develop significant weight loss in the absence of laboratory abnormalities. This weight loss may be due to increases in the energy costs of breathing secondary to accessory muscle use and performing the activities of daily living, coupled with a reduced caloric intake. When significant weight loss occurs, skeletal and presumably diaphragmatic muscle mass is reduced, leading to diminished muscle performance and a reduced ability to cope with any increased respiratory workload that might occur with respiratory infection or cardiac failure.

2. Patients with so-called pulmonary cachexia must increase caloric intake in order to increase muscle bulk and improve performance, often a difficult task in the outpatient setting. Patients may be placed on supplemental feedings and high-caloric diets but in general should not receive nasogastric feedings or peripheral parenteral nutrition. The use of high-lipid, low-carbohydrate diets has been advocated, based on the theory that less carbon dioxide would be produced as the end product of metabolism and the respiratory quotient would be lowered. The clinical benefit of such diets has never been proven, and altering fat/carbohydrate ratios in the diet is not presently advocated.

3. Emphysematous patients who are hypercapnemic and overweight should endeavor to lose weight to reduce the respiratory workload (nonelastic loading of the chest wall).

    4. No current evidence indicates that dietary formulations designed to decrease endogenous carbon dioxide production and reduce P_{CO_2} in chronically hypercapnemic patients are useful.

IV. Surgical therapy (38–40)

  A. Lung reduction surgery

    1. At present, volume reduction surgery for non-uniform emphysema is the only known therapy that can improve function (FEV_1, FVC, arterial blood gases, exercise capacity) in carefully selected patients with moderate-to-severe emphysema. Current medical therapies—bronchodilators, oxygen, portable home ventilator devices (continuous positive airway pressure [CPAP] and bilevel positive airway pressure [BiPAP])—only marginally improve symptoms and quality of life for this group of patients. These therapies neither improve pulmonary function nor reduce hospital admissions. Lung reduction surgery is performed to remove parenchyma that does not contribute to ventilation but occupies space in the thorax. Usually, upper lobe tissue is removed either through a thoracoscope or via a thoracotomy or median sternotomy, depending on the volume of tissue to be removed. However, lung reduction surgery should still be considered an experimental procedure because the long-term results are not known, morbidity and mortality are potentially high, and the procedure is quite expensive.

    2. Improvements in FEV_1 and FVC in the range of 50% to 100% after lung reduction surgery have been documented in some studies. The physiologic mechanism by which FEV_1 is improved after lung reduction is not yet clear, but the improvement may be due to increases in elastic recoil as the remaining lung ascends the volume–pressure curve or to restoration of normal diaphragmatic curvature and mechanics when tissue is removed from the hemithorax.

    3. Careful selection of patients is essential, even though exact guidelines for selection are not clear. Patients who meet the following criteria may be considered candidates for lung reduction:

      a. FEV_1 $\geq$25% predicted.

      b. Demonstrable preoperative motivation to have the surgery with agreement to participate in 4–6 weeks of pulmonary rehabilitation (the duration of rehabilitation varies among centers that perform the surgery).

      c. Excellent cardiac performance with left ventricular ejection fractions >45%.

      d. No other comorbidities.

    4. Lung perfusion or ventilation scanning, CT studies, and other imaging studies are not clearly useful in guiding the thoracic surgeon as to which or how much lung should be removed.

    5. Morbidity is due to the following factors:

      a. Persistent postoperative air leaks.

      b. Difficulty with postoperative weaning from the ventilator.

      c. Postoperative nosocomial pulmonary infections.

  B. Lung Transplantation

    1. Single lung transplantation is now considered the definitive surgical treatment for end-stage emphysema, since it does not require cardiac bypass and is technically much easier than double-lung or heart–lung transplants. However, concerns still exist about mediastinal shift in single-lung-transplanted patients with emphysema due to the increased compliance of the remaining lung.

    2. Single lung transplantation is usually reserved for younger patients with α_1-protease inhibitor deficiency, since donor lungs are in short supply. The predicted VC of the donor lung must be about 1.5 times larger than the volume of the recipient lung. Studies have shown subsequent improvement in exercise performance and arterial blood gases (39). Generally, patients must be <60 years of age.

    3. The selection criteria for lung transplantation for emphysematous patients are listed in Table 14-4.

      a. Significant coronary, hepatic, or renal disease is an absolute contraindication to lung transplantation. Patients with diabetes or long-standing hy-

Table 14-4. Selection criteria for lung transplantation in emphysema

Age <60 years, life expectancy limited only by lung disease
Disease limited to lungs, no multisystem disease
No multidrug-resistant infections
Good nutrition
Highly motivated patient with otherwise good quality of life
Lack of active psychiatric disease
Current corticosteroid use is a relative contraindication
Previous thoracic surgery is a relative contraindication
Previously treated malignancy is a relative contraindication

---

pertension may be considered only after extensive evaluation of end-organ function. Patients with connective tissue disease (eg, systemic lupus erythematosus) may also be considered when the disease is limited to the lungs.

   b. Patients being considered for transplantation should be evaluated at a recognized transplantation center, so that tests need not be repeated.

C. **Giant bullous disease.** Patients selected according to the criteria listed above should have resectional surgery. This should be performed through as small an incision as possible. Follow-up should include complete interval pulmonary function testing and CT scanning to assess the rate of new bullous formation.

D. **Spontaneous pneumothorax**

   1. Spontaneous pneumothorax is common in emphysema and usually due to the rupture of thinned parenchyma. **Acute severe dyspnea and respiratory failure** often result, depending on the amount of pulmonary reserve. Spontaneous pneumothorax may be difficult to diagnose by physical examination because good breath sounds are often lacking in severely emphysematous patients; it may also be difficult to distinguish from a giant bulla. Evidence of **tension** by vital signs and physical examination warrants emergent decompression of the pleural space.

   2. **Emergency inspiratory and expiratory chest radiographs** should be obtained. The expiratory film minimizes the size of the lungs and will show no change during expiration in the setting of a giant bulla. Comparison with previous films may be used to make the distinction.

   3. The pneumothorax may be difficult to treat because the pulmonary parenchyma is thin and does not heal rapidly. **Persistent air leaks** and **bronchopulmonary fistula** may develop.

   4. Treatment involves chest tube placement and **waterseal drainage**, or placement of a smaller, more comfortable **Heimlich valve** if the pneumothorax is small without compromise of vital signs or a mediastinal shift. If waterseal drainage does not result in resolution, replacement with negative-pressure suction to -20 to -30 cm H_2O for 48–72 hours is indicated to achieve reexpansion. When lung reexpands, the chest tube should be placed to waterseal drainage for another 24 hours, and the chest radiograph should be repeated to insure that the lung has not collapsed, prior to removing the chest tube. If the pneumothorax is large, suction should immediately be applied through a large-bore chest tube.

   5. **Surgical consultation** should always be obtained in emphysematous patients with spontaneous pneumothorax. If the lung does not reexpand with chest tube thoracoscopy, thoracotomy will be needed to perform pleurodesis or parietal pleurectomy.

   6. Repeated pneumothoraces on the same side may require **chemical sclerotic pleurodesis** through a large-bore chest tube. This should be performed by a respiratory specialist or thoracic surgeon.

V. Preoperative assessment in the emphysematous patient

A. General considerations (4,41–43).

1. The preoperative work-up of patients with emphysema who need surgery depends on the severity of the emphysema, the presence of other comorbidities, and the type of surgery being considered. No pulmonary work-up need be done if the surgery is emergent and thought to be life-saving. No work-up need be done if the patient has mild emphysema and the surgery is nonthoracic or upper abdominal. Patients with moderate-to-severe emphysema who require elective or semielective thoracic or upper abdominal procedures should be evaluated by a respiratory physician. As a general principle, the farther the operative site from the diaphragm, the lower the risk. When possible, the use of other methods of anesthesia (epidural, local block) should be attempted. The use of sedatives and narcotics should be minimized in all patients with emphysema.

2. **Assessment for nonthoracic procedures**

   a. **Upper abdominal procedures**

      i. Patients who smoke and/or have respiratory symptoms should have a chest film to rule out respiratory tract infection. Cough should not be suppressed, except perhaps when ophthalmologic surgery is to be done. Patients who are to have upper abdominal procedures or procedures in which anesthesia is to be lengthy should have preoperative pulmonary function testing including measurement of arterial blood gases. Patients with FEV_1 <1 L are at increased risk of pulmonary complications and death; patients with carbon dioxide retention at baseline also are at increased risk; these patients may require lengthy postoperative ventilatory support but should not have difficulty weaning unless the FEV_1 <800 mL. Patients with comorbid conditions, such as morbid obesity or heart disease, and the elderly have very high morbidity (70% to 80%) and mortality (3% to 5%).

      ii. Preoperative respiratory therapy for elective upper abdominal surgery is designed to reduce the risk of postoperative pulmonary complications. Therapy includes discontinuation of smoking, the use of bronchodilators to minimize airway resistance, antibiotics to treat associated bronchitis, mucolytics, deep-breathing (incentive spirometry) exercises every 2 hours to improve respiratory muscle performance, and evaluation and treatment of comorbidities involving major organ systems (cardiac, renal, gastrointestinal, neurologic). Laparoscopic surgical resections are preferred to laparotomies.

   b. **All other nonthoracic procedures**

      i. Ophthalmologic, urologic, gynecologic, and colorectal procedures are much less risky in patients with moderate-to-severe emphysema. Patients who smoke or have respiratory symptoms should have a chest film to rule out respiratory tract infection. Cough should not be suppressed, except perhaps when ophthalmologic surgery is to be done. Preoperative pulmonary function testing or measurement of arterial blood gases are generally not required. Patients with FEV_1 >1 L are not at substantially increased risk of pulmonary complications. However, patients with an FEV_1 <1 L who have comorbid conditions, such as morbid obesity or heart disease, or are elderly are at higher risk for postoperative morbidity and mortality.

      ii. Preoperative respiratory therapy for non–upper abdominal, nonthoracic procedures need not be quite as intensive as for patients undergoing elective upper abdominal surgery. Therapy would still include the discontinuation of smoking, the use of bronchodilators to minimize airway resistance, antibiotics to treat associated bronchitis, mucolytics, some deep-breathing (incentive spirometry) exercises, and evaluation and treatment of comorbidities involving major organ systems (cardiac, renal, gastrointestinal, neurologic).

      iii. Therapy should be continued for a period of time postoperatively. Incentive spirometry can be used to reduce atelectasis but is probably not very effective. It is relatively inexpensive and makes the patient think about deep breathing and coughing.

   iv. Postoperative pain after thoracotomy can be managed with regional (epidural) anesthetics. Laparoscopic approaches should be used whenever possible, as their effectiveness in reducing pulmonary complications in the nonemphysema patient has been proven; less pain medication is usually required.

   v. Thoracoscopy for lung biopsy through small incisions would appear to be the procedure of choice whenever possible in the emphysema patient.

3. **Assessment for intrathoracic procedures**
   a. **Cardiac procedures**
      i. The preoperative management of patients with mild-to-moderate emphysema may be carried out by the primary care physician. Chest films and pulmonary function testing are required. All patients with emphysema undergoing cardiac procedures should discontinue smoking for a minimum of 8 weeks prior to the procedure. Patients should have preoperative management with inhaled β_2-adrenergic agonists and inhaled corticosteroids to optimize pulmonary function. Immediate postoperative care should be delivered in the intensive care unit setting because most patients will require mechanical ventilation. At this point, responsibility for care should be transferred to an intensivist. Patients with moderate-to-severe emphysema should be seen by the pulmonary physician prior to the operation. These individuals present special problems and are likely to require lengthy periods of ventilatory support and specialized expertise in weaning.
   b. **Pulmonary procedures**
      i. The preoperative management of patients with emphysema who need lung surgery usually requires the expertise of the pulmonary physician. Patients meeting the following criteria should have further testing: FEV_1 <2 L or <50% predicted, maximal voluntary ventilation <50% predicted, or D_LCO <50% predicted who require a pneumonectomy.
      ii. An assessment must be made to predict the effect of resection on the amount of functional lung that will remain after surgery. This can be done by ventilation or perfusion scanning and measuring the distribution of ventilation or perfusion. Since pulmonary function (FEV_1) correlates with the distribution of either ventilation or perfusion, an estimate the remaining function (FEV_1) can be made by subtracting the ventilation or perfusion that will be lost from the total due to resection. If the remaining lung has >40% of the normal predicted value, then the surgery is feasible. This will not be the case for many patients with moderate-to-severe emphysema. In such patients, cycle ergometric exercise testing can be done to measure the oxygen transport ability of the cardiopulmonary system by measuring oxygen consumption (Vo_2) as a function of workload. If the Vo_2 is <10–15 mL O_2/min/kg body weight, then the proposed surgery is associated with a high risk of postoperative pulmonary complications. If the value is <10 mL O_2/min/kg, an increased mortality is associated with the surgery. If patients are undergoing lung resectional surgery for lung cancer, bronchoscopy is often necessary to determine the extent of disease and the type of surgery indicated.
      iii. As above, all individuals undergoing elective lung resectional surgery should discontinue smoking for a minimum of 8 weeks prior to the procedure. Preoperative management should include inhaled β_2-adrenergic agonists and inhaled corticosteroids to optimize pulmonary function. Postoperative care should be delivered by the pul-

monologist, since most patients will require mechanical ventilation and some will have difficulty weaning.

VI. **Outpatient ventilatory support for emphysematous patients**

   A. **Indications**

      1. **Carbon dioxide retention.** Patients with FEV_1 <1 L may begin to develop carbon dioxide retention due to irreplaceable loss of alveolar surface area. This development will not be alleviated by standard medical therapies. Eventually, when the FEV_1 has decreased to <600–800 mL, patients will be severely disabled and not capable of performing the activities of daily life. Such individuals have a high rate of hospitalization secondary to the development of hypercapnemic ventilatory failure.

      2. **Resting of respiratory muscles.** Studies of elective mechanical ventilation using both positive- and negative-pressure ventilators with the objective of resting ventilatory muscles have not provided definitive evidence of the utility of this modality. Devices have included the cuirass (turtle shell), the pneumowrap (raincoat), and nasal CPAP, all of which decrease respiratory muscle activity but do not reduce carbon dioxide retention. Respiratory muscle strength has not shown consistent improvement with the use of these devices, and they are not currently recommended for routine outpatient home use in ambulatory patients.

   B. **Technique.** See section on home oxygen and ventilation (Chapters 35 and 36).

VII. **Sleep** (44,45)

   A. Emphysema patients have a higher prevalence of sleep disorders, including insomnia, daytime sleepiness, and nightmares. Oxygen desaturation during sleep is common in patients with COPD as is reduced ventilation and carbon dioxide retention. Drops in Sao_2 associated with rapid eye movement (REM) sleep lead to increases in pulmonary artery (PA) pressures. Whether such nighttime increases in PA pressures lead to sustained daytime increases in PA pressure is unknown, but it is likely that nighttime desaturation alone can lead to chronic pulmonary hypertension. Therefore, emphysema patients who complain of sleep disorders should undergo a baseline nighttime oximetry to examine whether saturation decreases during sleep and to measure the frequency of apneas and/or hypopneas. Patients who desaturate to <88% or who have frequent apneas lasting longer than 10 seconds should undergo full sleep studies to study sleep architecture.

   B. Nighttime oxygen should be given to patients with nocturnal desaturations of <88% (mean Sao_2 or nadir of desaturation during REM sleep).

   C. Hypnotics should be used with caution in emphysema patients with sleep disorders, since they may increase carbon dioxide retention.

   D. Measurement of nocturnal Sao_2 is not recommended in the routine emphysema patient, and sleep studies are not necessary in any patient with a daytime Pao_2 >60 Torr.

VIII. **Obstructive sleep apnea** (OSA). OSA is not more common in patients with emphysema than in the general population. Full sleep studies should be performed in patients with emphysema who have symptoms consistent with OSA, because therapy may prevent pulmonary hypertension and cor pulmonale (28).

IX. **Prognosis** (46–48)

   A. **FEV_1. The prognosis for patients with emphysema depends on the FEV_1**, which correlates with the amount of functioning lung. The FEV_1 of nonsmokers declines 25–30 mL/year, beginning at age 35. The decline in FEV_1 in smokers is greater and is directly related to the amount of smoking. Some smokers lose FEV_1 at a rate >100 mL/yr or 1 L per decade, and hence some smokers will have a FEV_1 ≤1 L by age 60–65 and will experience dyspnea on exertion at this time. When the FEV_1 declines to <800 mL, individuals will be dyspneic while performing activities of daily life. The rate of decline is variable from person to person but correlates with the initial FEV_1, age, and the current number of cigarettes smoked. The lower the initial FEV_1, the more rapid will be the decline in function. Cessation of smoking after age 50 will not restore lost function, but the rate of future loss will approximate that of the age-adjusted nonsmoking population.

    B. Other indicators of poor prognosis are resting hypercapnia and the degree of hypoxemia. Reversibility of airflow obstruction by treatment with bronchodilators or corticosteroids is a positive prognostic sign.

    C. When the FEV_1 <750 mL, the mortality rate is 30% at 1 year and 95% at 10 years. Mortality may be reduced by the institution of continuous low-flow oxygen and appropriate medical therapy of intercurrent respiratory infections, respiratory failure, cardiac arrhythmias, or cardiac failure.

X. Air travel (49–52)

    A. Preflight evaluation. The degree of hypoxemia that will occur at altitude and the extent of comorbid conditions must be evaluated prior to the flight. Documentation of the relevant issues may be required, and a prescription for oxygen must be delivered to the airline for in-flight oxygen to be provided. Counseling should be done by the physician. Estimation of the degree of hypoxia expected at altitude may be made by exposing the patient to a hypoxic gas mixture adjusted to provide a fraction of inspired oxygen (FiO_2) equivalent to that at 8000 feet (15.1% of sea level FiO_2) for a minimum of 15 minutes. The clinical status, electrocardiogram, and SaO_2 should be monitored. This test is not recommended for routine use because of its variability and cost. Patients who may require this test include those with severe coronary artery disease and angina that develops with hypoxia, persons symptomatic during previous air travel, those who retain carbon dioxide with additional oxygen, and those with lower than normal PO_2 due to an acute condition (bronchitis/pneumonia).

    B. Regression equations based on preexisting pulmonary function, arterial blood gases, and comorbidities are available to estimate the effect of altitude on PO_2, but their use is not predictive of the development of symptoms or signs at altitude. Two equations are:

        1. PO_2 at altitude = 22.8 − 2.74X + 0.68Y,
        where X = anticipated altitude
        Y = arterial PO_2 at sea level.

        2. PO_2 at 8000 feet = 0.453 (Y) + 0.386 (FEV_1% predicted) + 2.44.

    C. In general, the PO_2 should be kept >50 mm Hg during the flight. This will usually require 1–3 L/min of 100% oxygen delivered by nasal cannula. Patients who require oxygen at sea level will need additional oxygen; the correct level can usually be achieved by increasing the normal flow rate by 1–2 L/min. Patients with stable emphysema who have completed flights without problems in the past may travel without receiving supplemental oxygen. Individuals who require in-flight oxygen must contact the airline well in advance of the flight; each airline has different requirements of the physician and patient.

XI. When to refer to a specialist. Patients should be evaluated by a specialist in respiratory medicine under the following conditions:

    A. Oxygen therapy. When the criteria for oxygen therapy are present, the patient should be evaluated by a specialist to determine the optimal delivery system. Most patients will be able to use a cannula system, some will require a pendant system, others may need intratracheal delivery.

    B. Acutely ill individuals or those in respiratory failure

        1. Patients with emphysema who are acutely ill and have not responded to routine medical management including use of bronchodilators, antibiotics, and oxygen should be evaluated by a respiratory specialist. In particular, steroid-dependent patients and those acutely treated with high doses of steroids who do not tolerate a taper should be seen. Patients with new-onset hypercapnemia or those suddenly requiring oxygen at a concentration >50% should also be evaluated by a respiratory specialist.

        2. Patients who have previously experienced respiratory failure requiring mechanical ventilation or who appear likely to require mechanical ventilation in the near term by exhibiting a rising PCO_2 at rest should be referred to a respiratory specialist. Acutely ill patients with emphysema admitted to an intensive care unit with neurologic symptoms and either hypoxic or hypocapnic respiratory failure with worsening respiratory acidosis (pH >7.25) should be evaluated by a respiratory specialist.

3. The decision to intubate and mechanically ventilate patients with severe emphysema is difficult, given the immediate life-saving benefits of mechanical ventilation versus the poor prognosis of such patients, utilization of expensive resources, patient discomfort and morbidity, and the likelihood of dependency on the ventilator.

4. Clinical evaluation alone is insufficient to determine the likelihood of survival after intubation, and objective markers of the severity of emphysema do not have any predictive value. Clinical data indicate that outcome after respiratory failure correlates with the severity of emphysema and the level of physical activity when well. Comorbidities contribute to poor patient outcome. From 75% to 90% of patients with emphysema and acute respiratory failure on mechanical ventilation will survive to discharge, and the 2-year survival of this group is 28% to 70%. The long-term survival of patients with emphysema who experience an episode of mechanical ventilation is the same as that of patients with an equal degree of emphysema who do not experience acute respiratory failure. Given this prognosis, most patients should be mechanically ventilated when indicated.

5. Patients with extremely poor baseline pulmonary function and poor quality of life prior to needing mechanical ventilation probably should not be intubated under any circumstances, and this should ideally be discussed with the patient and family well before the onset of acute illness. In these patients, a trial of noninvasive nasal positive-pressure ventilation (CPAP, BiPAP) may prove useful in improving oxygenation, reducing P_{CO_2}, and gaining time while other treatment modalities are being used.

C. Nighttime ventilation. Patients who require nighttime ventilation delivered via a positive-pressure (home ventilator, CPAP, BiPAP) or negative-pressure device should be under the care of a respiratory specialist.

D. Dyspnea evaluation. Distinguishing between pulmonary and cardiac dyspnea is often difficult; pulmonary exercise testing can help determine whether dyspnea is due to respiratory system limitations. Such testing is performed by the respiratory specialist.

E. Disability evaluation. Pulmonary function testing is often required in the evaluation of disability (see chapter 33).

References

1. U.S. Surgeon General: *The health consequences of smoking: chronic obstructive lung disease.* Washington DC: US Department of Health and Human Services, 1984; DHHS publication 84-50205.
2. Snider GL, Kleinerman J, Thurlbeck WM, Bengali ZK: The definition of emphysema: report of a National Heart, Lung, and Blood Institute, Division of Lung Diseases, workshop. *Am Rev Respir Dis* 1985;132:182–185.
3. American Thoracic Society: Chronic bronchitis, asthma, and pulmonary emphysema: a statement by the Committee on Diagnostic Standards for Nontuberculous Respiratory Diseases. *Am Rev Respir Dis* 1962;85:762–768.
4. American Thoracic Society: Standards for the diagnosis and care of patients with chronic obstructive pulmonary disease. *Am J Respir Crit Care Med* 1995;152(suppl):S78–S121.
5. Clausen JL: The diagnosis of emphysema, chronic bronchitis, and asthma. *Clin Chest Med* 1990; 11:405–416.
6. Bates DV: *Respiratory function in disease*, 3rd ed. Philadelphia: WB Saunders, 1989:172–187.
7. Heremans A, Verschaleken JA, Van Fraeyenhoven L, Demendts M: Measurement of mean lung density by means of quantitative CT scanning. A study of correlations with pulmonary function tests. *Chest* 1992;102:805–811.
8. Kinsella M, Muller NL, Abboud RT, et al.: Quantitation of emphysema by computed tomography using a density mask program and correlation with pulmonary function tests. *Chest* 1990;97: 315–321.
9. Klein JS, Gamsu G, Webb WR, et al.: High-resolution CT diagnosis of emphysema in symptomatic patients with normal chest radiographs and isolated low diffusing capacity. *Radiology* 1992;182:817–821.

10. Gould MA, MacNee W, McLean A, et al.: CT measurements of lung density in life can quantitate distal airspace enlargement—an essential defining feature of human emphysema. *Am Rev Respir Dis* 1988;137:380–392.
11. Sanders C, Nath PH, Bainley WC: Detection of emphysema with computed tomography: correlation with pulmonary function tests and chest radiography. *Invest Radiol* 1988;23:262–266.
12. Snider GL: Pulmonary disease in alpha$_1$-antitrypsin deficiency. *Ann Intern Med* 1989;111:957–959.
13. Brantly M, Nukiwa T, Crystal RG: Molecular basis of alpha$_1$-antitrypsin deficiency. *Am J Med* 1988;84:13–31.
14. Travis J: Alpha$_1$-proteinase inhibitor deficiency. In: Massaro M, ed. *Lung cell biology.* New York:Marcel Dekker, 1989:1227–1246.
15. Nickoladze GD: Functional results of surgery for bullous emphysema. *Chest* 1992;101:119–122.
16. Koltke TE, Battista RN, DeFriese GH: Attributes of successful smoking cessation interventions in medical practice: a meta-analysis of 39 controlled trials. *JAMA* 1988;259:2882–2889.
17. Fiore MC, Jorenby DE, Baker TB, Kenford SL: Tobacco dependence and the nicotine patch: clinical guidelines for effective use. *JAMA* 1992;268:2687–2694.
18. Fisher E, Haire-Joshu D, Morgan G, et al.: Smoking and smoking cessation. *Am Rev Respir Dis* 1990;142:702–730.
19. Schwartz JL: Methods for smoking cessation. *Clin Chest Med* 1991;12:737–753.
20. Camilli AE, Burrows B, Knudson RJ, Lyle SK, Lebowitz MD: Longitudinal changes in forced expiratory volume in one second in adults: effects of smoking and smoking cessation. *Am Rev Respir Dis* 1987;135:794–799.
21. Hudson LD, Tyler ML, Petty TL: Hospitalization needs during an outpatient rehabilitation program for severe chronic airway obstruction. *Chest* 1976;70:606–610.
22. Couser JI, Martinez FJ, Celli BR: Pulmonary rehabilitation that includes arm exercise reduces metabolic and ventilatory requirements for simple arm elevation. *Chest* 1993;103:37–41.
23. Petty TL, Nett LM, Finigan MM, Brink GA, Corsello PR: A comprehensive care program for chronic airway obstruction: methods and preliminary evaluation of symptomatic and functional improvement. *Ann Intern Med* 1981;70:1109–1120.
24. American Thoracic Society: Pulmonary rehabilitaton. *Am Rev Respir Dis* 1981;124:663–666.
25. Fishman AP: NIH workshop summary: pulmonary rehabilitation research. *Am J Respir Crit Care Med* 1994;149:825–833.
26. Hodgkin JE, Connors GL, Bell CW, eds.: *Pulmonary rehabilitation: guidelines to success.* Philadelphia: JB Lippincott, 1993.
27. Nocturnal Oxygen Therapy Trial Group: Continuous or nocturnal oxygen therapy in hypoxemic chronic obstructive lung disease. *Ann Intern Med* 1980;93:391–398.
28. Weitzenblum E, Sautegeau A, Ehrhart M, Mammosser M, Pelletier A: Long-term oxygen therapy can reverse the progression of pulmonary hypertension in patients with chronic obstructive pulmonary disease. *Am Rev Respir Dis* 1985;131:493–498.
29. Dunn WF, Nelson SB, Hubmayr RD: Oxygen-induced hypercarbia in obstructive pulmonary disease. *Am Rev Respir Dis* 1991;144:526–530.
30. Ferguson GT, Cherniack RM: Management of chronic obstructive pulmonary disease. *N Engl J Med* 1993;328:1017–1022.
31. Chapman KR: Therapeutic algorithm for chronic obstructive pulmonary disease. *Am J Med* 1991; 91:17S–23S.
32. Ziment I: Pharmacologic therapy of obstructive airway disease. *Clin Chest Med* 1990;11:461–486.
33. Anthonisen NR, Connett JE, Kiley JP, et al. for the Lung Health Study Group: The effects of smoking intervention and the use of an inhaled anticholinergic bronchodilator on the rate of decline of FEV_1: the Lung Health Study. *JAMA* 1994;272:1497–1505.
34. Hunter ABM, Carey MA, Larsh HW: The nutritional status of patients with chronic obstructive lung disease. *Am Rev Respir Dis* 1961;124:376–381.
35. Wilson DO, Rogers RM, Hoffman RM: Nutrition and chronic lung disease. *Am Rev Respir Dis* 1985;132:1347–1365.
36. Rogers RM, Donahue M, Constantino J: Physiologic effects of oral supplemental feeding in malnourished patients with chronic obstructive lung disease. *Am Rev Respir Dis* 1992;146:1511–1517.
37. Talpers SS, Romberger DJ, Bunce SB, Pingleton SK: Nutritionally associated increased carbon dioxide production: excess total calories vs. high proportion of carbohydrate calories. *Chest* 1992;102:551–555.

38. Cooper JD, Trulock EP, Triantafillou AN, et al.: Bilateral pneumonectomy (volume reduction) for chronic obstructive lung disease. *J Thorac Cardiovasc Surg* 1995;109:106–119.
39. American Thoracic Society. Lung transplantation. *Am Rev Respir Dis* 1993;147:772–776.
40. Low DE, Trulock EP, Kaiser LR, et al.: Morbidity, mortality, and early results of single versus bilateral lung transplantation for emphysema. *J Thorac Cardiovasc Surg* 1992;103:1119–1126.
41. Kearney DJ, Lee TH, Reilly JJ, DeCamp MM, Sugarbaker DJ: Assessment of operative risk in patients undergoing lung resection: importance of predicted pulmonary function. *Chest* 1994;105:753–759.
42. Markos J, Mullan BP, Hillman DR, et al.: Preoperative assessment as a predictor of mortality and morbidity after lung resection. *Am Rev Respir Dis* 1989;139:902–910.
43. Boysen PS: Perioperative management of the thoracotomy patient. *Clin Chest Med* 1993;14:321–333.
44. Douglas N, Flenley D: Breathing during sleep in patients with obstructive lung disease. *Am Rev Respir Dis* 1990;141:1055–1070.
45. Fletcher E, Donner C, Midgren B, et al.: Survival in COPD patients with a daytime Pa_{O_2} >60 mm Hg with and without nocturnal oxyhemoglobin desaturation. *Chest* 1992;101:649–655.
46. Fletcher C, Peto R: The natural history of chronic airflow obstruction. *BMJ* 1977;1:1645–1648.
47. Anthonisen NR: Prognosis in chronic obstructive lung disease: results from multicenter clinical trials. *Am Rev Respir Dis* 1989;133:S95–S99.
48. Postma DS, Sluiter HJ: Prognosis of chronic obstructive lung disease: the Dutch experience. *Am Rev Respir Dis* 1989;140:S100–S105.
49. Dillard TA, Berg BW, Rajagopal KR, Dooley JW, Mehm WJ: Hypoxemia during air travel in patients with chronic obstructive pulmonary disease. *Ann Intern Med* 1989;111:362–367.
50. Dillard TA, Beninati WA, Berg BW: Air travel in patients with chronic obstructive pulmonary disease. *Arch Intern Med* 1991;151:1793–1795.
51. AMA Commission on Emergency Medical Services: Medical aspects of transportation aboard commercial aircraft. *JAMA* 1982;247:1007–1011.
52. Berg BW, Dillard TA, Rajagopal KR, Mehm WJ: Oxygen supplementation during air travel in patients with chronic obstructive lung disease. *Chest* 1992;10:638–641.

15   Chronic Bronchitis and Bronchiectasis

David M.H. Wu and David M. Center

I. **Chronic bronchitis.** Chronic bronchitis is defined as the presence of productive cough greater than 250 mL per day for at least 3 months per year over 2 consecutive years, in the absence of other medical causes (eg, infection with *Mycobacterium tuberculosis*, congestive heart failure) (1,2). Sputum production may occur without airflow obstruction (simple bronchitis) or in conjunction with chronic airflow obstruction. If chronic airflow obstruction is present, then chronic bronchitis represents a form of chronic obstructive pulmonary disease (COPD).

A. **Presenting symptoms and signs**

1. The syndrome of chronic bronchitis develops insidiously over time. Unfortunately, the term *smoker's cough* has become synonymous with exposure to cigarette smoke. Thus, many affected individuals do not appreciate that they might have a medical condition until episodes of dyspnea begin to occur, by which time irreversible damage may be present. The cough rarely affects sleep or social discourse. Spontaneous improvement in cough frequently occurs early in the disease, but ultimately the cough becomes chronic and unrelenting by the sixth or seventh decade (3). In addition to the cough and sputum production that define the entity, most patients have a mixture of signs and symptoms that include wheezing, shortness of breath, and frequent bouts of acute infectious bronchitis complicating upper respiratory illnesses.

2. **Sputum production** is insidious; at the onset of disease, it often occurs only on arising from sleep. Over time, the most copious expectoration continues to be in the morning, likely due to pooling of secretions during sleep; lesser amounts of sputum are produced during the day. Sputum is usually mucoid, often with brownish discoloration. Increases in sputum volume or changes in color from whitish to yellow or green are reliable indicators of endobronchial infection that should be treated with antibiotics (3). **Hemoptysis** may occur during acute exacerbations, and bronchitis is now the most common cause of hemoptysis in the United States (2). **Bronchogenic carcinoma** must be ruled out in individuals with hemoptysis. **Chest pain** is not a common symptom. In individuals with coexisting emphysema, complaints of pleuritic pain should raise the possibility of pneumothorax or pneumonia when nonpulmonary causes of chest pain are eliminated.

3. **Signs**

a. Patients with bronchitis may appear normal or chronically ill. Examination of the chest may reveal decreased breath sounds, wheezes, or rhonchi. Hyperinflation and increased anteroposterior diameter of the thorax may be found after long-standing airway obstruction, especially with coexisting emphysema. At this stage, the accessory muscles of respiration (sternocleidomastoid, intercostal, etc) may be used during breathing. In severe obstructive disease, the latissimus dorsi or abdominal rectus muscles may be used as well to assist both inspiration and expiration. The forced expiratory time may be prolonged beyond the normal 4 seconds. Resting respiratory rate is usually greater than 16 breaths per minute and is proportional to disease severity (4). Rales or rhonchi may be heard over areas with bronchiectasis.

  b. In individuals with chronic airflow obstruction associated with chronic hypoxemia, **cor pulmonale and pulmonary hypertension** may develop. A resting tachycardia, atrial arrhythmias, murmurs of pulmonic or tricuspid valve insufficiency, and other signs of right ventricular failure (increased pulmonic component of the second heart sound, prominent right ventricular heave, right-sided third heart sound gallop, hepatojugular reflux, and peripheral dependent edema) may be observed (5). The electrocardiogram (ECG) is normal in individuals without airflow obstruction and those with only mild derangements in physiology. Characteristic ECG changes in patients with significant airflow obstruction are those of pulmonary hypertension and right ventricular hypertrophy, including rightward P and QRS axes, P pulmonale (prominent P waves in II, III, and aVF and biphasic P waves in I and/or aVL), right ventricular hypertrophy with an R:S ratio in V_1 >1, and an R:S ratio in V_6 <1 (6,7). Atrial fibrillation and complex atrial tachycardias are frequent in late disease.

  c. Individuals with chronic bronchitis without airflow obstruction have no laboratory abnormalities. With airflow obstruction and secondary hypoxemia, secondary erythrocytosis may be seen (8,9). Leukocytosis is a sign of acute infection or steroid therapy. Marked eosinophilia (>3000/mm³) should raise the suspicion of a complicating disorder such as allergic bronchopulmonary aspergillosis, eosinophilic pneumonia, or Churg-Strauss syndrome.

B. Etiology and pathogenesis

  1. In the United States, chronic airway irritation by inhaled cigarette smoke is the major etiologic factor in the development of chronic bronchitis. In other parts of the world (eg, eastern Germany, India, and China) and in certain parts of the United States, air pollutants are an additional cause. Occupational exposures (eg, nitrogen or sulfur oxides) may also be important. Nonspecific pathologic changes in the lung include infiltration of airway mucosa and submucosa with neutrophils and mononuclear cells, smooth muscle hypertrophy, and enlargement of the submucosal secretory glands. These mucus-secreting glands represent an increased percentage of the cross-sectional area of the airways of bronchitic individuals (the Reid Index). Many of these changes are also noted in asthma, cystic fibrosis, and pneumoconioses.

     a. When the airway lumen is occluded by secretions and narrowed by a thickened wall (increased submucosal glands, inflammatory cells, and smooth muscle hypertrophy), then patients have airflow obstruction and COPD. Emphysema almost always coexists in individuals with chronic bronchitis who exhibit airflow obstruction.

  2. The National Health Interview Survey in 1991 suggested that about 12.5 million men and women suffered from chronic bronchitis. The prevalence of chronic bronchitis is now estimated to be 51.5 per 1000 population (10). Chronic bronchitis can affect adults of all ages, its development depending on individual susceptibility and the level and duration of exposure to environmental toxins, including cigarette smoke. In the United States, the incidence is slightly higher in women and whites (10). Chronic bronchitis with airflow obstruction (COPD) is now the **fourth** leading cause of death among Americans (although these statistics include patients with emphysema as well). The trend over the past two decades indicates a 60% increase in the age-adjusted mortality from COPD. In contrast, mortality from vascular disease declined over the same period.

C. Pathogenesis (Table 15-1)

  1. The pathogenesis of chronic bronchitis is incompletely understood. Many injuries to the airways can result in chronic secretory processes. Experimental models in rodents and dogs have demonstrated secretory metaplasia, as well as alterations in the bronchial secretory apparatus on exposure to inhalational agents such as tobacco smoke, sulfur dioxide, or endotoxin (11,12). One mech-

Table 15-1. Pathology of chronic bronchitis

Secretory cell hyperplasia, hypertrophy, and ductal dilation of airways
Evidence of acute and chronic mucosal inflammation
Submucosal fibrosis and diverticula
Squamous metaplasia
Peripheral airway mucous plugging and secretory cell metaplasia
Smooth muscle hyperplasia

anism for the observed increase in mucus secretion involves enhanced ligand stimulation of epithelial cells mediated through cyclic AMP–dependent mechanisms. Under experimental conditions, exposure to ozone or nitrogen dioxide results in little injury to central airways but does cause bronchiolitis and injury to the ciliated and secretory cells of the membranous bronchioles as well as to type I epithelial cells (12,13). The relative contribution of oxidant injury is unclear. The causal role of viral or bacterial infections in chronic bronchitis also remains unclear. In individuals with existing chronic bronchitis, acute bacterial or viral infections can accelerate airway and parenchymal damage and impair mucociliary clearance, obstruct bronchioles, and contribute to chronic epithelial damage and bacterial colonization that further worsen symptoms and airway obstruction (14,15). Clearly, bacterial and viral infections play a role in acute exacerbations of chronic bronchitis. Further, acute viral infection can sometimes lead to chronic bronchitis in nonsmoking individuals; this suggests that virus infection alone can result in chronic airway inflammation and chronic sputum production.

2. A preponderance of neutrophils and mononuclear cells in areas of epithelial injury are characteristic features of chronic bronchitis (2,16,17). While the mechanisms of this inflammatory response are complex, all data from animals and humans implicate local secretion of chemoattractant cytokines from injured macrophages and epithelial cells (particularly interleukin-8 [IL-8]) that attract blood-derived leukocytes (neutrophils, monocytes, and activated T lymphocytes) to the airways (18–21).

3. As mentioned, chronic bronchitis with airflow obstruction (COPD) develops in a significant percentage of individuals with chronic bronchitis. To date, no definite hereditary or environmental factors have been found that predict the development of airflow obstruction in individuals with chronic bronchitis.

D. **Relevant physiology**

1. **Pulmonary function testing** is necessary to distinguish patients with and without airflow obstruction. No physiologic changes are observed in individuals with chronic bronchitis without airflow obstruction. Impaired gas exchange and abnormal pulmonary function will be observed in individuals with chronic bronchitis and airflow limitation. Early in obstructive disease, obstruction of small peripheral airways will be reflected by the finding of decreased flow rates at mid- to low-lung volumes (decreased mid–maximum expiratory flow rates [$FEF_{25\%-75\%}$ or $F_{75\%}$]), with a normal forced vital capacity (FVC) and forced expiratory volume in 1 second (FEV_1). Eventually, the FEV_1, the FEV_1/FVC ratio, the FVC, and the peak expiratory flow rate (PEFR) will all be reduced. These reductions do not distinguish chronic bronchitis with airflow obstruction from other obstructive lung diseases like asthma and emphysema. Patients with asthma will respond to inhalation of β_2-agonists, while patients with emphysema have characteristic airway collapse, as seen on flow-volume loops, and a decreased diffusing capacity for carbon monoxide ($D_L CO$).

2. One important caveat is that patients with chronic bronchitis and airflow obstruction often have features of asthma and emphysema as well. The total lung capacity (TLC) may be normal or increased in patients with concomitant em-

physema. There may be evidence of air trapping noted by an increased residual volume (RV) and RV/TLC ratio. The D_LCO may be decreased in proportion to the severity of coexisting emphysema in patients with bronchitis. Improvements of 15% to 25% in spirometric indices (FEV_1, FVC, and FEV_1/FVC) after treatment with a β_2-selective bronchodilator can be helpful in determining bronchial hyperreactivity (asthmatic component, asthmatic bronchitis) and indicates which patients may benefit from bronchodilator treatment (22).

3. **Arterial blood gases** may reveal hypoxemia without hypercapnia in the early stages of disease, with progression to hypercapnia in the later stages of COPD (23). Acute exacerbations, sleep, and exercise may also worsen blood gas abnormalities.

4. The diagnosis of chronic bronchitis is not based on radiographic criteria, and as many as 50% of patients may have no abnormalities on chest x-ray (24). The most common radiographic findings associated with chronic bronchitis are listed in Table 15-2. The chest radiograph is essential in excluding other pulmonary disorders (eg, pneumonia, pneumoconiosis, tuberculosis, and lung cancer) that present with symptom complexes identical to that of chronic bronchitis.

E. **Differential diagnosis**

1. The diagnosis of bronchitis is made by a clinical history of the presence of cough and sputum production. A detailed smoking and home- and work-exposure history is essential to determine potential environmental airway irritants. Pulmonary function tests are necessary to determine the extent and reversibility of airflow obstruction in order to rule out coexisting asthma or emphysema.

2. Systemic and local diseases that result in bronchiectasis must be ruled out, as the therapies for those diseases will be different from those for chronic bronchitis alone. If the history is suggestive of a disease associated with bronchiectasis, high-resolution computed tomography (HRCT) is necessary to define the location and extent of disease. If bronchiectasis is present on HRCT scans, other conditions must be considered.

F. **Specific approach to each diagnostic possibility**

1. The diagnosis of chronic bronchitis will be made by the appropriate clinical history (smoking) and associated pulmonary function test abnormalities. Sweat chloride testing should be obtained in individuals who are suspected of having cystic fibrosis because of an absence of smoking, younger age, or chest radiograph or CT abnormalities.

2. Individuals who are thought to be aspirating should be evaluated by barium swallow and neurologic and/or otolaryngologic examination.

G. **Management of the patient**

1. Patients with **chronic bronchitis without airflow obstruction** require no specific therapy. Treatment should focus on active prevention by helping patients stop smoking (smoking cessation programs), immunization against influenza virus and *Streptococcus pneumoniae*, and prompt antibiotic treatment of acute exacerbations caused by bacterial tracheobronchitis.

   a. **Smoking cessation.** Every effort should be made to institute a multidisciplinary approach to smoking cessation, including counseling, nicotine

Table 15-2. Radiographic findings in chronic bronchitis

Hyperinflation, with flattened diaphragms and subcardiac air

Thickened bronchial walls (mid-zone)

Increased bronchovascular markings

Periarterial edema

Prominence of the pulmonary artery (in pulmonary hypertension)

Right ventricular enlargement

gum or patch, and behavior modification techniques. Efforts are most successful when multiple interventions are practiced by several health care providers over many sessions; success rates vary from 25% to 77% at year after a program has begun (22,25).

   b. **Influenza virus vaccine.** The trivalent A and B influenza virus vaccine should be administered each fall in early to mid-November, before the usual arrival of influenza in December. Side effects are infrequent and usually self-limited but include fever, local erythema, pain at the injection site, myalgias, and malaise (26). The vaccine contains inactivated egg-grown virus, and patients allergic to egg proteins should **not** receive the vaccine.

   c. **Pneumococcal vaccine.** Patients with COPD and chronic bronchitis should receive the 23-valent pneumococcal vaccine once. The vaccine has been shown to protect against serotypes covering 87% of bacteremic pneumococcal infections and has been efficacious in 60% to 82% of high-risk healthy patients (26,27). We recommend revaccination of asplenic patients or those at risk for decline in antibody levels (transplantation patients, those with chronic renal failure, etc) every other year.

2. **Treatment of chronic bronchitis** is based on therapy with inhaled bronchodilators (β_2-adrenergic agents, anticholinergic agents, corticosteroids) and theophylline. Individuals with **chronic bronchitis with airflow obstruction** may be candidates for bronchodilator therapy if the pulmonary function tests improve (eg, 15% increase in FEV_1 or FVC, or 25% increase in $FEF_{25\%-75\%}$) following treatment. The major aims of drug therapy in chronic bronchitis with COPD are to reverse or control progression of airway obstruction and mucosal edema, lessen the volume of secretions, relieve bronchial smooth muscle spasm, and reduce airway inflammation.

   a. **β_2-Adrenergic bronchodilators** are useful and widely used in treating COPD (2) (Table 15-3). β_2-Selective agents such as albuterol, metaproterenol, terbutaline, fenoterol, bitolterol, and pirbuterol produce less tachycardia than nonselective adrenergic agonists and are therefore preferred. β-Agonists may enhance mucus clearance, decrease airway hyperresponsiveness, and improve respiratory muscle strength (2). Several studies have shown that hand-held metered-dose inhalers (MDIs) provide equivalent bronchodilatory effects to updraft powered nebulizers in stable COPD and during acute exacerbations .

   b. **Proper MDI technique** is imperative to ensure adequate drug administration. Extension devices or spacers should be used to improve delivery and minimize problems with hand–breath coordination. Oral β-agonists have an intrinsically higher risk of muscle tremor and tachycardia and

Table 15-3. Commonly used β_2-agonists for COPD and their dosages

Drug	Subcutaneous dose (mL)	MDI dose (mg) (puffs)	Nebulizer dose (mg)	Duration (h)
Albuterol		0.18–0.27 (2–6)	2.5–5.0	4–6
Metaproterenol		1.3–1.95 (2–6)	10–15	3–6
Terbutaline	0.25–0.5	0.4–0.6		4–6
Isoproterenol		0.16–1.02	0.63–3.8	1–2
Pirbuterol		0.4–0.8		4–6
Salmeterol		40 μg		12

MDI = metered = dose inhaler.

therefore should be reserved for those who fail a regimen of inhaled bronchodilators and theophylline or who are unable or refuse to use an MDI or home nebulizer (2).

3. **Anticholinergic agents.** The identification of significant airway inflammation and bronchial hyperreactivity in chronic bronchitis, as occurs in asthma, has led to an expanded role for anticholinergic agents. In addition, cholinergic stimulation has been shown to contribute to the bronchoconstriction found in both chronic bronchitis and bronchiectasis. Treatment is usually directed toward reducing smooth muscle contraction and mucus production.

   a. **Ipratropium bromide** is the most commonly used drug for this purpose in the United States. It is routinely administered by MDI (2–4 puffs q4–6h) and can also be delivered via powered nebulizer mist treatments.

   b. Recent studies have shown that anticholinergic therapy can be equally as effective as or more effective than the most potent β-adrenergic agents in chronic bronchitis and produce fewer side effects (14). Ipratropium can be initiated as front-line therapy when signs of fixed airway obstruction are present.

4. **Antibiotics** (Table 15-4)

   a. The major impact on survival and quality of life in patients with bronchitis and bronchiectasis has been achieved with effective antibiotic therapy and physical therapy. Prompt treatment of acute bacterial infections in both bronchitis and bronchiectasis reduces the frequency of exacerbations and improves pulmonary function (14,28).

   b. **Common bacterial pathogens** in patients with chronic bronchitis include *Haemophilus influenzae, H. parainfluenzae, S. pneumoniae, Moraxella catarrhalis, Klebsiella pneumoniae* and *Chlamydia trachomatis.* Commonly used and effective antibiotics include ampicillin, amoxicillin/clavulanate potassium, trimethoprim/sulfamethoxazole, doxycycline, ciprofloxacin, and ofloxacin. The newer macrolides, azithromycin and clarithromycin, can be used if there are resistant organisms (eg, *H. influenzae*) or if ampicillin cannot be tolerated. Patients should be given a course of 7–14 days and should be reevaluated if symptoms and physical findings do not return to baseline within 5–7 days.

5. **Mucolytics.** No clear evidence exists that mucolytics (eg, supersaturated potassium iodide, glyceryl guaiacolate) alter the rheology of the sputum in chronic bronchitis to an extent that airflow obstruction is reduced or clearance of secretions is enhanced. Thus, we do not recommend the use of mucolytics for the typical patient with chronic bronchitis.

   a. **Recombinant human deoxyribonuclease** (DNase) is currently approved by the Food and Drug Administration only for patients with cystic fibrosis, but not for routine use in patients with bronchitis or bronchiectasis. The increased sputum viscosity noted in bronchitis and bronchiectasis is caused by nuclear DNA from degraded cellular debris, so that theoretically solubilization of the DNA would improve the rheology of the sputum, making it easier to be expectorated. This hypothesis provides

Table 15-4. Antibiotic use in chronic bronchitis

Ampicillin 250–500 mg TID

Trimethoprim/sulfamethoxazole one double-strength tablet BID

Amoxicillin/clavulanate potassium 250 mg TID

Doxycycline 100 mg BID

Ciprofloxacin 500–750 mg BID

Ofloxacin 400 mg BID

Azithromycin 500 mg the first day, then 250 mg/d for 4 days

Clarithromycin 500 mg BID

the basis for the use of DNase in cystic fibrosis and by extension to bronchitis and bronchiectasis.

b. **Recombinant gelsolin**, an actin-depolymerizing protein, is also thought to reduce viscosity. Since cellular actin accounts for a much greater percentage of cellular debris than DNA, the utility of gelsolin may eventually be greater than existing mucolytics. When gelsolin will be available for clinical use is unknown.

6. **Corticosteroids.** Inflammation of the airways is a prominent feature of chronic bronchitis and bronchiectasis, especially when reversible bronchoconstriction is present. Anti-inflammatory agents such as inhaled corticosteroids have had favorable effects on improving airflow obstruction and symptoms. **The routine use of inhaled steroids is inappropriate in individuals without airflow obstruction and indicated only when reversible airflow obstruction can be documented.** In these individuals with reversible airflow obstruction, small increases in FEV_1 and decreased cough and sputum have been seen with long-term use of inhaled corticosteroids (29). Spacer devices should be used to enhance delivery and ease of use.

a. **Intravenous (IV) corticosteroids** are frequently prescribed during acute infectious exacerbations of chronic bronchitis. Efficacy in this setting is unproven, although the practice is now commonplace. If IV corticosteroids are to be used, we recommend using a high initial dose of 1–2 mg/kg/d for 1–5 days, with conversion to a course of an oral corticosteroid and a taper of 10 mg every 3 days.

7. **Supplemental oxygen.** Oxygen is the only effective treatment for cor pulmonale complicating chronic bronchitis with airflow obstruction. Measurement of oxygen tension (or saturation) during rest, exercise, and at night should be done to determine the level of supplemental oxygen necessary to correct hypoxemia (PaO_2 <55 mm Hg) (30).

H. **Problems and complications of therapy**

1. Therapies for chronic bronchitis and bronchiectasis are associated with a limited number of well described problems and complications. Smoking cessation is associated with weight gain. Attention must be paid to egg allergy before administration of influenza virus vaccine, which is also associated with occasional mild flu-like symptoms and painful local reactions. There are few contraindications to pneumococcal vaccine.

2. Tachyphylaxis develops to β_2-agonists, and deaths have been reported due to overuse, usually in asthmatics. Tachycardia, atrial arrhythmias, and restlessness are frequent pharmacologic side effects of theophylline and β-agonists. Anticholinergics are associated with dry mouth. It is rare for other signs of atropine overdose to appear.

3. The major problems with antibiotic use in chronic bronchitis include allergic responses, the emergence of resistant organisms, and the known side effects of antibiotic use (eg, diarrhea). Drug interactions are especially common with the macrolide antibiotics. Mucolytics are not generally recommended. Inhaled steroids are associated with pharyngeal candidiasis (thrush) and dysphonia. Some degree of adrenal suppression and osteoporosis can occur if inhaled steroids are chronically used in high doses. The effects of multiple courses of systemic corticosteroids are cumulative and include osteoporosis, cataracts, acne, exacerbation of existing hypertension and diabetes, and, if used in high doses for prolonged periods of time, immune suppression with susceptibility to *M. tuberculosis*, fungal infections, and other opportunistic infections.

I. **Specialist referrals.** We recommend that all individuals with the diagnosis of chronic bronchitis have complete pulmonary function evaluation including measurement of arterial blood gases to serve as a baseline. Individuals who have frequent acute exacerbations of chronic bronchitis, evidence of right heart failure, or hypoxemia at night or at rest should be evaluated by a pulmonologist for further detailed evaluation and therapy. Anyone with hemoptysis should be evaluated for the presence of lung cancer or tuberculosis and for possible bronchoscopy.

II. **Bronchiectasis.** Bronchiectasis is characterized by irreversible, localized or diffuse dilatation (>2 mm in diameter) and distortion of the bronchi. Destruction of the muscular and elastic components of the bronchial walls causes the dilatation, leading to impaired mucociliary clearance, chronic bacterial infection, and production of copious, purulent sputum (30). However, airway dilatation may occasionally occur without sputum production, and this pathologic process is termed *dry bronchiectasis*. Bronchiectasis is commonly associated with systemic conditions associated with recurrent lower respiratory infections, including cystic fibrosis, allergic bronchopulmonary aspergillosis, primary ciliary dyskinesia, and immunodeficiencies, particularly those associated with defects in bacterial microbicidal activity. Bronchiectasis can be indistinguishable from chronic bronchitis from both a clinical and pathologic perspective, and the two conditions overlap significantly (31). The dilatation occurs in one of several anatomic patterns. Cylindrical bronchiectasis is central in origin; this pattern is observed in association with pneumonia and is usually reversible. Persistent cylindrical bronchiectasis may also be noted in association with inflammatory conditions that affect central airways (allergic bronchopulmonary aspergillosis). Saccular bronchiectasis is a more advanced form of disease associated with pathologic processes that occur more distally in the lung. This pattern has no particular diagnostic significance, but the saccular type of dilatation predisposes to poorer clearance of secretions and more chronic infections. Cystic bronchiectasis refers to disease in which the dilatations are particularly large and are visible by routine chest roentgenograms.

   A. **Presenting symptoms and signs**

   1. **Symptoms.** Persistent sputum production following a necrotizing lower respiratory infection should alert the physician to possible permanent damage to the airways and bronchiectasis. Hemoptysis is the second most common symptom and can occur in the presence or absence of either chronic sputum production or active infection. In an individual with an appropriate history in whom lung cancer or other causes have been ruled out, the lower respiratory tract damage is generally assumed to be secondary to infection. Differentiating superimposed acute bacterial infection in areas of bronchiectasis from persistent chronic infections (eg, tuberculosis or aspergillosis) is sometimes difficult.

   2. **Signs.** The signs of bronchiectasis relate to local destructive processes in the lung producing mucus hypersecretion leading to airflow obstruction. Thus, localized areas of rales, rhonchi and wheezes may be found on auscultation of the chest. Clubbing, evidence of sinusitis, and nasal polyps are all associated findings. Chronically hypoxic individuals will exhibit signs of pulmonary hypertension and right-sided heart disease described in the section on chronic bronchitis.

   B. **Etiology and pathogenesis**

   1. Bronchiectasis occurs as a result of enzymatic destruction of airway walls in association with infection. Certain bacterial infections, particularly staphylococcal and gram-negative pneumonias, produce airway wall destruction, probably as a result of release of endogenous bacterial proteolytic enzymes. In addition, the chronic inflammatory process that accompanies infections associated with granuloma formation (eg, tuberculosis, fungal infections) is itself pathogenic to airways.

   2. In contrast to chronic bronchitis, a number of systemic syndromes associated with impaired upper and lower respiratory bacterial microbicidal activity also predispose to bronchiectasis. As a result, the presence of bronchiectasis should be suspected in any individual with chronic lower respiratory infection or a systemic disease that predisposes to recurrent bacterial infection (eg, cystis fibrosis, immunoglobulin deficiency, immotile cilia syndromes, neutrophil phagocytic, adherence, or motility defects, etc). Certain airway obstructive syndromes are also associated with bronchiectasis, the prototype being asthma due to chronic bronchopulmonary aspergillosis (Table 15-5).

   3. Since the introduction of antibiotics, bronchiectasis following parenchymal infection (pneumonia) has become much rarer in the United States, with an

Table 15-5. Major syndromes of obstructive lung disease

Chronic bronchitis
Emphysema
Asthma
Cystic fibrosis
Bronchiectasis
Pneumoconiosis

annual incidence of <1 per 10,000 people. Bronchiectasis following pneumonia may still be found in populations lacking access to health care and prescription antibiotics.

4. Abnormal dilation of the proximal subdivisions of bronchi that contain cartilage is seen pathologically. This is likely mediated by neutrophil elastase and the secretion of other inflammatory cytokines, such as IL-1, IL-8, and tumor necrosis factor, that recruit other cells (32). The resulting inflammation of the bronchial walls leads to destruction of the elastic and muscular components so that the supporting elastic alveolar walls can retract the now more compliant airways, resulting in dilatation. Chronic bronchial overdistention is associated with contraction, hypertrophy, and hyperplasia of surrounding normal airway musculature (30). These processes extend peripherally so that the conducting airways eventually become widened and distorted. Long-standing bronchiectasis is characterized by peribronchial fibrosis, squamous metaplasia, and obliteration of the distal bronchioles. The resulting impairment in tracheobronchial clearance predisposes patients to airway colonization and further infection, as in chronic bronchitis.

5. Patients with bronchiectasis have an increased risk of hemoptysis due to increased bronchial blood flow. Hemoptysis may be trivial or life-threatening, without any substantial predicting factors. The bleeding is almost always of bronchial artery origin and due to neovascularization in areas of granulation tissue associated with the underlying infectious process. In bronchiectatic areas where there is inflammation and increased bronchial blood pressure and flow, affected bronchial vessels may necrose and leak blood. Invasive infections in areas of bronchiectasis, such as those due to aspergillosis, are particularly prone to be associated with hemoptysis.

C. **Relevant physiology.** The relevant physiology of the airways was discussed in the section on chronic bronchitis. Pulmonary function abnormalities in bronchiectasis are similar to those found in chronic bronchitis.

D. **Differential diagnosis.** Table 15-6 lists a number of diseases associated with bronchiectasis, together with the primary characteristic of the bronchiectasis associated with each disease, the etiologic defect, and diagnostic work-up.

1. **Radiologic evaluation.** The evaluation of suspected bronchiectasis includes **chest roentgenography** to search for other causes of symptoms and signs. Dilated airway markings (tram tracks) and saccular cystic spaces with air-fluid levels are diagnostic. If no evidence of disease is observed on chest x-ray, **HRCT** is of value in identifying central bronchiectasis. While the routine use of CT is not necessary to establish the diagnosis in most cases, it may be of value in individuals with obscure causes of hemoptysis or chronic sputum production. A careful history to rule out any of the syndromes noted in Table 15-6, along with a diagnostic evaluation, is indicated in obscure cases. HRCT is also useful in assessing localized versus generalized bronchiectasis and is better than routine chest x-ray in the evaluation of large and small airway dilatation (33,34). The radiographic pattern of bronchiectasis holds some clues as to etiology.

   a. **Tuberculosis and sarcoidosis** produce bronchiectasis localized to the upper lung zones. Lower lung zone bronchiectasis suggests chronic aspiration, while bronchiectasis in the mid-lung zones in an individual with

Table 15-6. Diseases associated with bronchiectasis

Disease syndrome	Bronchiectasis	Defect	Diagnosis
Cystic fibrosis	Infections from childhood; upper lobes early, then all lobes; sinusitis common	Chloride channel resulting in inspissated secretions	Sweat chloride test; genetic screening
Immunoglobulin deficiency	Infections from childhood, diffuse distribution; other infections (skin, sinuses, otitis) common	Inadequate opsonization of respiratory pathogens	Immunoglobulin electrophoresis
Phagocyte defects	Infections from childhood; diffuse distribution (other infections common)	Multiple defects including absence of microbicidal activity, chemotactic and adhesion molecule defects	Screening requires special laboratories following elimination of other possibilities
Immotile cilia	Lower and upper respiratory infections; sinusitis; sterility; situs inversus viscerum	Cilia defects resulting in poor muco–ciliary clearance	Electron microscopy of ciliated mucosal surface or sperm
Allergic bronchopulmonary aspergillosis	Mid-lung zones; wheezing invariable	Chronic inflammation; secondary antigen–antibody complex–mediated inflammation	Elevated specific IgE and IgG levels
Complicating chronic tuberculosis or fungal disease	Upper lobe predominance	Destruction of airway walls from macrophage enzymes	Culture or polymerase chain reaction evidence of disease
Complicating bacterial pneumonia: aspiration	Lower lobes	Anaerobic necrotizing infection	Neurologic state, bacteriology, etc.
Complicating bacterial pneumonia: gram-negatives	Upper lobes	Destruction from leukocyte and bacterial enzymes	Bacterologic confirmation
Complicating bacterial pneumonia: necrotizing gram-positives	Lower lung zones if blood-borne staph (eg, in IV drug use); diffuse if following influenza infection	Bacterial enzymes	Blood and sputum cultures; appropriate history and characteristic pattern of chest x-ray

airflow obstruction should suggest allergic bronchopulmonary aspergillosis with asthma. Diffuse bronchiectasis is usually associated with systemic abnormalities.

2. **Pulmonary function evaluation.** Patients will have evidence of airway obstruction on pulmonary function testing, with the exception of mild, localized disease. In individuals with clinically significant but localized disease (by HRCT), resection of the involved area is occasionally recommended if the pulmonary function is good. Resectional surgery for bronchiectasis should not be undertaken without pulmonary consultation to rule out widespread disease, for which resection may result either in no improvement or respiratory failure.

3. It is no longer necessary to perform bronchography to make the diagnosis of bronchiectasis. Since this procedure can worsen bronchiectasis, it should not be done. It has provided insights into the characteristic anatomic changes of mucus gland filling and dilation of the submucosal glands in chronic bronchitis (35,36).

E. **Specific approach to each diagnostic possibility**

1. Table 15-6 lists the approaches to the differential diagnosis of bronchiectasis based on the history and the anatomic location of the lower respiratory disease. A history of past or recurrent infections is universal in patients with bronchiectasis and not particularly helpful. However, identification of the anatomic location of the lower respiratory infection may prove quite helpful. Recurrent infections limited to the same lobe are suggestive of a local process, either an obstructing lesion or localized airway destruction, but they may represent recurrent aspiration.

2. Widespread disease without bacterial infections in the skin or other organs suggests cystic fibrosis or immotile cilia syndrome. The presence of generalized infections of the lung, skin, and sinuses should prompt a search for immune deficiencies characterized by poor microbicidal function. This includes human immunodeficiency virus 1 infection, which is associated with an increased incidence of bacterial pneumonia.

3. In a young individual without smoking exposure, **cystic fibrosis** should be ruled out with sweat chloride measurements or genetic screening (Chapter 16).

4. **Immunoglobulin deficiencies** may be identified by immunoelectrophoresis followed by quantitative immunoglobulin subtype levels. Only IgG deficiencies should be treated with monthly IV replacement. Individuals with severe defects in ciliary motility can be identified by nasal mucosal biopsy. Assessment of phagocytic function requires a special laboratory equipped to determine the presence of phagolysosomes, the generation of halide-dependent H_2O_2 killing, and cell motility and adhesion molecule expression. Individuals with severe defects may require prophylactic antibiotic therapy. Complement deficiencies are determined by measurement of serum levels and individuals are treated according to the complex of recurrent infections developed.

F. **Management of the patient**

1. The management of the patient is completely dependent on the symptoms. General therapeutic measures include smoking cessation, influenza virus and pneumococcal vaccines, and treatment with bronchodilators, including β_2-agonists and anticholinergics if reversible airflow obstruction is present (37).

2. Individuals with recurrent or persistent lower respiratory infections or hemoptysis should be treated with chronic antibiotics as needed to suppress local superinfections. We recommend broad-spectrum antibiotics for patients with acute infections with or without hemoptysis for at least 3 months, followed by a close observation period. Individuals with recurrent infection or hemoptysis after such a course of antibiotics may require more prolonged antibiotic therapy or rotating courses of broad-spectrum antibiotics every 3–6 months. Individuals with underlying systemic diseases such as cystic fibrosis or immotile cilia syndrome will usually require lifelong therapy with antibiotics.

   a. Resectional surgery for recurrent infection in a single bronchiectatic area may be done in individuals who experience substantial morbidity from the recurrent infections or whose infection is resistant to all antibiotic therapy (*Mycobacterium avium-intracellulare* complex).

3. **Hemoptysis**

   a. With the exception of massive hemoptysis (>500 mL/d), bleeding should be evaluated by fiberoptic bronchoscopy to rule out endobronchial lesions and localize the site of bleeding to guide further therapy. Hemoptysis may stop if associated with bacterial infections that can be treated with antibiotics.

   b. **Resectional surgery** is the best therapy for individuals with localized disease associated with persistent or massive hemoptysis. Only individuals in whom the predicted FEV_1 following surgery is calculated to be >1.5 L or 35% of the normal predicted value can be brought immediately to surgery. Individuals with borderline pulmonary function tests in whom the FEV_1 following surgery is calculated to be >1.5 L or 35% of the normal predicted value should be evaluated with preoperative split-function ventilation–perfusion lung scans to determine the percentage of functional lung that will be removed during surgery. Patients with massive hemoptysis with poor pulmonary function whose postoperative FEV_1 is calculated to be <1 L may be respiratory cripples after surgery. These individuals may be treated by bronchial artery embolization.

   c. Bleeding can be temporized by **embolization of the bronchial artery** branch that supplies the bleeding vessel. The bronchial arteries originate in the aorta, and many branch from spinal arteries. Thus, paraplegia is a potential risk with embolization.

4. **Aspiration.** Aspiration should be evaluated by neurologic examination and pharyngeal and esophageal motility studies. Surgical closure of the vocal cords with tracheostomy can be performed to decrease aspiration if the problem becomes life-threatening.

G. **Problems and complications of therapy.** The major complication of chronic antibiotic therapy is emergence of resistant organisms. The complications of arterial embolization are those attendant to arteriography of the aorta, including cholesterol plaque embolization to the lower extremities and abdominal organs and paraplegia if a spinal artery branch is accidentaly embolized. The surgical complications are likewise those associated with general anesthesia and thoracic surgery. In particular, patients must be carefully assessed for pulmonary functional reserve, as the most serious postoperative complication is failure to sustain ventilation and oxygenation without mechanical ventilation.

H. **Specialist referrals.** We recommend that all individuals with hemoptysis be evaluated by a pulmonary specialist. When appropriate, bronchoscopy should be performed to rule out other causes of disease. Patients with chronic systemic diseases such as cystic fibrosis and immunoglobulin deficiencies are best cared for in centers prepared to address all the special problems of these patients. Anyone in whom surgery is anticipated should have a detailed evaluation by a pulmonary specialist to determine the risks of surgery and likelihood of postoperative respiratory failure.

References

1. American Thoracic Society: Chronic bronchitis, asthma and pulmonary emphysema. A statement by the Committee on Diagnostic Standards for Nontuberculous Respiratory Diseases. *Am Rev Respir Dis* 1962;85:762–768.
2. Snider GL, Faling LJ, Rennard SI: Chronic bronchitis and emphysema. In: Murray JF, Nadel JA, eds. *Textbook of respiratory medicine.* Philadelphia: WB Saunders, 1994;2:1331–1397.
3. Georgopulus D, Anthonisen NR: Symptoms and signs of COPD. In: Cherniack NS, ed. *Chronic obstructive pulmonary disease.* Philadelphia: WB Saunders, 1991:357–363.
4. Loveridge B, West P, Kryger M, Anthonisen NR: Alteration in breathing pattern with progression of chronic obstructive pulmonary disease. *Am Rev Respir Dis* 1986;134:930–934.
5. Hill NS: The cardiac exam in lung disease. *Clin Chest Med* 1987;8:273–285.
6. Hudson LD, Kurt TL, Geuton E: Arrhythmias associated with acute respiratory failure in patients with chronic airway obstruction. *Chest* 1973;63:661–665.

7. Calatayud JB, Abad JM, Khoi NB, et al.: P wave changes in chronic obstructive pulmonary disease. *Am Heart J* 1970;79:444–453.
8. Donahoe M, Rogers RM: Laboratory evaluation of the patient with chronic obstructive pulmonary disease. In: Cherniack NS, ed. *Chronic obstructive pulmonary disease.* Philadelphia: WB Saunders, 1991;373–386.
9. Golde DW, Hocking WG, Koeffler HP, Adamson JW: Polycythemia: mechanisms and management. *Ann Intern Med* 1981;95:71–87.
10. Adam PF, Benson V: Current estimates from the National Health Interview Survey, 1991. National Center for Health Statistics. *Vital Health Stat 10* 1992;10:184.
11. Reid L, Jones R: Experimental chronic bronchitis. *Int Rev Pathol* 1983;24:335–382.
12. Snider GL: Animal models of chronic airways injury. *Chest* 1992;101:74S–79S.
13. Lum H, Schwartz LW, Dungworth DL, et al.: A comparative study of cell renewal after exposure to ozone and oxygen. Response to terminal bronchiolar epithelium in the rat. *Am Rev Respir Dis* 1978;118:335–345.
14. Chodosh S: Treatment of acute exacerbations of chronic bronchitis :state of the art. *Am J Med* 1991;91(suppl 6A)Z:87S–92S.
15. Murphy TF, Sethi S: Bacterial infection in chronic obstructive pulmonary disease. *Am Rev Respir Dis* 1992;146:1067–1083.
16. Boucher RC, Van Scott MR, Willumsen N, et al.: Epithelial cell injury. *Am Rev Respir Dis* 1988;138:41–44.
17. Abramson SL, Malech HL, Gallin JI: Neutrophils. In: Crystal RG, West JB, eds. *The lung: scientific foundations.* New York: Raven Press, 1991:553–564.
18. Stockley RA: The role of proteinases in the pathogenesis of chronic bronchitis. *Am J Respir Crit Care Med* 1994;150(6, pt 1):S109–113.
19. Saetta M, Di Stefano A, Fabbri LM, et al.: Airway eosinophilia in chronic bronchitis during exacerbations. *Am J Respir Crit Care Med* 1994;150(6, pt 1):1646–1652.
20. Saetta M, Di Stefano A, Fabbri LM, et al.: Activated T lymphocytes and macrophages in bronchial mucosa of subjects with chronic bronchitis. *Am Rev Respir Dis* 1993;147:301–306.
21. Shelhamer N, et al.: Airway inflammation. *Ann Intern Med* 1995;123:288–304.
22. Kottke TE, Battista RN, De Friese GH, Brekke ML: Attributes of successful cessation interventions in medical practice: a meta-analysis of 39 controlled trials. *JAMA* 1988;259:2882–2889.
23. Bates DV: *Respiratory function in disease,* 3rd ed. Philadelphia: WB Saunders, 1989:172–187.
24. Fraser RG, Fraser RS, Pare PS: *Diagnosis of diseases of the chest,* 3rd ed. Philadelphia: WB Saunders, 1990:2116–2144.
25. Stokes J, Rigotti NA: The health consequences of cigarette smoking and the internist's role in smoking cessation. *Adv Intern Med* 1988;33:431–460.
26. Immunization Practices Advisory Commnitte: Update on adult immunization: pneumococcal disease. *MMWR* 1991;40:42–43.
27. Immunization Practices Advisory Committee: Pneumococcal polysaccharide vaccine. *MMWR* 1989;38:64–76.
28. Anthonisen NR, Manfreda J, Warren CPW, et al.: Antibiotic treatment in exacerbation of chronic obstructive pulmonary disease. *Ann Intern Med* 1987;106:196–204.
29. Griffith DE, Perkins RC: Changing strategies for treatment of chronic bronchitis. *Semin Respir Infect* 1994;9:49–57.
30. American Thoracic Society: Standards for the diagnosis and care of patients with chronic obstructive pulmonary disease. *Am J Respir Crit Care Med* 1995;152:S77–S120.
31. Luce JM: Bronchiectasis. In: Murray JF, Nadel JA, eds. *Textbook of respiratory medicine.* Philadelphia: WB Saunders, 1994;2:1331–1397.
32. Heard BE, Khatchatourov V, Otto H, et al.: The morphology of emphysema, chronic bronchitis and bronchiectasis: definitions, nomenclature, and classifcation. *J Clin Pathol* 1979;32:882–892.
33. Owen CA, Campbell EJ, Hill SL, Stockley RA: Increased adherence of monocytes to fibronectin in bronchiectasis. *Am Rev Respir Dis* 1992;145:626–631.
34. Barker AF, Bardana EJ: Bronchiectasis: update of an orphan disease. *Am Rev Respir Dis* 1988;137:969–978.
35. Stanford W, Galvin JR: The diagnosis of bronchiectasis. *Clin Chest Med* 1988;9:691–699.
36. Gamsu G, Forbes AR, Ovenfors CO: Bronchogenic features of chronic bronchitis in normal men. *AJR* 1981;36:317–322.
37. Fraser RG, Fraser RS, Renner JW, et al.: The roentgenologic diagnosis of chronic bronchitis: a reassessment with emphasis on parahilar bronchi seen end-on. *Radiology* 1976;120:1.

16

Cystic Fibrosis

Victor F. Tapson and Peter S. Kussin

Cystic fibrosis (CF) is a **common genetic disease characterized by severe bronchiectasis** (Table 16-1) **and exocrine pancreatic insufficiency**. Recurrent bacterial airway infections caused predominantly by *Staphylococcus aureus* and mucoid *Pseudomonas aeruginosa* account for substantial morbidity and mortality. The disease occurs in 1 in 2500 white births and less commonly in blacks and Asians (1). CF is an autosomal-recessive hereditary disease and heterozygotes are asymptomatic. Extensive basic research and numerous clinical trials have led to advances in understanding the pathophysiology of the disease (2). The defective chloride transmembrane regulator gene responsible for CF was isolated in 1989 (3–5). More than 100 CF centers in the United States are currently accredited by the Cystic Fibrosis Foundation. The major clinical manifestations of CF include respiratory and gastrointestinal disease, and these will be the primary focus of this chapter with particular emphasis on therapy of pulmonary disease.

I. **Etiology and pathogenesis** (6,7)
   A. **Genetics**
      1. CF results from mutations involving a single gene locus on the long arm of chromosome 7. The **most common mutation** involves a three-base-pair deletion that results in the absence of a phenylalanine residue at amino acid position 508 of the gene product. This deletion has been detected in approximately two-thirds of 17,000 CF patient chromosomes analyzed. Several hundred other mutations of the CF gene have been documented, but all occur infrequently.
      2. The **protein product** of the CF gene, the CF transmembrane conductance regulator (CFTR), functions as a cyclic AMP–regulated chloride channel, as well as a modulator of other plasma membrane channels. The abnormal CFTR changes sodium and chloride transport across epithelial surfaces in various organs and results in altered exocrine secretions, causing a broad array of manifestations in the respiratory, gastrointestinal, and reproductive tracts, as well as the sweat glands.
   B. **Pathogenesis of pulmonary disease** (8,9)
      1. **Electrolyte abnormalities and mucociliary clearance.** Failure to secrete chloride through the airway epithelial cells, as well as increased sodium resorption, results in dehydrated airway secretions. Abnormal mucociliary clearance contributes to airflow obstruction in CF, but the precise link between this and abnormal electrolyte transport remains unresolved. Failure to clear secretions establishes a milieu favorable for the development of chronic bacterial infection.
      2. **Airway inflammation and DNA**
         a. The influx of neutrophils into the lung results in a significant excess of proteinases and the release of large amounts of DNA from degenerating neutrophils into the airways and parenchyma. Excessive proteases and elastases may contribute to the destruction of airway and parenchymal connective tissue and may adversely affect antibody and complement-mediated phagocytosis and host immune response. Elastases may contribute to amplification of the inflammatory response and may also mediate mucus hypersecretion (7).

Table 16-1. Causes of bronchiectasis

Cystic fibrosis	Recurrent gastric aspiration
Bronchial obstruction	Chemical injury
Immotile cilia syndrome	Infection
Immunoglobulin deficiency	Yellow nail syndrome
Alpha$_1$-antitrypsin deficiency	Allergic bronchopulmonary aspergillosis
Sarcoidosis	Mounier-Kuhn syndrome
Obliterative bronchiolitis	Williams-Campbell syndrome
Diffuse panbronchiolitis	
Bronchocentric granulomatosis	

      b. The high DNA content in purulent CF sputum contributes to its abnormal viscoelastic properties (10).

   3. Bacterial infection (11,12)

      a. Chronic bacterial pulmonary infections are universal in CF patients. The primary organisms responsible include *P. aeruginosa* and *S. aureus*. Patients with CF are often colonized with *S. aureus* prior to colonization with *Pseudomonas*. Colonization with nonmucoid strains of *P. aeruginosa* is often followed by colonization or frank infection with mucoid strains.

      b. These organisms are rarely cleared from the airways despite the influx of neutrophils and the development of antipseudomonal antibodies. Chronic recurrent bacterial infections develop, with bronchiectasis and progressive deterioration in airflow. These concepts are the basis for antibiotic therapy in CF (see IV.C.1).

C. Pathogenesis of gastrointestinal disease (13,14). **Chronic pancreatic insufficiency** appears as a consequence of abnormal ion exchange, resulting in failure of sodium bicarbonate and water secretion into the pancreatic duct. The subsequent retention of pancreatic enzymes ultimately leads to the destruction of the gland. Inadequate chloride and water secretion through the intestinal epithelium impairs the clearance of intestinal macromolecules and may lead to intestinal obstruction. Defective hepatic duct chloride and water secretion leads to retention of biliary secretions with the resulting clinical manifestations described above.

D. Pathogenesis of abnormal sweat (15). The composition of sweat at the skin surface is regulated by the reabsorption of water and electrolytes by the sweat duct. Normally, sodium and chloride are actively reabsorbed, with a hypotonic fluid reaching the surface. The concentration of chloride in normal sweat is approximately 10–20 mEq/L. In CF, the sweat ductal epithelium is relatively impermeable to chloride so that the concentration of sweat chloride measured at the skin surface exceeds 60 mEq/L. This characteristic finding provides the basis for diagnostic sweat testing in CF (see III.B.3).

II. Presenting symptoms and signs. The majority of patients are diagnosed in the first year of life, but the disease can escape diagnosis until adolescence or adulthood.

  A. Lower respiratory tract

    1. Symptoms. Pulmonary symptoms occur during the first year of life in 90% of CF cases. Cough and wheezing are common and may be associated with severe bacterial bronchiolitis progressing to respiratory failure. In childhood or adulthood, patients often present with chronic cough and recurrent lower respiratory tract infections. Progression of pulmonary disease is associated with increasing frequency and severity of pulmonary symptoms and chronic productive cough. While massive hemoptysis (16) and spontaneous pneumothorax occur commonly in CF (17), these are not usually presenting symptoms.

    2. Physical examination. The lung examination may remain normal for a prolonged period in CF. Progressive disease is accompanied by hyperinflation, reduced air movement, and increased anteroposterior diameter of the chest. Musical rhonchi and crackles suggest bronchiectasis. CF should be considered in patients with respiratory disease associated with clubbing or *Pseudomonas* in the sputum. The presence of obstructive lung disease in a child or young adult, particularly with bronchiectasis, suggests the need for evaluation. Cor pulmonale eventually occurs.

3. **Pulmonary function tests** (9). Early changes in lung function include air trapping, suggested by increases in the residual volume, as well as the ratio of residual volume to total lung capacity. Airway obstruction occurs with a typical pattern of reduced forced expiratory flow between 25% and 75% of vital capacity and a reduced forced expiratory volume in 1 second (FEV_1). As pulmonary disease progresses, the carbon monoxide diffusing capacity decreases. Although deterioration in lung function is inevitable, the rate of decline is not easily predicted. End-stage lung disease is the most common cause of death in CF patients.

4. **Gas exchange** (9). Progressive obstructive lung disease due to infection, inflammation, and secretions eventually leads to significant **ventilation–perfusion mismatching** with hypoxemia. With continued deterioration, hypercarbia follows. Hypoxemia leads to increased pulmonary vascular resistance with pulmonary hypertension and right ventricular failure. Cor pulmonale ensues and is the most common cause of death. Despite hypoxemia, polycythemia is unusual in CF.

B. **Upper respiratory tract** (18). **Chronic sinusitis** is common with resulting rhinorrhea and nasal obstruction. Nasal polyps occur in as many as 20% of patients.

C. **Gastrointestinal tract**
1. In infancy, childhood, and adulthood, gastrointestinal symptoms are common. Approximately 10% of patients present within the first 24 hours of life with meconium ileus characterized by abdominal distention, obstipation, and emesis.
2. **Intestinal obstruction** (13)
   a. Distal intestinal obstructive syndrome (meconium ileus equivalent) occurs in children or adults and presents with anorexia, right lower quadrant pain, and emesis. Right lower quadrant fullness or a mass may be apparent by palpation. This syndrome may be confused with appendicitis.
   b. Constipation is common in CF patients.
   c. Rectal prolapse occurs in a significant minority of children with CF but is uncommon in adults.
3. **Exocrine and endocrine pancreatic insufficiency.** Pancreatic insufficiency and fat malabsorption are present in 85% of CF patients, resulting in bulky, greasy, foul-smelling stools. Malnutrition and vitamin deficiency adversely affect growth, and most patients with CF are underweight. Glucose intolerance is a late finding more common than previously suspected (19).
4. **Hepatobiliary disease** (14). An asymptomatic alkaline phosphatase elevation is the most common manifestation, while symptomatic biliary cirrhosis occurs in >5% of patients. These latter patients present with ascites, peripheral edema, and hyperbilirubinemia. Fatty changes in the liver are common. Hepatosplenomegaly may indicate cirrhosis with portal hypertension. Hematemesis may occur due to esophageal varices. Abdominal pain may suggest chronic cholecystitis or cholelithiasis.

D. **Genitourinary tract** (20,21). Male infertility is nearly always present due to obstructive azoospermia. As many as 20% of female patients are infertile. Abnormally thick cervical mucus inhibiting sperm migration, as well as the effects of significant chronic lung disease, may be important in female infertility. Delayed onset of puberty is common in both sexes.

III. **Differential diagnosis**
A. The differential diagnosis of CF is listed in Table 16-2.
1. The likelihood of CF in any individual presenting with bronchiectasis and gastrointestinal difficulties depends on age and exact presentation. Infants with meconium ileus are easily diagnosed, as are children or young adults with obstructive lung disease, particularly in the setting of bronchiectasis and/or *Pseudomonas* infection of the respiratory tract. Chronic sinusitis, nasal polyps, and male infertility make CF a consideration.

Table 16-2. Differential diagnosis of cystic fibrosis

Bronchiectasis
Chronic bronchial infection
Recurrent gastric aspiration
Immunoglobulin deficiency
Bronchial obstruction
Sarcoidosis
Alpha$_1$-antitrypsin deficiency
Immotile cilia syndrome
Chemical injury
Yellow nail syndrome
Obliterative bronchiolitis
Allergic bronchopulmonary aspergillosis
Mounier-Kuhn syndrome
Bronchocentric granulomatosis
Williams-Campbell syndrome
Diffuse panbronchiolitis

2. A number of entities other than CF may be associated with elevated sweat chloride levels. Most are rare diseases that are not confused with CF and do not warrant discussion here. Bronchiectasis in CF patients is generally diffuse and relatively symmetric with upper lobe predominance.

B. **Work-up and diagnosis.** The diagnosis of CF is based on a combination of clinical criteria and sweat chloride analysis. Patients with the appropriate clinical picture (bronchiectasis, pancreatic insufficiency) and the laboratory findings listed below are considered to have CF.

1. **Radiographic studies**

   a. A chest radiograph is necessary in the evaluation of patients with possible CF. Hyperinflation is apparent early in the course of CF lung disease. As the disease progresses, bronchial cuffing, mucous impaction, and ultimately bronchiectasis become evident with accompanying cystic and fibrotic changes. Radiographic abnormalities are most prominent in the upper lobes.

   b. Computed tomography of the chest is generally not necessary. Thin-section imaging, however, is sensitive for detection of bronchiectasis, cysts, mycetomas, and other abnormalities.

2. **Pulmonary function testing**

   a. Classic pulmonary function test findings are discussed in section II.A.3 Spirometry with lung volumes should be performed in all patients to obtain baseline measurements and confirm the presence of obstructive lung disease. After confirmation of the diagnosis, future testing of symptomatic but stable patients is necessary both to follow the rate of progression of disease and to facilitate the appropriate timing of referral for lung transplantation (see section VI.).

   b. Arterial blood gases should be obtained as a baseline and as clinically necessary thereafter. These measurements will be necessary in the determination of the need for transient or chronic oxygen therapy.

3. **Sweat chloride testing** (15)

   a. Despite the availability of genetic testing, an **elevated sweat chloride** remains the gold standard test for the diagnosis of CF. At least 100 mg of sweat collected after pilocarpine iontophoretic stimulation should be analyzed for sodium and chloride concentrations.

    b. Chloride values in normal sweat fall in the range of 10–20 mEq/L. The diagnosis of CF requires a sweat chloride **>60 mEq/L,** although patients with the disease often have levels >90 mEq/L. Occasionally, patients with classic pulmonary disease and pancreatic insufficiency will have sweat chloride values of 45–60 mEq/L, and these individuals are considered to have CF. A **false-negative** result can be found in the presence of hypoproteinemia or edema, while a false-positive result may occur with malnutrition or certain endocrine and metabolic abnormalities. The diagnosis can be confirmed with analysis of the CFTR gene, although this is seldom necessary.

IV. Acute pulmonary exacerbation

  A. **Symptoms and signs.** Exacerbations are characterized by malaise, fever, and a cough that is initially nonproductive but soon produces thick, tenacious, purulent sputum. The lungs may be clear or demonstrate hyperinflation, reduced air movement, musical rhonchi, and crackles suggestive of bronchiectasis. Consolidation can be seen when pneumonia is present.

  B. **Laboratory testing**

    1. In the setting of a typical uncomplicated flare, the **chest film** does not generally change from baseline. The presence of new infiltrates, atelectasis, or pneumothorax usually requires additional evaluation.

    2. **Sputum cultures** may reveal *S. aureus* or *Haemophilus influenzae* but eventually nearly always reveals *P. aeruginosa*, particularly mucoid strains. Several strains with differing sensitivities may be present. With more advanced disease, *Burkholderia cepacia* may be cultured. Other gram-negative rods, *Streptococcus pneumoniae*, and *Aspergillus* may also be present. Atypical mycobacteria may be cultured.

    3. **Peripheral blood analysis** may reveal leukocytosis. Severe exacerbations can be accompanied by prerenal azotemia secondary to intravascular volume depletion. Blood cultures should be sent when high fever is present, particularly when patients have permanent vascular access, even though they are rarely positive in CF. Isolated elevations of alkaline phosphatase are often present at baseline.

  C. **Therapy of acute exacerbation** (Table 16-3). Major therapeutic goals for pulmonary exacerbations include promoting clearance of respiratory secretions and managing pulmonary infection. The therapeutic approaches to other complications of CF are discussed in section IX.

    1. **Antibiotic therapy** (22–24)

      a. **Intravenous (IV) and oral antibiotics.** Infectious exacerbations are treated with antibiotics aimed primarily at *P. aeruginosa* and *S. aureus*. Previous sputum cultures may be helpful in guiding specific antibiotic choices. There should be a low threshold for admission to the hospital, with IV antibiotic coverage being administered over a 2–3-week period.

Table 16-3. Current therapeutic options for cystic fibrosis

Antibiotics

Chest physiotherapy

Bronchodilator therapy

Deoxyribonuclease I

Oxygen

Mechanical ventilation

Lung transplantation

Nutrition

Vitamin supplementation

When resources are available, therapy can often be completed at home. Cultures can be sent to centers where synergy testing is performed. This approach may be useful in guiding therapy in patients with resistant organisms. Failure to respond to appropriate coverage suggests the need for repeat sputum culture with antibiotic sensitivities. The antibiotic approach in pregnant patients does not generally vary from the usual approach, except that currently available quinolones are not utilized (25).

b. **β-Lactam and quinolone antibiotics.** An oral semisynthetic penicillin or cephalosporin (cephalexin 250–500 mg PO QID) may be useful in mild flares to treat *S. aureus* infection. Ciprofloxacin (500–750 mg PO QID) offers both staphylococcal and pseudomonal coverage, but resistance may develop relatively rapidly. Quinolone antibiotics, while often very useful, have been associated with arthropathy. *P. aeruginosa* generally requires double antibiotic coverage. A quinolone or β-lactam antibiotic such as piperacillin (3 g IV q4h) or ceftazidime (2 g IV q8h) may be used with an aminoglycoside.

c. **Aminoglycoside** dosing is generally aggressive because the pharmacokinetics of these drugs vary from normal in patients with CF, with lower serum concentrations following standard dosing. This may be explained by an increased total body clearance and/or larger volume of distribution, with the former being a more consistent finding. Gentamicin and tobramycin are generally initiated at 3 mg/kg IV q8h (26). Monitoring to keep peak levels near 10 µg/mL and troughs >2 µg/mL is important. Aminoglycoside nephrotoxicity may be manifested by reduced glomerular filtration, proteinuria, and tubular dysfunction, but renal compromise using the above approach is extremely uncommon. Ototoxicity may occasionally occur and may progress after discontinuation of therapy due to accumulation of the antibiotic in the labyrinth.

d. **IV colistimethate therapy** may be of benefit in patients with highly resistant *P. aeruginosa* infections. This drug is very active against this organism, and development of resistance is rare. Colistimethate has no activity against gram-positive organisms; *B. cepacia* is resistant. Toxicities include dose-related nephrotoxicity, neurotoxicity, pain at the site of injection, and allergic reactions such as fever and skin rash.

e. **Aerosolized antibiotics** may offer advantages, but precise indications are less standardized (27). Aerosolized aminoglycosides may be useful in controlling infections in CF patients. Potential indications for use include enhancing the effect of IV antipseudomonal antibiotics, chronic treatment to reduce acute exacerbations, and prevention of colonization with *P. aeruginosa*. Dosing with tobramycin has generally ranged from 80 mg PO TID to as high as 600 mg PO TID. Outcome measures have included improvement in airflow or clinical score, and reduction in sputum bacterial density. Precise indications for aerosolized aminoglycosides remain controversial. Aerosolized antibiotics of the polymyxin class (2.5 mg/kg/d) have been shown to reduce the rate of colonization and even pneumonia caused by *P. aeruginosa* but may result in an increased risk of pneumonia caused by polymyxin-resistant bacteria including *B. cepacia* (28). This form of therapy should be individualized.

2. **Chest physiotherapy.** Chest physiotherapy should be performed on a regular basis. Chest percussion and postural drainage have been the standard modality, but alternative maneuvers such as autogenic drainage, the high-frequency compression vest, and the use of an oscillating flutter device appear effective (29).

3. **Bronchodilator therapy.** Bronchodilators should be aggressively employed during acute exacerbations.
   a. **β-Adrenergic agents** should be administered by nebulizer at 4–6-hour intervals and may be continued at home by either metered-dose inhaler (MDI) or nebulizer (30). More β_2-specific agents such as albuterol or metaproterenol are preferred. Occasionally, patients do not exhibit improved flow rates with bronchodilators and may not benefit. Oral β-ago-

nists are no more effective than the inhaled form but increase the risk of adverse effects.

   b.   Although large clinical trials are not available, the anticholinergic agent **ipratroprium bromide** appears to be safe and effective and can be administered by MDI or nebulizer at the same intervals as the β-agonists (30).

   c.   More limited data are available for nebulized **sodium cromoglycate**, although it appears to be an effective adjunct in selected patients.

   d.   While **theophylline** may be used, it is sometimes poorly tolerated and should not be used as a first-line therapy.

4.   **Mucolytics**

   a.   **Deoxyribonuclease I (DNase)** is a human enzyme that degrades extracellular DNA. A recombinant form, commercially available for administration in aerosolized form, has been shown to reduce the incidence of respiratory tract infections requiring parenteral antibiotics and to improve pulmonary function in CF patients (31). The majority of clinical trials have involved patients with mild or moderate disease (FEV_1 ≥40% predicted), although improvement in airflow has been demonstrated after prolonged administration in patients with more severe pulmonary function abnormalities (32). The initial dose should be 2.5 mg/d. Continued use appears necessary to maintain clinical improvement. The optimal dose depends on careful assessment of the clinical response, and certain individuals may benefit from 2.5 mg BID. The drug is generally well tolerated, although upper airway irritation manifested as voice alteration, pharyngitis, and laryngitis may occur. These symptoms are generally mild and resolve spontaneously.

   b.   Other mucolytic agents such as acetylcysteine are generally not recommended.

5.   **Oxygen and mechanical ventilation**

   a.   Patients with hypercapnia should be monitored for further carbon dioxide retention by arterial blood gas analyses when oxygen is initiated during an acute exacerbation. In the event of a sudden deterioration, intubation with mechanical ventilation is used in CF as in any lung disease. While the need for intubation is an ominous sign, patients can sometimes be weaned and extubated if chest physiotherapy, suctioning, and antibiotics are aggressively employed.

   b.   Patients with relentlessly progressive disease who ultimately require mechanical ventilation rarely do well. In certain patients, aggressive supportive therapy may buy enough time to proceed to lung transplantation (33) (see section VI.).

6.   **Corticosteroid therapy.** Corticosteroids may be briefly employed in patients with significant airway inflammation, in addition to appropriate antibiotic therapy being instituted. Treatment of allergic bronchopulmonary aspergillosis should also include steroids (see section IX.F.). In general, steroids should be avoided in the long-term treatment of CF.

7.   **Anti-inflammatory therapy.** High-dose ibuprofen may slow the progression of lung disease without adverse effects in CF patients with mild-to-moderate disease (FEV_1 >60%), although safety profiles in more severely affected patients have not been established. Pharmacokinetic monitoring is recommended to optimize dosing and avoid deleterious peak effects.

V.   Routine therapy of cystic fibrosis

   A.   Routine therapy of CF includes use of all the modalities listed above that are used for acute exacerbations. Antibiotics are not generally prescribed on a routine basis without evidence of infection. Chest physiotherapy and treatment with bronchodilators, oxygen, and mucolytics may all be carried out in the home setting.

   B.   **Other considerations**

   1.   **Immunizations.** Administration of appropriate immunizations is crucial. Pertussis and measles vaccines should be administered early in life, and influenza virus vaccine should be given yearly. Amantadine can be given early in the setting of respiratory symptoms during influenza A epidemics. Pneumococcal infections are uncommon, and immunization is not mandatory.

2. The **"care-map" approach**, in which a problem list is outlined with desired outcomes, may streamline care. In this approach, laboratory tests, chest physiotherapy, medications, rehabilitation goals, teaching, and consultations are performed on a scheduled basis. Algorithms are available for various problems that arise.

3. **Future therapy** (34). Newer therapeutic modalities include gene therapy (35), amiloride (36) and antiprotease therapy. These are not yet standard practice and will not be discussed.

VI. **Lung transplantation in cystic fibrosis.** The outcome for CF patients undergoing lung transplantation has improved dramatically over the past decade. Actuarial survival may be as high as 87% at 1 year and 67% at 2 years (37).

A. **Indications and selection criteria** (38). Patients with CF should be considered for transplantation when there is progressive deterioration of lung function, with the FEV_1 approaching 30% of the predicted value. Selection criteria for transplantation are listed in Table 16-4 and are similar to criteria for transplantation for other pulmonary conditions.

B. **Evaluation for transplantation**

1. Patients meeting criteria should be referred to a transplantation center. An extensive evaluation of cardiac and pulmonary function will be completed at the center. Extensive serologic testing for hepatitis, cytomegalovirus (CMV), and human immunodeficiency virus is performed, and psychosocial factors are explored in detail to ensure patient compliance and psychological stability.

2. Bilateral lung transplantation is nearly always the procedure of choice for CF patients, even when severe cor pulmonale is present. Heart–lung transplantation is rarely necessary.

C. **Transplantation**

1. Immunosuppressive therapy is initiated at the time of transplantation, as well as antibacterial prophylaxis and prophylaxis against CMV infection. Details of the postoperative course are beyond the scope of this chapter. Patients with uncomplicated courses are generally hospitalized for 10–14 days. Infection and rejection are the most frequent complications.

2. Acute rejection generally responds to augmentation of immunotherapy. Chronic rejection (obliterative bronchiolitis) may progress relentlessly and is a common cause of death.

VII. **Therapy of gastrointestinal disease**

A. **Pancreatic insufficiency** (39). **Treatment is enzyme replacement**. The newer enteric-coated microsphere forms of pancreatic enzyme supplements do not completely normalize absorption but are sufficient to control symptoms and promote adequate nutrition in most cases. Dosage is titrated to the degree of symptoms, often in the range of 2–3 capsules per meal. Water-soluble vitamin replacement is also required (see section VIII. Nutrition).

Table 16-4. Selection criteria for lung transplantation in patients with cystic fibrosis

Age <50 years

FEV_1 <30% of predicted*

Life expectancy estimated to be ≤24 months

No malignancy in past 5 years

Normal serum creatinine

No significant hepatic disease

Medically compliant

Psychologically stable

Participation in extensive pulmonary rehabilitation

Absence of panresistant organisms in sputum

*Patients who undergo transplantation often have FEV_1 values closer to 20% of predicted.

B. **Small and large intestine** (14)
   1. **Treatment of constipation** with bulk laxatives and docusate may be effective for constipation if administered early (13). Pancreatic enzymes and fluid administration should be optimized.
   2. The development of **distal intestinal obstruction** syndrome must be differentiated from acute appendicitis, chronic appendicitis with abscess formation, and intussusception. Nonsurgical treatment is usually effective (40,41), and high-volume oral balanced electrolyte solutions (eg, Go-Lytely) are often effective. Patients not tolerating the above measures may be given hydrophilic enemas (meglumine diatrizoate). Some patients may respond to cisapride (10 mg PO before meals and at bedtime) (42).
   3. **Intussusception** may be effectively treated by hydrostatic reduction with contrast enemas, but recurrent episodes may occasionally require surgery. Pancreatic enzyme therapy should be optimized.
   4. **Rectal prolapse** is often effectively treated with manual reduction by gentle pressure. Again, appropriate pancreatic enzyme therapy should be addressed.
C. **Hepatobiliary disease. Treatment of cholelithiasis** is usually cholecystectomy, if the underlying pulmonary disease is stable. Biliary cirrhosis can present with the manifestations of portal hypertension, including symptomatic esophageal varices. Treatment is supportive with aggressive treatment of variceal bleeding. The approach to symptomatic hepatobiliary disease is discussed in more detail in other sources (14).

VIII. **Nutrition.** Patients with CF generally have a high caloric need due the increased work of breathing. As chronic infection progresses and weight loss becomes more refractory to increases in oral intake, nocturnal tube feeding may be required to supplement oral intake. A balanced diet is important. Nearly all patients require supplementation with pancreatic enzymes at meals. Dosing will require adjustments depending on weight gain, presence of abdominal cramping, and stool character. Standard daily multiple vitamins provide sufficient amounts of vitamins A and D, and vitamin E (200 U) should be administered daily. Other vitamins and minerals may be supplemented as needed.

IX. **Therapy of pulmonary complications**
   A. **Respiratory failure** (see Chapter 19).
   B. **Cor pulmonale.** Diuretic therapy (furosemide or spironolactone), limited sodium intake, and oxygen therapy may be helpful in reducing edema. Aggressive management of secretions and infection is crucial. Nutrition must be addressed as hypoalbuminemia may contribute to worsening edema. Vasodilator therapy and digoxin are rarely useful.
   C. **Massive hemoptysis**
      1. Massive hemoptysis, defined as 300–500 mL of blood expectorated over a 24-hour period, may occur in the setting of an acute bacterial infection and often resolves spontaneously. If the bleeding lung can be identified, the patient should be positioned with that side down to prevent aspiration into the remaining uninvolved lung. Because infection is often the stimulus for bleeding, antibiotics are often initiated if hemoptysis occurs.
      2. The intake of aspirin or other drugs that interfere with hemostasis should be monitored carefully. Functional vitamin K deficiency can result from inadequate intake, malabsorption of fat, decreased synthesis by bowel flora after prolonged antibiotic therapy, and cirrhosis.
      3. **Chest physiotherapy** can be carefully continued in CF patients who have blood-streaked sputum or small amounts of hemoptysis.
      4. **Therapy of refractory hemoptysis**
         a. **Bronchoscopy.** Bronchoscopy is rarely helpful during massive hemoptysis because of the difficulty in localizing the source of bleeding in the airways. An endobronchial occlusion balloon may be placed within a bleeding airway when localization is possible as a temporizing measure till more definitive therapy (embolization, lobectomy) can be performed.
         b. **Bronchial artery embolization** (43). This technique is initially very effective in controlling massive hemoptysis unresponsive to standard measures. The procedure should be performed cautiously to avoid embolization of a spinal artery.

    c. **Lobectomy** may be advised in extraordinarily rare cases of persistent, significant bleeding in spite of embolization.

D. Pneumothorax

   1. Pneumothorax may be treated with chest tube placement and talc pleurodesis. A limited thoracotomy and pleural abrasion may be necessary if the pneumothorax is large and symptomatic. Many experts recommend a sclerosing procedure after the first pneumothorax large enough to require chest tube drainage. (44,45).

   2. Sudden clinical deterioration with suspicion of a tension pneumothorax is an indication for immediate bedside needle insertion into the pleural space followed by chest tube placement. Smaller pneumothoraces without tension may resolve spontaneously. Occasionally, an expiratory film is necessary to document the presence of a small pneumothorax.

E. Atelectasis. Lobar atelectasis is generally due to thick, often infected secretions occluding the airways. The best approach utilizes aggressive IV antibiotics, bronchodilators, and chest physiotherapy. While bronchoscopy may be attempted, it rarely impacts significantly.

F. Allergic bronchopulmonary aspergillosis (ABPA)

   1. *Aspergillus fumigatus* (and other *Aspergillus* species) may be cultured in sputum from CF patients (46). Isolation of this organism does not necessitate treatment, but the possibility of ABPA should be considered. Major and minor criteria have been established but are more difficult to apply in the CF patient than in individuals with asthma.

   2. The optimal treatment for this intense hypersensitivity reaction is not clear. In non-CF patients, prolonged steroid therapy may be successful; steroid therapy may occasionally be indicated in CF patients with severe infiltration and worsening cough and/or dyspnea. Various corticosteroid regimens have been suggested (eg, 0.5 mg/kg/d with taper to an alternate-day regimen continued for several weeks). However, the precise dose and duration of steroid therapy is not standardized. While data on the natural history of ABPA in CF patients are scant, the prognosis generally appears to be good.

G. Atypical mycobacterial infections. While these organisms may be cultured from patients with CF, they are not necessarily responsible for episodes of clinical deterioration. Thus, routine therapy with four to six antituberculous drugs is not currently recommended for these organisms.

X. Specialist referral

A. Referral to CF centers. Patients with CF should be referred on a periodic basis to a CF center. This is useful for monitoring the clinical and nutritional status of the patient, informing patients of new treatment modalities and investigative protocols, and determining when patients may be suitable transplantation candidates.

B. Massive hemoptysis.

C. Pneumothorax.

D. Respiratory failure or oxygen requirement.

E. Recalcitrant acute exacerbations.

References

1. Fiel SB, FitzSimmons S, Schidlow D: Evolving demographics of cystic fibrosis. *Semin Respir Crit Care Med* 1993;15:349.

2. Ramsey BW, Boat T: Outcome measures for clinical trials in cystic fibrosis. *J Pediatr* 1994;124:177.

3. Rommens JM, Iannuzi MC, Kerem B, et al.: Identification of the cystic fibrosis gene: chromosome jumping and walking. *Science* 1989;245:1059–1065.

4. Riordan JR, Rommens JM, Kerem B, et al.: Identification of the cystic fibrosis gene: cloning and characterization of complementary DNA. *Science* 1989;245:1066–1073.

5. Kerem BS, Rommens JM, Buchanan JA, et al.: Identification of the cystic fibrosis gene: genetic analysis. *Science* 1989;245:1073–1080.

6. Cutting GR: Genotype defect: its effect on cellular function and phenotypic expression. *Semin Respir Crit Care Med* 1994;15:356.
7. Marshall BC: Pathophysiology of lung disease in cystic fibrosis. *Semin Respir Crit Care Med* 1994;15:364.
8. Davis PB: *Cystic fibrosis.* New York: Marcel Dekker, 1993.
9. Davis PB: Pathophysiology of the lung disease in cystic fibrosis. In: Davis PB, ed. *Cystic fibrosis.* New York: Marcel Dekker, 1993.
10. Lethem MI, James SL, Marriot C, Burke JF: The origin of DNA associated with mucus glycoproteins in cystic fibrosis sputum. *Eur Respir J* 1990;3:19–23.
11. Ramphal R, Vishwanath S: Why is *Pseudomonas* the colonizer and why does it persist? *Infection* 1987;15:281.
12. Hoiby N: Microbiology of lung infections in cystic fibrosis patients. *Acta Paediatr Scand Suppl* 1982;301:33.
13. Rubinstein S, Moss R, Lewiston N: Constipation and meconium ileus equivalent in patients with cystic fibrosis. *Pediatrics* 1986;78:473.
14. Stern RC: Cystic fibrosis and the gastrointestinal tract. In: Davis PB, ed. *Cystic fibrosis.* New York: Marcel Dekker, 1993.
15. Quinton PM, Reddy MM: The sweat gland. In: Davis PB, ed. *Cystic fibrosis.* New York: Marcel Dekker, 1993.
16. diSant'Agnese PA, Davis PB: Cystic fibrosis in adults. *Am J Med* 1979;66:121.
17. Huang NN, Schidlow DV, Szatrowski TH, et al.: Clinical features, survival rate, and prognostic factors in young adults with cystic fibrosis. *Am J Med* 1987;82:871–879.
18. Kerrebijn JDF, Poublon RML, Overbeek SE: Nasal and paranasal disease in adult cystic fibrosis patients. *Eur Respir J* 1992;5:1239.
19. DeSchepper J, et al.: Oral glucose tolerance testing in cystic fibrosis: correlations with clinical parameters and glycosylated haemoglobin determinations. *Eur J Pediatr* 1991;150:403.
20. Anguiano A, Oates RD, Amos JA, et al.: Congenital bilateral absence of the vas deferens: a primarily genital form of cystic fibrosis. *JAMA* 1992;267:1794–1797.
21. Cohen LF, di Sant'Agnese PA, Friedlander J: Cystic fibrosis and pregnancy: a national survey. *Lancet* 1980;2:842–844.
22. Lietman PS: Pharmacokinetics of antimicrobial drugs in cystic fibrosis: beta-lactam antibiotics. *Chest* 1988;94:115S.
23. Geddes DM: Antimicrobial therapy against *Staphylococcus aureus, Pseudomonas aeruginosa,* and *Pseudomonas cepacia. Chest* 1988;94:140S.
24. Strandvik B: Antibiotic therapy of pulmonary infections in cystic fibrosis: dosage schedules and duration of treatment. *Chest* 1988;94:146S.
25. Canny GJ, Corey M, Livingstone RA, et al.: Pregnancy and cystic fibrosis. *Obstet Gynecol* 1991; 77:850.
26. Hendeles L, Iafrate RP, Stillwell PC, Mangos JA: Individualizing gentamicin dosage in patients with cystic fibrosis: limitations to a pharmacokinetic approach. *J Pediatr* 1987;110:303–310.
27. Fiel SB: Aerosol delivery of antibiotics to the lower airways of patients with cystic fibrosis. *Chest* 1995;107:61S.
28. Feeley TW, Du Moulin GC, Hedley-Whyte J, et al.: Aerosol polymyxin and pneumonia in seriously ill patients. *N Engl J Med* 1975;293:471–475.
29. Thomas J, Cook DJ, Brooks D: Chest physical therapy management of patients with cystic fibrosis: a meta-analysis. *Am J Respir Crit Care Med* 1995;153:846.
30. Weintraub SJ, Eschenbacher WL: The inhaled bronchodilators ipratroprium bromide and metaproterenol in adults with CF. *Chest* 1989;95:861.
31. Fuchs HJ, Borowitz DS, Christiansen DH, et al.: Effect of aerosolized recombinant human DNase on exacerbations of respiratory symptoms and on pulmonary function in patients with cystic fibrosis. *N Engl J Med* 1994;331:637–642.
32. Hodson ME: Aerosolized dornase alpha (rhDNase) for therapy of cystic fibrosis. *Am J Respir Crit Care Med* 1995;151:S70.
33. Massard G, Shennib H, Metras D, et al.: Double-lung transplantation in mechanically ventilated patients with cystic fibrosis. *Ann Thorac Surg* 1993;55:1087–1091.
34. Knowles MR: New therapies for cystic fibrosis. *Chest* 1995;107:59S.
35. Rosenfeld MA, Collins FS: Gene therapy for cystic fibrosis. *Chest* 1996;109:241.
36. Knowles MR, Olivier KN, Hohneker KW, et al.: Pharmacologic treatment of abnormal ion transport in the airway epithelium in cystic fibrosis. *Chest* 1995;107:71S–76S.

37. Egan TM, Detterbeck FC, Mill MR, et al.: Improved results of lung transplantation for patients with cystic fibrosis. *J Thorac Cardiovasc Surg* 1995;109:224–234.
38. Tapson VF, Baz M: Lung transplantation. In: Baum G, Crapo J, Celli B, Karlinsky J, eds. *Textbook of pulmonary diseases*. Boston: Little, Brown, 1997.
39. diSant'Agnese PA, Hubbard VS: The pancreas. In: Taussig LM, ed. *Cystic fibrosis*. New York: Thieme-Stratton, 1984.
40. Cleghorn GJ, Stringer DA, Forstner GG, Durie PR: Treatment of distal intestinal obstruction in cystic fibrosis with a balanced intestinal lavage solution. *Lancet* 1986;1:8–11.
41. Kerem E, Corey M, Kerem B, et al.: Clinical and genetic comparisons of patients with cystic fibrosis, with or without meconium ileus. *J Pediatr* 1989;114:767–773.
42. Koletzko S, Corey M, Ellis L, et al.: Effects of cisapride in patients with cystic fibrosis and distal intestinal obstruction syndrome. *J Pediatr* 1990;117:815   822.
43. Cohen AM, Doershuk CF, Stern RC: Bronchial artery embolization to control hemoptysis in cystic fibrosis. *Radiology* 1990;175:401.
44. McLaughlin FJ, Matthews WJ Jr, Streider DJ, et al.: Pneumothorax in cystic fibrosis: management and outcome. *J Pediatr* 1982;100:863–869.
45. Penketh AR, Knight RK, Hodson ME, Batten JC: Management of pneumothorax in adults with cystic fibrosis. *Thorax* 1982;37:850–853.
46. Voss MJ, Bush RK, Mischler EH, Peters ME: Association of allergic bronchopulmonary aspergillosis and cystic fibrosis. *J Allergy Clin Immunol* 1982;69:539–546.

17

Pulmonary Hypertension and Pulmonary Vascular Disease

Samuel I. Hammerman and
Krista K. Graven

Diseases of the pulmonary vasculature comprise a variety of disorders that may arise in the pulmonary blood vessels themselves or are the consequence of systemic diseases. The disorders covered in this chapter include primary pulmonary hypertension, pulmonary thromboembolic disease (pulmonary embolism, deep venous thrombosis, chronic thromboembolic disease, and other forms of pulmonary emboli), and abnormal pulmonary vascular communications.

I. **Primary pulmonary hypertension** (PPH) is an idiopathic disease characterized by an increase in pulmonary vascular resistance (PVR) that ultimately leads to right ventricular (RV) failure. Although symptoms, physical examination, and noninvasive studies may suggest the diagnosis, right-sided cardiac catheterization is necessary for a definitive diagnosis. PPH is defined as the presence of a mean pulmonary artery pressure (PAP) >25 mm Hg or a PA systolic pressure >30 mm Hg with a normal PA wedge pressure (PAWP) and the absence of secondary causes of pulmonary hypertension (1,2).
   A. **Presenting signs and symptoms**
      1. The most frequently reported symptom is dyspnea, initially on exertion but eventually at rest (1,2). Other symptoms include fatigue, angina, near syncope, syncope, edema, and palpitations. By the time patients present with symptoms, the disease is usually far advanced with an elevation in RV pressures. Late in the course of the disease, hemoptysis, hoarseness (caused by compression of the recurrent laryngeal nerve by the main PA), abdominal pain secondary to hepatic congestion, and cyanosis occur. The symptoms of Raynaud's phenomenon are only slightly more common than in the general population (2).
      2. The most common signs are those of elevated PAP and decreased cardiac output (1,2). Signs include a prominent a wave in the jugular venous pulse, a left parasternal lift, a loud pulmonic component of the second heart sound, a right-sided fourth heart sound, and occasionally a murmur of pulmonary insufficiency. Eventually, signs of right heart failure are present, including cyanosis, leg edema, elevation of the jugular venous pressure with a prominent v wave and a pulsatile liver, a right-sided third heart sound, and the holosystolic murmur of tricuspid regurgitation. Clubbing is not present in patients with PPH and suggests other diseases.
   B. **Etiology and pathogenesis**
      1. PPH is a diagnosis of exclusion, and a number of secondary causes must be ruled out (Table 17-1). Its etiology is unknown. Several factors appear to contribute to a common final pathway that gives rise clinically and pathologically to PPH. Abnormalities in vasoconstriction are suggested by the response of some patients to vasodilators and the demonstration of medial hypertrophy of the pulmonary arterioles early in the pathology of PPH. However, vasoconstriction may not be the primary event. Certain stimuli (eg, hypoxia, autoimmunity, drugs, toxins, pregnancy, lung injury) may damage the pulmonary endothelium and lead to an imbalance in vasoreactive mediators and/or coagulation factors (1–5). The latter is suggested by the frequent finding of microthromboemboli at autopsy.

Table 17-1. Secondary causes of pulmonary hypertension

Pulmonary embolic disease
Pulmonary venous thrombosis
Pulmonary venous obstruction
  Mediastinal fibrosis
  Congenital stenosis
  Tumor
  Takayasu's disease
Parasitic disease
  Schistosomiasis
  Filariasis
Hemoglobinopathies, eg, sickle cell disease
Collagen vascular diseases and vasculitides
  Systemic lupus erythematosus
  Scleroderma
  Polymyositis/dermatomyositis
Interstitial lung disease
  Pneumoconioses
  Rheumatoid arthritis
  Sarcoidosis
Disorders of pulmonary ventilation
  Sleep apnea
  Chest wall abnormalities
Congenital lung disease
Hypoxia due to residence at high altitude
Chronic obstructive pulmonary disease
Exogenous substances
  Dietary agents (eg, aminorex, fenfluramine)
  L-tryptophan
  Toxic rapeseed oil
  Cocaine
Talc emboli
Increased left atrial pressure
  Secondary to mitral or aortic valve disease
  Secondary to left ventricular dysfunction
Congenital heart disease causing left-to-right shunts and increased pulmonary blood flow
Portal hypertension (eg, cirrhosis)
HIV infection

2. PPH occurs most commonly in young adults (mean age is 36 years in the National Institutes of Health registry) but can present relatively late in life (9% of cases presenting during or after age 60 years) (1,2). The reported female:male incidence ratio varies between 1.7:1 and 2.5:1. A subgroup of patients (7%) have familial PPH, with an autosomal-dominant pattern of inheritance with variable penetrance (6).
3. The majority of patients with idiopathic pulmonary hypertension have diffuse structural abnormalities on the arterial side of the pulmonary circulation and are classified as having PPH. A small percentage of patients have changes primarily in the venous circulation that are classified as pulmonary veno-occlusive disease (PVOD). Although controversial, PVOD is felt to be a distinct disease entity along with another potential subset of PPH, pulmonary capillary hemangiomatosis (1,7).
4. Pathologically, all forms of PPH demonstrate a pulmonary arteriopathy that

features medial hypertrophy of the muscular arteries and arterioles, frequently of an onion-skin pattern. Three histologic patterns have been identified: (a) isolated medial hypertrophy, (b) plexogenic pulmonary arteriopathy, and (c) thrombotic pulmonary arteriopathy. The clinical usefulness of this classification is controversial. Patients with thrombotic lesions are thought to have a better prognosis; however, many patients have both plexogenic and thrombotic changes (1,7).

C. Relevant physiology

1. The pulmonary circulation is a high-flow, low-resistance system. With exercise, blood flow increases and PVR falls due to distention of blood vessels and recruitment of unopened vessels. This prevents significant increases in PAP, although blood flow increases 3–5-fold. The RV is thin-walled and distensible and can accommodate variations in systemic venous return without large changes in filling pressures.

2. When obliteration and narrowing of pulmonary vessels occur (whether due to endothelial dysfunction, vasoconstriction, or thrombosis), PAP increases and the RV subsequently hypertrophies. The RV functions normally early in the course of PPH because the decrease in pulmonary vessel cross-sectional area and distensibility is small. As the disease progresses, PVR increases significantly, and the RV eventually is unable to increase cardiac output with exercise despite an increase in filling pressures. Blood flow to the RV may be compromised by an increase in RV pressures and heart rate leading to RV ischemia. RV failure will also affect left ventricular (LV) diastolic function by increasing LV end diastolic pressure and decreasing LV filling. PAWP may then increase. Syncopal episodes may be related to the inability to increase cardiac output as necessary.

D. Differential diagnostic possibilities. Since PPH is a diagnosis of exclusion, secondary causes of pulmonary hypertension must be ruled out (see Table 17-1). Numerous drugs and toxins are associated with pulmonary hypertension, including anorectic agents (dexfenfluramine, fenfluramine), L-tryptophan, toxic rapeseed oil, and crack cocaine. Pulmonary hypertension is associated with numerous systemic conditions, including human immunodeficiency virus (HIV) infection, portal hypertension, autoimmune disorders, platelet storage pool disease, and pregnancy (1–5, 8,9). In addition, various cardiac and pulmonary parenchymal diseases must be excluded.

E. Diagnostic evaluation

1. Many diseases that directly produce secondary hypertension can be excluded on the basis of history, physical examination, and appropriate laboratory tests. Other diseases, such as cirrhosis, HIV infection, and certain collagen vascular diseases, are only associated with pulmonary hypertension.

2. Potentially treatable causes of pulmonary hypertension must be ruled out. Cardiac catheterization must be performed to confirm the diagnosis of pulmonary hypertension and document a normal pulmonary capillary wedge pressure. After cardiac catheterization is performed to confirm the diagnosis of pulmonary hypertension and secondary causes are excluded, certain patients will require open lung biopsy to establish an accurate diagnosis. This will depend on the condition of the patient and the likelihood that the results will lead to a significant change in management.

3. **In most cases of PPH, the chest x-ray shows evidence of increased PAP**, including prominence of the main PA, hilar vessel enlargement, and/or pruning of the peripheral vessels with generalized hyperlucency of the lung periphery (1,2). The chest x-ray will be normal in 6% of patients.

4. **The electrocardiogram (ECG) frequently shows right-axis deviation (QRS axis >90°), tall and peaked P waves, tall anterior R waves, and ST-segment depression and/or T-wave inversion anteriorly.** Neither ECG nor chest x-ray abnormalities correlate with the severity of the pulmonary hypertension (1,2).

5. Patients with PPH frequently have an elevated antinuclear antibody level with no specific pattern or titer. No definite link between PPH and collagen vascu-

lar disease (CVD) has been established. CVDs are associated with pulmonary hypertension, and patients with specific findings of a CVD (eg, skin, muscle, or tissue biopsies; esophageal motility studies; complement levels) should be considered to have secondary pulmonary hypertension (1,2,4).

6. **Pulmonary function tests may be normal or show a slight decrease in vital capacity and lung compliance with a mild decrease in the diffusing capacity for carbon monoxide ($D_L CO$).** Pulmonary function testing is useful for ruling out other pulmonary diseases such as chronic obstructive pulmonary disease (COPD) or severe restrictive disease. Arterial blood gases are normal initially but eventually show mild hypoxemia with a chronic respiratory alkalosis (P_{CO_2} 30–35 mm Hg, P_{O_2} 65–85 mm Hg). The P_{O_2} may be normal at rest but decrease with exercise.

7. **Echocardiography** should be performed to assess the progression of pulmonary hypertension and exclude other conditions that cause similar symptoms, such as mitral stenosis, patent foramen ovale, atrial or ventricular septal defects, or patent ductus arteriosus (10,11). The typical echocardiogram shows RV enlargement and paradoxical septal motion. Right atrial enlargement and regurgitation of the pulmonic and tricuspid valves may be present. With tricuspid regurgitation, Doppler ultrasound is helpful to estimate PAP. The accuracy of an echocardiogram, particularly the estimation of PAP, will vary among institutions and with the experience of the user. A normal echocardiogram does not rule out PPH (11).

8. A **ventilation–perfusion (V/Q) lung scan should be performed to rule out chronic thromboembolic disease** (1,2,12). In PPH, the scan is either normal or shows small, patchy defects (low probability for embolic disease). In thromboembolic disease, the lung scan demonstrates at least one large V/Q mismatch. An indeterminate scan does not rule out thromboembolic disease. When the diagnosis is in question, angiography is indicated to differentiate PPH from large-vessel thromboembolic disease or occlusion of the pulmonary vessels from acquired or congenital lesions.

9. The presence of one or more segmental defects on the V/Q scan necessitates a **pulmonary arteriogram** to document chronic thromboembolic disease (1,2,13). The diagnosis of chronic thromboembolic disease is often problematic because emboli may spontaneously resolve or become incorporated into the blood vessel wall and render the angiogram inconclusive. A pattern of peripheral vascular pruning is characteristic of PPH but may not always be present. Pulmonary hypertension is not a contraindication for pulmonary angiography, since the safety of this test has been improved with the use of nonionic dye and the ability to limit dye loads through angiograms selective to areas of defects on lung scans.

10. **Right-sided cardiac catheterization** should be performed to document pressures, cardiac output, and the presence of congenital heart disease (1, 2,14). PAP can be accurately documented and can be used to assess efficacy of treatment.

11. **Cardiopulmonary exercise tests** are helpful in assessing the cause of dyspnea in an undiagnosed patient. Certain patterns of ventilatory and cardiac responses suggest either pulmonary hypertension or other causes for dyspnea, although these patterns are neither sensitive nor specific for PPH. Exercise testing is not considered mandatory for evaluation of PPH (15). These tests should be performed in specialized centers experienced in cardiopulmonary exercise testing.

12. The need for an **open lung biopsy** to diagnose PPH is controversial. Open lung biopsy can be used to make a definite diagnosis of PPH when the clinical picture is unclear. In most patients, it is not essential to make an accurate diagnosis, since therapy is not usually affected. Some specialists advocate open lung biopsy with all patients for both prognosis and assessment of treatment options. However, sufficient data are not available to support this approach, given the risks. Transbronchial lung biopsy has no role in diagnosing PPH and may be especially risky given the increased PAP.

F. **Management.** Treatment of patients with PPH is challenging (Table 17-2), and no consensus has been reached on the best therapeutic approach. Patients should be referred to a center with expertise in this area. Patients should avoid circumstances that exacerbate the symptoms of the disease, such as severe exercise or ascent to altitude. Exercise should be guided by symptoms; airplane travel may require supplemental oxygen. High altitudes worsen pulmonary hypertension by causing vasoconstriction of the pulmonary bed and therefore should be avoided. Pregnancy has caused deterioration in PPH, and patients considering childbearing should consult with the appropriate specialists. Oral contraceptives may also worsen PPH; other forms of contraception should be used (1).

1. **Supplemental oxygen.** Most patients with PPH do not have resting hypoxemia and do not require supplemental oxygen at rest. Patients who have oxygen desaturation with exercise benefit from ambulatory oxygen therapy. Patients with severe RV failure and decreased cardiac output with resting hypoxemia should be treated with continuous oxygen therapy maintaining arterial oxygen saturation >90% to 92% at rest and with exercise.

2. **Diuretics.** Use of diuretics can improve the edema and ascites of right heart failure. Excess diuresis should be avoided because the RV is dependent on preload (intravascular volume). Initial diuretic therapy should consist of furosemide (10–40 mg/d, increased as needed) with careful monitoring of volume status, electrolytes, and renal function. Metolazone may be required in patients who are refractory to furosemide doses >160 mg/d.

3. **Cardiac glycosides.** Studies do not support the use of cardiac glycosides (eg, digoxin) in PPH. Some authors advocate the use of digoxin to offset the negative inotropic effects of high-dose calcium channel blockers (1,16).

4. **Anticoagulant therapy.** Thrombosis occurs *in situ* in pulmonary arteriolar vessels and may play a significant role in the pathophysiology of PPH. Additional risk for thrombotic events is due to sedentary lifestyle, right heart failure, and low cardiac output. The efficacy of anticoagulants in the treatment of PPH remains controversial. Anticoagulation significantly improved survival in patients with PPH who failed to respond to high-dose calcium channel blockers (16). Current histologic and clinical data suggest that careful use of warfarin is recommended in patients with PPH, unless a significant contraindication exists (1,16–18). Various levels of anticoagulation have been recommended (international normalized ratio [INR] 1.5–2.5 vs. 2.0–3.0). The best anticoagulant and the appropriate level of anticoagulation are unknown at this time. Adjusted-

Table 17-2. Treatment of primary pulmonary hypertension

Avoid:	pregnancy, oral contraceptives, high altitudes, exercise that causes hypoxemia
Diuretics (if peripheral edema):	**furosemide,** initial dose of 10–40 mg/d, increase as needed; add **metolazone,** 5–10 mg/d if refractory to 160 mg/d of furosemide
Oxygen therapy:	if hypoxemic at rest, with exertion, when sleeping or if signs of right heart failure
Anticoagulation:	**warfarin,** unless contraindicated, adjust dose to INR of 1.5–2.5; alternative: **heparin** SC BID–TID, adjust dose to keep PTT 1.3–1.5 ×control
Calcium channel blockers:	(high dose) after testing in ICU. Exact dose will depend on results of ICU testing; alternative: prostacyclin IV after testing in ICU
Transplantation:	consider heart–lung, single or double lung transplant, especially if NYHA functional class III or IV

BID = twice a day; ICU = intensive-care unit; INR = international normalized ratio; IV = intravenous; NYHA = New York Heart Association; PTT = partial thromboplastin time; SC = subcutaneous; TID = three times a day.

dose heparin is an alternative for those patients who cannot tolerate warfarin (keeping partial thromboplastin time [PTT] 1.3–1.5 times control).

5. **Vasodilators.** Various vasodilators have been used to treat PPH, because pulmonary vasoconstriction contributes to the pathophysiology of PPH and even small reductions in RV afterload should improve RV output. Conflicting or disappointing results have been obtained with the long-term use of acetylcholine, phentolamine, tolazoline, isoproterenol, hydralazine, and captopril (1,17,18). High-dose calcium channel blockers (eg, diltiazem, nifedipine) are beneficial (improved hemodynamics, symptomatology, and survival) in approximately 25% of patients (16). This subset of patients, studied in a closely monitored intensive care unit setting, had large decreases in both PAP and PVR in response to increasing doses of calcium channel blockers. Such testing should be recommended to all appropriate PPH patients, since 25% may have significant improvement in survival and symptoms. Invasive monitoring and testing is associated with complications (hypotension, hypoxemia, worsened right heart failure) and requires careful baseline studies and interpretation of the data. Unmonitored empiric therapy with vasodilators is strongly discouraged. Prostacyclin is used for both acute testing and/or long-term therapy. The short half-life requires continuous intravenous infusion and necessitates the placement of a chronic indwelling catheter and daily preparation of solutions (1,17,18). Inhaled nitric oxide may prove to be an efficacious treatment option in the future (18,19).

6. **Transplantation.** Combined heart–lung transplantation has been used in PPH for a decade (1,18). Successful single- and double-lung transplantations have been performed more recently. Transplantation should be considered for all patients who have severe functional impairment (New York Heart Association [NYHA] class III or IV), meet age and psychosocial criteria, and are free of systemic disease. Three-year survival for heart–lung transplantation recipients has improved to 65%. Complications include a high incidence of bronchiolitis obliterans in transplanted lungs, organ rejection, and opportunistic infections. Acute pulmonary edema may occur in the single transplanted lung in patients who undergo this procedure.

G. **Problems and complications of therapy.** Overdiuresis will decrease cardiac output and compromise other therapies (eg, vasodilator therapy). An increased incidence of digitalis toxicity was reported in patients with PPH, perhaps related to hypoxemia and/or diuretic-induced hypokalemia. An increase in cardiac output without a concomitant decrease in PAP may worsen RV ischemia. The use of calcium channel blockers and other vasodilators may worsen RV failure and cause hypotension, hypoxemia, and/or salt and water retention.

H. **Prognosis.** The estimated median survival for PPH is <3 years. Actuarial survival at 1 year is approximately 68% to 77%; at 2 years, 52% to 58%; and at 5 years, 22% to 38%. The most frequent cause of death is RV failure, followed by pneumonia and sudden death. Occasionally, spontaneous regression of the disease may occur, and patients will live for many years. Poor prognostic indicators include PAP ≥85 mm Hg, lack of response to vasodilator therapy, NYHA functional class III or IV, mean right atrial pressure >20 mm Hg, and cardiac index <2.0 L/min/m² (1,20).

I. **Other pertinent information**

1. Pulmonary hypertension occurs in PVOD and pulmonary capillary hemangiomatosis (PCH) (1,3,21). PCH is a rare disease that can be familial and is characterized by a proliferation of microvessels infiltrating the peribronchial and perivascular interstitium, the pulmonary parenchyma, and the pleura. The presentation is similar to PPH, and a lung biopsy is usually required for diagnosis (1,3).

2. PVOD is slightly more common but accounts for <10% of patients with unexplained pulmonary hypertension. The signs and symptoms are similar to PPH. However, a slight male predominance exists, and the presentation tends to be earlier in life and affects infants, children, and young adults more often than PPH. The etiology is unknown, with some cases familial and others associated with viral syndromes, toxins, and chemotherapy. Pathologic abnormalities are

found in the pulmonary veins and venules. Abnormalities are also found in the muscular arteries in approximately 50% of cases. The veins and venules are obstructed by organized or recanalized thrombi and eccentric intimal fibrosis, and the veins also show medial hypertrophy and arterialization. The physiology and hemodynamics approximate PPH, although the PAWP may be elevated. The differential diagnosis is similar that for PPH, and most diagnostic tests will have similar results. The chest x-ray may reveal Kerley's B lines without other evidence of congestive heart failure, and the V/Q scan may show a diffuse patchy pattern. The definitive diagnostic test is an open lung biopsy. Therapeutic options are not well studied, and lung transplantation is the only consistently effective treatment.

II. **Venous thromboembolism.** Venous thromboembolism (VTE) is responsible for 300,000 hospitalizations per year and ranks as the third most common cause of death due to cardiovascular disease in the United States (22,23). Since death from VTE commonly occurs within 1 hour of symptoms, the reduction of morbidity and mortality depends on early recognition, diagnosis, and institution of appropriate therapy. The diagnosis was not initially considered in approximately 50% of deaths due to VTE (24).

A. **Presenting signs and symptoms**

   1. **Deep venous thrombosis (DVT)** may be asymptomatic. Classically, patients report the sudden onset of pain and/or swelling of the proximal or distal lower extremity that may be relieved with elevation. Less commonly, cyanosis of the skin may be noted in the dependent position. Physical examination may reveal tenderness to gentle palpation in the calf, popliteal, or femoral region, and a hard cord over the affected vein. Swelling of the involved extremity is commonly noted, particularly when comparative measurements of bilateral extremities are performed. Dilated superficial collateral veins are present in the setting of iliofemoral thrombosis. Pain on dorsiflexion of the ankle with the knee extended (Homan's sign), found in >20% of patient with DVT, may also be observed with musculoskeletal disease and therefore is a nonspecific finding (25,26). A normal physical examination does not rule out DVT.

   2. **Pulmonary embolism (PE)**

      a. Common symptoms include sudden onset of dyspnea and chest pain that is often pleuritic in nature (27). The duration and intensity of dyspnea are dictated by the extent of embolization. Cough, hemoptysis, and a sense of apprehension may occur during the course of illness. Syncope and substernal chest pain are more characteristic of massive embolic events.

      b. Tachypnea is the most common sign associated with PE. Tachycardia is found in >50% of cases and may be transiently associated with tachypnea. Localized rales or wheezing may be noted on auscultation, and a low-grade fever is found in 40% of cases (28). Massive PE with resultant RV strain and pulmonary hypertension may be marked by the development of hypotension, an increase in the pulmonic component of the second heart sound (P_2), RV lift or gallop, and prominent jugular venous pulsations.

B. **Etiology and pathogenesis**

   1. PE is frequently a complication of DVT, and these entities have common clinical risk factors. As shown in Table 17-3, the most common predisposing conditions are prolonged immobilization and vascular injury (29,30). Age >50 years, obesity, surgery, or trauma are associated with increased risk of VTE. DVT occurs with increased frequency following orthopedic procedures involving the hips and knees, as well as with extensive abdominal, pelvic, and thoracic surgery (31). Additional risk factors for VTE include underlying heart failure, malignancy (especially lung, pancreas, breast, gastrointestinal, and genitourinary), pregnancy, a history of thrombotic disease, and the use of oral contraceptives (32). Less commonly, the deficiency of a coagulation cascade component, such as antithrombin III, protein C, protein S, or plasminogen activators, can increase the incidence of VTE (33).

   2. The pathogenesis of DVT involves stasis (as reflected in the above risk factors), injury to the vascular endothelium, and/or perturbations in the coagula-

Table 17-3. Risk factors for venous thromboembolism

Age >50 years

Immobilization

Paralysis due to stroke

Surgery
    Especially major abdominal and pelvic surgery and major orthopedic
      surgery (hip and knee replacement and hip fracture)

Multiple trauma

Malignancy

Pregnancy (including postpartum period)

Previous deep venous thrombosis

Hypercoagulable states
    Deficiency of antithrombin III, protein C or protein S
    Antiphospholipid syndrome
    Excessive plasminogen-activator inhibitor

---

tion cascade. Thrombosis frequently develops in the vicinity of venous valves or at sites of intimal injury. The majority of clinically significant PEs result from above-knee thrombi; most of the latter represent extension of calf vein thrombi (24,34). However, only 15% of calf vein thrombi will extend, and such extension seldom occurs after 10 days (35,36).

C. Relevant physiology

    1. DVT. The presence of lower extremity edema and cyanosis is related to the degree of vessel occlusion and the ability to utilize collaterals. DVT may be clinically silent because thrombosis is limited to a single vessel and has little impact on the extensive venous drainage of the lower extremity.

    2. PE

        a. PE results in physiologic alterations within both the vascular and parenchymal regions of the lung. Hemodynamically, embolic obstruction results in loss of a portion of the pulmonary vascular bed, regional hypoxic vasoconstriction, and consequent elevation in PVR. Marked increases in PAP, particularly in patients with underlying cardiopulmonary disease, may lead to RV failure (37). Acute cor pulmonale associated with massive PE results in hypotension and shock.

        b. The pulmonary parenchymal sequelae of significant vascular obstruction include increased alveolar dead space (V/Q mismatch) and arterial hypoxemia. Loss of pulmonary surfactant, which occurs approximately 24 hours after the initial event, results in focal atelectasis and edema.

        c. Pulmonary infarction develops in <10% of patients with PE; 70% to 80% of this group have underlying cardiopulmonary disease or malignancy (38). Infarction is probably secondary to an inadequate bronchial arterial supply and airway patency in the portion of lung compromised by PE.

D. Differential diagnostic possibilities

    1. DVT. Clinical findings associated with DVT are nonspecific and potentially attributable to other diagnoses including musculoskeletal causes (plantaris tendon rupture, gastrocnemius muscle injury), impaired venous or lymphatic flow, and popliteal inflammatory cysts (Baker's cysts).

    2. PE. The constellation of findings associated with PE, including dyspnea and/or pleuritic chest pain, are likewise nonspecific and may be attributed to processes such as viral pleuritis, pneumothorax, bacterial or viral pneumonitis, atelectasis, asthma, angina, myocardial infarction, dissecting aortic aneurysm, and hyperventilation syndrome.

E. Diagnostic evaluation

1. **DVT.** Despite the nonspecific clinical manifestations of DVT, the diagnosis can often be made with noninvasive testing. When a DVT is not detected by the initial noninvasive tests and the clinical suspicion remains high, further evaluation is required, including serial noninvasive imaging or venography.

    a. **Impedance plethysmography (IPG)** indirectly detects venous obstruction through measured changes in electric impedance. The sensitivity and specificity of this procedure are highest in symptomatic patients with occluding proximal thrombi (39). Since nonocclusive thrombi cannot be detected, IPG is not useful for screening of asymptomatic patients at high risk. A positive IPG in a patient with a clinical suspicion of DVT establishes the diagnosis; however, a normal study does not exclude the presence of nonocclusive, proximal vein thrombi or calf vein thrombosis.

    b. **Ultrasonography. Doppler ultrasonography** uses variations in flow sounds to identify thrombi. This test is operator dependent and lacks sensitivity for nonocclusive proximal and calf vein thrombi, and therefore should be supplemented by real-time ultrasonography **(duplex scanning)** in the initial evaluation of suspected DVT. Duplex scanning is the most appropriate initial test in the evaluation of patients with suspected DVT because of safety and overall sensitivity and specificity (40). **Real-time ultrasound** imaging, utilizing B-mode scanning, detects echogenic densities and determines the compressibility of the deep venous system. Failure to compress the vein indicates thrombus. The sensitivity is equivalent to IPG for proximal DVT in symptomatic patients; it is not useful for diagnosis of calf or inguinal thrombi (41).

    c. **Venography** remains the gold standard for the diagnosis of both distal and proximal thrombi. The specific disadvantages include the risk of contrast-induced peripheral vein thrombosis (2% to 3%), anaphylactic reactions, inability of the test to be readily repeated, and cost. Venography is indicated for suspected DVT not demonstrated by noninvasive testing and for the differentiation of acute recurrent disease from chronic venous outflow obstruction.

    d. **D-dimer.** Plasma D-dimer, a product of plasmin digestion of cross-linked fibrin, is elevated in the presence of DVT or PE. While the sensitivity of plasma D-dimer levels (as measured by enzyme-linked immunosorbent assay) is high, the test lacks specificity (42). Although a low D-dimer level suggests that VTE is not present, additional testing to exclude thrombosis is required.

2. **PE.** The diagnosis of PE requires a high index of suspicion and the identification of significant abnormalities on V/Q scan and/or pulmonary angiogram (Fig. 17-1).

    a. **ECG.** The ECG is frequently abnormal, with sinus tachycardia, PR-interval depression, and nonspecific T-wave changes being the most common findings. The classic S1Q3T3 pattern occurs in only 15% of patients and usually in the setting of massive PE (24).

    b. **Chest x-ray.** The chest x-ray is helpful in the exclusion of other conditions responsible for the clinical syndrome. While the chest x-ray in patients with PE is frequently normal, consolidation, atelectasis, and pleural effusion may be present, particularly when pulmonary infarction has occurred. More subtle radiographic signs of PE include regional oligemia (Westermark's sign), enlargement of the descending PA, and elevation of the diaphragm.

    c. **Laboratory abnormalities** such as elevations in lactate dehydrogenase and indirect bilirubin are inconsistent and not helpful in establishing the diagnosis.

    d. **Arterial blood gases** usually reveal hypoxemia, hypocarbia, and a widened alveolar-arterial oxygen gradient (>20 mm Hg). However, normal arterial blood gases are found in up to 20% of patients with PE (28). PE should be suspected in patients with underlying COPD and chronic

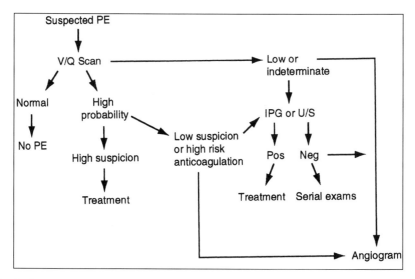

Fig. 17-1. Approaches to the diagnosis of pulmonary embolism (PE) in the clinically stable patient (V/Q = ventilation–perfusion scan, IPG = impedance plethysmography, U/S = ultrasound, Pos = positive, Neg = negative. (From Libman H, Witzburg RA. *HIV infection*, 3rd ed. Boston: Little, Brown, 1996.)

carbon dioxide retention whose P_{CO_2} falls below the established baseline level.

e. **Thoracentesis** usually reveals nonspecific findings. Bloody effusions occur infrequently but are suggestive of the diagnosis.

f. **Echocardiography** may demonstrate RV dysfunction, intraluminal thrombi, and elevated PAP. A normal echocardiogram does not rule out PE, and this test plays a minor role in the diagnosis of PE (43).

g. **Computed tomography (CT)** may demonstrate thromboemboli in second-to-fourth division vessels when spiral volumetric techniques are used. This test requires further study before recommendation as a standard diagnostic tool in the evaluation of PE (44).

h. **V/Q scanning** is the initial procedure of choice in patients with suspected PE. A normal perfusion scan rules out the diagnosis of PE. Abnormal perfusion scans may be difficult to interpret without a synchronous chest x-ray and ventilation scan. Criteria for diagnosis of PE using V/Q scanning have been derived from several large clinical studies and are based on size and number of defects, chest x-ray findings, and distribution of ventilation (45). High-probability scans are generally sufficient to establish the diagnosis of PE if causes of false-positive scans are excluded (eg, pneumonia, pulmonary edema). The interpretation of an indeterminate or low-probability scan is more difficult and strongly influenced by clinical suspicion. For example, low-probability scans coupled with low clinical suspicion accurately predict the absence of PE. Nondiagnostic scans (low or indeterminate) in patients with significant clinical suspicion for PE require further diagnostic evaluation (see Fig. 17-1). High-probability scans in patients who are at high risk for anticoagulation or in whom clinical suspicion is low require further evaluation.

i. **Pulmonary angiography** is the gold standard for the diagnosis of acute PE (46). Demonstration of a filling defect or abrupt cutoff of a vessel is considered sensitive for diagnosis, and the test may be delayed up to 7 days after the embolic episode without losing diagnostic accuracy. Complications such as cardiopulmonary arrest, PA perforation, arrhythmias, and contrast allergy are rare. Severe pulmonary hypertension is not a contraindication to angiography, but the test should be performed by highly experienced personnel. The use of selective angiograms (ie, unilateral pulmonary vasculature) adds to the safety of this test. Angiography is most frequently utilized in the setting of a nondiagnostic V/Q scan and a significant clinical suspicion of PE. Angiography should be the initial study in patients who require urgent diagnosis due to severe hypoxemia or may require thrombolytic therapy, vena caval interruption, or embolectomy.

F. **Management.** In general, all patients with DVT or PE should receive anticoagulation therapy. Standard approaches to acute VTE currently include the use of unfractionated heparin, warfarin, and inferior vena caval interruption. The role of low-molecular-weight heparin, thrombolytics, pulmonary embolectomy, and transvenous catheter extraction is controversial and remains individualized. Patients with calf vein thrombosis should either receive anticoagulation or undergo serial noninvasive testing over 2 weeks to exclude proximal extension.

1. **Anticoagulation**

   a. **Heparin** is considered first-line therapy in the treatment of acute DVT or PE. Absolute contraindications to anticoagulation with heparin include documented hypersensitivity, heparin-induced thrombocytopenia, active bleeding or a significant risk of bleeding (eg, cerebrovascular accident, surgery within 2 weeks of the event, underlying bleeding diathesis, a platelet count <150,000/µL). Inferior vena cava (IVC) filter placement should be considered for these patients. Suspected DVT or PE requires empiric therapy with 5,000 U heparin IV pending diagnostic studies, because failure to establish adequate anticoagulation within the first 24 hours of treatment is associated with progression or recurrence of VTE. Upon confirmation, the level of anticoagulation should be targeted to an activated PTT of 1.5–2.0 times control; suggested dosing guidelines based on published nomograms, including a weight-based protocol, are listed in Table 17-4 (47,48). Heparin requirements are greatest within the first 72 hours of the event and frequent PTT monitoring is imperative.

   b. **Warfarin** inhibits synthesis of vitamin K–dependent coagulation factors and is an effective oral agent for long-term therapy in VTE. Contraindications to warfarin include documented hypersensitivity, severe active bleeding, and pregnancy. Because its onset of action is 4–5 days, treatment with warfarin should begin on day 1 of heparin therapy. A daily dose of 5–10 mg should be given to achieve an INR of 2.0–3.0 (prothrombin time [PT] 1.5–2.5 times control) by day 5–7 of heparin infusion. Heparin is discontinued 24–36 hours after an INR of 2.0–3.0 has been established. Since drug and diet interactions with warfarin are common and may cause significant alterations in the INR, the frequency of testing and dosing regimens must be individualized. Minimum duration of therapy with warfarin for VTE is 3–6 months. Chronic therapy may be required in patients with persistent risk factors such as prolonged immobilization, malignancy, or deficiencies of antithrombin III, protein C, or protein S.

   c. **Subcutaneous (SC) unfractionated heparin** may be utilized as an alternative in the acute and long-term therapy of VTE. This is the treatment of choice for patients unable to take warfarin (eg, pregnancy). The total daily dose given SC in divided doses (eg, q8h) in the acute setting ranges from 30,000 to 40,000 U. After 5–7 days, long-term therapy is initiated with 7500–10,000 U q12h, and the dose adjusted to maintain a PTT of 1.5–2.0 times control.

   d. **Low-molecular-weight heparin** is an emerging alternative therapy in the treatment of acute VTE. Superior bioavailability and longer plasma half-life allow SC dosing once or twice daily without monitoring. Al-

Table 17-4. Guidelines for anticoagulation with heparin therapy in venous thromboembolism (VTE)

Dosing regimen	Alternative
VTE suspected	
5,000 U IV (pending diagnostic studies)	Weight-based protocol: bolus 80 U/kg; maintain at 18 U/kg/h
VTE confirmed	
Readminister bolus of 5,000–10,000 U IV; begin maintenance infusion at 1300 U/h (reduce rate to 25,000 U/24 h in patients with high risk of bleeding)	Bolus 80 U/kg; maintain at 18 U/kg/h
Determine PTT 6 h after initial bolus	
Adjust dosing to maintain PTT 1.5–2.5 × control or 46–70 sec	
Check PTT 6 h after dosage change	
When two consecutive PTTs are therapeutic, check PTT (and adjust dose) every 24 h	
Check CBC and platelet count daily	
Begin warfarin on day 1 of heparin therapy at 10 mg/d (use lower dose [2–5 mg] if patient is elderly, malnourished, has liver disease, on warfarin-potentiating drug)	
On day 2 check INR; if ≤ 1.5, give same dose; if ≥ 1.5, give lower dose	
On day 3 check INR and adjust maintenance dose, keeping INR 2.0–3.0	
Discontinue heparin once INR has reached 2.0–3.0 for 24–36 hr (4–7 days)	

CBC = complete blood cell count; INR = international normalized ratio; PTT = partial thromboplastin time.

though recent studies suggest effectiveness and safety in the treatment of acute VTE, excessive cost is the primary limitation (49). Further studies to clarify the role of this therapy in acute VTE are ongoing.

2. **IVC filters.** Indications for placement of an IVC filter include PE or acute proximal DVT, a contraindication to anticoagulation, complications of early treatment, documented recurrent PE despite therapeutic anticoagulation, massive PE with a high risk of recurrence, and prophylaxis in patients at high risk for DVT or PE (50). Although long-term patency of most devices is >95%, anticoagulation should be continued for 3 months if not contraindicated.

3. **Thrombolytic therapy.** The current roles of urokinase, streptokinase, and tissue plasminogen activator in the treatment of VTE remain controversial. Early use of thrombolytic agents may reduce the incidence of postphlebitic syndrome in DVT, but further studies to confirm an advantage over conventional treatment are needed. For PE, thrombolysis results in earlier resolution of lung scan abnormalities and improved RV dysfunction, but studies have not shown an improvement in survival (50). This treatment should be considered in the setting of acute, massive PE with hemodynamic instability. Contraindications include cerebrovascular accident within 2 months of the event, other active intracranial processes, active bleeding, surgery within 10 days of the event, recent labor and delivery, trauma, or severe hypertension. Relative contraindications include minor trauma, left heart thrombus, pregnancy, hemorrhagic retinopathy, and endarterectomy. No difference in effectiveness or risk of bleeding has been shown among individual agents; in addition, directed de-

livery offers no advantage over systemic infusion via a peripheral line. Consideration for thrombolytic therapy requires consultation with a pulmonologist or cardiologist.

4. **Pulmonary embolectomy** is associated with significant mortality and should be limited to those patients with massive PE and hemodynamic compromise who have a contraindication to thrombolytic therapy. **Transvenous catheter extraction** of emboli may provide an alternative to surgical embolectomy. Currently, the procedure is associated with a mortality of 27%, and further investigation is required.

G. Problems and complications of therapy

1. **Heparin.** The major complications of heparin therapy include excessive bleeding and **thrombocytopenia**. Baseline laboratory studies should include PT, PTT, and complete blood cell count. Platelet counts should be monitored. Heparin therapy should be discontinued if the platelet count falls to <100,000/µL. Development of arterial thromboembolism and progression of existing VTE may be associated with heparin-induced thrombocytopenia. Transient elevation of liver enzyme levels may occur during the first week of therapy, but resolve spontaneously and are not associated with chronic liver injury.

2. **Warfarin.** Bleeding is the most common complication of warfarin therapy. Anticoagulation can be reversed in 1–2 days using vitamin K (10 mg/d SC for 3 days); life-threatening episodes of bleeding require fresh frozen plasma. Warfarin-induced skin necrosis, a rare complication of therapy, occurs shortly after initiation of therapy and has been associated with protein C deficiency and malignancy.

3. **IVC filters.** Complication rates are low and primarily involve technical difficulties during placement. Long-term patency rates are >90% (50).

4. **Thrombolytic therapy.** Intracranial or retroperitoneal hemorrhage are the most worrisome bleeding complications with thrombolytic agents (1,51). Prior to administration, a careful neurologic history and physical examination should be performed. If an intracranial hemorrhage is suspected, immediate consultation with a neurologist or neurosurgeon is recommended. Though retroperitoneal hemorrhage is difficult to diagnose, a precipitous fall in blood pressure and hematocrit without obvious source of blood loss should raise suspicion for this entity and prompt further investigation.

H. Prognosis

1. **DVT.** Patients receiving anticoagulants for 3 months have >90% resolution of abnormal venous flow 1 year after the diagnosis. The recurrence rate of DVT is approximately 15% within the first 5 years of the event and is associated with a history of VTE and age >65 years. Symptoms of pain, discoloration, or swelling are reported in 42% of patients at 6–8 years of follow-up (52). In patients with isolated calf vein thrombosis, withholding treatment and monitoring proximal thrombus extension with serial noninvasive tests appear to be safe and are associated with low rates of recurrence when evaluated at 6 months of follow-up.

2. **PE.** Most patients experiencing a PE suffer no significant long-term effects. The earliest resolution of angiographic and hemodynamic abnormalities in patients receiving heparin therapy is 14 days (53). Longitudinal studies (using V/Q scans) of patients who received heparin followed by oral anticoagulation revealed that 50% to 70% of defects resolved 3 months after the event and 75% to 100% were resolved at 1 year (51,54). Thrombus persists in <2% of patients, leading to chronic pulmonary hypertension and cor pulmonale.

I. Prevention of VTE. Prophylaxis is the cornerstone of the management of thrombotic disease. The majority of patients with fatal PE die within 1 hour of presentation, and therefore no treatment is more influential in the prevention of morbidity and mortality than prophylaxis. Effective prophylactic therapy should be instituted immediately upon patient admission to the hospital and guided by identification of risk factors listed in Table 17-5.

J. Chronic thromboembolic disease. Chronic thromboembolic disease is a complication of large PEs of the central vessels (main, lobar, segmental arteries) that fail to resolve.

Table 17-5. Recommended prophylaxis of venous thromboembolism (VTE)

Procedure/condition	Prophylaxis
General surgery	
Age <40, duration <60 min	Elastic stockings, early ambulation
Age <40, duration >60 min	Heparin 5000 U SC BID, Low-molecular-weight heparin or external pneumatic compression device
with h/o VTE	Increase heparin to 5000 U SC TID; add external pneumatic compression device
Orthopedic surgery	
Hip arthroplasty/fracture	Low-molecular-weight heparin or warfarin (adjusted to INR 2.0–3.0)
Knee arthroplasty	Low-molecular-weight heparin or external pneumatic compression
Neurosurgery	External pneumatic compression device with or without elastic stockings
Trauma	
Multiple; extensive soft tissue or fractures	External pneumatic compression device or warfarin (adjusted) or low-molecular-weight heparin
Acute spinal cord injury	Warfarin (adjusted) or low-molecular-weight heparin or heparin 5000 U SC TID
Stroke	
Lower extremity paralysis (nonhemorrhagic)	Heparin 5000 U SC TID or low-molecular-weight heparin
(hemorrhagic)	External pneumatic compression device
Myocardial infarction	Heparin 5000 U SC BID or low-molecular-weight heparin or external pneumatic compression device
Medical conditions with risk factors for VTE	Heparin 5000 U SC BID or low-molecular-weight heparin

BID = twice a day; SC = subcutaneous; TID = three times a day.

1. **Signs and symptoms.** Symptoms are nonspecific and similar to those of PPH. Half of patients have a history of documented PE or DVT. Physical findings are likewise similar to PPH. Patients may have a flow murmur over the narrowed PA, and approximately 25% will have evidence of chronic venous stasis in the lower extremities (54).

2. **Etiology and pathogenesis.** The reasons emboli fail to resolve in some patients are unknown. Abnormalities of coagulation or fibrinolysis have not been documented. If chronic thromboemboli are not treated, symptoms will slowly progress to dyspnea at rest and right heart failure, most likely a result of progressive arterial hypertension in lung regions not affected directly by the arterial occlusion (54,55).

3. **Relevant physiology.** Physiologic abnormalities are similar to those in PPH, with eventual right heart failure from a progressive increase in PAP.

4. **Differential diagnostic possibilities.** Early in the disease, the differential diagnosis includes fibrosing mediastinitis with obstruction of the PA, congenital PA stenosis or agenesis, primary or metastatic tumors that cause obstruction of the PA, and Takayasu's arteritis. In more advanced disease, the differential diagnosis includes primary and secondary PPH.

5. **Diagnostic evaluation.** The initial diagnostic evaluation is similar to that for PPH. The ECG, chest x-ray, pulmonary function tests, arterial blood gases, and

echocardiogram will all have similar findings to those seen in PPH. Unlike PPH, however, imaging of the lower extremity venous system will reveal abnormalities in 75% of patients, and the V/Q scan will show bilateral segmental or larger perfusion defects in areas with normal ventilation (54). The V/Q scan is less reliable in detecting central obstruction (56,57). Definitive diagnosis requires right heart catheterization (to document hemodynamics) and pulmonary angiography. Angiography is particularly important to document operability.

6. **Treatment.** The patient should be referred to an institution experienced in the surgical treatment (thromboendarterectomy) of this disease (54). If symptoms are more consistent with acute embolism, a trial of anticoagulation followed by repeat lung scan may be warranted prior to referral. An IVC filter should be placed in all patients due to the severe consequences of PE in an already compromised pulmonary vascular bed.

7. **Complications of treatment.** The overall surgical mortality is 10%, with mortality occurring more frequently in those patients in NYHA functional class IV (54). Pulmonary edema may occur in the immediate postoperative period in the regions served by the previously occluded vessel (58). All patients should be anticoagulated with warfarin for life.

K. **Other forms of embolism.** The pulmonary circulation acts as a sieve for all particles entering the venous system. Many different agents may be trapped in the pulmonary circulation and result in obstruction or exposure of the lung. In addition, embolic events associated with schistosomiasis and talc embolization from IV drug abuse may produce discrete clinical syndromes (59,60).

1. **Air embolism.** This form of nonthrombotic embolism is usually seen as a result of invasive medical and surgical procedures or trauma (61,62) and is particularly problematic during placement of central venous catheters. A change in sensorium, coma or seizures resulting from cerebral embolism, or cardiac ischemia resulting from coronary embolism are the most serious symptoms. Thrombocytopenia may also occur. Prevention is the most important approach, especially during high-risk surgeries and placement and accessing of a central line. Treatment requires recompression in a hyperbaric chamber.

2. **Fat embolism.** Dyspnea, confusion, petechiae, and hypoxemia represent the characteristic syndrome of fat embolism (63,64). The most common cause is fracture of long bones; pulmonary symptoms are delayed 24–48 hours. Diagnosis is made by the characteristic clinical presentation. The chest x-ray may show diffuse patchy infiltrates. Finding fat droplets on bronchoalveolar lavage suggests the diagnosis but is neither sensitive nor specific (65). Treatment is supportive, and mechanical ventilation may be necessary. Corticosteroid prophylaxis in high-risk patients may be helpful, but steroids are not indicated once the syndrome has developed. With aggressive supportive care, the prognosis is good.

3. **Amniotic fluid embolism.** This form of embolism occurs during or after delivery (vaginal or surgical) (66). Amniotic fluid enters the venous system and results in sudden severe respiratory distress and hypotension. The amniotic fluid activates the coagulation cascade, causing fibrin deposition in the lungs and a consumptive coagulopathy. Diagnosis is suggested by the clinical presentation, laboratory tests showing consumptive coagulopathy and hypoxemia, and a chest x-ray showing diffuse infiltrates. The diagnosis can be confirmed by the demonstration of fragments of the vernix caseosa in PA blood. Treatment is supportive, with aggressive pulmonary and hemodynamic care in an intensive care unit.

4. **Septic embolism.** The most common causes of septic emboli are indwelling venous catheters and IV drug use. Septic pelvic thrombophlebitis is a less common cause. Symptoms and signs include dyspnea, cough, pleuritic chest pain, intermittent fevers, chills and/or sweats, and hemoptysis. Scattered rales may be present on pulmonary examination. The chest x-ray typically shows scattered infiltrates that eventually cavitate. Blood and sputum cultures should be performed, although negative cultures do not rule out the diagnosis. An

echocardiogram may show evidence of an infected pulmonic or tricuspid valve. Treatment includes removal of any indwelling catheters and administration of appropriate antibiotics guided by culture results whenever possible. Surgical treatment is frequently required for management of septic thrombophlebitis and endocarditis (67,68).

III. **Pulmonary vascular abnormalities.** The most common pulmonary vascular abnormalities are communications between branches of the PA and pulmonary vein, most notably pulmonary arteriovenous malformations (AVMs). The general category of pulmonary vascular abnormalities will be discussed first, followed by systemic–venous communications (including bronchopulmonary sequestration) and PA aneurysms.

A. **Pulmonary vascular communications (including AVMs).** These communications may be acquired or congenital (usually in association with hereditary hemorrhagic telangiectasia [HTT]) and cause right-to-left shunts resulting in hypoxemia. Communications are usually found within the lung parenchyma and range in size from microscopic to large aneurysmal malformations.

1. **Presenting signs and symptoms**
   a. In adult patients, AVMs may be asymptomatic or present as worsening dyspnea (69–71). Symptoms may develop at any age and include hemoptysis (which may be massive), platypnea (breathlessness that worsens when sitting upright and improves when lying flat), and symptoms related to hemothorax (which may occur suddenly). Headache, tinnitus, seizures, transient ischemic attacks, and hemiplegia occur in 30% of patients, probably as a result of paradoxical emboli or *in situ* thrombosis secondary to polycythemia. Patients with HHT may also present with symptoms related to AVMs elsewhere in the body (eg, gastrointestinal, genitourinary, central nervous system), the most common being epistaxis (70).
   b. Classically, patients with AVMs present with cyanosis, clubbing, and a murmur over the AVM, although none of these signs needs to be present. Hypoxemia on exertion or at rest is frequently present and usually related to shunt size. Dyspnea does not correlate with the degree of hypoxemia and may be a late feature even with large right-to-left shunts. Orthodeoxia (a fall in oxygen saturation when the patient changes from a supine to upright position) may occur. Patients with HTT may have normal physical examinations, except for papular, ruby-red, round skin lesions that do not blanch with pressure. Presenting signs may include neurologic findings related to stroke or brain abscess from paradoxical emboli (69–71).

2. **Etiology and pathogenesis**
   a. The most common acquired cause of AVMs in the United States is hepatic cirrhosis (usually secondary to alcohol abuse or viral infection) (69, 71,72). Other causes of acquired AVMs include mitral stenosis, trauma, pulmonary infections (including schistosomiasis and actinomycosis), metastatic tumors, thoracic surgery, and Fanconi's syndrome. Congenital pulmonary AVMs are frequently associated with HHT, also known as Osler-Weber-Rendu disease. Patients with HHT may have many AVMs in the lungs and other tissues. This disorder has an autosomal-dominant pattern of inheritance with incomplete penetrance. Approximately 50% of pulmonary AVMs are not associated with HHT. Two-thirds of these patients have single lesions, and one-third have multiple lesions. The etiology of these lesions and HHT is unknown (69–71).
   b. Most pulmonary AVMs are 1–5 cm in diameter and occur peripherally in the lower lobes, adjacent to the visceral pleura. The blood supply is usually from branches of the pulmonary arteries. Approximately 80% of AVMs are supplied by a single feeding artery and are drained by a single vein. Drainage is usually to the left atrium (69,73).

3. **Relevant physiology.** AVMs cause right-to-left shunts and arterial hypoxemia. The magnitude of the hypoxemia is dependent on the size of the shunt, which is usually dependent on the size and number of AVMs. Hypoxemia will not correct with supplemental oxygen. Platypnea and orthodeoxia are thought

to be due to an increase in blood flow to the lung bases, where most AVMs are located (69–72).

4. **Differential diagnostic possibilities.** Patients with AVMs present with symptoms related to their pulmonary lesion(s) or to AVMs elsewhere; asymptomatic lesions may be found incidentally on an chest x-ray (69–71).

   a. For patients with pulmonary symptoms, the differential diagnosis includes parenchymal lung disease (eg, COPD, interstitial lung disease, pulmonary hypertension) and cardiac disease (eg, coronary vascular disease, congestive heart failure, valvular heart disease, intracardiac shunts). The diagnosis of pulmonary AVM may be more apparent in patients with HHT who have symptoms related to AVMs elsewhere.

   b. In asymptomatic patients with chest x-ray abnormalities, the differential diagnosis includes those entities that produce nodular lesions, such as primary or metastatic lung malignancies, infectious granulomatous disease (eg, tuberculous, parasitic, or fungal), other congenital abnormalities (eg, bronchogenic cyst or sequestration), and, less commonly, sarcoidosis, Wegener's granulomatosis, or pulmonary infarct.

5. **Specific approach to each diagnostic possibility.** Symptomatic patients should be initially evaluated with a chest x-ray, ECG, and arterial blood gases. On chest x-ray, an AVM classically appears as a peripheral lower lobe mass with an enlarged feeding artery radiating to the hilum and a draining vein extending into the right atrium (69–71). A high-resolution CT scan with IV contrast may demonstrate the architecture of vessels in an AVM, while defining other potential pulmonary abnormalities. Other tests that may suggest the diagnosis of AVM but are not diagnostic include (a) echocardiography with contrast that shows the indicator dye appearing in the left atrium or aorta prematurely and (b) a perfusion scan that shows rapid collection of the radioisotope in the left heart and early distribution to the extrathoracic organs. Classic findings on chest x-ray, supported by hypoxemia on arterial blood gases either at rest or with exertion, or suggestive findings from other tests should lead immediately to a pulmonary angiogram.

   a. Pulmonary angiography should be performed in all patients with suspected pulmonary AVMs to make the diagnosis reliably and to determine the vascular supply necessary for obliterative therapy or resection (72–74).

   b. Changes on the ECG and/or chest x-ray may suggest cardiac disease and guide further evaluation in that direction. Pulmonary function tests may show a decreased $D_L CO$ or an increased minute ventilation, but they are nondiagnostic (73,74). They may help define other pulmonary problems.

6. **Management**

   a. The natural history of untreated AVMs is unknown. Asymptomatic AVMs may not alter life expectancy, and thus prophylactic therapy is controversial. Since such patients theoretically run the risk of paradoxical emboli and/or massive hemoptysis, treatment of all patients with pulmonary AVMs has been proposed. If a pulmonary AVM is left untreated, antibacterial prophylaxis should be used at the time of dental or surgical procedures (69–71).

   b. The treatment of AVMs has been evolving. Several recent studies have shown good results with percutaneous catheter embolization of pulmonary AVMs using steel coils or detachable balloons (74,75). The use of detachable balloons runs the risk of balloon deflation, and the use of steel coils appears to be more durable, although migration of the coil is a potential complication. Nonetheless, this treatment option is rapidly replacing surgery as the treatment of choice for this disease. Surgical treatment involves local segmental resection. Simple ligation of feeder vessels is not recommended because of the potential for either collateral blood supply to the lesion or thrombosis of the venous side of the lesion with subsequent systemic embolization. Both forms of treatment risk worsening pulmonary hypertension in a patient with elevated PAP at baseline.

PAP should thus be measured at the time of angiography, and, if elevated, the post-treatment hemodynamics should be assessed by occluding the blood supply to the AVM with a balloon-tipped catheter and measuring the resulting PAP. If the PAP increases during transient occlusion, further treatment should be reconsidered. Both surgical resection and embolization provide symptomatic and physiologic improvement with minimal morbidity and mortality in properly selected patients (73–75).

B. Systemic–pulmonary vascular communications. This category of pulmonary vascular abnormalities is much less common than AVMs but still results in a right-to-left shunt. The systemic vessel that penetrates the lung usually arises from the coronary arteries, intercostal arteries, or internal mammary arteries. Most such communications are traumatic in origin but may also be due to thoracic neoplasms, bronchopulmonary sequestrations, and chronic inflammatory disorders including bronchiectasis (76,77).

1. **Presenting signs and symptoms.** Most such lesions, including extralobar sequestrations, are asymptomatic and discovered on a chest x-ray performed for other reasons (76–78). Intralobar sequestrations may cause recurrent pneumonia with cough, fever, and occasionally hemoptysis (79). They frequently become symptomatic in adolescence. These and other forms of systemic–pulmonary vascular communications will cause dyspnea if large right-to-shunts are present. Physical examination may be normal or reveal clubbing, cyanosis, and/or a continuous murmur over the chest (76–80).

2. **Etiology and pathogenesis**
    a. Bronchopulmonary sequestrations are probably due to an abnormality in development of the embryonic foregut (77,79). The pathology shows masses of rubbery tissue with an orderly or disorderly arrangement of normal lung tissue. Intralobar sequestrations share a common visceral pleural investment with normal adjacent lung, and extralobar sequestrations have their own pleural lining that separates them completely from the remaining lung tissue. Extralobar sequestrations are rare and occur more often in men. Often associated with other congenital malformations (especially diaphragmatic hernias), they occur more frequently in the lower chest, are twice as common on the left as on the right, and rarely contain air. The arterial supply is from the aorta, while venous drainage is through the azygos or hemizygos systems. Thus, they are not true systemic–pulmonary vascular communications.
    b. Intralobar sequestrations are more common and occur equally in males and females. Other congenital abnormalities are usually not present. The most common locations are the medial or posterior basal segments of the lower lobes, more often on the left. Air is often present, and intralobar sequestrations can become secondarily infected.

3. **Relevant physiology.** With the exception of extralobar sequestrations, these lesions cause right-to-left shunts. The degree of hypoxemia and severity of the symptoms depend on the size of the shunt. The hypoxemia does not correct with supplemental oxygen.

4. **Differential diagnostic possibilities.** The differential diagnostic possibilities for asymptomatic lesions are similar to those for AVMs. The classic basilar location of sequestrations should suggest the diagnosis. Infected intralobar sequestrations may be confused with pyogenic lung abscesses, although the location should suggest sequestration. The differential diagnosis also includes bronchogenic cysts or infectious granulomatous disease (eg, tuberculosis or fungal infection), although the location for the latter would be unusual.

5. **Specific approach to each diagnostic possibility.** A CT scan with IV contrast will define the anatomy and density of the lesion precisely. If these are suggestive, further evaluation with angiography will demonstrate the aberrant artery and confirm the diagnosis. Multiple lesions on CT scan, diffuse pulmonary parenchymal disease, and mediastinal adenopathy suggest other diagnoses, such as malignancy or granulomatous disease.

6. **Management.** Surgery is the usual treatment for symptomatic lesions. The natural history of untreated, asymptomatic vascular communications is unknown. Extralobar sequestrations can be removed without disturbing the surrounding lung parenchyma. Intralobar sequestrations and other systemic–pulmonary communications require lobectomy. The prognosis for those who undergo treatment is excellent.

C. **Pulmonary artery aneurysms.** These are rare vascular anomalies frequently associated with congenital cardiac disorders such as patent ductus arteriosus, ventricular septal defects, tetralogy of Fallot, and pulmonary valvular stenosis. Pseudoaneurysms may be caused by infection, trauma, and neoplasms (80–83).

1. **Presenting signs and symptoms.** These lesions are frequently asymptomatic (80). Large lesions can cause dyspnea or chest pain. If the lesion is associated with other congenital abnormalities, the symptoms may be related to cardiac or great vessel abnormalities. Lesions caused by infection (eg, tuberculosis, septic emboli) may present with symptoms of fever, chills, sweats, weight loss, fatigue, or dyspnea. Rupture will cause massive hemoptysis and hypotension (81–83). Physical examination may be normal or reveal the underlying congenital or infectious processes.

2. **Etiology and pathogenesis.** Approximately 40% of PA aneurysms are associated with congenital defects that cause right-to-left shunting. Patent ductus arteriosus is the most common. The other major causes of PA aneurysms or pseudoaneurysms include infection (eg, syphilis, tuberculosis causing Rasmussen's aneurysms, septic emboli), pulmonary hypertension (primary or secondary), trauma (eg, right heart catheterization), cystic medial necrosis, atherosclerosis, Marfan's syndrome, and large vessel vasculitides such as giant cell arteritis, Takayasu's arteritis, and Behçet's syndrome.

3. **Relevant physiology.** Aneurysms due to infection or trauma result in abnormalities in PA flow and occasionally PA hypertension. The relevant physiology of aneurysms associated with congenital heart defects will relate primarily to the specific cardiac defects.

4. **Differential diagnostic possibilities.** The differential diagnosis includes pulmonary valvular defects, bacterial or fungal endocarditis, and metastatic or primary tumors of the PA.

5. **Specific approach to each diagnostic possibility.** Chest CT scan can define potential aneurysm anatomy. Echocardiography will define PA anatomy and image possible valvular lesions (eg, vegetations). Blood cultures are mandatory to rule out endocarditis and determine other infectious etiologies of PA aneurysms. Angiography provides the definitive diagnosis of possible aneurysms suggested by echocardiogram or CT scan.

6. **Management.** The prognosis of PA aneurysms is unknown since many remain asymptomatic. In autopsy series, approximately one-third of patients with PA aneurysms died of rupture, while two-thirds died of right heart failure, PE, or unrelated causes. Since aneurysms are inherently unstable, treatment is recommended, especially if hemoptysis occurs. Treatment should also target the underlying disease or infection. Embolization with steel coils or inflatable balloons has been used successfully, as has resection of the aneurysm (81–83).

References

1. Rubin LJ: Primary pulmonary hypertension. *Chest* 1993;104:236–250.
2. Rich S, et al.: Primary pulmonary hypertension: a national prospective study. *Ann Intern Med* 1987; 107:216–223.
3. Higgenbottam T: Pathophysiology of pulmonary hypertension: a role for endothelial dysfunction. *Chest* 1994;105(suppl):72S–74S.
4. Rich S, et al.: Antinuclear antibodies in primary pulmonary hypertension. *J Am Coll Cardiol* 1986; 8:1307–1311.

5. Nelson DM, Main E, Crafford W, Ahumada GG : Peripartum heart failureq due to primary pulmonary hypertension. *Obstet Gynecol* 1983;62:58S–63S.
6. Langleben D: Familial primary pulmonary hypertension. *Chest* 1994;105(suppl):13S–16S.
7. Pietra GG: The histology of primary pulmonary hypertension. *Chest* 1994;105(suppl):2S–6S.
8. Mani S, Smith GJW: HIV and pulmonary hypertension. *South Med J* 1994;87:357–362.
9. Robalino BD, Moodie DS: Association between primary pulmonary hypertension and portal hypertension: analysis of its pathophysiology and clinical, laboratory and hemodynamic manifestations. *J Am Coll Cardiol* 1991;17:492–498.
10. Berger M, Haimowitz A, Van Tosh, Berdoff RL, Goldberg E: Quantitative assessment of pulmonary hypertension in patients with tricuspid regurgitation using continuous wave Doppler ultrasound. *J Am Coll Cardiol* 1985;61:359–365.
11. Chen WJ, Chen JJ, Lin SC, Hwang JJ, Lien WP: Detection of cardiovascular shunts by transesophageal echocardiography in patients with pulmonary hypertension of unexplained cause. *Chest* 1995;107:8–13.
12. Rich S, et al.: Primary pulmonary hypertension: radiographic and scintigraphic patterns of histologic subtypes. *Ann Intern Med* 1986;105:499–502.
13. Nicod P, et al.: Pulmonary angiography in severe chronic pulmonary hypertension. *Ann Intern Med* 1987;107:565–568.
14. Sleeper JC, et al.: Primary pulmonary hypertension: review of clinical features and pathologic physiology with a report of pulmonary hemodynamics derived from repeated catheterization. *Circulation* 1962;26:1358–1369.
15. Wasserman K et al.: *Principles of exercise testing and interpretation.* Philadelphia: Lea and Febiger, 1987.
16. Rich S, Kaufmann E, Levy PS: The effect of high doses of calcium-channel blockers on survival in primary pulmonary hypertension. *N Engl J Med* 1992;327:76–81.
17. Rich S: The medical treatment of primary pulmonary hypertension: proven and promising strategies. *Chest* 1994;105(suppl):17S–20S.
18. Butt AY: New therapies for primary pulmonary hypertension. *Chest* 1994;105(suppl):21S–25S.
19. Sitbon O, Brenot F, Denjean A, et al.: Inhaled nitric oxide as a screening vasodilator agent in primary pulmonary hypertension. *Am J Respir Crit Care Med* 1995;151:384–389.
20. D'Alonzo GE, et al.: Survival in patients with primary pulmonary hypertension: results from a national prospective registry. *Ann Intern Med* 1991;115:343–349.
21. Wagenvoort CA, Wagenvoort N, Takahashi T: Pulmonary veno-occlusive disease: involvement of pulmonary arteries and review of the literature. *Hum Pathol* 1985;16:1033–1041.
22. Goldhaber SZ: Thrombolysis for pulmonary embolism. *Prog Cardiovasc Dis* 1991;34:113–134.
23. Ansari A: Acute and chronic pulmonary thromboembolism: current perspectives. Part I: glossary of terms, historic evolution and prevalence. *Clin Cardiol* 1986;9:398–402.
24. Wilson JE III: Pulmonary embolism: diagnosis and treatment. *Clin Notes Respir Dis* 1981;19:3–7.
25. Haeger K: Problems of acute deep venous thrombosis. I. The interpretation of signs and symptoms. *Angiology* 1969;20:219–223.
26. Kakkar VV, et al.: Deep vein thrombosis of the leg: is there a "high risk" group? *Am J Surg* 1980; 120:527–530.
27. Moser KM: Pulmonary embolism: state of the art. *Am Rev Respir Dis* 1977;115:829–852.
28. Bell WR, Simon TL, DeMets DL: The clinical features of submassive and massive pulmonary emboli. *Am J Med* 1977;62:355–360.
29. Hull RP, et al.: Prophylaxis of venous thromboembolism: an overview. *Chest* 1986;89:374S–406S.
30. Carter C, Gent M: The epidemiology of venous thrombosis. In: Coleman RW et al., eds. *Hemostasis and thrombosis: basic principles and clinical practice.* Philadelphia: JB Lippincott, 1982: 805–819.
31. Manucci PM, et al.: Low-dose heparin and deep vein thrombosis after total hip replacement. *Thromb Haemost* 1976;36:157–164.
32. Salzman EW, Hirsh J: Prevention of venous thromboembolism. Coleman RW et al., eds. *Hemostasis and thrombosis: basic principles and clinical practice.* Philadelphia: JB Lippincott, 1982: 986–999.
33. Schafer A: The hypercoagulable states. *Ann Intern Med* 1985;102:814–828.
34. Moser KM, LeMoine JR: Is embolic risk conditioned by location of deep venous thrombosis? *Ann Intern Med* 1981;94:439–444.
35. Kakkar VV et al.: Natural history of post-operative deep venous thrombosis. *Lancet* 1969;2: 230–232.

36. Huisman MV, Buller HR, ten Cate JW, Vreeken J: Serial impedance plethysmography for suspected deep venous thrombosis in outpatients. *N Engl J Med* 1986;828:823–828.
37. McIntyre KM, Sasahara AA: Determinants of right ventricular function and hemodynamics after pulmonary embolism. *Chest* 1974;65:534–543.
38. Tsao MS, Schraufnagel D, Wang NS: Pathogenesis of pulmonary infarction. *Am J Med* 1982; 72:599–608.
39. Wheeler HB: Diagnosis of deep vein thrombosis: review of clinical evaluation and impedance plethysmography. *Am J Surg* 1985;150:7–13.
40. White RH, McGahan JP, Daschbach MM, Hartling RP: Diagnosis of deep vein thrombosis using duplex ultrasound. *Ann Intern Med* 1989;111:297–304.
41. Lensing AWA, Prandoni P, Brandjes D, et al.: Detection of deep-vein thrombosis by real-time B-mode ultrasonography. *N Engl J Med* 1989;320:342–345.
42. Bounameaux H, de Moerloose P, Perrier A, Reber G: Plasma measurements of D-dimer as diagnostic aid in suspected venous thromboembolism: an overview. *Thromb Haemost* 1994;71:1–6.
43. Kasper W, Meinertz T, Henkel B, et al.: Echocardiographic findings in patients with proved pulmonary embolism. *Am Heart J* 1986;112:1284–1290.
44. Remy-Jardin M, Remy J, Wattinne L, Giraud F: Central pulmonary thromboembolism: diagnosis with spiral volumetric CT with the single-breath-hold technique: comparison with pulmonary angiography. *Radiology* 1992;185:381–387.
45. PIOPED Investigators: Value of the ventilation/perfusion scan in acute pulmonary embolism: results of the prospective investigation of pulmonary embolism diagnosis (PIOPED). *JAMA* 1990; 263:2753–2759.
46. Dalen JE, Brooks HL, Johnson LW, et al.: Pulmonary angiography in acute pulmonary embolism: indications, techniques, and results in 367 patients. *Am Heart J* 1971;81:175–185.
47. Cruickshank MK, Levine MN, Hirsh J, Roberts R, Siguenza M: A standard heparin nomogram for the management of heparin therapy. *Arch Intern Med* 1991;151:333–337.
48. Raschke RA, Reilly BM, Guidry JR, Fontana JR, Srinivas S: The weight-based heparin dosing nomogram compared with a "standard care" nomogram: a randomized controlled trial. *Ann Intern Med* 1993;119:874–881.
49. Harenberg J, Huck K, Bratsch H, et al.: Therapeutic application of subcutaneous low-molecular-weight heparin in acute venous thrombosis. *Haemostasis* 1990;20(suppl 1):205–219.
50. Greenfield LJ, Michna BA: Twelve-year clinical experience with the Greenfield vena cava filter. *Surgery* 1988;104:706–712.
51. National Heart, Lung, and Blood Institute: Urokinase pulmonary embolism trial: phase 2 results. *JAMA* 1970;214:2163–2172.
52. Beyth RJ, Cohen AM, Landefeld CS: Long-term outcomes of deep-vein thrombosis. *Arch Intern Med* 1995;155:103–107.
53. Dalen JD, et al.: Resolution rate of pulmonary embolism in man. *N Engl J Med* 1969;280: 1194–1197.
54. Moser KM, Auger WR, Fedullo PF, Jamieson SW: Chronic thromboembolic pulmonary hypertension: clinical picture and surgical treatment. *Eur Respir J* 1992;5:334–342.
55. Moser KM, Bloor CM: Pulmonary vascular lesions occurring in patients with chronic major vessel thromboembolic pulmonary hypertension. *Chest* 1993;103:685–692.
56. Fishman AJ, Moser KM, Fedullo PF: Perfusion lung scan versus pulmonary angiography in evaluation of suspected primary pulmonary hypertension. *Chest* 1983;84:679–683.
57. Ryan KL, Fedullo PF, Davis GB, Vasquez TE, Moser KM: Perfusion findings understate the severity of angiographic and hemodynamic compromise in chronic thromboembolic pulmonary hypertension. *Chest* 1988;93:1180–1185.
58. Levinson RM, Shure D, Moser KM: Reperfusion pulmonary edema after pulmonary artery thromboendarterectomy. *Am Rev Respir Dis* 1986;134:1231–1235.
59. Jawalurz KI, Karpas CM: Pulmonary schistosomiasis: a detailed clinicopatholgical study. *Am Rev Respir Dis* 1965;88:517–524.
60. Robertson CH Jr, Reynolds RC, Wilson JE III: Pulmonary hypertension and foreign body granulomas in intravenous drug abusers. *Am J Med* 1976;61:657–662.
61. Peters JL, Armstrong R, Bradford R, Gelister JK: Air embolism: a serious hazard of central venous catheter systems. *Intensive Care Med* 1984;10:261–262.
62. Yee ES, et al.: Management of air embolism in blunt and penetrating thoracic trauma. *J Thorac Cardiovasc Surg* 1993;85:661–668.
63. Levy DL: The fat embolism syndrome: a review. *Clin Orthop* 1990;261:281–286.

64. Fabian TC: Unraveling the fat embolism syndrome. *N Engl J Med* 1993;329:961–963.
65. Vedrinne JM, Guillaume C, Gagnieu MC, et al.: Bronchoalveolar lavage in trauma patients for diagnosis of fat embolism syndrome. *Chest* 1992;102:1323–1327.
66. Morgan M: Amniotic fluid embolism: a review. *Anesthesiology* 1979;34:20–31.
67. Julander I: Staphylococcal septicaemia and endocarditis in 80 drug addicts. *Scand J Infect Dis* 1983;41:49–54.
68. Hershey CO, Tomford JW, McLaren CE, Porter DK, Cohen DI: The natural history of intravenous catheter-associated phlebitis. *Arch Intern Med* 1984;144:1373–1375.
69. Burke CM, Safai C, Nelson DP, Raffin TA: Pulmonary arteriovenous malformations: a critical update. *Am Rev Respir Dis* 1986;134:334–339.
70. Guttmacher AE, Marchuk DA, White RI Jr: Hereditary hemorrhagic telangiectasia. *N Engl J Med* 1995;333:918–924.
71. Dines DE, Arms RA, Bernatz PE, Gomes MR: Pulmonary arteriovenous fistulas. *Mayo Clinic Proc* 1974;49:460–465.
72. Krowka MJ: Pulmonary aspects of chronic liver disease and liver transplantation. *Mayo Clinic Proc* 1985;60:407–418.
73. White RI Jr, Mitchell SE, Barth KH, Kaufman SL, et al.: Angioarchitecture of pulmonary arteriovenous malformations: an important consideration before embolotherapy. *AJR* 1983;140:681–686.
74. Chilvers ER, Whyte MK, Jackson JE, Allison DJ, Hughes JM: Effect of percutaneous transcatheter embolization on pulmonary function, right-to-left shunt and arterial oxygenation in patients with pulmonary arteriovenous malformations. *Am Rev Respir Dis* 1990;142:420–425.
75. Pennington DW, et al.: Treatment of pulmonary arteriovenous malformations by therapeutic embolism. Rest and exercise physiology in eight patients. *Am Rev Respir Dis* 1992;145:1047–1051.
76. Savic B, et al.: Lung sequestration: report of seven cases and review of 540 published cases. *Thorax* 1979;34:96–101.
77. Zumbro GL, et al.: Pulmonary sequestration: a broad spectrum of bronchopulmonary foregut abnormalities. *Ann Thorac Surg* 1975;20:161–169.
78. Kristo DA, Pluss JL, Chantelois A: Asymptomatic extralobar sequestration in a 43-year-old woman. *South Med J* 1995;88:225–226.
79. Rubin EM, Garcia H, Horowitz MD, Guerra JJ Jr: Fatal massive hemoptysis secondary to intralobar sequestration. *Chest* 1994;106:954–955.
80. Tami LF, McElderry MW: Pulmonary artery aneurysm due to severe congenital pulmonic stenosis: case report and literature review. *Angiology* 1994;45:383–390.
81. Remy J, Lemaitre L, Lafitte JJ, Vilain MO, et al.: Massive hemoptysis of pulmonary arterial origin: diagnosis and treatment. *AJR* 1984;143:963–969.
82. Williams JE, et al.: Pulmonary artery aneurysms. *J Thorac Cardiovasc Surg* 1971;62:63–66.
83. Santelli ED, Katz DS, Golsschmidt AM, Thomas HA: Embolization of multiple Rasmussen aneurysms as a treatment of hemoptysis. *Radiology* 1994;193:396–398.

18

Pulmonary Rehabilitation

Bartolome R. Celli

The Council of Rehabilitation has stated that the goal of rehabilitation is the restoration of the individual's maximum possible medical, mental, emotional, social, and vocational potential. Rehabilitation programs must be *individualized*, tailored to the needs of each patient. Variations in therapy from one patient to another make objective evaluation and comparison of different rehabilitation programs very difficult.

I. Definition, objectives, and goals of pulmonary rehabilitation

    A. Definition

        1. Pulmonary rehabilitation is a broad therapeutic concept that has recently been redefined by an National Institutes of Health workshop (1) as "A multidisciplinary continuum of services directed to persons with pulmonary diseases and their families, usually by an interdisciplinary team of specialists, with the goal of achieving and maintaining the individual's maximum level of independence and functioning in the community."

        2. Because pulmonary rehabilitation is multidisciplinary and utilizes different therapeutic components, it is difficult to attribute improved global outcomes to the effect of individual elements of a program. Independent of the study design used, conventional measurements of pulmonary function have failed to reveal any changes after pulmonary rehabilitation.

    B. Objectives. Pulmonary rehabilitation has two major objectives:

        1. Control, alleviate, and reverse the symptoms and pathophysiologic processes leading to respiratory impairment.

        2. Improve the patient's quality of life, and attempt to prolong survival.

    C. Goals. In the broadest sense, pulmonary rehabilitation attempts to provide good, comprehensive respiratory care for patients with pulmonary disease (2,3). Practically, comprehensive care is best provided by a multidisciplinary approach through a structured *rehabilitation program*. The goals of such a program are listed in Table 18-1.

    D. Benefits. Although the mechanism by which pulmonary rehabilitation may be effective remains debatable, a consensus exists that a comprehensive rehabilitation program improves the quality of life and the capacity to complete daily activities (3,4). Certain modalities of therapy have been shown to prolong life (oxygen therapy) (5,6) and diminish the rate of decline of lung function (smoking cessation) (7,8). Others, like exercise conditioning, are associated with an improved lifestyle, while patient and family education often increase cooperation and compliance. Each of these modalities likely has a role in the beneficial outcomes of pulmonary rehabilitation.

II. Components of pulmonary rehabilitation

    A. Patient selection

        1. Any individual with symptomatic respiratory disease is a candidate for rehabilitation. Patients with moderate to moderately severe disease are preferentially chosen for rehabilitation. The intense effort and cost of a rehabilitation program may not be justified for persons with mild disease. Severely compromised individuals cannot perform the tasks necessary to benefit from the program. Factors that may hinder the ultimate success of rehabilitation include the presence of other disabling diseases such as severe heart failure or arthritis, the pa-

Table 18-1. Practical goals of a pulmonary rehabilitation program

Reduce work of breathing
Improve pulmonary function
Normalize arterial blood gases
Alleviate dyspnea
Increase efficiency of energy utilization
Correct nutrition
Improve exercise performance and activities of daily living
Restore a positive outlook in patients
Improve emotional state
Decrease health-related costs
Improve survival

tient's educational level, a lack of family support or other resources, and, above all, a lack of patient motivation.

2. While patients with cancer are not generally considered candidates for rehabilitation, selected patients with limited exercise performance who are under consideration for surgery may be entered. Pulmonary rehabilitation may also be used for the preoperative conditioning of patients undergoing lung transplantation or lung volume reduction surgery.

B. **Components of a pulmonary rehabilitation program.** Pulmonary rehabilitation programs require a coordinator to organize the following components into a functioning unit:

1. An **educational program** that teaches the basics of respiratory anatomy and physiology, respiratory pathophysiology, and concepts of therapy.
2. Teaching of **practical respiratory therapy** (equipment and techniques).
3. **Physical therapy** (breathing techniques, chest physical therapy, postural drainage).
4. **Exercise conditioning** of both upper and lower extremities to increase the ability to perform activities of daily living (work simplification, energy conservation).
5. Ability to evaluate nutritional, psychological, and vocational needs (2,9).

C. **Structure of the program.** The decision whether to have an inpatient or an outpatient program depends on several factors, including reimbursement, patient population, available personnel, and hospital policy. The ideal program would include an in-hospital arm that allows a patient to begin the program while recovering from an acute illness in the hospital, followed by an outpatient arm that completes the program. This arrangement helps assure continuity of care. Recent evidence also suggests the benefits of *at-home* rehabilitation (1).

III. **Therapeutic modalities involved in pulmonary rehabilitation**

A. **Modalities that increase survival**

1. **Smoking cessation** (Chapter 31). Tobacco dependence occurs by a mechanism similar to that of other substances such as alcohol or drugs (10). Therefore, treatment programs for cigarette smoking employ the same strategies that have been successful in the treatment of drug-dependent persons and should be an integral part of a comprehensive pulmonary rehabilitation program. The typical success rate of smoking cessation programs at 1 year after treatment varies from 14% to 35% (10,11). Some question whether patients who smoke should be included in a rehabilitation program. We have not denied the beneficial effects of a comprehensive program solely on the basis of continuation of smoking.

a. **Smoking cessation treatment** should be individualized and should begin with the first physician contact. Clinical counseling rendered through a smoking cessation program can help most patients to consider quitting or to actually quit. The physician can reinforce concepts and help sustain an initial success and avoid frequent relapses. Most patients in a smoking cessation program will abstain temporarily but will resume smoking with time. Those who stop abruptly (cold turkey) within the first 2 weeks of a program are less likely to relapse than those who gradually reduce (taper) consumption. Therefore, programs should aim for complete cessation of smoking at a specific date and time that is mutually agreed on.

    b. The high tendency to relapse (60% to 70%) underscores the importance of follow-up mechanisms, including reminders and repeated telephone conversations with close physician reinforcement.

    c. The addition of nicotine substitution through patches or gum increases the success rates of comprehensive programs (12). Nicotine substitution should never be used as the single therapeutic modality. Self-help packages available from the American Lung Association can be used as a supplement. Besides improving pulmonary function, abstinence from cigarettes results in decreased influenza infections, as well as a reduction in pulmonary symptoms such as cough and phlegm. The beneficial effects on other organs, such as the oropharynx, upper airways, heart, and urinary tract, are also well recognized and provide further reasons to promote abstinence.

2. **Oxygen therapy.** Oxygen therapy has been shown to prolong life in hypoxemic patients with severe chronic airflow obstruction (5,6). Hypoxemia is frequently secondary to ventilation–perfusion mismatching and thereby amenable to correction by oxygen administration. A Pa_{O_2} <60 mm Hg has been shown to induce pulmonary hypertension that may result in fixed hypertenson if chronically sustained. Lower Pa_{O_2} levels lead to erythropoietin release and secondary polycythemia; increased blood viscosity worsens vascular resistance, heart failure, and decreases cerebrovascular perfusion. Furthermore, since a Pa_{O_2} of 60 mm Hg is on the shoulder of the oxyhemoglobin dissociation curve, further small drops with exercise or with sleep can result in profound hypoxemic events with severe consequences such as ventricular arrhythmias or cardiac ischemia.

    a. The evaluation of patients for continuous oxygen therapy is discussed in detail in chapter 35. Arterial blood gases should be assessed during stable maintenance on optimal medical therapy. If the Pa_{O_2} is ≤55 mm Hg, continuous (24-hour) supplemental oxygen is recommended. If the Pa_{O_2} is 55–59 mm Hg and the patient has polycythemia, heart failure, or "P" pulmonale on electrocardiogram, supplemental oxygen to raise the Pa_{O_2} to >60 mm Hg is indicated. Since increasing the Pa_{O_2} may induce hypoventilation in these individuals, blood gases should be measured during oxygen therapy to insure adequate oxygen dosing. Since patients with chronic obstructive pulmonary disease (COPD) and adequate resting Pa_{O_2} may develop hypoxemia during exercise or sleep, they may require long-term supplemental oxygen only during these activities. Like any other drug, oxygen should be titrated according to individual needs. The actual method of oxygen administration varies; nasal cannulas are the most accepted modality.

    b. The recent introduction of the technique of **transtracheal oxygen** administration using a small transtracheal catheter has gained some popularity because it is cosmetically more appealing and makes patients feel better. While the work of breathing is reduced, this technique is associated with significant complications such as mucous balls and infection.

    c. Other oxygen-conserving devices that may include reservoirs deliver oxygen only during inspiration, thereby decreasing oxygen waste and prolonging the useful life of oxygen tanks (see chapter 34). Since the objective of rehabilitation is optimal patient independence, any system that helps achieve this goal is worthwhile.

    d. Oxygen may be supplied in the form of cylinders of compressed gas or liquid oxygen or by an electrically powered concentrator. Care must be taken to provide each patient with the dose, delivery system, and supply method to allow maximal exercise capacity. The patient and the family must be instructed on the long-term goals of oxygen therapy, as well as the importance of compliance, particularly since the symptoms may not be immediately relieved and the benefits may not be noticeable in the short term (13).

B. Modalities that improve performance

1. Exercise conditioning. Exercise conditioning is based on three physiologic principles: training specificity, which improves performance of only the muscles used in the exercise practiced; training intensity, by which only a load higher than baseline will induce a training effect; and training reversal, whereby training effects disappear over time with discontinuation of the exercise. The first two have been extensively applied in the rehabilitation of patients with COPD. Little is known about the long-term follow-up of patients who have completed rehabilitation or whether maintenance exercise programs are efficacious in these patients.

2. Lower extremity exercise. Casaburi (14) pooled the results of 36 uncontrolled studies with over 900 patients with COPD that evaluated the effect of endurance training on exercise capacity and demonstrated that aerobic training resulted in an increase in exercise endurance. This observation is supported by the results of eight controlled trials (15–22). Further, O'Hara et al. (20) enrolled 14 patients with COPD in a home program to evaluate the effect of strength training on exercise capacity. The individuals in this study were randomized to daily walking while carrying a light backpack (controls) or to the same regime with additional weightlifting (wrist and arms curls, partial leg squats, calf raises, and supine dumbbell press). After training, the weightlifting group experienced reduced minute ventilation and an increased ergometry endurance (16%), when compared with the control group. This study suggested that strength training can achieve results similar to those of specific endurance training. A recent European trial confirmed that exercise training can be successfully implemented at home (21).

a. The mechanism by which exercise improves endurance remains unclear. Since lung and respiratory muscle function does not objectively change, a mechanical explanation is very unlikely. As exercise training progresses, patients with COPD may become desensitized to the dyspnea induced by the ventilatory load. This hypothesis is supported by studies, such as the one by Belman and Kendregan (23). These authors randomized patients to upper or lower extremity exercise, and muscle biopsies of the trained limbs were obtained before and after training. In spite of a significant increase in exercise endurance, no changes in the oxidative enzyme content of the trained muscle were noted. In contrast, support for a true training effect is provided by the study of Casaburi et al. (24), which showed a reduction in exercise lactic acidosis proportional to the intensity of the training and a reduction in minute ventilation after training.

b. Patients with severe COPD have been shown to accrue benefits from lower extremity exercise training. ZuWallack et al. (25) evaluated 50 individuals with COPD whose forced expiratory volume in 1 second (FEV_1) ranged from 0.38 L to 3.24 L before exercise training; in FEV_1 measurements after exercise, they found an inverse relationship between the baseline 12-minute walk distance and oxygen uptake.

3. Upper extremity exercise. Most knowledge of exercise conditioning is unfortunately derived from programs utilizing leg training, even though the performance of many everyday tasks requires not only the hands but also the concerted action of other muscle groups used in positioning the upper torso and arms. Some of these serve a dual function (respiratory and postural); thus, arm exercises will decrease the capacity of the shoulder girdle muscles to participate in ventilation (26). These observations suggest that if the arms are trained to perform more work or if the ventilatory requirement for the same work is decreased, the capacity to perform activities of daily living would be improved. Several studies have shown that arm training results in improved performance, which for the most part is task specific (26–30), and may be a more effective way to train COPD patients to perform activities that resemble those of daily living.

C. **Physical modalities.** These modalities consist of controlled-breathing techniques (diaphragmatic breathing exercise, pursed-lip breathing, and bending forward) and chest physical therapy (postural drainage, chest percussion, and vibration position). The former are aimed at decreasing dyspnea and the latter at enhancing drainage of secretions. The benefits of these modalities include less dyspnea, increased exercise tolerance, decreased anxiety and panic attacks, and an improved sense of well-being. Careful instruction by specialists that have familiarity with the techniques is required. These modalities should be initiated as soon as possible and repeated often with close supervision until the patient shows a thorough understanding of the techniques. Most of these modalities require two persons (eg, chest percussion), and therefore the involvement of family members is critical.

1. **Breathing training.** Breathing training employs techniques aimed at controlling the respiratory rate and breathing pattern, thereby decreasing air trapping and the work of breathing and improving the position and mechanical function of the diaphragm and other muscles of respiration (31).

   a. **Pursed-lip breathing** is the easiest of these methods; patients inhale through the nose and exhale over a 4–6-second interval through lips pursed in a whistling or kissing position. Reflex elevation of the levator palatini can cause occlusion of the nasopharynx, and air is exhaled by the mouth. The exact mechanism by which this technique decreases dyspnea is unknown. Functional residual capacity and oxygen uptake are not changed, but respiratory frequency is decreased, while tidal volume increases.

   b. **Bending-forward posture** has been shown to result in a decrease in dyspnea in some patients with severe COPD, both at rest and during exercise. These changes can also be seen in the supine or Trendelenburg's position. Recent observations indicate that diaphragmatic function improves as the increased gastric pressure in these positions places the diaphragm in a better contracting position to decrease the use of accessory muscles and reduce dyspnea. Most patients report symptomatic improvement, including reduced dyspnea.

   c. **Diaphragmatic breathing** is a technique aimed at changing the breathing pattern from one in which the rib cage muscles are the predominant pressure generators to a more normal one where pressures are generated with the diaphragm. This training technique has to be taught by a skilled individual and must be practiced for at least 20 minutes two to three times daily. The patient should start training in the supine position and advance to the upright posture. Patients are instructed to inspire while attempting to outwardly displace a hand that is placed on the abdomen. Patients then exhale through pursed lips while using abdominal musculature to return the diaphragm to a more lengthened resting position. Four to ten pounds of abdominal weight may help assist the training by increasing muscle strength. The respiratory rate and minute ventilation usually fall, and the tidal volume usually increases. It must be emphasized that although most patients report improvement in dyspnea, this technique results in minimal, if any, changes in oxygen uptake and resting lung volume and no improvement in gas exchange. Recent reports actually suggest that the work of breathing might actually be increased. More research is needed to understand the mechanical effects of this technique.

2. **Chest physical therapy.** The goal of these techniques is to remove airway secretions, thereby decreasing airflow resistance and the possibility of bronchopulmonary infection. Techniques include postural drainage, chest percussion, chest vibration, and directed cough.

   a. **Postural drainage** uses gravity to help drain the individual lung segments. The position angles range from 10° to 50°, but some patients become dyspneic when placed in very acute angles. Fortunately, most patients with COPD will tolerate a 10–20° decrement from the horizontal without important changes in lung volume and oxygen saturation. This angle can be comfortably obtained at home by employing pillows on the floor or on the bed. Physical therapy should be done in several positions for a total of 20–30 minutes twice daily. Most benefit will occur in the morning. Coupled with adequate hydration (2–3 L/d) and inhalation of bronchodilators, postural drainage can result in an increase in sputum removal.

b. **Percussion** is performed by gently striking the rib cage with cupped hands or by using a mechanical percussor. It should be taught by a specialist familiar with the technique and should be administered by a trained person for 2–5 minutes over the area of the chest that is thought to benefit from the drainage. Care must be taken in patients with osteoporosis or bone problems. Vibrations can be applied with the use of crossed hands as pressure is applied over a drainage zone, or a mechanical vibrator using a 10–20 Hz vibrating frequency. This frequency is within the range of the ciliary beating rhythm of the respiratory epithelium and is thought to result in a significant increase in sputum clearance.

c. **Cough** is also an effective technique for removing excess mucus from the larger airways. Unfortunately, patients with COPD have impaired cough mechanisms, maximum expiratory flow is reduced, ciliary beat is impaired, and the mucus itself has altered viscoelastic properties. Since cough spasms may lead to dyspnea, fatigue, and worsened obstruction, directed cough may be helpful by modulating the beneficial effect and preventing the untoward ones. With controlled coughs, patients are instructed to inhale deeply, hold their breath for a few seconds, and then cough two or three times with mouth open. They are also instructed to compress their upper abdomen to assist in the cough. Two of these maneuvers are then followed by a 3 minute resting period before the cough is repeated again.

d. The results of all these maneuvers are difficult to ascertain. It seems clear that pulmonary functions do not improve with any of these techniques. On the other hand, programs that include a combination of postural drainage, percussion, vibration, and cough do increase the clearance of inhaled radiotracers and increase sputum volume and weight. The single most important criterion that suggests a need for these techniques is the presence of important sputum production.

IV. **Ventilatory muscle training.** Leith and Bradley (32) first demonstrated that, like their skeletal counterparts, the respiratory muscles of normal individuals could be specifically trained to improve their strength or endurance. Following that observation, multiple studies have shown that a training response will occur if there is enough of a stimulus. An increase in inspiratory muscle strength (and perhaps endurance) should result in improved respiratory muscle function. Since reduced inspiratory muscle strength is evident in patients with COPD, considerable effort has been made to define the role of respiratory muscle training in these patients. The extensive data available indicate that ventilatory muscle training with resistive breathing results in improved ventilatory muscle strength and endurance and has marginal effects on overall exercise performance. It is not clear whether this effort results in decreased morbidity or mortality or offers any other clinical advantage.

A. **Strength training.** Inspiratory muscles are trained by performing inspiratory maneuvers against a closed glottis or shutter. Studies have shown an increase in maximal inspiratory pressures when the respiratory muscles have been specifically trained for strength (33). However, respiratory muscle strength has also been shown to increase as a byproduct of endurance training. It is therefore possible that some of the observed benefits reported after endurance training may relate to increased strength.

B. **Endurance training.** Flow-resistive loading, threshold loading, and voluntary isocapneic hyperpnea have been used to endurance-train the respiratory muscles.

1. **Flow-resistive loading.** The load consists of breath-holding at different resistive loads. Frequency, tidal volume, and inspiratory time are held constant. Although most studies in patients with COPD have shown an improvement in the time that a given respiratory load can be maintained (ventilatory muscle en-

durance), the results have to be interpreted with caution since endurance can be increased with changes in the pattern of breathing.

2. **Threshold loading** is a method where the inspired pressure is high enough to ensure training independent of inspiratory flow rate. When threshold devices are used, the breathing pattern (inspiratory time and respiratory rate) is not critically important. Many studies of threshold training have been uncontrolled, so that results are very difficult to interpret. Several controlled studies have shown an increase in the endurance time that the ventilatory muscles could tolerate a known load (34–41). Some have shown a significant increase in strength and a decrease in dyspnea during inspiratory load and exercise. In the studies in which systemic exercise performance was evaluated, there was a minimal increase in walking distance. The pressure required to achieve training has to exceed 30% of maximal inspiratory pressure (34,41).

V. **Respiratory muscle resting.** Pertinent to rehabilitation is the concept of respiratory muscle resting in patients with severe COPD whose diaphragm is thought to be near or at fatigue.

   A. The use of **negative-pressure body-respiratory** (iron lung) **ventilation** or **facial** (nasal or mouth) **positive-pressure ventilation** results in a decrease in the electric activity of the diaphragm and other respiratory muscles. If respiratory muscle resting is to be considered, the specialist should be very familiar with the technique.

   B. Ventilated patients may complain of claustrophobia, back pain, and anxiety. All patients to be placed on noninvasive nasal positive-pressure ventilation (NPPV) should have a sleep study, since some patients may develop upper airway obstruction while ventilated. Experience suggests that the COPD patients who may benefit from NPPV are those with very low FEV_1 (<30% predicted) who have hypercapnia ($Paco_2$ >45 Torr) and manifest clinical evidence of diaphragmatic fatigue (tachypnea of 30 breaths per minute or chest–abdomen dyssynchrony).

VI. **Nutritional evaluation.** It has long been perceived that many patients with severe emphysema are cachectic. These individuals not only are thinner than normal controls but may also be protein-calorie malnourished. Poor nutrition has been shown to adversely influence lung repair after injury and reduce the mechanical capabilities of the ventilatory muscles.

   A. Most authorities agree that an attempt should be made to correct nutritional deficiencies that may be present. Correction of factors such as anemia (to improve oxygen carrying capacity) and electrolyte imbalances (sodium, potassium, phosphorous, and magnesium) could result in improved cardiopulmonary performance. Similarly, simple measures such as encouraging patients to take small amounts of food at more frequent intervals would result in less abdominal distention and may decrease the frequent complaint of dyspnea after meals.

   B. Evaluating oxygen saturation during meals might also be recommended. If desaturation occurs with meals, supplementary oxygen should be added at that time. Finally, it is theoretically possible that meals high in carbohydrates result in increased carbon dioxide production that in turn increases minute ventilation and decreases exercise tolerance. It has been suggested that high carbohydrate meals may increase the risk of ventilatory failure in patients with severely compromised states. This is not a frequent problem in stable patients undergoing rehabilitation.

VII. **Psychological support.** Most patients with severe lung disease experience psychological problems, mainly reactive depression and anxiety. Fortunately, these problems are likely to improve as the patients become involved in a rehabilitation program that improves physical performance. Simple measures such as being able to exercise under the supervision of supportive specialists frequently results in reduced symptoms. Breathing retraining allows the patient to be in a position to have some control of the variables that induce dyspnea. The setting of reasonable goals and their achievement improves self-image. It has been shown that 15–20 rehabilitation sessions that include education, exercise, the use of modalities of physical therapy, breathing techniques, and relaxation are more effective in reducing anxiety than a similar number of psychotherapy sessions (42). Occasionally, patients will have major psychological problems that will require primary psychiatric evaluation and treatment.

References

1. Pulmonary rehabilitation research. N.I.H. workshop summary. *Am Rev Respir Dis* 1994;49:825.
2. Petty T, Nett LM, Finigan MM, et al.: A comprehensive program for chronic airway obstruction: methods and preliminary evaluation of symptomatic and functional improvement. *Ann Intern Med* 1969;70:1109.
3. Celli BR: Pulmonary rehabilitation. *Am J Respir Crit Care Med* 1995;152:361–364.
4. Make BJ: Pulmonary rehabilitation: myth or reality? *Clin Chest Med* 1986;7:519–540.
5. Medical Research Council Working Party: Long-term domiciliary oxygen therapy in chronic hypoxic cor pulmonale complicating chronic bronchitis and emphysema. *Lancet* 1981;1:681–686.
6. Nocturnal Oxygen Therapy Trial Group: Continuous or nocturnal oxygen therapy in hypoxemic chronic obstructive lung diseases: a clinical trial. *Ann Intern Med* 1980;92:391–398.
7. Buist AS, Sexton GJ, Nagy JM, Ross BB: The effect of smoking cessation and modification on lung function. *Am Rev Respir Dis* 1976;114:115–122.
8. Anthonisen N, Connet J, Kiley J, et al.: The effect of smoking intervention and the use of an inhaled anticholinergic bronchodilator on the rate of decline in FEV_1: the Lung Health Study. *JAMA* 1994;272:14971–15055.
9. Hodgkin JE, Connors GL, Bell C: *Pulmonary rehabilitation: guidelines to success*, 2nd ed. Philadelphia: JB Lippincott, 1993.
10. Herningfield JE, Nemeth-Coslet R: Nicotine dependence: interface between tobacco and tobacco-related disease. *Chest* 1988;93:375–555.
11. Koltke TE, Battista R, Del Friese G: Attributes of successful smoking cessation interventions in medical practice: a meta-analysis of 39 controlled trials. *JAMA* 1988;259:2882–2889.
12. Prochaska J, Goldstein M: Process of smoking cessation. *Clin Chest Med* 1991;12:7267–7354.
13. Celli BR: Long-term oxygen therapy. *N Eng J Med* 1995;333:710–714.
14. Casaburi R: Exercise training in chronic obstructive lung disease. In: Casaburi R, Petty TL, eds. *Principles and practice of pulmonary rehabilitation*. Philadelphia: WB Saunders, 1993.
15. Crockoft AE, Saunders MJ, Berry G: Randomized controlled trial of rehabilitation in chronic respiratory disability. *Thorax* 1981;36:2003.
16. Sinclair DJ, Ingram CG: Controlled trial of supervised exercise training in chronic bronchitis. *BMJ* 1980;1:519.
17. Reardon J, Awad E, Normandin E, et al.: The effect of comprehensive outpatient pulmonary rehabilitation on dyspnea. *Chest* 1994;105:1046.
18. O'Donnell DE, Webb HA, McGuire MA: Older patients with COPD: benefits of exercise training. *Geriatrics* 1993;48:59.
19. Ries AL, Kaplan R, Linberg T, Prewitt L: Effects of pulmonary rehabilitation on physiologic and psychosocial outcomes in patients with chronic obstructive pulmonary disease. *Ann Intern Med* 1995;122;823–832.
20. O'Hara WJ, Lasachuk BP, Matheson P, et al.: Weight training and backpacking in chronic obstructive pulmonary disease. *Respir Care* 1984;29:1202.
21. Wykstra PJ, Van Altens R, Kraan J, et al.: Quality of life in patients with chronic obstructive pulmonary disease improves after rehabilitation at home. *Eur Respir J* 1994;7:269.
22. Goldstein RS, Gork EH, Stubbing D, et al.: Randomized controlled trial of respiratory rehabilitation. *Lancet* 1994;344:1394.
23. Belman M, Kendregan BE: Exercise training fails to increase skeletal muscle enzymes in patients with chronic obstructive pulmonary disease. *Am Rev Respir Dis* 1981;123:256.
24. Casaburi R, Patessio A, Joli F, et al.: Reductions in exercise lactic acidosis and ventilation as a result of exercise training in patients with obstructive lung disease. *Am Rev Respir Dis* 1991;143:9.
25. ZuWallack RL, Patel K, Reardon JZ, et al.: Predictors of improvement in the 12-minute walking distance following a six-week outpatient pulmonary rehabilitation program. *Chest* 1991;99:805.
26. Celli BR: The clinical use of upper extremity exercise. *Clin Chest Med* 1994;15:339.
27. Ries AL, Ellis B, Hawkins RW: Upper extremity exercise training in chronic obstructive pulmonary disease. *Chest* 1988;93:688.
28. Keens TG, Krastins IR, Wannamaker EM, et al.: Ventilatory muscle endurance training in normal subjects and patients with cystic fibrosis. *Am Rev Respir Dis* 1977;116:853.
29. Lake ER, Henderson K, Briffa T, et al.: Upper limb and lower limb exercise training in patients with chronic airflow obstruction. *Chest* 1990;97:1077.

30. Martinez FJ, Vogel PD, Dupont DN, et al.: Supported arm exercise vs. unsupported arm exercise in the rehabilitation of patients with chronic airflow obstruction. *Chest* 1993;103:1397.
31. Faling LJ: Pulmonary rehabilitation: physical modalities. *Clin Chest Med* 1986;7:599–618.
32. Leith DE, Bradley M: Ventilatory muscle strength and endurance training. *J Appl Physiol* 1976; 4:508.
33. Reid WD, Warren CP: Ventilatory muscle strength and endurance training in elderly subjects and patients with chronic airflow limitation: a pilot study. *Physio Canada* 1984;36:305.
34. Larson JL, Kim MJ, Sharp JT: Inspiratory muscle training with a pressure threshold breathing device in patients with chronic obstructive pulmonary disease. *Am Rev Respir Dis* 1988;138:689.
35. Harver A, Mahler D, Daubenspeck J: Targeted inspiratory muscle training improves respiratory muscle function and reduces dyspnea in patients with chronic obstructive pulmonary disease. *Ann Intern Med* 1989;111:117.
36. Belman M, Shadmehr R: Targeted resistive ventilatory muscle training in chronic obstructive pulmonary disease. *J Appl Physiol* 1988;65:2726.
37. Noseda A, Carpiaux J, Vandeput N, et al.: Resistive inspiratory muscle training and exercise performance in COPD patients: a comparative study with conventional breathing retraining. *Bull Eur Physiopathol Respir* 1987;23:457.
38. Weiner P, Azgad Y, Ganam R: Inspiratory muscle training combined with general exercise conditioning in patients with COPD. *Chest* 1992;102:1351.
39. Belman M, Mittman C: Ventilatory muscle training improves exercise capacity in chronic obstructive pulmonary disease patients. *Am Rev Respir Dis* 1980;121:273.
40. Wanke T, Formanek D, Lahrmann H, et al.: Effects of combined inspiratory muscle and cycle ergometer training on exercise performance in patients with COPD. *Eur Respir J* 1994;7:2205.
41. Lisboa C, Munoz V, Beroiza T, et al.: Inspiratory muscle training in chronic airflow limitation: comparison of two different training loads with a threshold device *Eur Respir J* 1994;7:1266.
42. Lustig FM, Hass A, Castillo R: Clinical and rehabilitation regimen in patients with COPD. *Arch Phys Med Rehabil* 1972;53:315–322.

19 Acute and Chronic Respiratory Failure

Charles Andrew Powell and
Martin F. Joyce-Brady

I. **Acute respiratory failure** is a sudden and life-threatening deterioration in the gas exchange function of the lung. Gas exchange can be directly assessed by measurement of arterial blood gases: the partial pressures of oxygen (Pao_2) and carbon dioxide ($Paco_2$), together with pH. Acute respiratory failure is defined as a Pao_2 <50 mm Hg or a $Paco_2$ >50 mm Hg with an arterial pH <7.35. Acute respiratory failure requires immediate intervention to correct or compensate for the gas exchange abnormality and identify the cause.

   A. **Presentation**
   1. Acute respiratory failure can present in multiple ways, varying from acute respiratory distress to acute delirium to coma. Frequent presenting symptoms include dyspnea, fatigue, and headache.
   2. Frequent signs include bradypnea (respiratory rate <8) or tachypnea (respiratory rate >20), altered mental status (somnolence, delirium, agitation), sternal retraction, nasal flaring, cyanosis (peripheral or central), and abnormal breath sounds (wheezes, rhonchi, or rales).

   B. **Physiology of acute respiratory failure**
   1. The lung functions to exchange gas between the blood and the lung alveoli. The partial pressure of carbon dioxide in the mixed venous blood ($Pvco_2$) exceeds that of the alveolus; hence, CO_2 diffuses from the blood to the alveolus. Alveolar CO_2 is then eliminated to the atmosphere by lung ventilation. The partial pressure of O_2 in mixed venous blood (Pvo_2) is less than that of the alveolus; hence, O_2 diffuses from the alveolus into the blood. The pressures of these gases may be measured in arterial blood.
   2. The **normal** $Paco_2$ is 40 mm Hg (range 36–44 mm Hg). This level is tightly regulated by the central nervous system. Inadequate CO_2 elimination is defined as a $Paco_2$ >44 mm Hg (hypercarbia). Excessive CO_2 elimination is defined as a $Paco_2$ <36 mm Hg (hypocarbia). The normal Pao_2 is 98–99 mm Hg and is a function of the partial pressure of O_2 in the alveoli (Pao_2), the ability of O_2 to diffuse into the blood of lung capillaries, and the ability of the lung to match ventilation and perfusion (V/Q ratio).
   3. **The adequacy of O_2 exchange can be assessed by calculation of the alveolar-arterial difference for O_2 (A-a)Do_2.** This may be done by first calculating the Pao_2 using the **alveolar air equation:**

   $$Pao_2 = Fio_2 (Pb - P_{H_2O}) - 1.25 (Paco_2)$$

   Since $Paco_2 = Paco_2$, the latter value may be obtained directly from blood gas measurements. The Pao_2 is also obtained directly from blood gas measurements. The (A-a)O_2 is then calculated:

   $$(A-a)O_2 = \text{calculated } Pao_2 - \text{measured } Pao_2$$

   The normal **(A-a)O_2 ≤10 mm Hg** is due to a combination of V/Q mismatch in the normal lung and venous admixture into the left atrium from bronchial veins of the airways and the thebesian veins of the heart. A value of $(A\text{-}a)O_2$ **>10 mm Hg** suggests the presence of pulmonary disease.

4. **The adequacy of O_2 delivery to tissues depends on the arterial O_2 content (Cao_2),** which in turn depends on the oxyhemoglobin dissociation curve. The Pao_2 of arterial blood influences the arterial O_2 content by determining the amount of O_2 bound to hemoglobin and the amount dissolved in blood.

$$Cao_2 \text{ (mL } O_2/dL) = \text{dissolved } O_2 + \text{oxyhemoglobin}$$

$$\text{Dissolved } O_2 \text{ (mL } O_2/dL) = Pao_2 \times 0.003 \text{ mL } O_2/dL \text{ blood/mm Hg}$$

Dissolved O_2 only accounts for 0.3 mL of O_2/dL of blood when the Pao_2 is 100 mm Hg. This would equal only 3 mL O_2/L of arterial blood. If the human body relied solely on this level of dissolved O_2, the cardiac output would have to be about 80 L/min to meet normal resting O_2 consumption requirements! Instead, hemoglobin functions as the main carrier of O_2 in the blood; the oxyhemoglobin dissociation curve relates the O_2 saturation of hemoglobin to the Pao_2. The oxyhemoglobin content of blood is calculated as

$$\text{Oxyhemoglobin} = 1.34 \times \% \text{ hemoglobin saturation} \times [\text{hemoglobin}]$$

This value is about 19.9 mL O_2/dL of blood when hemoglobin is 99% saturated with O_2 and is 15 g/dL. Hence, the O_2 content of normal arterial blood is

$$Cao_2 = 0.3 + 19.9 = 20.2 \text{ mL } O_2/dL \text{ blood}$$

and oxyhemoglobin accounts for 98.5% of the Cao_2.

a. As the Pao_2 falls, Cao_2 will be reduced and result in **hypoxemia**. For example, if the Pao_2 falls to 75 mm Hg, the $Cao_2 = 0.23 + 19.3 = 19.5$ mL O_2/dL blood. The Pao_2 has fallen by approximately 25%, but the Cao_2 has fallen only about 3% due to the **sigmoid shape of oxyhemoglobin dissociation** (Fig. 19-1).

b. The hemoglobin saturation ranges from 90% to 100% over the range of Pao_2 from 55 mm Hg to 100 mm Hg. As Pao_2 falls to <55 mm Hg, the oxyhemoglobin dissociation curve begins to steeply descend, and hemoglobin

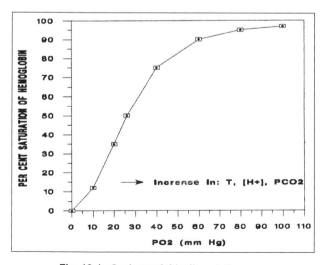

Fig. 19-1. Oxyhemoglobin dissociation curve.

saturation falls rapidly with further decreases in Pa_{O_2}. Hence, reductions in Ca_{O_2} will be mild until the Pa_{O_2} falls to <55 mm Hg, the inflection point of the oxyhemoglobin dissociation curve. When the Pa_{O_2} falls to <50 mm Hg, the reduction in the Ca_{O_2} becomes severe and life threatening.

C. **Respiratory failure and hypoxemia** result from five different pathogenetic mechanisms that can be distinguished by their effects on the A-a gradient.

   1. **Reductions in Pa_{O_2} associated with a normal A-a gradient, due to either a decrease in the ambient concentration of O_2 or $F_{I}O_2$** (mechanism 1) or to **alveolar hypoventilation that produces hypercarbia** (mechanism 2). In this circumstance, the Pa_{CO_2} increases by almost exactly the same amount as the Pa_{O_2} falls, and the sum total of both partial pressures in the alveoli does not change. Pa_{O_2} will fall by the same amount as does Pa_{O_2}, so the A-a gradient will not change. This type of respiratory failure is therefore not due to an intrinsic gas exchange problem or to parenchymal lung disease.

   2. **Reduced Pa_{O_2} associated with an increased A-a gradient suggests an intrinsic problem with gas exchange in the lung from either an increased barrier for O_2 diffusion, an increase in V/Q mismatch, or an increase in the fraction of cardiac output traversing a right-to-left shunt (shunt fraction [Q_s/Q_t]).**

      a. **V/Q mismatch is the most common cause of hypoxemia in acute respiratory failure** (mechanism 3). V/Q mismatch is accentuated in the diseased lung. In areas where this ratio approaches zero, Pa_{CO_2} and Pa_{O_2} mirror values found in mixed venous blood; in other areas where the V/Q ratio is high, the Pa_{CO_2} and Pa_{O_2} resemble end-capillary blood in lung alveoli.

      b. **Increased Q_s/Q_t is an extreme of V/Q mismatch where the V/Q ratio = 0** (mechanism 4) and may be seen in the settings of severe pneumonia, pulmonary edema, adult respiratory distress syndrome, arteriovenous malformations, and intracardiac right-to-left shunting. V/Q mismatch may be distinguished from a true increase in the Q_s/Q_t by measuring the response of hypoxemia to increasing $F_{I}O_2$ (1). **Hypoxemia from V/Q mismatch will correct when breathing 100% O_2; hypoxemia from shunt will not correct.**

         i.   The Q_s/Q_t is that proportion of blood that enters the left atrium without passing through oxygenated lung alveoli. The Q_s/Q_t can be calculated from the O_2 content of arterial blood (Ca_{O_2}), mixed venous blood (Cv_{O_2}), and end-capillary blood ($Cc_{I}O_2$) according to the equation:

         $$Q_s/Q_t = Cc_{I}O_2 - Ca_{O_2}/Cc_{I}O_2 - Cv_{O_2}$$

         The $C_{c}O_2$ may be measured using blood obtained from a wedged pulmonary artery catheter or estimated using the $P_{A}O_2$. The normal Q_s/Q_t is <2% of the cardiac output and results from both anatomic and normal physiologic shunting due to the normal distribution of V/Q ratios from a high value (lung apex) to a low value (lung base) in the upright lung.

         ii. The Q_s/Q_t will increase if collapsed alveolar units continue to be perfused (V/Q = 0). It will also increase in the presence of intracardiac right-to-left anatomic shunts (atrial septal defect, patent foramen ovale, ventricular septal defect complicating interventricular septal rupture after myocardial infarction) or intrapulmonic right-to-left shunts (arteriovenous malformation).

      c. **Alveolar-capillary diffusion abnormalities** (mechanism 5) alone almost never account for significant elevation of the (A-a)O_2 gradient.

      d. Hypoxemia can also result from nonrespiratory causes such as anemia, where hemoglobin and O_2 carrying capacity is reduced, or impaired oxyhemoglobin formation, as seen in CO poisoning, methemoglobinemia, or sulfhemoglobinemia. Tissue hypoxia can also result when the Ca_{O_2} is normal, under conditions of shock from any cause when tissue perfusion is reduced.

D. Etiologies of acute respiratory failure
   1. **Hypoxemia with normal A-a gradient** (Table 19-1).
   2. **Hypoxemia with increased A-a gradient** (Table 19-2).
E. Approach and management. A history, physical examination, chest x-ray, sputum examination, pulmonary function testing, and selected blood tests are necessary to determine the etiology of acute hypoxemic respiratory failure. Table 19-3 delineates the key clinical findings, key diagnostic tests, and specific therapies for the common causes of acute respiratory failure.
F. Therapeutic goals. The therapeutic goals for the management of acute respiratory failure are to increase Pao_2 by increasing F_IO_2 and to normalize pH by increasing minute ventilation. The definitive interventions for accomplishing these objectives are endotracheal intubation and mechanical ventilation. The initial assessment of the patient and the decision to initiate mechanical ventilation should be completed rapidly to minimize the life-threatening complications associated with prolonged hypoxemia, such as cardiac arrhythmias and anoxic encephalopathy.
   1. **Endotracheal intubation should be performed by the most experienced operator available.** Proper placement of the endotracheal tube should be confirmed immediately by auscultation of breath sounds, examination of a chest x-ray, and assessment of end-tidal CO_2 excretion. All intubated patients should be placed on either assist control or intermittent mandatory ventilation at a rate of 10–15 breaths per minute, tidal volume of 5–10 mL/kg, and a F_IO_2 of 100%. An arerial blood gas reading should be obtained within 20 minutes of initiation of mechanical ventilation, and settings should be adjusted to maintain arterial blood oxygen saturation (Sao_2) >90% and to normalize pH status.
   2. **Ventilatory alternatives to endotracheal intubation for management of acute respiratory failure by noninvasive positive-pressure mask ventila-**

Table 19-1. Etiology of hypoxemia with normal alveolar-arterial oxygen gradient

Reduced Fio_2	Alveolar hypoventilation
High-altitude	Diseases affecting the respiratory center (eg CVA) Medulla oblongata abnormality Neuromuscular dyscoordination Phrenic nerve dysfunction Diaphragm and intercostal muscle weakness/paralysis

Table 19-2. Etiology of hypoxemia with increased alveolar-arterial oxygen

Lung disease	Airway dysfunction	Vascular disease	Lymphatic disease
Pulmonary edema	Asthma	Pulmonary embolism	Lymphangitic carcinomatosis
Pneumonia	Chronic obstructive pulmonary disease	Arteriovenous malformation	
Adult respiratory distress syndrome	Foreign body		
Alveolar hemorrhage			
Pleural effusion			
Atelectasis			
Pulmonary infarction			
Pneumothorax			

Table 19-3. Evaluation and management of common causes of acute respiratory failure

Etiology	Key clinical findings	Key diagnostic tests	Specific therapy
Normal alveolar-arterial gradient			
Reduced FIO_2	Geographic location (altitude)	Ambient FIO_2	Change location
CNS depression	History of drug overdose, head trauma, or anoxic encephalopathy	Response to naloxone	Naloxone, charcoal
		Toxicology screen	Correct electrolytes
	Comatose	Electrolytes (glucose, calcium, sodium)	Neurologic evaluation
		CT head, EEG	
Neuromuscular dysfunction	Neck trauma or neuromuscular disease	Cervical spine films	Stabilize cervical spine
	Received paralytic medications (2)	Review medications	Discontinue paralytics
		CXR: elevated hemidiaphragms	Noninvasive ventilation
		Upright/supine PFTs (reduced VC, NIF, PEF in supine position)	
Increased alveolar-arterial gradient			
1. Alveoli/interstitium			
Cardiogenic pulmonary edema	Rales, diaphoresis	CXR: pulmonary edema PA line: elevated PCWP	Diuresis
		ECG, echocardiogram	Reduce LVEDP
Adult respiratory distress syndrome	Rales	CXR: pulmonary edema PA line: normal or low PCWP	Treat underlying cause
	PaO_2 <55 mm Hg with FIO_2 >60%		
Pneumonia	Fever	CXR: diffuse or lobar infiltrate	Antibiotics: empiric therapy tailored to likely pathogens
	Lung sounds: rales and/or egophony	CBC: leukocytosis	
		Sputum Gram's stain, blood culture	
Pleural effusion	Lung sounds: egophony	CXR: pleural effusion; contralateral mediastinal shift	Drainage
		Thoracentesis	Treat underlying cause
			Consider pleurodesis
Atelectasis	Diminished breath sounds	CXR: volume loss, ipsilateral mediastinal shift	Reduce sedation
	Postoperative		Pulmonary toilet
			Consider bronchoscopy
Pneumothorax	Diminished breath sounds	CXR: pneumothorax; contralateral mediastinal shift	Decompression: chest tube
	Chest wall asymmetry		
	Tracheal deviation		

Condition	Clinical features	Diagnostic findings	Management
Alveolar hemorrhage	Hemoptysis	CXR: localized or diffuse infiltrate; air bronchograms Sputum: hemosiderin-laden macrophages ANCA, antiGBM, sputum AFB, cytology, Gram's stain, urinalysis	Protect uninvolved lung Identify bleeding site and etiology If localized, consider resection, embolization
Pulmonary infarct	Tachypnea, tachycardia Pleuritic CP, hemoptysis Risk for DVT; hypercoagulable	CXR: wedge-shaped peripheral infiltrate Abnormal V/Q scan or PA gram	Heparin anticoagulation Consider thrombolysis and IVC filter
2. Airways Asthma	Wheezing (may be absent if severe airflow obstruction)	Reduced PEF	β-agonists Corticosteroid Theophylline Consider HELIOX
Chronic obstructive pulmonary disease	Wheezing: infrequent		Titrate oxygen carefully to Sao_2 >89% β-agonists Ipratropium bromide Corticosteroid Theophylline Antibiotics: if clinical evidence of infection
Acute airway obstruction Foreign body	Witnessed aspiration	CXR	Localize and remove foreign body via bronchoscope
Epiglottitis	Odynophagia, drooling	Lateral neck films	Racemic epinephrine, antibiotics, HELIOX
3. Vascular disease Pulmonary embolus	See pulmonary infarct	CXR: nonspecific Abnormal V/Q scan or PA gram	Heparin anticoagulation Consider thrombolysis and IVC

Table 19-3. (continued)

Etiology	Key clinical findings	Key diagnostic tests	Specific therapy
4. Lymphatic disease			
Lymphangitic carcinomatosis	History of neoplasm	CXR: reticular infiltrates Cytology from PA line	Treat underlying disease

AFB = acid fast bacilli; ANCA = anti neutrophilic cytoplasmic antibody; antiGBM = antiglomerular basement membrane antibody; CBC = complete blood cell count; CNS = central nervous system; CP = chest pain; CT = computed tomography; CXR: chest x-ray; DVT = deep venous thrombosis; ECG = electrocardiogram; EEG = electroencephalogram; HELIOX = helium and oxygen mixture; IVC = inferior vena cava; LVEDP = left ventricular end-diastolic pressure; NIF = negative inspiratory force; PA = pulmonary artery; PA gram = pulmonary arteriogram; PCWP = pulmonary capillary wedge pressure; PEF = peak expiratory flow; PEFR = peak expiratory flow rate; PFTs = pulmonary function tests; VC = vital capacity; V/Q = ventilation—perfusion. Data from Kass JE, Casstriotta RJ. Heliox therapy in acute severe asthma. *Chest* 1995;107:757–760; Nocturnal Oxygen Therapy Group. Continuous or nocturnal oxygen therapy in hypoxemic chronic obstructive lung disease. *Ann Intern Med* 1980;93:391–398; and Raschke RA, Reilly BM, Guidry JR et al. The weight-based heparin dosing normogram compared with a "standard care" normogram. *Ann Intern Med* 1993;119:874–881.

tion: continuous positive airway pressure (CPAP), bilevel positive airway
pressure (BiPAP), and pressure support. The principle advantage of mask
ventilation is the avoidance of complications associated with endotracheal intubation such as pneumonia, sinusitis, and injury to the trachea and larynx. The
principal disadvantages are leaving the airway unprotected, and the reliance on
patient–ventilator synchrony in order to adequately ventilate the patient. Usual
initial ventilator settings are CPAP 5 cm H_2O, BiPAP (8 cm H_2O inspiratory and 2
cm H_2O expiratory), and pressure support 15–20 cm H_2O. Two recent small,
prospective, randomized trials of noninvasive positive-pressure ventilation
(NPPV) in chronic obstructive pulmonary disease (COPD) patients with acute
respiratory failure demonstrated a decreased need for endotracheal intubation
and more rapid resolution of dyspnea in patients treated with 6–8 hours per day
of mask ventilation and standard therapy, as compared with patients treated
with standard therapy alone (2,3). A small mortality benefit was also seen in one
of the studies, but larger trials will be necessary before NPPV can be accepted as
standard therapy for patients with acute respiratory failure. We continue to advocate endotracheal intubation and mechanical ventilation as the definitive
means of ventilatory support for patients with acute respiratory failure.

   3. **Acute respiratory failure treatment always requires supplemental O_2.** The
   F_IO_2 is usually started at 100% and is gradually decreased while a SaO_2 >90% is
   maintained. There is little toxicity associated with brief periods of high concentrations of O_2. At an FIO_2 of 100%, resorption atelectasis will occur due to nitrogen washout. Prolonged exposure (>24 hours) to high concentrations of O_2
   (>60%) can cause alveolar inflammation and fibrosis. O_2 toxicity appears to be
   mediated by O_2 metabolites and free radicals. It is time- and concentration-
   dependent and can be minimized by reducing the F_IO_2 to <60%.
   4. **Hypoxemia in patients with COPD must be treated aggressively but
   cautiously.** A rapid increase in PaO_2 will cause an increase in $PaCO_2$, placing
   the patient at higher risk for respiratory arrest. Multiple mechanisms are
   likely responsible for CO_2 retention in this setting, including an increase in
   CO_2 production or an increase in the alveolar dead space ventilation (V_D/V_T),
   which is associated with rapid shallow breathing and a reduction in the hypoxemic drive to breath (4). Hence, in this group of patients, supplemental O_2
   should be titrated upward very carefully using O_2 administered through low-
   flow nasal cannulas or via Venturi mask, while SaO_2 and pH are closely monitored. If adequate oxygenation (>89%) cannot be achieved without a progression of respiratory acidosis, intubation and mechanical ventilation should be
   performed.
G. **Specific therapies**
   1. **Hypoxemia with normal A-a gradient.** Recognition of reversible causes of
   hypoventilatory respiratory failure can lead to rapid improvement. These reversible causes include hypoglycemia, medication overdose, and toxin ingestion causing central nervous system depression or neuromuscular blockade
   (Table 19-4).
      a. Opiates are the most common class of medications causing respiratory
      failure; barbiturates and benzodiazepines are less common. All narcotic
      overdoses should be treated with intravenous naloxone, a specific opioid
      antagonist, as well as activated charcoal for oral ingestions. Flumazenil,
      a benzodiazepine antagonist, is not effective in reversing respiratory fail-
      ure. Barbiturate antagonists are not currently available, but barbiturate
      excretion can be enhanced by alkalinization of the urine.
      b. Neuromuscular blockade is being utilized with increasing frequency in
      the critical care setting (5). Depolarizing agents such as succinylcholine
      are rarely the cause of respiratory failure, given their brief duration of ac-
      tion. Nondepolarizing agents such as pancuronium, atracurium and ve-
      curonium have relatively long durations of action that can be prolonged
      by hepatic or renal dysfunction. Neostigmine, an anticholinesterase, can
      be employed to assess for a reversible neuromuscular blockade induced
      by nondepolarizing agents. However, the duration of blockade caused by

Table 19-4. Specific therapies for acute respiratory failure due to hypoventilation

Condition	Drug	Mechanism of Action	Usual Dose	Adverse Effects
Hypoglycemia	Hypertonic dextrose (D50)		50 mL of 50% Dextrose (D50) IV	
Narcotic overdosage	Activated charcoal	Adsorption	1 g/kg, can repeat 0.5–1 g/kg q4h	Abdominal cramping, vomiting, aspiration pneumonitis
	Naloxone	Opiate antagonist	2 mg IV	
	Flumazenil	Benzodiazepine antagonist	2.5 mg IV slow infusion, then 1 mg/min up to 5 mg	
Neuromuscular blockade	Neostigmine	Anticholinesterase	1 mg over 1 min up to 3 mg/h	May lengthen blockade produced by succinylcholine

succinylcholine can be prolonged as the result of plasma cholinesterase activity.

2. **Hypoxemia with increased A-a gradient.** Supplemental O_2 will readily increase Pao_2 in acute respiratory failure caused by disease that predominantly causes V/Q mismatching. On the other hand, hypoxemia will persist in the presence of shunt despite high concentrations of supplemental O_2. In any case, attention must be given to specific therapies that can decrease Q_s/Q_t (Table 19-5).

   a. **Positive end-expiratory pressure (PEEP)** serves to decrease Q_s/Q_t by at least two mechanisms: redistributing alveolar fluid into the interstitium and maintaining patency of alveoli that would otherwise be collapsed due to disease. The optimal PEEP allows a decrease in F_IO_2, while avoiding or minimizing the alveolar overdistention that causes decreased lung compliance and alveolar damage. Other adverse effects of PEEP include an increased risk for barotrauma (pneumothorax, pneumomediastinum, interstitial emphysema) and decreased cardiac output.

   b. **Pressure-control ventilation (PCV) with its decelerating flow-volume waveform has been demonstrated to reduce Q_s/Q_t to a larger extent than traditional volume ventilation with constant flow.** The main disadvantages to PCV are the variability in tidal volume and the usual requirement for neuromuscular blockade.

   c. **Inverse-ratio ventilation improves oxygenation by increasing mean alveolar pressure and decreasing dead space.** As the I:E ratio increases, dynamic hyperinflation (auto-PEEP) occurs. Auto-PEEP will increase peak alveolar pressure during volume-cycled ventilation and decrease tidal volume during PCV. Of course, the same adverse effects of set (extrinsic) PEEP occur with intrinsic auto-PEEP.

H. **Specialist referrals.** Patients requiring mechanical ventilation for hypoxemic respiratory failure in the setting of an increased A-a gradient are likely to require a prolonged duration of ventilation and should be evaluated by a pulmonary or critical care specialist who can optimize ventilator settings and identify and treat the complications of acute respiratory failure (6). Patients in whom neurologic disease is thought to be the precipitant of hypercapneic respiratory failure should be evaluated by a neurologist. Cardiology consultation should be obtained for patients who have respiratory failure secondary to cardiogenic pulmonary edema.

Table 19-5. Specific therapies for acute respiratory failure with elevated alveolar-arterial oxygen gradient

Condition	Drug	Usual dose	Adverse effects
Cardiogenic pulmonary edema	Furosemide	10–80 mg IV	Hypotension, ototoxicity
	Morphine sulfate	2–4 mg IV, 5–10 IM	Hypotension, respiratory depression
	Nitroglycerin	varies sl, po, iv	Hypotension, headache
Pulmonary infarct, pulmonary embolism	Heparin consider thrombolysis	Use weight-based normogram	Bleeding, thrombocytopenia
Asthma	β-agonists	Nebulizer	Tachycardia
	Steroids	Methylprednisolone sodium succinate 40 mg IV TID	Tachycardia
	Aminophylline	6 mg/kg over 30 min, then 0.5 mg/kg/h; decrease by 50% if patient on theophylline	Gastrointestinal symptoms
Chronic obstructive pulmonary disease	Same as asthma except Ipratropium bromide	Metered-dose inhaler or nebulizer solution (500 μg in 2.5 mL of saline)	Mucous impaction
Epiglottitis/ laryngospasm	Racemic epinephrine	Nebulize 0.5 mL in 3 mL of saline	Tachycardia

From Raschke RA, Reilly BM, Guidry JR et al. The weight-based heparin dosing normogram compared with a "standard care" normogram. *Ann Intern Med* 1993;119:874–881.

I. **Other pertinent information.** The Pao_2 declines and the A-a gradient increases with aging because of age-related increases in V/Q mismatch. The changes appear to be linear from age 30–70 years and at age 70 the A-a gradient is about 15 mm Hg. The A-a gradient may be used to assess the etiology of acute respiratory failure at the time of presentation but cannot be used to follow the course of illness because the FIo_2 cannot be determined accurately in the nonintubated patient receiving O_2.

II. **Chronic respiratory failure** can be defined as a deterioration in the gas exchange function of the lung that has either developed insidiously or has persisted for a prolonged period of time following an episode of acute respiratory failure. Chronic respiratory failure may arise from a nonacute or subacute process, such as a progressive neuromuscular disease. Chronicity is suggested by the absence of acute symptoms such as shortness of breath and by the presence of chronic respiratory acidosis. Arterial blood gas analysis usually reveals a Pao_2 repeatedly <55 mm Hg or a $Paco_2$ >50 mm Hg with the pH <7.35.

  A. **Presentation.** Chronic respiratory failure, by definition, develops slowly. The presenting signs and symptoms are similar to those of acute respiratory failure, the difference being in the timing of the onset of the signs and symptoms. Although pulmonary hypertension may occur in acute hypoxemic respiratory failure, it is more likely to progress to cor pulmonale (right-sided heart failure) in chronic hypoxemic respiratory failure.

   1. **Frequent symptoms** include dyspnea, fatigue, and headache.
   2. **Signs**
      a. Cor pulmonale.
         i. Pedal edema.
         ii. Increased jugular venous distention.
         iii. Loud pulmonic valve component of the second heart sound on cardiac auscultation.

    b. Bradypnea or tachypnea.

    c. Altered mental status: somnolence, delirium, agitation.

    d. Sternal retraction.

    e. Nasal flaring.

    f. Cyanosis.

    g. Abnormal breath sounds: wheezes, rhonchi, rales.

B. Physiology

  1. Chronic respiratory failure ensues when alveolar ventilation is not sufficient to maintain a $Paco_2$ that allows pH to be >7.35. In chronic respiratory diseases, the path toward respiratory failure usually involves an interaction between the inspiratory properties of the lung, such as compliance, and the neuromuscular system that controls respiration. In normal individuals, the neuromuscular system or "pump" interacts efficiently with the compliant lung, resulting in adequate minute ventilation and a normal $Paco_2$. However, an increase in the work of breathing caused by an increased inspiratory load of the lung (decreased compliance, stiffer lung) that cannot be compensated for by the neuromuscular system will lead to pump failure and respiratory acidosis (7,8).

  2. An increased work of breathing (inspiratory load) can be due to multiple conditions but will always result in the need to generate a higher inspiratory pressure per tidal breath (P_T) to overcome the effects of decreased compliance.

    a. Pathophysiology

      i. Decreased compliance of chest wall, eg, kyphoscoliosis, thoracoplasty, flail chest, obesity, neuromuscular disease, pleural disease.

      ii. Mechanical disadvantage of inspiratory muscle, eg, COPD (hyperinflation).

      iii. Increase of airway resistance, eg, COPD, obstructive sleep apnea, and upper airway obstruction.

      iv. Lung compliance, eg, atelectasis, interstitial lung disease (rarely a cause of ventilatory failure).

      v. Hypoxemia (see causes of acute respiratory failure).

    b. As the P_T increases, fatigue ensues. The first compensatory step for increased P_T is a decrease in the tidal volume (V_T). In order to maintain a stable minute ventilation (V_E), the respiratory rate must be increased (rapid, shallow breathing), a step that increases the work of breathing. Finally, the decrease in V_T leads to an increase in the relative ventilation of dead space per tidal volume (V_D/V_T), which will lead to an increased $Paco_2$ and a further increase in the work of breathing due to the need for increased V_E. Eventually, this vicious cycle culminates in respiratory failure.

C. Etiology and pathogenesis

  1. Increased work of breathing.

  2. Diminished pump function

    a. Pathophysiology

      i. Central hypoventilation, eg, drug overdose, central nervous system disease, Ondine's curse.

      ii. Motor neuron dysfunction, eg, amyotrophic lateral sclerosis, postpoliomyelitis muscular atrophy.

      iii. Neuromuscular transmission defect, eg, diaphragmatic paralysis, traumatic quadriplegia, myasthenia gravis, Eaton-Lambert syndrome.

      iv. Peripheral neuron dysfunction, eg, Guillain-Barré syndrome.

      v. Muscle weakness, eg, Duchenne's muscular dystrophy, myotonic dystrophy.

    b. Respiratory muscle fatigue is rarely the primary cause of failure in conditions other than myopathies. Fatigue certainly contributes to progression of ventilatory failure, especially in the presence of comorbid conditions such as hypoxemia, cardiac failure, sepsis, and malnutrition. Prompt identification and treatment of these comorbid conditions may prevent or reverse chronic respiratory failure.

D. **Management**
1. **Mechanical ventilation and supplemental O_2 are the mainstays of therapy for chronic respiratory failure.** As in acute respiratory failure, $Paco_2$ must be closely monitored, even with low-flow O_2 administration. A recent report from the Mayo Clinic described an increase in the mean $Paco_2$ of 28 Torr in eight patients with neuromuscular disease or diaphragmatic dysfunction after low-flow O_2 treatment (9).
2. There is growing literature on the use of alternative modes of noninvasive ventilation in patients with chronic respiratory failure and adequate bulbar function (Table 19-6). There is likely to be an increased interest in these alternatives, as they tend to be more comfortable for patients than ventilation via tracheotomies. Further, noninvasive modes may be used in the community and may result in lower costs; complication related to chronic trachectomies may also be avoided (10–13). In some patients, intermittent periods of mechanical ventilation (eg, nocturnal ventilation) allow for ventilator-free periods; many patients with chronic respiratory failure will require full-time mechanical ventilation.

E. **Complications of chronic respiratory failure**
1. Inability to wean.
2. Pulmonary embolism.
3. Respiratory tract infections
   a. Pneumonia.
   b. Tracheobronchitis.
4. Mucous plugging.
5. Tracheotomy complications.
   a. Tracheomalacia.
   b. Tracheal stenosis.
   c. Tracheoesophageal fistulas.

Table 19-6. Options for noninvasive ventilation modes

Option	Advantages	Disadvantages
Negative-pressure chest shell (cuirass)	Comfortable, allows access to oropharynx	May cause upper airway obstruction, especially in chronic obstructive pulmonary disease or during sleep
Glossopharyngeal breathing (tongue and pharyngeal muscles used to project air boluses past glottis)	Safe and effective means of supplementing tidal volume during ventilator-free periods (breath = 6–9 gulps of 60–100 mL each); enhances cough force	Rarely taught; not useful in presence of tracheotomy
Rocking bed	Comfort	Not as effective as negative-pressure ventilators
Intermittent abdominal pressure ventilator (4-inch-wide belt containing air bladder)	Augments tidal volumes up to 300 mL	Must be sitting; ineffective in scoliosis and obesity
Electrophrenic respiration	Unilateral phrenic stimulation often adequate	Expensive; patients usually require tracheostomy
Intermittent positive-pressure ventilation (IPPV)	Custom mouthpieces and nasal IPPV allow leak-proof ventilation during sleep	Discomfort, nasal bridge skin breakdown, orthodontic deformities

6. Psychiatric disorders.
    a. Depression.
    b. Agitation.
F. **Specialty referrals.** All patients with chronic respiratory failure and a preserved mental status should be evaluated by a pulmonary specialist for the feasibility of using noninvasive modes of ventilation or intermittent periods of mechanical ventilation so as to potentially improve quality of life and allow care outside of a chronic care facility. Depressed or agitated patients should be evaluated for antidepressant medication or psychotherapy. Finally, a comprehensive team approach to managing the multiple medical and psychosocial problems manifested by these patients is vital to a successful outcome.

References

1. Hall JB, Schmidt GA, Wood LDH: Principles of critical care for the patient with respiratory failure. In: Murray JF, Nadel JA, eds. *Textbook of respiratory medicine.* Philadelphia: WB Saunders, 1994:2545–2588.
2. Kramer N, Meyer TH, Meharg J, et al.: Randomized, prospective trial of noninvasive positive pressure ventilation in acute respiratory failure. *Am J Respir Crit Care Med* 1995;151:1799–1806.
3. Brochard L, Mancebo J, Wysocki M, et al.: Noninvasive ventilation for acute exacerbations of chronic obstructive pulmonary disease. *N Engl J Med* 1995;333:817–822.
4. Aubier M, Murciano D, Milic-Emili J, et al.: Effects of the administration of O_2 on ventilation and blood gases in patients with chronic obstructive pulmonary disease during acute respiratory failure. *Am Rev Respir Dis* 1980;122:747–754.
5. Hunter JM: New neuromuscular blocking drugs. *N Engl J Med* 1995;332:1691–1698.
6. Pingleton SK: Complications of acute respiratory failure. *Am Rev Respir Dis* 1988;137:1463–1493.
7. Begin P, Grassino A: Inspiratory muscle dysfunction and chronic hypercapnia in chronic obstructive pulmonary disease. *Am Rev Respir Dis* 1991;143:905–912.
8. Roussos C, Fixley M, Gross D, Macklem PT: Fatigue of inspiratory muscles and their synergic behavior. *J Appl Physiol* 1979;46:897–904.
9. Gay PC, Edmonds LC: Severe hypercapnia after low-flow oxygen therapy in patients with neuromuscular disease and diaphragmatic dysfunction. *Mayo Clinic Proc* 1995;70:327–330.
10. Bach JR, Intintola P, Alba AS, Holland IE: The ventilator-assisted individual: cost analysis of institutionalization vs. rehabilitation and in-home management. *Chest* 1992;101:26–30.
11. Bach JR: Updates and perspectives on noninvasive respiratory muscle aids. *Chest* 1994;105:1230–1240.
12. Bach JR, Alba AS, Saporito LR: Intermittent positive pressure ventilation via the mouth as an alternative to tracheostomy for 257 ventilator users. *Chest* 1993;103:174–182.
13. Bach JR, Alba AS: Noninvasive options for ventilatory support of the traumatic high-level quadriplegic patient. *Chest* 1990;98:613–619.

20

Obstructive Sleep Apnea

Daniel J. Gottlieb

Obstructive sleep apnea syndrome is characterized by repeated episodes of decreased to no airflow during sleep, caused by collapse of the pharyngeal airway and commonly accompanied by reduced oxygen saturation and multiple repetitive arousals from sleep. This syndrome is part of a spectrum of obstructive sleep-disordered breathing that includes **snoring**; **obstructive sleep apnea (OSA)**, defined as the presence of episodic reduction (hypopnea) or cessation (apnea) of airflow during sleep; and **obstructive sleep apnea** *syndrome* **(OSAS)**, defined as OSA plus a variety of symptoms, of which excessive sleepiness is the most common (1). In some individuals, periodic increases in resistance to airflow in the upper respiratory tract are associated with arousal despite the absence of an observed reduction in airflow. When associated with daytime sleepiness, this is known as the upper airways resistance syndrome (2).

I. **Epidemiology**
   A. **Prevalence.** Sleep-disordered breathing is frequently encountered in clinical practice. The prevalence of habitual snoring among adults age 30–60 years in the United States has been estimated to be 44% in men and 28% in women, and increases with age (3). The prevalence of OSA in this population, defined as ≥5 apneas or hypopneas per hour of sleep, is 24% in men and 9% in women. Like snoring, OSA prevalence also increases with age, from 17% of men and 7% of women in the fourth decade of life to 31% and 16%, respectively, in the sixth decade. Based on the presence of OSA plus the self-report of excessive sleepiness, at least 4% of men and 2% of women in this population had OSAS.
   B. **Risk factors.** As noted above, the prevalence of OSA increases with age, at least through the sixth decade of life, and is more common in men. The prevalence of OSA in women is greater after menopause, a finding independent of the effect of age (4). **Obesity** is the most important and treatable risk factor for OSA. This association was identified in the earliest clinical reports of this condition and has been confirmed in many subsequent epidemiologic studies (5). **Cigarette smoking** is associated with an increased risk of OSA, although the mechanism underlying this association is unknown (6).
II. **Presenting signs and symptoms.** Sleepiness and snoring are the most common presenting complaints of patients with OSAS. Given the high prevalence of OSAS, these symptoms should be included in the review of systems of a general health history.
   A. **Symptoms.** The most common symptom for which patients with OSAS seek medical attention is **excessive daytime sleepiness**. The presence of OSAS should be considered in any patient who complains of excessive sleepiness. This should be distinguished from fatigue or lethargy on the basis of questions about the likelihood of falling asleep, as opposed to just feeling tired, in a variety of situations, such as reading, watching television, or being a passenger in or the driver of a motor vehicle (7). An objective measure of sleepiness can be obtained from the multiple sleep latency test, although this expensive test is rarely justified in the routine assessment of sleepiness. **Snoring** is usually present in patients with OSAS, although many people are unaware of their own snoring; physicians must rely on the report of a roommate or bed partner (8). Frequent, loud, and irregular snoring is more likely to be associated with OSA than is occasional, soft, regular snoring. The occurrence of gasping, choking, or snorting noises during sleep is also suggestive of OSA, as is awakening with a choking sensation. The **nocturnal dyspnea** associated with OSA

typically resolves within a few breaths after awakening and can thus be distinguished from congestive heart failure or asthma. **Periods of apnea** witnessed by a bed partner are a fairly specific, although insensitive, marker of OSA. Although less common than sleepiness and snoring in patients with OSAS, morning headaches, memory loss, difficulty concentrating, irritable mood, and impotence may be present (1).

B. **Signs**

1. There are few signs of OSAS. If daytime sleepiness is extreme, the patient may be observed to fall asleep during history taking or physical examination. The uvula and soft palate may be inflamed and swollen from the barotrauma of loud snoring, but this finding will not distinguish between snorers with and without sleep apnea. OSAS is associated with a high prevalence of hypertension (9), although this is of little diagnostic value. Pulmonary hypertension may occur in OSAS, most commonly in those patients who have resting daytime hypoventilation and hypoxemia, and may lead to cor pulmonale. Left ventricular failure may also complicate OSAS, and occult OSA should be considered in the differential diagnosis of dilated cardiomyopathy (10).

2. Although the physical examination is of little use in identifying patients with OSAS, it may identify potentially reversible factors associated with this disorder. Obesity is the most important modifiable factor associated with OSA. Attention should be paid to the presence of craniofacial and oropharyngeal abnormalities associated with OSA that may be surgically correctable, such as adenotonsillar enlargement, deviated septum, macroglossia, and retrognathia. Evidence of hypothyroidism or neuromuscular disorders, which may be complicated by OSAS, may also be detected on physical examination.

III. **Etiology and pathogenesis.** The upper airway from the velopharynx to the larynx is a partially collapsible structure. Patency is maintained by the action of dilator muscles that contract either tonically throughout the respiratory cycle (eg, tensor palatini) or phasically with inspiration (eg, genioglossus). Obstructive apneas and hypopneas during sleep result from airway narrowing due to mechanical factors, as well as reduced activity of these dilator muscles. While a wide variety of medical conditions is associated with an increased risk of OSA (Table 20-1), the relative importance of static and dynamic factors in producing OSA in a given adult patient is usually unknown. Adenotonsillar enlargement is the cause of most cases of pediatric OSAS.

A. **Mechanical factors.** Reduced size of the upper airway is a common feature of patients with OSAS and leads to increased upper airway resistance and a predisposition to airway collapse. Airway narrowing may occur at any point along the upper airway, including the nose (septal deviation, rhinitis, nasal polyps), velopharynx (long soft palate, large uvula), and oropharynx (adenotonsillar enlargement, macroglossia, fat

Table 20-1. Conditions associated with obstructive sleep apnea

Endocrine disorders
  Obesity
  Hypothyroidism
  Acromegaly

Developmental abnormalities
  Retrognathia
  Micrognathia

Nasal obstruction

Adenotonsillar enlargement

Macroglossia

Neuromuscular disorders
  Muscular dystrophy
  Postpolio syndrome
  Myasthenia gravis
  Amyotrophic lateral sclerosis

deposition in pharyngeal muscles). Craniofacial abnormalities such as retrognathia and micrognathia can narrow the posterior airway space and predispose to OSA.

B. Dynamic changes in the upper airway during sleep. Despite these anatomic abnormalities, apneas and hypopneas typically do not occur during wakefulness in OSAS patients. Waking airway patency is maintained in part by a compensatory increase in the activity of phasic dilator muscles of the upper airway (11) that is lost with sleep onset (12). Activity of tonic dilator muscles of the upper airway is reduced during sleep in both normal subjects and patients with OSAS (13). These sleep-related changes in muscle activity result in increased upper airway collapsibility, allowing airway closure to occur in response to the small negative pharyngeal pressure needed to generate inspiratory airflow; in severe OSAS, airway closure during sleep may occur at pressures above atmospheric (14). The importance of pharyngeal muscle tone is further reflected in the greater severity of OSA during rapid eye movement (REM) sleep, when muscle tone is lowest. OSA is also associated with other conditions that reduce pharyngeal muscle tone, such as neuromuscular disease and the acute ingestion of alcohol and sedative hypnotic medications.

IV. Relevant physiology
A. Sleep consequences. Fragmented sleep (multiple cycles of apnea and hypopnea terminated by brief arousals) is the principal cause of excessive sleepiness in individuals with OSAS (15). Such patients typically have reduced proportions of both REM sleep and the deeper (slow-wave) stages of non-REM sleep. Although the neurophysiologic role of REM sleep remains controversial, its role in memory formation may be important. The relatively greater deprivation of REM sleep may contribute to the impaired cognitive function noted in OSAS. One important consequence of excessive sleepiness is an increased risk of motor vehicle accidents; patients with untreated OSAS have a risk of accidents estimated at seven times greater than the general population (16).

B. Cardiovascular and pulmonary consequences. Patients with OSAS have a high prevalence of hypertension and an increased risk of myocardial infarction and stroke (9,17). While these associations result in part from the shared risk factor of obesity, OSA may be an independent risk factor for cardiovascular disease. Several mechanisms may contribute to this association. Although transient and unlikely to cause sustained pulmonary hypertension in the absence of daytime hypoxemia, **nocturnal hypoxemia** in OSA may promote atherogenesis and predispose to cardiac ischemia or arrhythmias in patients with underlying cardiac disease (18). **Sympathetic nervous system activity** increases at apnea termination, and sustained daytime increases in catecholamine excretion have been demonstrated in patients with OSAS, contributing to atherogenesis and the development of systemic hypertension (18). Large negative swings in intrathoracic pressure occur during respiratory effort against an obstructed airway, thereby **increasing cardiac preload and afterload**. Together with changes in sympathetic nervous system activity, these factors can eventually cause left ventricular dysfunction. Treatment of OSA often leads to improvement in left ventricular ejection fraction in patients with OSAS and dilated cardiomyopathy (10). **Chronic alveolar hypoventilation** occurs in approximately 10% to 20% of patients with OSAS, usually those with concomitant chronic obstructive lung disease or morbid obesity (19–21). The resultant chronic hypoxemia may cause **pulmonary hypertension**. Treatment of OSAS may lead to reversal of the pulmonary hypertension and daytime hypoventilation.

V. Diagnosis. The diagnosis of OSAS is based on a combination of characteristic clinical features plus compatible polysomnographic findings. Physical findings are generally nonspecific but may help to guide therapy.

A. Radiographic and laboratory evaluation. Radiographs and blood tests are generally not useful in the diagnosis of OSAS. Formal **cephalometric roentgenograms** may reveal evidence of a decreased posterior airway space, long soft palate, or maxillary or mandibular deficiency (22). These measurements are useful in the preoperative evaluation of patients for whom surgical intervention is contemplated but are not warranted in the routine evaluation of the patient with suspected sleep apnea. Assessment of **thyroid function** is useful to exclude the diagnosis of hypothyroidism in the patient with documented OSAS. **Arterial blood gases** will reveal chronic alveolar hypoventilation in 10% to 20% of patients with OSAS, particularly those with morbid obesity or coexistent obstructive lung disease, and should be obtained if resting hypoxemia or pulmonary hypertension is suspected. Polycythemia is uncommon.

B. **Polysomnography.** The principal laboratory test in the diagnosis of OSAS is polysomnography (PSG).

   1. **Technique.** PSG should be performed during a single full night of sleep in a sleep laboratory, with continuous monitoring by a trained PSG technician who can observe the patient, adjust or replace malfunctioning sensors, and initiate therapy if appropriate. The study typically includes assessment of **sleep state and stage** via electroencephalography (EEG), electro-oculography, and chin electromyography (the latter two measures helping to distinguish REM from non-REM sleep); **respiratory airflow** via thermistry, pneumotachography, or thoracic and abdominal strain gauges; **respiratory effort** via strain gauges or esophageal pressure manometry; **arterial oxygen saturation** via pulse oximetry; and **body position** via a position sensor or recording by the technician (23). These signals are used to characterize the nature and severity of sleep apnea. **Heart rate and rhythm** are commonly monitored via electrocardiography to identify apnea-associated arrhythmias, and **leg movements** via electromyography or actigraphy to identify periodic leg movements. Snoring sounds may be recorded, although there is no accepted objective definition of snoring and many sleep laboratories therefore rely on the technician's assessment of snoring (8). Esophageal pH monitoring may be used to assess gastroesophageal reflux. Esophageal pressure manometry, although not routinely employed in most laboratories, is the optimal method to detect increased upper airway resistance and discriminate between central and obstructive respiratory events. The shape of the inspiratory airflow–time curve may be analyzed to identify airflow limitation from increased upper airway resistance.

   2. **Scoring.** The typical PSG report contains summary measures of both sleep and respiratory variables, including total sleep time, percentage of sleep time spent in each stage of sleep, baseline oxygen saturation, and number and frequency of apneas, hypopneas, leg movements, and oxygen desaturations. **A commonly used summary measure of sleep apnea is the apnea–hypopnea index (AHI), defined as the number of apneas plus hypopneas per hour of sleep.** Although the staging of sleep is well standardized (24), the scoring of respiratory disturbances is complicated by the lack of both reliable measures and standardized operational definitions for apnea and hypopnea. The commonly used techniques for measuring airflow are only semiquantitative, and the percentage reduction of airflow used to define hypopnea varies considerably, as does the requirement for an associated reduction in oxygen saturation or for EEG evidence of arousal (25). Typically, apneas are defined as a cessation of airflow lasting for at least 10 seconds. Apneas are classified as **obstructive** if respiratory effort continues throughout the apnea, **central** if no respiratory effort is present during the apnea, and **mixed** if both central and obstructive components are present. Mixed apneas appear to have the same clinical significance as obstructive apneas. Hypopneas are not typically classified as obstructive or central, since this differentiation is usually not possible in the absence of esophageal pressure manometry.

   3. **Interpretation.** The diagnosis of sleep apnea on the basis of PSG results is complicated by a lack of consensus about the frequency of apneas and hypopneas that should be considered abnormal (24), reflecting both technical and biologic factors. Because sleep laboratories employ sensors of varying sensitivity and utilize varying definitions of apnea and hypopnea, normal ranges will vary considerably. More important, the correlation between AHI and symptoms is poor: Some patients with an AHI <5, a level generally considered to be within the normal range, may be quite sleepy due to sleep fragmentation resulting from increased upper airway resistance, while other patients with severely elevated AHI may be free of symptoms. Whether the increase in AHI

that occurs with advancing age is a physiologic or pathologic feature of aging is unknown.

    a. **These caveats notwithstanding, a general guideline for interpretation of the summary respiratory disturbance measures from PSG is as follows: AHI <5, normal; AHI 5–19, mildly elevated; AHI 20–39, moderately elevated; AHI ≥ 40, severely elevated.**

    b. Remember that the diagnosis of OSAS requires the presence of OSA plus symptoms attributable to the OSA. For the purpose of clinical decision making, the absolute frequency of respiratory events is less important than the severity of symptoms, especially sleepiness. The severity of obstructive apnea varies from night to night, dependent only in part on readily identifiable factors such as body position and alcohol consumption. When the clinical suspicion of OSAS is high, a repeat PSG study may be warranted if the initial study is normal (26); instrumentation capable of detecting increased upper airway resistance should be used.

C. **Limited sleep studies.** While the standard, in-laboratory PSG study remains the accepted diagnostic test for sleep apnea, limited portable sleep studies are being performed with increasing frequency due to convenience and lower cost. The American Sleep Disorders Association recognizes three levels of limited sleep study, based on the intensity of monitoring (27): **comprehensive portable PSG**, which differs from standard PSG primarily by the absence of a technician to monitor the study and initiate therapeutic interventions (level II); **modified portable sleep-apnea testing**, in which respiratory effort and airflow, heart rate, and oxygen saturation are recorded, but sleep stage is not measured (level III); and **continuous single or dual bioparameter recording**, such as overnight oximetry recording (level IV).

    1. When the diagnosis of OSA is urgent and standard PSG is unavailable or impractical, level II and level III studies are acceptable diagnostic alternatives; however, these studies will not allow diagnosis and initiation of therapy on a single night, as is often possible with standard PSG (28).

    2. Limited studies are also useful for the assessment of adequacy of treatment in patients with a diagnosis of OSA previously established by standard PSG. Single-parameter studies, such as overnight oximetry, have insufficient sensitivity to be recommended as diagnostic tests for OSA.

D. **Multiple sleep latency test (MSLT).** The MSLT is designed to provide an objective assessment of sleepiness and identify abnormal sleep-onset REM episodes (29). Using a standard protocol, the patient is asked to attempt to sleep during a series of four or five 20-minute naps taken at 2-hour intervals. The test is usually performed on the day following a night of monitoring in the sleep laboratory, as the results will be greatly affected by the quality and quantity of any preceding sleep. An average latency to sleep onset of <5 minutes is considered pathologically short, while most normal controls have an average score of 10–20 minutes. Intermediate values are in a diagnostic gray area. The presence of REM sleep during more than one nap is considered pathologic, usually reflecting either narcolepsy or severe REM sleep deprivation. While not indicated in the routine evaluation of excessive sleepiness, the MSLT is critical to the diagnosis of narcolepsy and may provide a useful objective measure in the patient for whom no cause of sleepiness can be identified.

VI. **Differential diagnosis.** OSAS must be distinguished from other conditions associated with excessive sleepiness including disorders of sleep and respiration, nonrespiratory sleep disorders, and a variety of miscellaneous conditions that may cause sleepiness (Table 20-2).

A. **Insufficient sleep time.** Insufficient sleep time, which may result from insomnia or poor sleep hygiene, is the most common cause of excessive daytime sleepiness. Virtually all individuals are affected occasionally, although for some this can be a chronic condition. A detailed sleep history is critical to obtain in the sleepy patient and should include the usual bedtime and waking times, the time it takes to fall asleep, sleep continuity, and the presence and frequency of insomnia. Potential causes of sleep disruption should be sought, including light or noise in the bedroom, such as a television, small children, pets, or a snoring bed partner; the pres-

Table 20-2. Differential diagnosis of excessive sleepiness

Sleep-associated respiratory disorders
  Obstructive sleep apnea syndrome
  Upper airways resistance syndrome
  Central sleep apnea
Insufficient sleep time
  Poor sleep hygiene
  Insomnia
Narcolepsy
Limb-movement disorders
  Periodic leg movements of sleep
  Restless legs syndrome
Circadian rhythm disorders
  Advanced or delayed circadian rhythm
  Jet lag
Depression
Hypothyroidism
Idiopathic hypersomnia
Medication effect
  Anticonsulvants (eg, benzodiazepines, barbiturates)
  Antidepressants (eg, amitriptyline, doxepin)
  Antihistamines (H_1-antagonists)
  Antihypertensives (eg, β-blockers, clonidine, methyldopa)
  Neuroleptics (eg, chlorpromazine, clozapine)
  Opioid analgesics
  Sedatives, hypnotics, ethanol

---

ence of anxiety, depression, or chronic pain; and the use of caffeine or medications that may affect sleep quality.

B. **Central sleep apnea (CSA).** CSA is characterized by repetitive episodes of breathing cessation during sleep that, in contrast to OSA, result from an absence of respiratory effort (30). CSA is less common than OSA and comprises a heterogeneous group of disorders. Because respiratory drive is lower during sleep than during wakefulness, hypopnea or apnea at sleep onset is fairly common; however, this is rarely a clinically significant phenomenon. The most common form of CSA is Cheyne-Stokes respiration, seen in patients with severe congestive heart failure, bilateral medullary lesions, or diffuse neurologic disease. In Cheyne-Stokes respiration, arousal may occur during the hyperventilatory phase of the periodic breathing cycle, with resultant daytime sleepiness. CSA and OSA may cause identical patterns of repetitive, transient oxygen desaturation on overnight oximetry but are easily distinguished polysomnographically.

C. **Narcolepsy.** Narcolepsy is a condition characterized by excessive sleepiness that is variably associated with other features including cataplexy (sudden loss of skeletal muscle tone during wakefulness, often precipitated by strong emotions), sleep paralysis, and hypnogogic hallucinations, which are felt to represent the abnormal intrusion of features of REM sleep (muscle atonia, dream content) into wakefulness (31). Symptoms of narcolepsy typically begin by early adulthood, although medical attention may not be sought until later in adult life. A family history of similar symptoms is often present. Diagnosis is not difficult when the full-blown clinical syndrome is present, but narcolepsy may be confused with OSAS when excessive sleepiness is the only symptom. The diagnosis is made by the demonstration on MSLT of an abnormally short sleep latency and REM sleep latency (REM sleep occurring during at least two of five naps), after a night of documented normal sleep. The preceding normal sleep must be carefully documented, as sleep deprivation will cause a short sleep latency, and REM sleep deprivation will cause a short REM latency. Many patients with untreated OSAS often have sleep fragmentation that is most severe during REM sleep and consequently have MSLT results consistent with narcolepsy. Worsening of narcolepsy during adulthood should raise the suspicion of OSAS, as the latter is a relatively common condition and will exacerbate the symptoms of narcolepsy.

D. **Periodic limb movements of sleep and restless legs syndrome.**
1. **Periodic limb movements of sleep (PLMS)** is a condition of unknown etiology characterized by repetitive involuntary flexion of the lower extremities during sleep. The movements occur periodically at intervals of 10–40 seconds and are often accompanied by a brief arousal (32). The prevalence of this condition is uncertain but appears to increase with advancing age and may affect as many as 10% of adults >60 years of age. Although often asymptomatic, the repetitive arousals lead to profound daytime sleepiness in some patients. Diagnosis is made by PSG demonstration of periodic limb movements and arousals; because the occurrence of PLMS may vary considerably from night to night, more than a single night's recording may be warranted if the clinical suspicion is high.
2. **Restless legs syndrome (RLS)** is characterized by poorly described paresthesias primarily affecting the lower extremities and associated with an uncontrollable urge to keep the legs in motion (32). This is most severe at rest, particularly upon retiring to bed, and can thereby cause difficulty in sleep initiation. RLS occurs as an idiopathic condition but is also commonly associated with other medical illnesses, including chronic renal failure and diabetic peripheral neuropathy. The diagnosis of RLS is made by clinical history. Many patients with RLS will also have PLMS, although they are distinct entities.
E. **Circadian rhythm disorders.** Circadian rhythm disorders are characterized by a dissociation between the endogenous sleep–wake cycle and the solar dark–light cycle, with a normal total sleep requirement (33). In a **delayed circadian rhythm,** sleep onset occurs later than is desired, which may result in sleepiness if the time of awakening is not allowed to be similarly delayed. In an **advanced circadian rhythm,** the need for sleep occurs early, and awakening occurs similarly early. This may manifest as excessive afternoon and evening sleepiness and is a cause of "sundowning" in the elderly. **Jet lag** is a common, if short-lived, form of circadian rhythm disorder. The diagnosis of circadian rhythm disorders is based primarily on the clinical history and may be confirmed by PSG demonstration of normal sleep architecture occurring at an abnormal time of day.
F. **Other disorders. Depression** is a common medical disorder associated not only with fatigue and decreased volitional activity but also with an objective increase in sleepiness, as determined by MSLT, despite normal or increased total sleep time. Sleepiness improves with effective treatment of the depression. **Hypothyroidism** may cause excessive sleepiness in the absence of sleep apnea. Idiopathic hypersomnia is an uncommon condition in which the subjective complaint of excessive sleepiness is confirmed by short sleep latency on MSLT despite normal sleep time and sleep architecture on overnight PSG and the absence of other conditions known to cause sleepiness. Sleepiness is a common medication side effect that may accompany the use of certain antihistamines, antidepressants, anticonvulsants, and antihypertensives, among others (34) (see Table 20-2).

VII. **Treatment**
A. **Behavioral therapies.** Behavioral interventions are inexpensive and noninvasive and should always be recommended in the treatment of OSAS (Table 20-3). Although these measures will not eliminate OSAS in most cases, they may reduce the severity of symptoms and will frequently improve the efficacy of other treatments. In all cases of OSAS, **abstinence from alcohol** should be recommended, particularly in the evening hours. **Benzodiazepines should be avoided**; when they are necessary for the treatment of anxiety disorders, short-acting agents are preferable, with morning or afternoon rather than evening doses. **Weight loss**, while difficult to achieve and sustain, has been clearly demonstrated to reduce the severity of OSAS (5). In mild cases, this may be successful monotherapy. In more severe dis-

Table 20-3. Therapeutic options in obstructive sleep apnea

Behavior modification
    Weight loss
    Avoidance of alcohol and sedative hypnotics
    Good sleep hygiene
Positive airway pressure
    Continuous positive airway pressure
    Bilevel positive airway pressure
Surgical modification of upper airway
    Tracheotomy
    Tonsillectomy and adenoidectomy
    Uvulopalatopharyngoplasty
    Tongue reduction
    Glossopharyngeal or maxillomandibular advancement
Oral appliances
Medication
    Protriptyline
    Fluoxetine

ease, weight loss is an important adjunctive therapy likely to improve the efficacy of other therapies such as positive airway pressure. Because OSA is usually most severe in the supine position, **avoidance of the supine position** may improve sleep quality and reduce symptoms; however, patients who have not already adopted a nonsupine sleep position by the time of diagnosis are often unable to do so, even with the aid of a tennis or golf ball sewn into the back of a nightshirt. Sleep deprivation may worsen the severity of OSA, and **good sleep hygiene** is particularly important in the OSAS patient: a regular sleep schedule with adequate sleep time, a dark, quiet bedroom, comfortable bedclothes, and avoidance of alcohol and caffeine or other stimulants. Although state and national regulations vary in regard to the implications of OSAS for licensure to operate a motor vehicle, driving and operation of heavy equipment should be discouraged in any patient with excessive sleepiness (35).

B. **Continuous positive airway pressure (CPAP).** The most widely used therapy for OSAS is nasal CPAP, in which a constant pressure is applied to the nasal inlet throughout the respiratory cycle via a nasal mask or nasal prongs (36,37). Most current CPAP devices deliver this pressure with blowers that generate a bias flow at rates of 20–60 L/min and provide maximum mask pressures of up to 20 cm H_2O (36). Rebreathing of expired gases is prevented by venting the dead space through a valve near the mask or through a small hole in the mask or the mask fitting. The appropriate CPAP level is usually determined during the course of nocturnal PSG by gradually increasing the pressure to a level that markedly reduces or eliminates obstructive respiratory events. This is between 5 cm H_2O and 15 cm H_2O pressure for most patients. The efficacy of the CPAP level should ideally be demonstrated for each stage and position of sleep, but this is often impractical. Because a full night of PSG may be required for the diagnosis of OSAS, a second night is often necessary to administer and adjust the level of CPAP. However, split-night PSG studies have become increasingly common, during which the diagnosis of OSAS is made during the first half and nasal CPAP administered and titrated during the second half of the study (28). Although criticized as potentially increasing the likelihood of misdiagnosis or ineffective CPAP titration, split-night PSG studies appear to be an efficient approach to the diagnosis and treatment of appropriately selected patients, including those with severe OSAS.

1. **Efficacy and compliance.** CPAP is very effective in decreasing the frequency of obstructive events, with reduction of AHI to normal levels achievable in up to 90% of patients; however, long-term compliance with CPAP therapy appears

to be obtained in only 50% to 85% of patients (36,38–39). Although some patients are unable to tolerate CPAP due to claustrophobia or discomfort from the positive pressure, the most important determinant of compliance is the perception of an improvement in daytime sleepiness. Symptomatic improvement is often noted after only a single night of effective CPAP therapy. Patients who continue to feel sleepy after several weeks of therapy may warrant further evaluation to document that effective CPAP pressure is being delivered and to exclude coexisting illnesses such as narcolepsy or PLMS.

2. **Complications.** Minor complications of CPAP therapy are fairly common and include vasomotor rhinitis with nasal congestion and rhinorrhea, drying of the nasal and oral mucosa, skin irritation from contact with the mask, and eye irritation from air leaks directed toward the eyes. Nasal symptoms can often be reduced with antihistamines or by adding a humidification system to the CPAP device. Dry mouth often results from air leaking from the mouth, which may be prevented by means of a chin strap. If an intractable mouth leak prevents effective use of nasal CPAP, a full-face mask covering both nose and mouth can be used to deliver CPAP (40). Elimination of air leaks between the mask and face can usually be achieved by choosing a better fitting mask from among the wide array of commercially available mask shapes and sizes, although on occasion a custom-fitted mask may be needed.

3. **Newer modalities.** Other modalities of positive airway pressure administration are less frequently employed. The most commonly used is **bilevel positive airway pressure**, in which a higher pressure is applied during inspiration than during expiration. The expiratory pressure is typically set approximately 4 cm H_2O less than the inspiratory pressure but must be sufficiently high to prevent airway closure in late expiration. The difference between inspiratory and expiratory pressures allows the bilevel device to function as a nasal pressure–support ventilator, which may be useful in those OSAS patients with chronic alveolar hypoventilation. The lower expiratory pressures are also perceived to be more comfortable than CPAP, although present evidence does not suggest greater compliance with the use of bilevel devices (36). Several **self-adjusting positive airway pressure** devices have been recently introduced, in which the inspiratory flow contour is used to identify airflow obstruction, allowing continuous adjustment of the positive pressure level as need varies (eg, with changes in sleep position or sleep stage) (41). The utility of such devices is presently unknown.

C. **Surgery.** Various surgical procedures have been developed for the treatment of OSAS. They vary greatly in complexity and associated disfigurement and, hence, in patient acceptability. The clear potential advantage of surgical therapy is the assurance of patient compliance; however, the most widely employed surgical treatments for sleep apnea appear less effective than CPAP, while other surgical interventions are of limited availability or have not been subjected to adequate clinical investigation to establish efficacy (42).

1. **Tracheotomy.** Tracheotomy with permanent tracheostomy was the first highly efficacious therapy available for OSAS and remains definitive therapy for patients with severe disease who are unable to tolerate or do not benefit from other therapies. Tracheotomy effectively bypasses the collapsible portion of the upper airway and has been demonstrated to eliminate obstructive apneas, improve daytime sleepiness, and reverse chronic alveolar hypoventilation in patients with severe OSAS (43). Although it is effective, the associated disfigurement has generally limited the use of tracheotomy to those patients with severe disease accompanied by respiratory failure, cardiovascular complications, or disabling sleepiness.

2. **Uvulopalatopharyngoplasty (UPPP).** The most widely employed surgical procedure for treatment of OSAS has been UPPP, in which the uvula, posterior portion of the soft palate, and redundant tissue of the lateral pharyngeal walls are resected.

   a. **Efficacy and patient selection.** UPPP is of variable efficacy in the treatment of OSAS. The average short-term reduction in AHI is approximately

40% (43). When response is defined as a reduction in AHI of at least 50% to a level <20 per hour, the overall response rate to UPPP is approximately 40% (43), although normalization of AHI is obtained in <25% of patients (44). The low overall success rate for UPPP may reflect the fact that airflow obstruction is relieved only in the retropalatal area, while obstruction may be present at multiple sites. Attempts have been made at preoperative identification of the site of obstruction, most often by fiberoptic nasopharyngoscopy during the performance of a Müller's maneuver or cephalometric roentgenograms. The site of airway collapse during awake maneuvers may not reflect the site of obstruction during sleep, and the elimination of one site of obstruction may unmask obstruction elsewhere in the upper airway. Thus, while the presence of retrolingual collapse or airspace narrowing predicts a poor response to UPPP, the response rate in patients with collapse or narrowing limited to the retropalatal region is only approximately 50% (43). A poor response to UPPP has been noted in patients with morbid obesity, which is likely to be associated with multiple sites of airway collapse, and in patients with normal body weight who may be more likely to have OSA on the basis of mandibular deficiency. Notwithstanding these limitations, UPPP does lead to a dramatic reduction in AHI and symptomatic improvement in some patients with OSAS and should be considered in patients who do not respond to conservative measures and cannot tolerate nasal CPAP.

   b.   Complications. Moderate-to-severe postoperative pain is common but generally resolves within 2 weeks (44). Perioperative mortality is approximately 1%, resulting primarily from airway obstruction (43). Potential long-term complications of UPPP include the development of nasal speech and velopharyngeal insufficiency. The reported incidence of velopharyngeal insufficiency varies from 3% to 20%, usually manifest as mild nasal regurgitation of liquids (43).

   c.   Modifications of UPPP

   i.   Uvulopalatopharyngoglossoplasty. This procedure is a modification of UPPP that includes a partial resection of the tongue base in an effort to relieve retrolingual obstruction. The benefits of this approach have not been adequately demonstrated.

   ii.   Laser-assisted uvulopalatoplasty (LAUP). LAUP is an office-based procedure performed under local anesthesia, in which a carbon-dioxide laser is used to excise parts of the uvula and soft palate. By removing these tissues, which are important in generation of the snoring sound, LAUP is effective in substantially reducing the severity of snoring in approximately 75% of patients (44). LAUP is a much less extensive procedure than traditional UPPP, and the morbidity appears to be lower; for the same reason, however, LAUP is likely to be less effective than UPPP in treatment of OSAS. LAUP has not been demonstrated to be efficacious in the treatment of OSAS and is not indicated for this condition (44).

3.   Tongue reduction surgery. The limited tongue resection of **laser midline glossectomy** and the more extensive **linguoplasty** attempt to prevent retrolingual airway collapse by removing a strip of tissue from the posterior tongue. Although the latter procedure in particular has had good initial results, insufficient data are available regarding the efficacy of either of these procedures (42).

4.   Glossopharyngeal advancement with hyoid myotomy and suspension. In this procedure, the retrolingual airway is enlarged by means of a limited mandibular osteotomy to isolate the genioid tubercle (anterior attachment of the tongue), which is then fixed to the mandible in a more anterior position. The hyoid bone is freed from its inferior muscular attachments and fixed to the anterior mandible or thyroid cartilage (43). This procedure is often combined with UPPP. The rate of response, defined as a 50% reduction in AHI to a postoperative level of <20 per hour, was approximately 65% in several series. The principal complication is transient anesthesia of the lower anterior teeth.

At experienced centers, this procedure is an acceptable alternative therapy for patients intolerant of nasal CPAP.

5. **Maxillomandibular advancement (MMO).** Surgical advancement of the maxilla, mandible, and hyoid bone has been advocated for the treatment of OSAS in patients who fail therapy with CPAP and have a hypopharyngeal site of airway collapse (45). This surgery was found to be an effective alternative to nasal CPAP in patients with severe OSAS for whom CPAP was effective but not tolerated and in whom UPPP was ineffective. In these patients, MMO led to a 90% reduction in RDI from baseline. This aggressive surgical technique requires jaw fixation for 2–3 weeks and orthodontic treatment to correct changes in occlusion. Other postoperative morbidity is limited primarily to chin and cheek anesthesia that resolves within 6–12 months in >80% of patients. When a surgeon experienced in the technique is available, this procedure may be considered for appropriate patients with severe OSAS who are intolerant of CPAP.

6. **Tonsillectomy and adenoidectomy.** In children, OSAS is usually the result of adenotonsillar enlargement and is often cured by tonsillectomy and adenoidectomy. This procedure may also be beneficial in adults with OSAS and marked adenotonsillar enlargement (46).

7. **Septoplasty.** Chronic nasal obstruction may increase the severity of OSAS, as well as interfere with the effective application of nasal CPAP. Most chronic nasal obstruction results from perennial allergic or nonallergic rhinitis; however, when obstruction is the result of a severely deviated nasal septum, septoplasty may result in improvement of OSAS and an improved response to nasal CPAP administration.

D. **Oral appliances.** A variety of oral appliances are available for the treatment of OSAS. These appliances fall into two general categories: **mandibular advancement devices**, which advance the mandible while rotating it downward, and **tongue-retaining devices**, which hold the tongue anteriorly in the oral cavity. Both types of appliance attempt to modify upper airway anatomy to increase airway caliber and decrease collapsibility. Most oral appliances require fitting and construction in a dental laboratory and may require frequent adjustments early in the course of therapy. Although not well studied, oral appliances appear to reduce the AHI by at least 50% in approximately two-thirds of patients and to normal levels in as many as one-half (47). Patient and device characteristics that predict successful therapy are unknown. Discomfort and excessive salivation are common early complaints, which often subside with adjustment of fit and continued use. Temporomandibular joint discomfort and occlusive changes can be late complications of oral appliance use. Oral appliances appear less effective than nasal CPAP for treatment of OSAS and should be reserved for those patients with primary snoring or mild OSAS unresponsive to behavioral measures or for those with more severe OSAS who are intolerant of nasal CPAP.

E. **Oxygen.** Supplemental oxygen has little effect on apnea frequency or severity and no significant effect on daytime sleepiness, and therefore is not recommended as primary therapy for OSAS. In patients with asymptomatic OSA and severe nocturnal arterial oxygen desaturation, nocturnal supplemental oxygen may be administered to prevent desaturation, although the risks associated with transient nocturnal hypoxemia of this type have not been established. Because sleep is associated with some degree of decreased arterial oxygen saturation, OSA patients with borderline daytime hypoxemia are likely to have sustained hypoxemia at night, even with effective control of apnea by nasal CPAP; in these patients, supplemental oxygen may be added to the nasal CPAP system to maintain adequate oxyhemoglobin saturation (48).

F. **Medication.** Various pharmacologic agents have been employed for treatment of OSAS, although most have had limited success and are reserved primarily for patients who have failed other forms of therapy. The most commonly used is **protriptyline**, usually given as a bedtime dose of 10–30 mg, which theoretically might improve OSA by increasing both respiratory drive and upper airway dilator muscle tone, while decreasing REM sleep as a percentage of total sleep time. In small and mostly uncontrolled trials, protriptyline appeared to cause a moderate (20% to 30%) reduction in the RDI in patients with moderate to severe OSAS and similar reductions in percentage oxygen desaturation (49,50). Interestingly, subjective improvement in daytime sleepiness was reported despite a lack of effect on arousal frequency. This might result from a direct stimulant effect of protriptyline, leading some to employ morning or BID dosing. Anticholinergic side effects are common. A single study found the serotonin-reuptake inhibitor **fluoxetine** at a dose of 20 mg/d to have a similar effect on OSA, with fewer side effects (50). The respiratory stimulants **medroxyprogesterone** and **acetazolamide** have been recommended for treatment of OSAS associated with chronic alveolar hypoventilation, although the benefit of these agents has not been well established. **Theophylline** increases respiratory drive and respiratory muscle strength and may be effective in the treatment of CSA but does not appear effective in the treatment of OSAS. Aggressive treatment of nasal congestion is likely to improve sleep quality in the patient with mild OSAS and the efficacy of therapy with nasal CPAP.

VIII. Specialist referrals
   A. Snoring and asymptomatic OSA. Many patients with snoring are otherwise asymptomatic and do not require specialized evaluation. If the snoring is socially disruptive and refractory to conservative measures (weight loss, change in sleep position, alcohol and benzodiazepine avoidance, treatment of nasal congestion), surgical referral should be considered. In such cases, documentation of the lack of significant OSA should be obtained via PSG, as the presence of significant OSA might lead to an alternative choice of therapy (CPAP) or different surgical approach (eg, UPPP rather than LAUP). Patients with truly asymptomatic OSA (eg, that witnessed by a bed partner) should also be instructed in conservative measures. While more aggressive treatment of OSA might theoretically reduce the risk of cardiovascular disease, little evidence supports this position, and the inconvenience and discomfort of nasal CPAP usually lead to noncompliance in the asymptomatic patient.
   B. Unexplained sleepiness and suspected OSAS. Many patients who complain of excessive daytime sleepiness have an etiology easily gleaned from the medical history, such as depression, insomnia or poor sleep hygiene. In those for whom sleepiness remains unexplained, referral to a sleep specialist is warranted, as the diagnosis and treatment of most other disorders of excessive sleepiness, including OSAS, narcolepsy, and PLMS, require the specialized diagnostic tools of the sleep laboratory.

References

1. Krieger J: Obstructive sleep apnea: clinical manifestations and pathophysiology. In: Thorpy MJ, ed. *Handbook of sleep disorders*. New York: Marcel Dekker, 1990:259–284.
2. Guilleminault C, Stoohs R, Clerk A, et al.: From obstructive sleep apnea syndrome to upper airway resistance syndrome: consistency of daytime sleepiness. *Sleep* 1992;15:S13–S16.
3. Young T, Palta M, Dempsey J, et al.: The occurrence of sleep disordered breathing among middle-aged adults. *N Engl J Med* 1993;328:1230–1235.
4. Block AJ, Wynne JW, Boysen PG, et al.: Menopause, medroxyprogesterone and breathing during sleep. *Am J Med* 1981;70:506–510.
5. Strobel RJ, Rosen RC: Obesity and weight loss in obstructive sleep apnea: a critical review. *Sleep* 1995;19:104–115.
6. Wetter DW, Young TB, Bidwell TR, et al.: Smoking as a risk factor for sleep-disordered breathing. *Arch Intern Med* 1994;154:2219–2224.
7. Johns MW: A new method for measuring daytime sleepiness: the Epworth Sleepiness Scale. *Sleep* 1991;14:540–545.
8. Hoffstein V: Snoring. *Chest* 1996;109:201–222.
9. Fletcher EC: The relationship between systemic hypertension and obstructive sleep apnea: facts and theory. *Am J Med* 1995;98:118–128.
10. Malone S, Liu PP, Holloway R, et al.: Obstructive sleep apnoea in patients with dilated cardiomyopathy: effects of continuous positive airway pressure. *Lancet* 1991;338:1480–1484.
11. Mezzanotte WS, Tangel DJ, White DP: Waking genioglossal electromyogram in sleep apnea patients versus normal controls (a neuromuscular compensatory mechanism). *J Clin Invest* 1992; 89:1571–1579.

12. Remmers JE, DeGroot WJ, Sauerland EK, Anch AM: Pathogenesis of upper airway occlusion during sleep. *J Appl Physiol* 1978;44:931–938.
13. Tangel DT, Mezzanotte WS, White DP: The influence of sleep on tensor palatini EMG and upper airway resistance in normal subjects. *J Appl Physiol* 1991;70:2574–2581.
14. Gleadhill IC, Schwartz AR, Schubert N, et al.: Upper airway collapsibility in snorers and in patients with obstructive hypopnea and apnea. *Am Rev Respir Dis* 1991;143:1300–1303.
15. Kribbs NB, Getsy JE, Dinges DF: Investigation and management of daytime sleepiness in sleep apnea. In: Saunders NA, Sullivan CE, eds. *Sleep and breathing*, 2nd ed. New York: Marcel Dekker, 1994:575–604.
16. Findley LJ, Unverzagt ME, Suratt PM: Automobile accidents involving patients with obstructive sleep apnea. *Am Rev Respir Dis* 1988;138:337–340.
17. Guilleminault C, Stoohs R, Partinen M, Kryger M: Mortality and morbidity of obstructive sleep apnea syndrome. In: Saunders NA, Sullivan CE, eds. *Sleep and breathing*, 2nd ed. New York: Marcel Dekker, 1994:557–574.
18. Hedner JA, Wilcox I, Sullivan CE: Speculations on the interaction between vascular disease and obstructive sleep apnea. In: Saunders NA, Sullivan CE, eds. *Sleep and breathing*, 2nd ed. New York: Marcel Dekker, 1994:823–846.
19. Martin TJ, Sanders MH: Chronic alveolar hypoventilation: a review for the clinician. *Sleep* 1995; 18:617–634.
20. Shepard JWJ: Cardiorespiratory changes in obstructive sleep apnea. In: Kryger MH, Roth T, Dement WC, eds. *Principles and practice of sleep medicine*, 2nd ed. Philadelphia: WB Saunders, 1994:657–666.
21. Weitzenblum E, Krieger J, Apprill M, et al.: Daytime pulmonary hypertension in patients with obstructive sleep apnea syndrome. *Am Rev Respir Dis* 1988;138:345–349.
22. Guilleminault C: Clinical features and evaluation of obstructive sleep apnea. In: Kryger MH, Roth T, Dement WC, eds. *Principles and practice of sleep medicine*, 2nd ed. Philadelphia: WB Saunders, 1994:667–677.
23. American Thoracic Society: Indications and standards for cardiopulmonary sleep studies. *Am Rev Respir Dis* 1989;139:559–568.
24. Rechtschaffen A, Kales A: A manual of standardized terminology: techniques and scoring system for sleep stages of human subjects. Los Angeles: UCLA Brain Information Service/Brain Research Institute, 1968.
25. Moser NJ, Phillips BA, Berry DTR, Harbison L: What is hypopnea, anyway? *Chest* 1994;105:426–428.
26. Meyer TJ, Eveloff SE, Kline LR, Millman RP: One negative polysomnogram does not exclude obstructive sleep apnea. *Chest* 1993;103:756–760.
27. Ferber R, Millman R, Coppola M, et al.: Portable recording in the assessment of obstructive sleep apnea. *Sleep* 1994;17:378–392.
28. Iber C, O'Brien C, Schluter J et al.: Single-night studies in obstructive sleep apnea. *Sleep* 1991; 14:383–385.
29. Carskadon MA, Dement WC, Mitler MM, et al.: Guidelines for the multiple sleep latency test (MSLT): a standard measure of sleepiness. *Sleep* 1986;9:519–524.
30. Bradley TD, Phillipson EA: Central sleep apnea. *Clin Chest Med* 1992;13:493–505.
31. BroughtoRJ: Narcolepsy. In: Thorpy MJ, ed. *Handbook of sleep disorders*. New York: Marcel Dekker, 1990:197–216.
32. Coccagna G: Restless legs syndrome/periodic leg movements in sleep. In: Thorpy MJ, ed. *Handbook of sleep disorders*. New York: Marcel Dekker, 1990:457–478.
33. Roehrs T, Roth T: Chronic insomnias associated with circadian rhythm disorders. In: Kryger MH, Roth T, Dement WC, eds. *Principles and practice of sleep medicine*, 2nd ed. Philadelphia: WB Saunders, 1994:477–481.
34. Nicholson AN, Bradley CM, Pascoe PA: Medications: effect on sleep and wakefulness. In: Kryger MH, Roth T, Dement WC, eds. *Principles and practice of sleep medicine*, 2nd ed. Philadelphia: WB Saunders, 1994:364–372.
35. Pakola SJ, Dinges DF, Pack AI: Review of regulations and guidelines for commercial and noncommercial drivers with sleep apnea and narcolepsy. *Sleep* 1995;18:787–796.
36. American Thoracic Society: Indications and standards for use of nasal continuous positive airway pressure (CPAP) in sleep apnea syndromes. *Am J Respir Crit Care Med* 1994;150:1738–1745.
37. Sullivan CE, Grunstein RR: Continuous positive airway pressure in sleep-disordered breathing. In: Kryger MH, Roth T, Dement WC, eds. *Principles and practice of sleep medicine*, 2nd ed. Philadelphia: WB Saunders, 1994:694–705.

38. Hoffstein V, Viner S, Mateika S, Conway J: Treatment of obstructive sleep apnea with nasal continuous positive airway pressure. *Am Rev Respir Dis* 1992;145:841–845.
39. Kribbs NB, Pack AL, Kline LR, et al.: Objective measurement of patterns of nasal CPAP use by patients with obstructive sleep apnea. *Am Rev Respir Dis* 1993;147:887–895.
40. Sanders MH, Kern NB, Stiller RA, et al.: CPAP therapy via oronasal mask for obstructive sleep apnea. *Chest* 1994;106:774–779.
41. Bradley PA, Mortimore IL, Douglas NJ: Comparison of polysomnography with ResCare Autoset in the diagnosis of the sleep apnoea/hypopnoea syndrome. *Thorax* 1995;50:1201–1203.
42. American Sleep Disorders Association: Practice parameters for the treatment of obstructive sleep apnea in adults: the efficacy of surgical modifications of the upper airway. *Sleep* 1995;19:152–155.
43. Sher AE, Schechtman KB, Piccirillo JF: The efficacy of surgical modifications of the upper airway in adults with obstructive sleep apnea syndrome. *Sleep* 1995;19:156–177.
44. American Sleep Disorders Association: Practice parameters for the use of laser-assisted uvulopalatoplasty. *Sleep* 1994;17:744–748.
45. Riley RW, Powell NB, Guilleminault C: Maxillofacial surgery and nasal CPAP, a comparison of treatment for obstructive sleep apnea syndrome. *Chest* 1990;98:1421–1425.
46. Mangat D, Orr WC, Smith RO: Sleep apnea, hypersomnolence, and upper airway obstruction secondary to adenotonsillar enlargement. *Arch Otolaryngol* 1977;103:383.
47. Schmidt-Nowara W, Lowe A, Wiegand L, et al.: Oral appliances for the treatment of snoring and obstructive sleep apnea: a review. *Sleep* 1995;18:501–510.
48. Sanders MH: Medical therapy for sleep apnea. In: Kryger MH, Roth T, Dement WC, eds. *Principles and practice of sleep medicine,* 2nd ed. Philadelphia: WB Saunders, 1994:678–693.
49. Smith PL, Haponik EF, Allen RP, Bleecker ER: The effects of protriptyline in sleep-disordered breathing. *Am Rev Respir Dis* 1983;127:8–13.
50. Hanzel DA, Proia NG, Hudgel DW: Response of obstructive sleep apnea to fluoxetine and protriptyline. *Chest* 1991;100:416–421.

21 Neuromuscular Diseases of the Chest

Fernando J. Martinez

The respiratory system is driven by a series of complex interactions between the central nervous system, peripheral nervous system, and respiratory musculature. Each of these components may be evaluated using one or more pulmonary function tests which will aid in the diagnosis and management of neuromuscular diseases.

I. **Pulmonary function tests** are described in detail in Chapter 2. The specific features applicable to neuromuscular disorders are detailed below.

   A. **Spirometry**

      1. Measurement of the vital capacity (VC) is widely used to diagnose and follow neuromuscular diseases because the extent of muscular involvement is generally mirrored by reductions in VC. The test is simple to perform, inexpensive, and reproducible. However, the VC is much less sensitive than measurement of respiratory muscle pressures in assessing neuromuscular dysfunction. Respiratory muscle strength must fall to <50% of predicted values before the VC is significantly impaired (1,2). Abnormalities in gas exchange (Pa_{O_2}, Pa_{CO_2}) will be seen when the VC falls to <55% of predicted values (1).

      2. Flow-volume loops can also be obtained with a spirometer. Typical changes seen in neuromuscular disease include a decreased peak expiratory flow (<70% predicted), delayed rise to peak expired flow (slope <4.05 in men and 2.57 in women), abrupt vertical drop in expired flow near residual volume, and impaired inspiratory flow generation (decreased $FIF_{50\%}$ <3 L/sec) (3). An abnormality in any of these parameters, although not specific, should lead to consideration of respiratory muscle weakness in a patient.

   B. **Lung volumes**, especially the residual volume (RV) and the total lung capacity (TLC), are typically reduced in neuromuscular diseases. Decreases in RV linearly correlate with decreases in expiratory pressures (PE_{max}).

   C. **Arterial blood gas** values are neither sensitive nor specific in the diagnosis and management of neuromuscular disease. The presence and/or degree of hypoxemia with neuromuscular disease depends on many factors, including the presence of diaphragmatic involvement, atelectasis, aspiration, and other associated diseases (2). Hypercarbia is a late finding in neuromuscular disease, generally seen when respiratory muscle strength is <30% of normal or VC is <55% of predicted (1).

   D. **Respiratory pressures**

      1. **Mouth static pressures. Extensive experience has confirmed that measurement of maximal inspiratory mouth pressures (PI_{max}) and expiratory pressures (PE_{max}) are the most sensitive indices of respiratory muscle weakness** (2,4,5). There is no correlation between generalized muscle strength and respiratory muscle strength (2,6). As such, measure of respiratory muscle strength should be performed early in the evaluation of possible respiratory neuromuscular disease. In general, respiratory failure occurs when PI_{max} falls to <-230 cm H_2O.

      2. **The PEmax, with its larger range, may be a particularly sensitive indicator of respiratory muscle weakness.** PE_{max} is affected to a greater extent in myopathic rather than neuropathic processes (Table 21-1) and in proximal

323

Table 21-1. Neuromuscular diseases classified by site of involvement

Site of involvement	Disease state
Motor nerves	Peripheral neuropathy*
	Trauma
Spinal cord	Trauma*
	Amyotrophic lateral sclerosis*
	Poliomyelitis
	Syringomyelia
Neuromuscular junction	Myasthenia gravis*
	Eaton-Lambert syndrome
	Poisoning
Muscle	Dystrophy*
	Myopathy*

*Discussed in text.

versus distal skeletal muscle involvement (6). Cough efficiency is impaired when PEmax falls to <40 cm H_2O.

3. **Transdiaphragmatic pressure.** Static mouth pressures are obtained during voluntary maneuvers and, as such, suffer from a lack of specificity. Very low values and normal values may be interpreted easily, but intermediate values are difficult to interpret. Furthermore, low mouth pressures suggest that global respiratory muscle strength is reduced, but offer no information as to the specific muscle group involved. Additional information can be obtained from the simultaneous measurement of pleural (via transnasal esophageal catheter) and abdominal pressure (via transnasal gastric catheter), and the difference between the two, the transdiaphragmatic pressure (Pdi). **Pdi measurement during a sharp sniff maneuver (Pdi$_{sniff}$) is a reproducible and sensitive measure of diaphragm strength** (7). The addition of transcutaneous phrenic nerve stimulation at the neck provides valuable information largely independent of artifacts due to patient effort. This measurement also provides information on phrenic nerve versus diaphragm muscle involvement by disease (8).

II. **Diaphragmatic paralysis.** The diaphragm is the major inspiratory muscle and receives innervation from the phrenic nerves, which can be involved by unilateral (unilateral diaphragm paralysis [UDP]) or bilateral disease (bilateral diaphragm paralysis [BDP]).
   A. **Unilateral diaphragm paralysis**
      1. **Presenting signs and symptoms.** More than 50% of patients with UDP present with no symptoms. The diagnosis is usually suggested by an abnormal chest x-ray demonstrating elevation of a hemidiaphragm (9). The remaining patients present with breathlessness, orthopnea, persistent cough, chest pain, or a combination of these symptoms. The symptoms are more frequent and severe if there is concomitant obesity or a primary lung disease (10). Physical signs are nonspecific and include unilateral decreased excursion of the diaphragm, decreased breath sounds, or symmetric excursion of the abdominal wall on the affected side, particularly when the patient is supine.
      2. The **etiology** of UDP can be identified in 40% to 50% of cases (Table 21-2); most cases of UDP are thus idiopathic. Neoplasm, thoracic or neck surgery, trauma, or neurologic disease make up the majority of identified cases. Lung cancer can involve the phrenic nerve along any part of its course. Surgical procedures can result in a similar injury, with cardiac surgery being the most common. UDP likely occurs in as many as 10% of cardiac procedures (11).
      3. **Relevant physiology.** The hemidiaphragms function relatively independently so that physiologic effects of UDP are less than those of BDP. Forced vital capacity (FVC) decreases mildly, while PI_{max} is reduced to about 60% of predicted and the maximal Pdi is reduced to about 50% of normal P (10).

Table 21-2. Causes of unilateral diaphragm paralysis

Postsurgical
  Cervical operations (inadvertent)
  Thoracic operations (inadvertent)
  Intentional phrenic crush or transection
Neoplastic
  Direct invasion of phrenic nerve
  Metastatic to phrenic nerve
Neuromuscular
  Sequelae of degenerative neurologic illness
  Myelitis, encephalitis, poliomyelitis
Post-traumatic
Mechanical compression
  Substernal thyroid
  Vascular aneurysm
Infectious
  Sequelae of bacterial, viral, syphilitic, or tuberculous infection
Miscellaneous
Idiopathic

From Piehler J, Pairolero P, Gracey D, Bernatz P. Unexplained diaphragmatic paralysis: a harbinger of malignant disease? *J Thorac Cardiovasc Surg* 1982;84:861–4.

4. **Differential diagnosis.** One clue that suggests the diagnosis of UDP is an elevated hemidiaphragm on chest x-ray, although this finding can be due to diaphragmatic eventration (a congenital failure of muscular development of part or all of the hemidiaphragm usually seen in infancy [10]), subpulmonic fluid, or other subdiaphragmatic disease.

5. **Diagnostic approach.** In patients with the appropriate history and an elevated hemidiaphragm, further imaging should be performed to rule in DP and rule out subpulmonic pleural fluid and malignancy. Fluoroscopic visualization of the hemidiaphragm during the performance of a sharp sniff maneuver can easily confirm asymmetric diaphragm movement. Decubitus films can exclude subpulmonic pleural fluid. If no lesions are seen on routine chest films, computed tomography (CT) of the neck, chest, and upper abdomen would be indicated to exclude malignancy. CT of the chest would be particularly important in patients with vocal cord paralysis and left UDP, given the likelihood of carcinoma. Pulmonary function abnormalities are usually present in UDP but are not diagnostic. If no obvious etiology is found during this initial evaluation, further testing rarely proves cost effective (9,10). As most patients with UDP have no cardiopulmonary symptoms, consideration of coexisting cardiopulmonary disease is warranted if significant symptoms exist.

6. **Management.** Asymptomatic individuals with UDP require no specific management. In those patients with symptoms, coexisting cardiopulmonary disease should be treated and weight loss initiated in those with obesity. If symptoms persist, plication of the hemidiaphragm should be considered. This surgical procedure results in long-term improvement in symptoms, pulmonary function, and gas exchange (12).

7. **Specialist referral.** In those individuals with confirmed UDP due to carcinoma of the lung or neck, referral is indicated for diagnosis and treatment. If no obvious etiology is found after an initial evaluation and the patient is asymptomatic, referral is not indicated. Referral is warranted in symptomatic individuals who may require plication.

B. **Bilateral diaphragm paralysis**
  1. **Presenting symptoms and signs**

    a. BDP results in much greater symptomatic and physiologic derangement and is usually seen in the context of generalized skeletal muscle weakness. As such, the underlying disease may dictate the presenting symptoms. The most common respiratory symptoms are breathlessness and, more specifically, orthopnea. This latter symptom may be so severe that the patient cannot lie supine, and the resultant sleep disturbance may be quite prominent.

    b. The physical examination typically reveals tachypnea and respiratory distress, particularly when the patient is supine. Decreased breath sounds at the bases and bilaterally impaired diaphragmatic excursion are usually observed. The most specific finding is abdominal wall paradoxical movement, particularly noted in the supine position.

2. Etiology and pathogenesis. BDP is generally seen in the setting of diffuse neuromuscular disease. Many disorders have been shown to involve the diaphragm. A partial list is presented in Table 21-3.

Table 21-3. Disorders associated with bilateral diaphragm paralysis

Spinal cord
Trauma above C-5
Cervical disc surgery
Cervical spondylosis
Multiple sclerosis
Motor neuron disease
Amyotrophic lateral sclerosis
Poliomyelitis
Spinal muscular atrophy
Phrenic nerves
Charcot-Marie-Tooth polyneuropathy
Critical illness polyneuropathy
Guillain-Barré polyneuropathy
Hypothyroidism
Malignant invasion
Neuralgic amyotrophy
Paraneoplastic syndrome
Toxins
Trauma
Neuromuscular junction
Myasthenia gravis
Poisoning
Drugs
Eaton-Lambert syndrome
Diaphragmatic muscle
Acid maltase deficiency
Amyloid infiltration
Dermatomyositis
Malnutrition
Metabolic
Mitochondrial myopathies
Mixed connective tissue disease
Muscular dystrophies
Myositis
Sarcoidosis
Systemic lupus erythematosus
Systemic sclerosis

3. **Physiology.** Impairment in diaphragm function has significant effects on inspiratory muscle function. Patients demonstrate moderate restriction in lung volume with preserved gas exchange (when the diffusing capacity for carbon monoxide is corrected for alveolar volume). There is a >25% drop in FVC from the sitting to the supine position in patients with significant diaphragm weakness. PI_{max} is reduced, while PE_{max} is generally preserved in isolated BDP. Pdi_{sniff} is decreased in proportion to the extent of diaphragm weakness. Mild hypoxemia is common, although hypercarbia is felt to be rare in isolated BDP (13). The presence of significant hypercarbia should raise suspicion of generalized muscle disease or associated lung disease (2). Sleep related hypoxemia and hypercarbia have been described (2).

4. **Differential diagnosis.** Cardiac disease must be excluded in patients presenting with orthopnea and dyspnea on exertion. Restriction of lung volumes must be evaluated in the context of parenchymal lung disease, as well as respiratory muscle weakness. Once a diagnosis of BDP is made, the diagnostic possibilities in Table 21-3 must be entertained.

5. **Specific diagnostic approach**

   a. Cardiovascular disease must be excluded in all patients with dyspnea and orthopnea. Subsequent diagnostic studies indicated to rule out BDP include chest radiography, which typically reveals reduced lung volumes, and pulmonary function studies, which demonstrate restriction. Fluoroscopy is less helpful than in UDP, as apparently normal diaphragm excursion can be seen with passive descent after relaxation of the abdominal musculature, which may contract during the preceding inspiration (10). A drop in sitting to supine VC is a useful screening test for diaphragmatic weakness. Documenting a decrease in PI_{max} is usually adequate to confirm significant diaphragmatic weakness in this setting. Measurement of Pdi can confirm the diagnosis but is indicated only in patients with suspected isolated or disproportionate weakness of the diaphragm. If the cause of paralysis is uncertain after an initial clinical evaluation, phrenic nerve stimulation with measurement of Pdi can isolate the problem to the phrenic nerve or the diaphragm muscle.

   b. Consideration must be given to ruling out diseases enumerated in Table 21-3. Thyroid function should be measured, cervical spine imaging with CT or magnetic resonance (MR) imaging should be performed to exclude cervical lesions, and electromyography (EMG) with nerve conduction velocities should be performed to exclude systemic neuromuscular disease.

6. **Management.** The management of BDP is determined by the underlying condition. Unfortunately, most of the disorders listed in Table 21-3 have no specific therapy. In occasional patients with phrenic injury in the upper cervical cord or brainstem, pacing of the phrenic nerves may be appropriate (10). With generalized muscle weakness, nocturnal ventilatory assistance may improve not only sleep quality but also daytime respiratory muscle function. Both negative-pressure ventilation and positive-pressure ventilation with a nasal mask have been utilized for this purpose (14).

7. **Problems and complications of therapy**

   a. Negative-pressure ventilation with tank ventilators, cuirass, or wrap ventilators are limited by patient tolerance. Problems include limitations in patient mobility, musculoskeletal back and shoulder pain and discomfort and pressure sores at points of skin contact.

   b. Nasal positive-pressure ventilation has become more acceptable with the development of relatively comfortable nasal masks. Despite this, nasal congestion or dryness, skin ulcers over the bridge of the nose, and aerophagia impede patient compliance. These can be minimized by humidification of inspired air, reducing mask pressure, placing protective materials at sites of skin contact, or using custom-fitted nasal masks. Air leakage around the mask or through the mouth can be minimized by refitting the mask or the use of chin straps or mouthpiece ventilation (14).

8. Specialist referral. Much of the initial evaluation for BDP can be performed by the primary care physician. Specific diaphragmatic testing and initiation of nocturnal ventilatory assistance is best performed in conjunction with consultants familiar with neuromuscular respiratory disease.

III. Guillain-Barré syndrome (GBS) is the most common cause of acute generalized paralysis (15).

A. Presenting symptoms and signs (15,16)

1. **GBS usually presents with a typical pattern of fine paresthesias in the toes or fingertips.** Within days, leg weakness follows in an ascending fashion. Variable facial, arm, and oropharyngeal weakness may be seen as the paralysis ascends. Pain may be a prominent symptom, particularly early in the syndrome, with sciatica or myalgia in the upper legs, flanks, and back. Preceding events including viral infections, vaccinations, surgery, and *Mycoplasma* and *Campylobacter* infections are seen in two-thirds of patients. GBS occurs more frequently in patients with lymphoproliferative illness or systemic lupus erythematosus.

2. **The hallmark clinical signs in GBS are weakness and decreased or absent tendon reflexes.** The weakness is usually symmetric and associated with minimal loss of sensation despite the paresthesias. With progressive disease, the weakness proceeds proximally and in severe cases involves the muscles of respiration. Affected individuals will exhibit alveolar hypoventilation and hypoxemia, but the alveolar-arterial oxygen difference will be normal, unless preexisting lung disease is present. The nadir of weakness is seen in 50% of cases within 2 weeks, in 80% within 3 weeks, and in 90% within 4 weeks (16). The severity of disease varies, with about one-third of patients experiencing significant respiratory muscle weakness (16). The overall mortality varies between 3% and 6%, while mortality in those patients requiring mechanical ventilation can reach 30% (16). Recovery over a period of weeks to months is typical; 85% of patients have residual neurologic deficits.

B. Etiology and pathogenesis. GBS is thought to be an inflammatory peripheral neuropathy. A primary T lymphocyte–mediated process in response to a precipitating infection or immunologic stimulus is thought to be the etiology (15).

C. Physiology

1. The **clinical signs** depend on the extent and location of nerve involvement. Respiratory failure requiring mechanical ventilation is seen with respiratory muscle weakness or denervation of the bulbar musculature, leading to inability to swallow and subsequent aspiration. Weakness of laryngeal musculature can also impair cough. As respiratory muscle weakness progresses, the ability to generate intermittent sighs is lost, and the effectiveness of cough is further impaired. Progressive microatelectasis occurs with associated hypoxemia. With progressive loss of respiratory muscle force, hypoventilation and hypercapnia result. This sequence of events is illustrated in Fig. 21-1.

D. Differential diagnosis. The differential diagnosis of acute weakness in a critically ill individual is listed in Table 21-4. The differential diagnosis of GBS, in order of clinical importance, includes spinal cord lesions, transverse myelitis, myasthenia gravis, basilar artery occlusion (simulating Fisher syndrome variant with ophthalmoplegia, ataxia, areflexia with little weakness), critical illness polyneuropathy, neoplastic meningitis, vasculitic neuropathy, myositis, metabolic myopathies, paraneoplastic neuropathy, hypophosphatemia, heavy-metal intoxication, neurotoxic fish poisoning, botulism, poliomyelitis, and tick paralysis (15).

E. Diagnostic approach. A detailed history and physical examination emphasizing the diagnostic clues suggested in Table 21-4 is the initial diagnostic step. Neurologic examination should include detailed analysis of muscle strength, sensory deficits, cranial nerve findings, and reflexes. Abnormalities of nerve conduction velocity are the most sensitive and specific criteria for the diagnosis of GBS (15). Characteristic electrodiagnostic changes suggesting early demyelination include conduction block, abnormal temporal dispersion, and conduction slowing. Cerebrospinal fluid analysis serves as confirmatory when normal pressure is identified along with few or no cells and a protein concentration >0.55 g/L after the first week of illness (15).

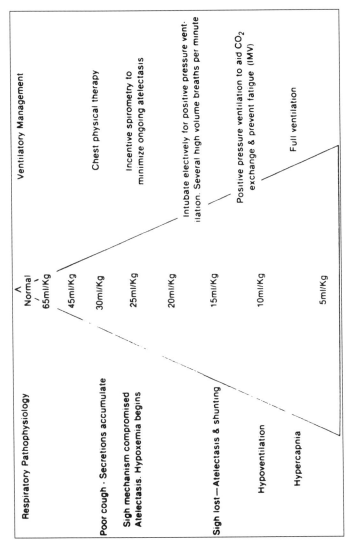

Fig. 21-1. Relationship between VC, pathophysiology of lung function, and suggested therapy in Guillain-Barré syndrome. (Adapted from Ropper AH. ICU management of acute inflammatory-postinfectious polyneuropathy. In: Ropper AH, Kennedy SF, eds. *Neurological and neurosurgical intensive care*, 2nd ed. Rockville, Md: Aspen Publishers, 1988, with permission.)

Table 21-4. Neuroanatomic differential of severe weakness in critically ill individuals

Site and diagnoses	Diagnostic clues
Spinal cord	
Transverse myelitis	Reflexes and tone; profound limb weakness
Compression/ischemic cord injury	Absence of facial involvement
	Sensory level
	Urinary incontinence
Anterior horn disease	
Poliomyelitis	Rare in U.S.; consider in immigrants; viral prodrome; meningeal signs; CSF pleocytosis
Rabies	History is appropriate
Paraneoplastic syndrome	History or primary tumor
Multiple radiculopathy	
Carcinomatous meningitis	Patchy reflex loss, cranial nerve dysfunction
Lymphomatous meningitis	CSF protein; CSF pleocytosis; positive CSF cytology
Peripheral nerves	
Critical illness polyneuropathy	Sensorimotor polyneuropathy; distal atrophy and hyporeflexia; axonal neuropathy
Guillain-Barré syndrome	Rapidly ascending weakness and hyporeflexia; sensory symptoms prominent early; autonomic dysfunction prominent; demyelination; CSF protein
Acute intermittent porphyria	Psychiatric and abdominal manifestations; prophyrins in urine
Neuromuscular junction	
Persistent neuromuscular blockade	Nondepolarizing agents used; liver and/or renal disease; delayed recovery of neuromuscular function with decremental conduction after repetitive nerve stimulation
Myasthenia gravis	Weakness and fatigability increasing with exercise; extraocular muscle involvement common; positive anti–acetylcholine receptor antibodies in 85%; anticholinesterase response in many
Hypermagnesemia	Flaccidity, areflexia; hypermagnesemia
Botulism	Prominent early bulbar symptoms; appropriate exposure
Muscle	
Acute myopathy syndrome	Rapid quadriparesis; nondepolarizing neuromuscular blocking agents; high-dose steroids; +/− aminoglycoside agents, atrophy and/or necrosis on muscle biopsy
Hypokalemia	Rapidly progressive quadriparesis; hypokalemia

CSF = cerebrospinal fluid.

F.   Management. Almost all patients with GBS should be observed in the hospital for several days. Very mild cases with distal paresthesias and mild weakness need no treatment. Two weeks of observation are required before it can be concluded that there will be no progression (15). Progressive disease requires both supportive and specific management.

1. **Supportive management**
   a. **Respiratory failure.** As respiratory complications can be life-threatening, close attention should be paid to respiratory muscle function. VC should be monitored every 4–6 hours. A fall in VC to <15 mL/kg has been generally accepted as an indication of severe respiratory muscle involvement requiring elective intubation (see Fig. 21-1) (15–17). Similarly, airway protection is another indication for early intubation. Elective intubations should always be performed in a controlled environment, since this procedure may be complicated in patients with GBS. Numerous reports

have documented marked cardiovascular lability during intubation, partly due to the dysautonomia that can be prominent in the early part of the syndrome. In addition, fatal hyperkalemia has been reported with the use of succinylcholine in these patients (16).

  b. With profound respiratory muscle weakness, close attention must be paid to adequate bronchial hygiene and possible pneumonia. The course of illness should be determined to identify those patients who require tracheostomy. The decision to perform tracheostomy should be delayed until the end of the second week of mechanical ventilation. Tracheostomy at this time is generally desirable in individuals with apparently severe GBS in whom mechanical ventilation is more likely to be prolonged (16). Weaning is successful in almost all patients, although the time to extubation varies. Initiation of weaning should begin when VC is >7 mL/kg (17). The optimal mode of weaning has not been defined; weans can be performed by the classic T-piece technique (17), by decreasing the IMV rate (16), or by using pressure support.

  c. **Pulmonary embolism** is a consideration, given the possible prolonged muscle weakness and prolonged period of mechanical ventilation. Unless obvious contraindication exists, subcutaneous heparin (5000 U sc q12h) should be administered.

  2. **Specific therapy**
     a. **Plasma exchange.** Several randomized controlled trials have established the benefit of plasma exchange in acute GBS. These studies demonstrated improved ability to walk and decreased requirement for mechanical ventilation (15). The benefit is optimal if treatment is begun within 2 weeks of the onset of illness.

     b. **Immune globulin infusion.** A recent controlled trial comparing plasma exchange and intravenous immune globulin infusion (0.4 g/kg/d given for a mean of 5 days) demonstrated improved strength with globulin infusion. In addition, this group had fewer complications and less need for mechanical ventilation (18). However, questions remain about relapse rate after immune globulin therapy, so that plasmapheresis currently remains the therapy of choice.

  G. **Problems and complications of therapy.** The problems and complications of mechanical ventilation with or without tracheostomy are well known. Plasma exchange is contraindicated in individuals with cardiovascular instability, myocardial infarction, unstable angina, or active sepsis (15). Administration of immune globulin is associated with mild side effects, including hematuria, liver function abnormalities, and transient hypotension (18).

  H. **Specialist referral.** The management of respiratory complications in GBS will require the input of a specialist. Optimal respiratory care is provided in an intensive care unit (ICU) setting with experience in the monitoring and treatment of patients with neuromuscular respiratory failure. Specific therapy is best provided with the aid of consultants familiar with plasmapheresis and immune globulin administration.

IV. **Critical illness polyneuropathy (CIP)**
  A. **Presenting symptoms and signs.** CIP presents in critically ill individuals as a sensorimotor polyneuropathy with limb weakness in a distal predominant distribution, muscle atrophy, reduced or absent reflexes, and a relative preservation of cranial nerve function. CIP is the most common cause of neuropathy in the ICU (19,20). In a recent prospective study, 70% of patients in an ICU demonstrated electrophysiologic evidence of CIP, half of whom demonstrated clinically significant weakness. Failure to wean from mechanical ventilation is commonly due to this condition (19).

  B. **Etiology and pathogenesis.** The etiology of CIP remains unclear, but it has a high association with the multiple organ failure syndrome (MOFS) (19). The possible relation of this syndrome to use of an antibiotic (aminoglycosides) or neuromuscular blocking agent remains controversial. CIP injury is most likely due to the same fundamental defect that affects all organ systems in MOFS (19).

C. **Differential diagnosis.** Severe muscle weakness in a critically ill patient must be recognized and rapidly evaluated. The cause may lie anywhere in the neuroaxis. A neuroanatomic differential is shown in Table 21-4. Diagnostic clues are provided.

D. **Diagnostic approach.** The optimal diagnostic approach involves quick clinical evaluation and judicious use of diagnostic studies. Such an approach includes a detailed exposure history and assessment of the following:

1. The **pattern of muscle weakness** including a determination of proximal versus distal involvement, facial muscle and cranial nerve involvement. An assessment of diaphragm weakness should be performed by measuring pressures.

2. The **pattern of sensory involvement.** Lack of sensory involvement points to GBS or a spinal cord problem.

3. **Laboratory parameters** including electrolytes, thyroid function, and cerebrospinal fluid studies (cell count, differential, and protein level).

4. **Electrophysiologic testing.** Nerve conduction velocity studies can assess axonal and/or demyelinating processes or neuromuscular junction diseases. Repetitive nerve stimulation can be useful in identifying neuromuscular transmission abnormalities. EMG can identify an early axonal or myopathic process.

E. **Management.** Optimal therapy of CIP consists of excluding other treatable processes (see Table 21-4), since improvements in symptoms and signs require resolution of underlying critical illnesses. If these illnesses resolve, then the majority of patients with CIP will demonstrate clinical improvement. The degree of resolution is inversely related to the extent of neuropathy; more severely involved individuals have a higher mortality and more residual weakness (19).

F. **Specialist referral.** The finding of severe weakness in the critically ill patient poses a substantial diagnostic and therapeutic challenge. This is best managed in conjunction with an intensivist and/or neurologic consultant.

V. **Diseases of the spinal cord**

A. **Trauma**

1. **Presenting signs and symptoms** of spinal cord injuries depend mainly on the location and extent of injury (incomplete or complete) (21). Lesions above C-3 are more likely to result in profound respiratory muscle weakness and respiratory failure. Lesions below C-5 will produce variable inspiratory and expiratory muscle problems.

2. **Etiology and pathogenesis.** Traumatic injury to the spinal cord is most commonly due to motor vehicle, athletic, or industrial accidents. Pulmonary complications, predominantly pneumonia, are the leading causes of death (22). Other complications can directly or indirectly contribute to death, including hypotension, hypoxemia, hypocarbia/hypercarbia, respiratory failure, increased intracranial pressure, thromboembolic disease, and concomitant injury to other organs (21). **Spinal shock occurs secondary to sudden withdrawal of descending excitatory influences from higher nerve centers and is characterized by hypotension, paraplegia or quadriplegia, and absent cord reflexes below the level of illness.**

3. **Relevant physiology.** The effects of cervical spinal cord injury are generally separated into two categories:

   a. **High cervical injury (C1-2).** As the diaphragm is innervated by C3-5, high cervical injuries result in almost total respiratory muscle paralysis. Sternocleidomastoid, trapezius, platysma, myohyoid, and sternohyoid muscle activity cannot compensate for diaphragmatic loss and produce only limited inspiratory effects. Ventilatory support is therefore required in these patients.

   b. **Mid- or lower cervical cord injury (C3-8).** Most quadriplegics have injuries at this level. After mid- or lower cervical injury, the VC decreases to 1200–1500, along with decrements in both PImax and PEmax (23). The VC becomes greatly dependent on posture, and values will be greatest in the supine position. Pulmonary function improves as the initial muscle flaccidity of spinal shock changes to spasticity. As a result, the VC may sometimes double within 3 months of injury (22).

4. **Management.** Management of the neurologic problem includes assessment and

treatment of any associated injuries, usually requiring consultation with neurosurgical and orthopedic specialists. Management of medical complications falls to the primary care and/or respiratory physician. Medical complications are usually respiratory in nature and include the following:

a. **Hypersecretion of tenacious mucus occurs in 20% of quadriplegics** (21). The key to prevention of atelectasis and pneumonia is close attention to pulmonary (bronchial) hygiene. The use of standardized protocols to aid in removal of secretions has been shown to improve respiratory status and possibly decrease death (24). These techniques are likely of greatest value between the third and fifth days after injury, a particularly high risk period for respiratory complications (22).

b. **Pneumonia is the principal cause of death** in patients with spinal cord injuries (21). *Staphylococcus, Enterobacter,* and *Pseudomonas* species most commonly colonize the oropharynx in these hospitalized patients and are the most common pathogens in pneumonia. **Prophylactic antibiotics appear to increase resistance without a change in outcome and are thus not recommended.** When pneumonia is clinically felt to be present, intensification of bronchial hygiene is indicated, and appropriate antibiotics should be utilized. The choice of agents should be dictated by the findings of sputum examination but should include broad-spectrum antibiotics to cover the gram-negative organisms found in the particular institution.

c. **The incidence of deep venous thrombosis (DVT) and pulmonary embolism after spinal cord injury is thought to be approximately 16%** (25). Most cases of DVT occur within the first month, are more common in patients with thoracic spine injuries, and, for unclear reasons, tend to occur predominantly in the left leg. Clinical detection of DVT in these patient is notoriously difficult; only about 15% of patients with confirmed DVT are identified clinically. The optimal prophylactic regimen remains controversial, although anticoagulation should likely be withheld for at least 48 hours after injury to minimize risk of bleeding in the cord at the site of damage (21). Subsequently, low-dose heparin (5000 U sc q12h) is a reasonable and effective therapy. If anticoagulation is contraindicated, pneumatic compression boots may be adequate (21).

d. **Endotracheal intubation with positive-pressure ventilation should be initiated promptly after injury, when clinically indicated.** Controversy exists regarding the optimal method of intubation in the presence of cervical spine injury. **Nasotracheal intubation** has largely been felt to be the method of choice, although it is contraindicated in the presence of facial fractures. However, oral intubation with manual in-line axial traction or with guidance by fiberoptic bronchoscopy may achieve a similar goal. The experience of the physician should dictate the modality chosen.

e. Most quadriplegics with intact diaphragm function can be weaned from mechanical ventilation. The majority of patients with C-4 or lower lesions fall in this category. Some patients with C-2 and C-3 lesions may successfully be weaned from the ventilator for part of the day. Since pulmonary function improves for up to 4 months after injury, weaning may require a prolonged period of time. Whether a particular mode of weaning is more efficacious is not known; most authors use a T-piece approach. If weaning is not successful despite improved pulmonary function, home ventilation may be a good alternative in selected patients (14,21,22).

B. **Amyotrophic lateral sclerosis** (ALS) is a progressive, neurodegenerative disorder of the voluntary motor system that affects both the upper and lower motor neurons and is invariably fatal. Most patients die of respiratory muscle involvement and failure.

1. **Presenting symptoms and signs.** ALS may begin anywhere in the neuroaxis and presents with a combination of muscle weakness, wasting, fasciculations, spasticity, and hyperreflexia. All skeletal muscles can be affected with the exception of the extraocular muscles and sphincters. The respiratory muscles are involved in all patients at some point in the illness. Occasionally, ALS pre-

sents with respiratory muscle involvement leading to respiratory symptoms and respiratory failure.

2. The **signs and symptoms** of ALS clearly relate to the involvement of neurons along the neuroaxis. Upper motor neuron involvement leads to spasticity, hyperreflexia, clonus, or Babinski's signs. Lower motor neuron involvement leads to muscle wasting, weakness, and fasciculations. When the neurons controlling inspiratory respiratory muscle function become involved, respiratory failure ensues. This usually occurs in the setting of established limb and bulbar involvement (26). In those patients presenting with diaphragm weakness, pathologic lesions involving the phrenic motor neurons have been demonstrated. Clinical staging criteria related to the degree of muscle involvement are listed in Table 21-5.

3. **Physiology.** As expected, most patients with ALS demonstrate characteristic abnormalities in pulmonary function tests that are more likely to be found in patients with respiratory symptoms. In general, progressive decrements in pulmonary and respiratory muscle function are found with worsening disease. PI_{max} and PE_{max} are decreased before other pulmonary function parameters (26,27) and a linear decrease in VC and respiratory muscle function occur over time. The slope of this decline is quite variable in a given patient (27). In end-stage disease, the VC falls at an accelerated rate (26).

4. **Differential diagnosis.** The clinical diagnosis of ALS is usually straightforward, as there is no other condition that causes the unique combination of upper and lower motor neuron findings (28). The main differential diagnostic considerations include cervical spondylotic myelopathy and multifocal motor neuropathy with conduction block. Cervical spondylosis can cause a spastic paraplegia with no sensory loss, although, as a rule, there is some sensory loss that distinguishes it from ALS. Motor neuropathy with conduction block progresses more slowly, is more likely to affect the hands first, and is usually more asymmetric (28). In contrast to ALS, benign fasciculations are not associated with significant weakness.

5. **Specific diagnostic approach.** ALS is usually suspected on the basis of clinical findings indicating both upper and lower motor neuron disease. EMG should be performed to look for signs of denervation in at least three body segments that would support the clinical impression. Motor neuropathy with conduction block typically will have a different EMG pattern with evidence of multiple conduction blocks. Measurement of levels of antibody to ganglioside GM_1 are also more common in motor neuropathy (75% of patients demonstrate these antibodies compared with 10% of ALS patients) (28). Cervical MR imaging should be performed to exclude spondylotic myelopathy, if evidence of denervation is limited to the cervical segments.

6. **Management.** There is currently no treatment that reverses the progressive deterioration seen in ALS. Supportive measures include:

   a. **Assisted cough** is necessary to help mobilize secretions as expiratory muscle weakness worsens and cough is further impaired (PE_{max} <40 cm H_2O). The push-assist techniques used with spinal cord injury patients can be utilized. Patients with bulbar involvement suffer from impaired swallowing and are at increased risk of aspiration. Anticholinergic agents

Table 21-5. Clinical staging of amyotrophic lateral sclerosis (ALS)

Stage I	Symptoms limited to one limb, bulbar or respiratory musculature
Stage II	Symptoms in an additional site
Stage III	Inability to walk, work or involvement of all limbs
Stage IV	Wheelchair-bound >50% of time
Stage V	Bed-bound
Stage VI	Death from ALS

From Schiffman P, Belsh J. Pulmonary function at diagnosis of amyotrophic lateral sclerosis: rate of deterioration. *Chest* 1993;103:508–513.

(eg, imipramine) can be used to decrease oral secretions (29). In addition, all patients should take food while upright with the neck flexed. Modifying the diet to include soft or pureed foods may decrease the risk of aspiration (26). Eventually, a percutaneous endoscopic gastrostomy can be utilized to maintain nutrition.

   b. **Pulmonary infections** should be treated early and vigorously. All patients should receive polyvalent pneumococcal vaccine and yearly influenza virus vaccination.

   c. All patients with ALS will eventually develop respiratory failure, and thus **monitoring pulmonary function studies** every 3–6 months is advised. Early in the disease, severe sleep desaturation can be seen. Theophylline therapy can be used to improve respiratory muscle strength and possibly endurance (30). Both negative and positive noninvasive ventilation has been shown to be useful in patients with PI_{max} <30 cm H_2O, $Paco_2$ >45 mm Hg, or FVC <1 L (14,29). Long-term ventilatory assistance via tracheostomy is controversial, given the inexorable progression of disease. Its use should be discussed with the patient and family early in the course of disease so that an informed decision can be made.

  7. **Specialist referral.** Management of many aspects of care can be coordinated by a well informed primary physician. As respiratory muscle weakness worsens, referral to a specialist with expertise in neuromuscular disease and noninvasive ventilatory support is appropriate. This is also the case in those patients wishing to pursue long-term ventilatory support at home.

VI. **Myasthenia gravis** (MG) is an acquired autoimmune disorder caused by antibodies directed against the acetylcholine receptor at the neuromuscular junction. The prevalence of MG is 50–125 cases per million people (31).

 A. **Presenting symptoms and signs**

  1. MG has no race predominance but has a female-to-male ratio of 2:1 (32). The cardinal features are weakness and fatigability of skeletal muscles. These symptoms tend to increase with exercise and decrease with rest. The onset may be abrupt or more insidious, and the course is variable.

  2. The most common initial presentation is extraocular muscle weakness, producing ptosis and diplopia. In 15% to 25% of cases, these are the only muscles involved. Other muscles innervated by cranial nerves can be involved, resulting in facial weakness with a typical flattened smile (variably described as snarling), everted lips, and jaw drop, as well as nasal speech and difficulty chewing and swallowing (32). In 85% of cases, generalized weakness develops, often with a proximal predominance. The diaphragm can be involved as the initial manifestation.

  3. The clinical severity is usually graded regionally and by severity of involvement (Osserman classification):

Grade

I: Ocular—isolated ocular involvement.

IIA: Mild generalized weakness—insidious, mild generalized disease.

IIB: Severe generalized weakness—more rapid, generalized disease.

III: Acute fulminant—severe generalized weakness with early respiratory muscle involvement.

IV: Late severe—severe disease developing after initial grades I and II (31,32).

  4. **Myasthenic crises** are severe exacerbations of muscle weakness that often involve the respiratory musculature. Crises are usually seen with reduction or discontinuation of anticholinesterase medications and occur in grade IIB, III or IV MG. Crises are most commonly precipitated by operative stress (33), infection, emotional trauma, or other complications, including medications (32). Myasthenic crises must be distinguished from other similar events:

   a. **Cholinergic crises** seen in response to an excess of anticholinergic medication. In addition to increased muscle weakness, muscarinic and nicotinic side effects occur, including colic, diarrhea, lacrimation, increased oropharyngeal secretions, fasciculations, and cramps.

   b. **Brittle crises** seen when myasthenic and cholinergic crises rapidly alternate in an individual.

B. Etiology and pathogenesis. The basic abnormality in MG is a decrease in the number of acetylcholine receptors, thought to result from an antibody-mediated process. The majority of patients demonstrate a circulating antibody directed against acetylcholine receptors. Those with antibody-negative MG are felt to have antibodies directed against epitopes not present in the current assays (31). The thymus may be the source of antibody, as 75% of patients have thymic abnormalities (hyperplasia, 85%; thymoma, 15%) (31).

C. Differential diagnosis. Conditions causing weakness of the cranial and somatic musculature are listed in Table 21-6.

D. Diagnostic approach

   1. Because of the extensive differential diagnosis, confirmation of MG is necessary before initiation of therapy, particularly in the case of immunosuppressive medications.

   2. The following series of diagnostic studies should be obtained (31):

      a. **Anticholinesterase testing.** Edrophonium chloride, with its rapid onset of action (30 seconds) and short duration (5 minutes), is commonly used to test for the presence of anticholinesterase activity. After a detailed evaluation of muscle strength is performed (including measure of PI_{max} and PE_{max}, atropine (0.4 mg IV) is given as a placebo control and to protect from the muscarinic side effects of edrophonium. Muscle strength is tested two minutes later. Edrophonium is given (2 mg IV), and muscular strength is reevaluated. If no response is seen, a second dose of 8 mg can be given. Unequivocal improvement in an objectively weak muscle is considered positive (31,32).

      b. **Repetitive nerve stimulation.** Electric stimulation at slow rates (2–5 Hz) are delivered, and action potentials are recorded with surface electrodes over the muscle. A rapid reduction of 10% to 15% in amplitude is considered positive (31,32).

      c. **Assay for anti–acetylcholine receptor antibody.** A positive test is specific for MG and is present in approximately 85% of patients (31). The titer does not correlate with severity of disease (32).

      d. **Single-fiber EMG.** This detects failed or delayed transmission of electric activity in pairs of muscle fibers supplied by single motor units. It is positive in 88% to 92% of patients with MG but has limited specificity.

      e. **Thyroid function** should be measured. History of drug use or appropriate exposure should be detailed. The presence of isolated ocular involvement or additional cranial nerve findings should prompt an exclusion of an intracranial mass process.

E. Management. The treatment approach depends on the stage of disease and the extent and severity of involvement. Therapeutic options include medical, surgical, and mechanical modalities (plasmapheresis and mechanical ventilation).

   1. **Medical treatment**

      a. **Anticholinesterase agents are the first line of therapy**. Pyridostigmine bromide is the most widely used agent. Its effect is seen within 30 minutes and peaks at 2 hours. The dosage and schedule are tailored to the patient, with the maximal dosage rarely exceeding 120 mg q3h (31). High doses can worsen weakness. Most patients improve with this therapy but rarely regain normal function (32).

      b. **Immunosuppressive therapy. Corticosteroids** are the most commonly used immunosuppressive therapy but have significant side effects. The most worrisome is transient worsening of weakness when therapy is initiated. Remissions can be induced in 80% of patients (32). Patients with moderate to severe generalized disease should be hospitalized to initiate therapy. The initial dose is 15–25 mg of prednisone; this dose should be increased by 5 mg every 2–3 days as tolerated. The rate of increase is guided

Table 21-6. Differential diagnosis of myasthenia gravis (MG)

Condition	Characteristics and symptoms	Comments
Lambert-Eaton syndrome	Weakness, fatigue, areflexia Pelvic girdle and thigh muscles *Increased* strength with sustained contraction	Incremental response on repetitive nerve stimulation Antibody to calcium channel present 60% Associated with small cell lung cancer
Drug-induced MG		
Penicillamine	Similar to MG	Recovery after drug withdrawal
Curare, procainamide, quinines, aminoglycoside antibiotics	Exacerbation in MG, weakness in normal subjects	Recovery after drug withdrawal
Hyperthyroidism	Exacerbation in MG	Abnormal thyroid function studies
Grave's disease	Diplopia	Exophthalmos present
Botulism	Generalized weakness, ophthalmoplegia	Incremental response on repetitive nerve stimulation Pupillary dilation Appropriate exposure history
Progressive external ophthalmoplegia	Ptosis, diplopia, occasional generalized weakness	Mitochondrial abnormality
Cranial nerve compression from intracranial mass	Ophthalmoplegia Cranial nerve weakness	Abnormal CT or MR imaging
Congenital myasthenic syndromes	Rare; onset in infancy Not autoimmune in origin	Electrophysiologic diagnosis Immunocytochemical testing

CT = computed tomography; MR = magnetic resonance.
Data from Drachman D. Myasthenia gravis. *N Engl J Med* 1994;330:1797–1810, and Zulueta J, Fanburg B. Respiratory dysfunction in myasthenia gravis. *Clin Chest Med* 1994;15:683–691.

by clinical response to a maximum dosage of 50–60 mg/d. Improvement usually is seen within 2–4 weeks and is maximal after 6–12 months or longer of therapy. After 3 months of high-dose daily therapy, the schedule is tapered to an every-other-day dosage regimen as tolerated. **Azathioprine** is reserved for those who have contraindications to steroid use, show insufficient response to steroids, or are taking large doses of steroids. Azathioprine may be used in an effort to lower steroid dose. The therapeutic effect begins slowly, and a therapeutic trial may last 6 months to 1 year. Dosage is initiated with 50 mg/d for 1 week and is increased to a maximum dose of 2–3 mg/kg/d (32). Recently, **cyclosporine** has been used and appears to work more quickly than azathioprine. The dosage is usually 5 mg/kg/d in two divided doses.

2. **Surgical treatment.** Thymectomy can improve outcome in the majority of patients (32) and is widely recommended for patients between the ages of puberty and approximately 60 years (31). Thymectomy should be performed in centers with extensive experience, as complications can be severe (see F. below).

3. **Mechanical modalities**
   a. **Plasmapheresis** removes circulating antibodies and produces a clinical improvement in many patients. It is used primarily to stabilize an individual in myasthenic crisis or to improve function prior to surgery.
   b. **Mechanical ventilation** is often required in crises to treat established respiratory failure, as well as in patients with imminent respiratory failure (VC <10–15 mL/kg) or in those with bulbar MG to protect the airway. Most patients can be weaned from mechanical ventilation.

F. Problems and complications of therapy
   1. Medical treatment
      a. Anticholinesterase inhibition may be associated with muscarinic side effects including abdominal cramps, nausea, vomiting, diarrhea, diaphoresis, increased bronchial secretions, and bradycardia. These can be minimized by pretreatment with atropine or glycopyrrolate (32).
      b. Corticosteroids have well defined side effects and may produce transient worsening of weakness in individuals with MG.
      c. Azathioprine can be associated with an idiosyncratic flu-like illness that can be quite severe and includes fever, malaise, and myalgia (31). Another worrisome side effect is bone marrow suppression, and frequent monitoring of the complete blood cell and platelet count is indicated during initiation of therapy and with any change in dosage. Counts should be measured within 7–10 days of initiating therapy, biweekly for the next 6 weeks, and monthly thereafter. A white blood cell count <3500/mm^3 should prompt adjustment of dosage. Pancreatitis and hepatic toxicity are seen much less frequently. An increase in lymphoproliferative disorders and other teratogenic effects may be seen.
      d. Cyclosporine has well known side effects, including hypertension, nephrotoxicity, and central nervous system toxicity. Hirsutism and gingival hypertrophy are possible cosmetic side effects. Blood pressure and renal function should be followed, as well as trough cyclosporine levels.
   2. Surgical therapy. Thymectomy can be associated with a severe, transient deterioration in muscle strength. If the patient's preoperative status is optimized, the mortality is the same as for general anesthesia (31). Preoperative optimization of anticholinesterase and/or immunosuppressive medications and plasmapheresis (if VC <2 L) are indicated (31,32).
G. Specialist referral. The primary care physician should be familiar with the presentation and differential diagnosis of myasthenia. Evaluation and management should include neurologic consultation and referral to a pulmonologist if respiratory compromise is an issue.
VII. Diseases of muscle: inherited myopathic disorders. A wide spectrum of myopathic disorders can involve the respiratory muscles. The origin, clinical presentation, and subsequent therapy can vary significantly. Myopathic disorders are best separated into inherited and acquired disorders as illustrated in Table 21-7.
A. The **clinical characteristics** of the inherited disorders are presented in Table 21-8.
B. Etiology and pathogenesis
   1. Duchenne's muscular dystrophy is an X-linked recessive disorder caused by mutation of the gene for the cytoskeletal protein dystrophin.
   2. Myotonic dystrophy has been shown to result from an unstable expansion of a CTG triplet sequence on chromosome 19 (34).
   3. Nemaline myopathy results from the accumulation of rod-like bodies in muscle fibers.
   4. Acid maltase deficiency is an inherited deficiency of acid maltase causing a type II glycogen storage disease. Skeletal muscle is exclusively involved.
   5. Mitochondrial myopathies result from a variety of mitochondrial enzymatic defects. The inheritance pattern is unique, as mitochondrial DNA is separate from nuclear DNA. Mitochondrial genes are derived exclusively from maternal inheritance (34). Most of these disorders are characterized by ragged red fibers in biopsies of skeletal muscle.
C. Differential diagnosis. The differential features of each inherited disorder are enumerated in Table 21-8.
D. Diagnostic approach. The diagnosis of a myopathic disorder is generally based on a high index of suspicion.
   1. Duchenne's muscular dystrophy is suggested by its typical clinical features and is confirmed by EMG abnormalities, markedly elevated creatine phosphokinase (CPK) levels, and muscle biopsy.
   2. Myotonic dystrophy also has a typical clinical appearance. Serum CPK levels

Table 21-7. Myopathic disorders that can affect respiratory muscle function in adulthood

Inherited disorders
  Muscular dystrophies
    Duchenne's muscular dystrophy*
    Myotonic dystrophy*
    Facioscapulohumeral muscular dystrophy
    Limb-girdle dystrophy
    Oculopharyngeal dystrophy
  Congenital myopathies
    Nemaline rod myopathy*
  Metabolic myopathies
    Acid maltase deficiency*
    Mitochondrial myopathies*
  Periodic paralysis
    Hypokalemic*
Acquired myopathies
  Inflammatory myopathies
    Polymyositis*
    Dermatomyositis*
  Systemic lupus erythematosus*
  Endocrine myopathies
    Hypothyroidism*
    Hyperthyroidism*
    Hyperadrenocorticosteroid
  Acute steroid myopathy*
  Electrolyte disorders
    Hypokalemia
    Hypophosphatemia
    Rhabdomyolysis

*Discussed in text.
From Lynn D, Woda R, Mendell J. Respiratory dysfunction in muscular dystrophy and other myopathies. *Clin Chest Med* 1994;15:661–674.

    may be slightly elevated, and the electrocardiogram (ECG) may show brady-cardia with prolonged PR intervals. Needle EMG reveals typical findings.

3. **Nemaline myopathy** usually presents in adults with slowly progressive, mild proximal limb weakness. Prominent cardiac involvement is seen in some individuals. Laboratory evaluation is unremarkable, but the histopathology is typical (35).

4. **Acid maltase deficiency** is characterized by focal proximal muscle weakness. Respiratory muscle weakness may be out of proportion to limb weakness, and patients may present with respiratory failure (36). CPK levels are increased, and EMG demonstrates typical abnormalities. Muscle biopsies demonstrate periodic acid–Schiff-positive vacuoles. The enzymatic defect can be demonstrated to confirm the diagnosis.

5. **Mitochondrial myopathies** are suggested by the typical clinical scenarios in Table 21-9. Given that over 25 different mitochondrial enzymatic defects have been isolated, the clinical presentation can vary widely (37). In milder disease, distinct abnormalities on exercise testing, including reduced workload with rapid heart rate and elevated ventilation for given work rates, have been documented (37). Muscle biopsy demonstrates distinctive changes, with the enzymatic defect demonstrable in many patients (34).

E. **Management.** The specific treatment of these disorders is limited; therapy generally consists of supportive care.

1. **Duchenne's muscular dystrophy.** Supportive care consists of physiother-

Table 21-8. Clinical characteristics of inherited myopathic disorders involving the respiratory muscles in adults

Condition	Clinical features	Respiratory involvement
Muscular dystrophies Duchenne's muscular dystrophy	Onset in early childhood; proximal weakness; most wheelchair-bound by age 12, death around age 20	FVC $\neq$ in early teens then relentlessly $\varnothing$; PImax and PEmax decline; scoliosis worsens restriction Respiratory failure typical
Myotonic dystrophy	Progressive myotonia and weakness; cardiac conduction defects; endocrine abnormalities with infertility, early onset cataracts, premature frontal balding, and mild mental retardation	Respiratory insufficiency even with mild weakness; central hypoventilation during sleep; pharyngo-esophageal dysfunction with aspiration; myotonia of chest wall
Congenital myopathies Nemaline rod myopathy	Slowly progressive proximal weakness; prominent cardiac involvement in some	Respiratory muscle involvement can be seen
Metabolic myopathies Acid maltase deficiency	Proximal muscle weakness beginning in third or fourth decade, striking focality in weakness	Preferential involvement of respiratory muscles; sleep-related respiratory failure
Mitochondrial myopathies Kearns-Sayre syndrome	Ptosis, external ophthalmoplegia, heart block, retinal degeneration, ataxia, peripheral neuropathy	Respiratory muscle weakness; hypoventilation and decreased respiratory response to hypoxia and hypercarbia independent of muscle weakness
Myoclonic epilepsy and ragged red fibers (MERRF)	Myoclonic epilepsy, ataxia, central hypoventilation, myopathy	
Myopathy, encephalopathy, lactic acidosis, stroke-like syndromes (MELAS)	Episodic nausea and vomiting, migraine-like headaches, stroke-like episodes, generalized seizures	
Periodic paralysis Hypokalemic	Onset in second decade; attacks of severe weakness; hypokalemia (to 2–3 mEq/L); carbohydrate load can precipitate	Acute, severe respiratory muscle weakness with respiratory failure can result

apy, aggressive attention to bronchial hygiene, adequate but not excessive nutrition (obesity is a major problem), and prompt treatment of respiratory infections. Prednisone (0.75 mg/kg) has been shown to slow the decline of muscle strength in males between ages 5 and 15 years (38). Surgical spine fixation for scoliosis may improve comfort and endurance but does not appear to improve pulmonary function (34). Family and patient education is crucial, given the relentless nature of the disease. This should occur before the FVC drops to <30% of predicted. Nighttime ventilatory support can improve Pao$_2$ and Paco$_2$. Both negative-pressure and positive-pressure (via nasal mask or mouthpiece) ventilation have been utilized (14,34).

2. **Myotonic dystrophy.** Nighttime respiratory distress is common and should be considered when the FVC drops to <20–30 mL/kg. Treatment with nasal positive-pressure ventilation is particularly useful if nighttime oxygen satura-

tion drops to <85% or end-tidal carbon dioxide rises to >50 Torr (34). Close attention to possible aspiration risk should be considered. Myotonia of respiratory muscles can lead to dyspnea and may respond to antimyotonic medications such as phenytoin (100 mg TID), quinine, and procainamide (500 mg QID) (39). Cardiologic consultation should be obtained when these medications are prescribed to patients with cardiac conduction defects. Patients with myotonic dystrophy are exquisitely sensitive to general anesthesia, respiratory depressants, and neuromuscular blocking agents (34).

3. **Nemaline myopathy** has no specific therapy and is treated with supportive measures similar to those used for Duchenne's muscular dystrophy.

4. **Acid maltase deficiency** is associated with frequent sleep-disordered breathing and responds well to negative- or positive-pressure ventilatory support.

5. **Mitochondrial myopathies** may be treated with specific supplementation depending on the enzymatic defect present. Carnitine replacement is an example (40).

6. **Periodic paralysis.** Death from respiratory muscle weakness can occur with severe attacks of hypokalemic periodic paralysis. During attacks, the ECG should be closely monitored for hypokalemic conduction defects. Treatment consists of potassium supplementation orally or intravenously with 5% mannitol as the diluent. IV administration of glucose or physiologic saline can worsen hypokalemia. Interattack treatment includes oral potassium supplementation, a low-carbohydrate diet, and acetazolamide (34).

VIII. **Diseases of muscle: acquired myopathic disorders**

A. **Presenting symptoms and signs.** The acquired myopathies vary in clinical presentation and severity and are usually seen as a manifestation of systemic illness. As such, the primary disease may dictate the symptoms and signs. Acquired myopathies affecting respiratory function are presented in Table 21-9.

B. **Etiology and pathogenesis. Polymyositis** appears to result from cell-mediated, antigen-specific cytotoxicity, while **dermatomyositis** seems to result from aberrant humoral immune responses. Both are felt to represent the result of an immune response mounted against an environmental (possibly viral) antigen in genetically predisposed individuals (41). Respiratory muscle involvement in **hypothyroidism** likely reflects both a phrenic neuropathy and a myopathic process (42). In **hyperthyroidism**, the diaphragm weakness likely reflects a predominant myopathic process. In **systemic lupus erythematosus** (SLE), the "shrinking lung" syndrome reflects a myopathic rather than neuropathic process (34). The **acute steroid myopathy** recently described likely reflects the interaction of neuromuscular blocking agents and high-dose steroids used in the treatment of primary lung disease (obstructive or adult respiratory distress syndrome) (34,43).

C. **Differential diagnosis.** Diseases that can present with myopathic symptoms include the congenital disorders discussed earlier, as well as the acquired disorders described in Table 21-9.

D. **Diagnostic approach**

1. In the evaluation of suspected myopathic disorders, a careful history and physical examination may identify an associated primary illness (eg, SLE). Elevated muscle enzymes (CPK, aldolase, serum glutamic-oxaloacetic transaminase, serum glutamate pyruvate transaminase, and lactate dehydrogenase) will be found in most of these disorders, including the inflammatory myopathies and acute steroid myopathy. Measurement of antinuclear antibodies and thyroid function should be routine in the evaluation of these patients. Identification of myositis-specific auto-antibodies is useful in classifying the inflammatory myopathies (41). The presence of anti-Jo-1 antibodies identifies a syndrome in younger individuals with a relatively acute onset, fever, Raynaud's phenomenon, and a much higher incidence of interstitial lung disease. Antibodies against signal-recognition particles describes a syndrome with acute onset, severe weakness, and high incidence of dysphagia but little interstitial lung disease.

2. Any EMG or myopathic changes found will not be specific to a particular myopathy but may be valuable in classifying the distribution and severity of muscle involvement (41). A muscle biopsy is invaluable in establishing the diagnosis of an inflammatory myopathy (41).

Table 21-9. Selected acquired myopathies involving respiratory function

Condition	Clinical features	Respiratory involvement
Inflammatory myopathies		
Polymyositis	Insidious onset; weakness initially in shoulders and pelvic girdle; ocular muscles rarely involved; dysphagia and dysphonia seen; no rash	Respiratory involvement in 40% to 50%, interstitial lung disease most common, aspiration pneumonia second; respiratory muscle weakness occasionally; pulmonary vascular disease
Dermatomyositis	Similar to polymyositis; rash: heliotrope discoloration of eyelids, erythematous rash over face/neck, Grottron's sign	Similar to polymyositis
Systemic lupus erythematosus	Manifestations of primary disease, dyspnea out of proportion to chest x-ray, orthopnea; "shrinking lung"	Respiratory muscle weakness
Endocrine myopathies Hyperthyroidism	Manifestations of primary disease, dyspnea	Respiratory muscle weakness
Hypothyroidism	Manifestations of primary disease; dyspnea, fatigue	Respiratory muscle weakness; decreased diffusion capacity; pleural effusion
Acute steroid myopathy	Severe quadriparesis after steroid treatment; hypotonic weakness with difficulty weaning from ventilator; probable association with administration of neuro-muscular blocking agents	Decrements in PImax and PEmax

Data from Dickey B, Myers A. Pulmonary disease in polymyositis/dermatomyositis. *Semin Arthritis Rheum* 1984;14:60–76 and Douglas J, Tuxen D, Horne M. Myopathy in severe asthma. *Am Rev Respir Dis* 1992;146:517–9.

E. **Management**
1. **Inflammatory myopathies. Glucocorticoids are the first-line medications for idiopathic inflammatory myopathies.** Treatment is based on three principles: (a) the initial prednisone dose should be adequate (1–2 mg/kg but no more than 100 mg/d, and given in split doses in very severe cases); (b) this dose is continued until strength improves and CPK values have returned to normal, generally about 4–8 weeks; regular determinations of muscle enzymes should be performed; and (c) prednisone should be tapered gradually by reducing the dose no more than 10 mg/mo (41,44). It should be noted that muscle strength will lag behind CPK changes (44). Poor outcomes may be related to (a) early discontinuation of prednisone without appropriate low-dose maintenance therapy, (b) development of side effects forcing an early taper of prednisone dose, and (c) treatment for the wrong diagnosis (metabolic myopathy). Cytotoxic therapy with azathioprine or methotrexate should be used in the 25% to 50% of patients who do not respond to corticosteroids (41,44).
2. **SLE.** The treatment of SLE is beyond the scope of this chapter. The response of respiratory muscle dysfunction to treatment is highly variable (45).
3. **Endocrine myopathies.** The treatment of hypothyroidism and hyperthyroidism is also beyond the scope of this chapter. Respiratory muscle function can dramatically improve with appropriate therapy of these disorders (42).

4. **Acute steroid myopathy.** The treatment of this unusual complication of steroid therapy is supportive. In order to avoid this problem, steroid tapers should be as rapid as possible. Avoidance of neuromuscular blocking agents used in the intensive care setting (ICU) to ease endotracheal intubation and provide skeletal muscle relaxation during mechanical ventilation, as well as avoidance of other drugs that can affect neuromuscular function (eg, aminoglycoside antibiotics), will likely aid recovery in patients with steroid myopathy. Use of high-dose steroid therapy and concomitant neuromuscular blockade in the ICU should be avoided unless absolutely necessary. Acute steroid myopathy may take months to resolve.

F. **Complications of therapy.** The major complication of therapy of the inflammatory myopathies is the well documented myopathic effect of moderate-dose prednisone therapy. This should be suspected when proximal muscle strength continues to deteriorate or fails to improve despite normalization of muscle enzyme levels. Persistent or worsening neck flexor weakness is rare with steroid myopathy and implies continued inflammatory change (44). A provocative challenge with higher doses of prednisone or rapidly tapering the dosage is often the only way to determine the cause of clinical decline (41).

References

1. Braun N, Arora N, Rochester D: Respiratory muscle and pulmonary function in polymyositis and other proximal myopathies. *Thorax* 1983;38:616–623.
2. Rochester D, Esau S: Assessment of ventilatory function in patients with neuromuscular disease. *Clin Chest Med* 1994;15:751–763.
3. Vincken W, Elleker M, Cosio M: Flow-volume loop changes reflecting respiratory muscle weakness in chronic neuromuscular disorders. *Am J Med* 1987;83:673–680.
4. Black L, Hyatt R: Maximal static respiratory pressures in generalized neuromuscular disease. *Am Rev Respir Dis* 1971;103:641–650.
5. Griggs R, Donohoe K, Utell M et al: Evaluation of pulmonary function in neuromuscular disease. *Arch Neurol* 1981;38:9–12.
6. Vincken W, Elleker M, Cosio M: Determinants of respiratory muscle weakness in stable chronic neuromuscular disorders. *Am J Med* 1987;82:53–58.
7. Mier-Jedrzejowicz A, Brophy C, Moxham J, Green M: Assessment of diaphragm weakness. *Am Rev Respir Dis* 1988;137:877–883.
8. Mier A, Brophy C, Moxham J, Green M: Twitch pressures in the assessment of diaphragm weakness. *Thorax* 1989;44:990–996.
9. Piehler J, Pairolero P, Gracey D, Bernatz P: Unexplained diaphragmatic paralysis: a harbinger of malignant disease? *J Thorac Cardiovasc Surg* 1982;84:861–864.
10. Gibson G: Diaphragmatic paresis: pathophysiology, clinical features, and investigation. *Thorax* 1989;44:960–970.
11. DeLisser J, Grippi M: Phrenic nerve injury following cardiac surgery, with emphasis on the role of topical hypothermia. *J Intensive Care Med* 1991;6:195–301.
12. Graham D, Kaplan D, Evans C, et al.: Diaphragmatic plication for unilateral diaphragmatic paralysis: a 10-year experience. *Ann Thorac Surg* 1990;49:248–252.
13. Laroche C, Carroll N, Moxham J, Green M: Clinical significancce of severe isolated diaphragm weakness. *Am Rev Respir Dis* 1988;138:862–866.
14. Unterborn J, Hill N: Oqptions for mechanical ventilation in neuromuscular diseases. *Clin Chest Med* 1994;15:765–781.
15. Ropper A: The Guillain-Barré syndrome. *N Engl J Med* 1992;326:1130–1136.
16. Teitelbaum J, Borel C: Respiratory dysfunction in Guillain-Barré syndrome. *Clin Chest Med* 1994; 15:705–714.
17. Chevrolet J, Deleamont P: Repeated vital capacity measurements as predictive parameters for mechanical ventilation need and weaning success in the Guillain-Barré syndrome. *Am Rev Respir Dis* 1991;144:814–818.
18. van der Meche F, Schmitz P, DG-BS Group: A randomized trial comparing intravenous immune globulin and plasma exchange in Guillain-Barré syndrome. *N Engl J Med* 1992;326:1123–1129.
19. Witt N, Zochodne D, Bolton C, et al.: Peripheral nerve function in sepsis and multiple organ failure. *Chest* 1991;99:176–184.

20. Raps E, Bird S, Hansen-Flaschen J: Prolonged muscle weakness after neuromuscular blockade in the intensive care unit. *Crit Care Clin* 1994;10:799–813.
21. Slack R, Shucart W: Respiratory dysfunction associated with traumatic injury to the central nervous system. *Clin Chest Med* 1994;15:739–49.
22. Mansel J, Norman J: Respiratory complications and management of spinal cord injuries. *Chest* 1990;97:1446–1452.
23. Carter R: Respiratory aspects of spinal cord injury management. *Paraplegia* 1987;25:262.
24. McMihan J, Michel L, Westbrook P: Pulmonary dysfunction following traumatic quadriplegia. *JAMA* 1980;243:528–531.
25. Weingarden S: Deep venous thrombosis in spinal cord injury. *Chest* 1992;102(suppl):636S–639S.
26. Kaplan L, Hollander D: Respiratory dysfunction in amyotrophic lateral sclerosis. *Clin Chest Med* 1994;15:675–681.
27. Schiffman P, Belsh J: Pulmonary function at diagnosis of amyotrophic lateral sclerosis: rate of deterioration. *Chest* 1993;103:508–513.
28. Rowland L: Amyotrophic lateral sclerosis and related diseases. In: Mohr J, Gautiers, J, eds. *Guide to clinical neurology.* New York: Churchill Livingstone, 1995:795–798.
29. Sherman M, Paz H: Review of the respiratory care of the patient with amyotrophic lateral sclerosis. *Respiration* 1994;61:61–67.
30. Schiffman P, Belsh J: Effect of inspiratory resistance and theophylline on respiratory muscle strength in patients with amyotrophic lateral sclerosis. *Am Rev Respir Dis* 1989;139:1418–1423.
31. Drachman D: Myasthenia gravis. *N Engl J Med* 1994;330:1797–1810.
32. Zulueta J, Fanburg B: Respiratory dysfunction in myasthenia gravis. *Clin Chest Med* 1994;15:683–691.
33. Gracey D, Divertie M, Howard F: Mechanical ventilation for respiratory failure in myasthenia gravis: two-year experience with 22 patients. *Mayo Clinic Proc* 1983;58:597–602.
34. Lynn D, Woda R, Mendell J: Respiratory dysfunction in muscular dystrophy and other myopathies. *Clin Chest Med* 1994;15:661–674.
35. Bodensteiner J: Congenital myopathies. *Neurol Clin* 1988;6:499–512.
36. Rosenow E III, Engel A: Acid maltase deficiency in adults presenting as respiratory failure. *Am J Med* 1978;64:485–491.
37. Hooper R, Thomas A, Kearl R: Mitochondrial enzyme deficiency causing exercise limitation in normal-appearing adults. *Chest* 1995;107:317–22.
38. Fenichel G, Florence J, Pestronk A, et al.: Long-term benefit from prednisone therapy in Duchenne muscular dystrophy. *Neurology* 1991;41:1874–1877
39. Fitting J, Leuenberger P: Procainamide for dyspnea in myotonic dystrophy. *Am Rev Respir Dis* 1989;140:1442–1445.
40. DiMauro S, Bonilla E, Zeviani M, et al.: Mitochondrial myopathies. *J Inherit Metab Dis* 1987; 10(suppl 1):113–128.
41. Wortmann R: Inflammatory diseases of muscle. In: Kelley W, Harris E, Ruddy S, Sledges C, eds. *Textbook of rheumatology.* Philadelphia: WB Saunders, 1993:1159–1188.
42. Martinez F, Bermudez-Gomez M, Celli B: Hypothyroidism: a reversible cause of diaphragmatic weakness. *Chest* 1989;96:1059–1063.
43. Douglas J, Tuxen D, Horne M, et al.: Myopathy in severe asthma. *Am Rev Respir Dis* 1992;146:517–519.
44. Oddis C: Therapy of inflammatory myopathy. *Rheum Dis Clin North Am* 1994;20:899–918.
45. Wiedemann H, Matthay R: Pulmonary manifestations of collagen vascular disease. *Clin Chest Med* 1989;10:677–722.

22 Noninfectious Parenchymal Lung Diseases

Robert Paine III

Noninfectious diseases of the lung parenchyma constitute a diverse group of conditions in which the site of significant pathologic abnormality is the pulmonary alveolar wall or the alveolar space. The etiologies of these diseases are poorly understood. Conditions to be discussed here include idiopathic pulmonary fibrosis, bronchiolitis obliterans with organizing pneumonia, eosinophilic granuloma, lymphangioleiomyomatosis, and pulmonary alveolar proteinosis. The first two are sufficiently common that many primary care physicians will see patients with these diseases, but the others are far less common. A number of other specific conditions that might fall under this title are addressed in other chapters in this book: sarcoidosis, hypersensitivity pneumonitis, chronic eosinophilic pneumonia, occupational lung disease, drug-induced lung disease, pulmonary involvement in connective tissue diseases, and pulmonary vasculitides; these will be described only briefly in this chapter.

I. Idiopathic pulmonary fibrosis

A. Idiopathic pulmonary fibrosis (IPF), also known as cryptogenic fibrosing alveolitis, is the most common of the conditions discussed in this chapter and is the prototype of noninfectious parenchymal lung diseases. The reported incidence in the United States is approximately 5 cases per 100,000 population, although this probably underestimates the true incidence. IPF frequently presents in middle-aged individuals and in males more often than females (1).

B. Although the etiology of IPF is not yet understood, the syndrome has common clinical, physiologic, and pathologic patterns. Histologically, lung obtained from individuals with IPF exhibits increases in inflammatory cells, fibroblast proliferation, and collagen deposition within the alveolar wall and/or the alveolar space. The pattern of significant fibrosis with heterogeneous derangement of alveolar structures and relatively little intra-alveolar inflammation has been characterized as *usual interstitial pneumonitis* (UIP), whereas an extensive intra-alveolar inflammatory infiltrate has been described as *desquamative interstitial pneumonitis* (DIP) (2). While UIP and DIP patterns may represent different points within the temporal progression of IPF, both patterns have been found at the same time in different areas of the same lung. However, the terms still appear frequently in the literature.

C. Signs and symptoms

1. Typically, patients with IPF complain of the insidious onset of breathlessness with exertion (3,4). In some instances, patients may date their complaints from an illness similar to an upper respiratory tract infection. Dyspnea first limits exercise but is eventually present during minimal exertion or at rest. Patients commonly will have an irritating, nonproductive cough. Systemic symptoms, including fatigue, weight loss, malaise, fever, and arthralgias, are less common but may be prominent in some individuals.

2. Patients with IPF commonly have fine, late-inspiratory crackles on physical examination. These dry rales, best heard over the lower lung zones posteriorly, are relatively symmetric and classically described as resembling the sound of Velcro. Clubbing is common in IPF and suggests advanced disease. Signs of pulmonary hypertension, such as an increased pulmonic component of the second heart sound or a right ventricular lift or gallop, may develop as

345

the disease progresses. Florid cor pulmonale with right ventricular dilation and elevated venous pressures with edema and hepatic congestion may be present in advanced disease. Cyanosis is a late finding.

D. Etiology and pathogenesis

1.   The **etiology** of IPF has not been determined (5). Familial cases of IPF have been described, suggesting that the disease may have a genetic basis. However, in most instances, there is no familial association. Most investigators believe that IPF represents an abnormal response to an unknown and possibly prolonged insult in an appropriately susceptible individual (1). Viral infection, perhaps with cytomegalovirus or Epstein-Barr virus, may be involved in this initial insult.

2.   The **pathogenesis of IPF** appears to involve abnormal host immune and inflammatory responses. Increased numbers and activity of inflammatory cells within the lung parenchyma are a universal feature of this condition, as is deposition of immune complexes in the alveolar wall (1,6,7). The presence of these immune complexes correlates with disease activity and prognosis (8). Increased fibroblast proliferation and collagen production are a central pathologic feature of IPF. Whether these cellular responses represent the primary cause of IPF or are a consequence of other abnormalities is the subject of active investigation.

E. Physiology

1.   **Pulmonary function testing** typically demonstrates a restrictive ventilatory abnormality. The vital capacity is reduced, often out of proportion to the forced expiratory volume in 1 second (FEV_1). Thus, the FEV_1 percent (FEV_1/FUC) is normal or increased. Measurement of static lung volumes reveals a reduction in the total lung capacity (TLC) and its subdivisions. The elastic recoil of the lung is increased, so that the pulmonary compliance is significantly reduced, a change that may be reflected in an elevated FEV_1 percentage. Diminished lung volumes due to stiff and noncompliant lungs cause patients to compensate by shallow breathing (at decreased tidal volume) with a rapid respiratory rate. The single-breath diffusing capacity for carbon monoxide (DLCO), a sensitive measure of gas exchange, is often the first pulmonary function study found to be abnormal early in the disease. Measurement of arterial blood gases frequently reveals hypoxemia, with a widened alveolar-arterial oxygen difference [$(A-a)O_2$]. The PCO_2 is usually normal or reduced, and patients often have a mild respiratory alkalosis. Elevation of the PCO_2 to values above normal is an ominous finding seen only in advanced disease.

2.   **Cardiopulmonary exercise testing** reveals a number of additional abnormalities in patients with IPF (9). During exercise, normal individuals increase alveolar ventilation by increasing both tidal volume and respiratory rate. Patients with IPF are unable to augment tidal volume and must rely predominantly on increasing respiratory rate. Thus, exercise capacity is limited by ventilatory capacity in IPF. Furthermore, the ratio of physiologic dead space ("wasted ventilation") to tidal volume increases during exercise in patients with IPF, leading to progressively less efficient ventilation. Similarly, gas exchange almost always deteriorates during exercise, with further widening of the $(A-a)O_2$, in contrast to the expected fall in this difference in normal individuals. Individuals not requiring supplemental oxygen at rest may develop significantly reduced oxygen saturation even during mild exercise.

F. Differential diagnosis

1.   Many conditions mimic IPF and must be included in the differential diagnosis (Table 22-1): other fibrotic conditions of known cause, as well as nonfibrotic diseases encompassing diverse pathologic processes, including cardiovascular diseases, infectious diseases, noninfectious inflammatory diseases (including those associated with connective tissue diseases), diseases attributable to occupational and environmental exposures, and malignant diseases.

2.   The **diagnosis** of IPF involves a series of steps, during which the clinician attempts to exclude the diagnosis. The history, physical examination, pulmonary function studies and radiographic studies are required in all patients but will

Table 22-1. Differential diagnosis of interstitial pulmonary fibrosis (IPF)

Cardiac disease
  Left ventricular failure
  Mitral valve disease
Chronic infectious diseases
  Tuberculosis
  Histoplasmosis
  Bronchiectasis
  Allergic bronchopulmonary aspergillosis
  Pneumocystis carinii
Non-infectious inflammatory diseases
  IPF
  Sarcoidosis
  Hypersensitivity pneumonitis
  Rheumatoid arthritis
  Systemic lupus erythematosus
  Scleroderma
  Polymyositis/dermatomyositis
  Drug-induced lung disease (eg, bleomycin)
  Radiation pneumonitis
Occupational diseases
  Asbestosis
  Silicosis
  Talcosis
  Berylliosis
Malignancy
  Metastatic disease (lymphangitic spread)
  Bronchoalveolar cell carcinoma
Other
  Eosinophilic granuloma
  Lymphangioleiomyomatosis
  Pulmonary alveolar proteinosis
  Chronic pulmonary hemorrhage

only suggest the diagnosis. Serologic studies may be useful in excluding connective tissue diseases. Ideally, lung tissue should be examined to confirm the diagnosis.

  a. The **history** may provide useful information to help determine whether a patient with restrictive lung disease has IPF or another condition (see Table 22-1). The clinician must define the nature and duration of the patient's pulmonary complaints, recognizing that IPF usually has a subtle onset with a subacute or chronic presentation. A detailed history of exposures is critically important, including dusts known to cause interstitial lung disease, antigens that might be associated with hypersensitivity pneumonitis (hobbies, pets), and drugs (including over-the-counter medications). A history of chest pain, orthopnea, skin rashes, arthritis or arthralgias, and hemoptysis, among other complaints, may suggest the presence of cardiac disease, metastatic carcinoma, pulmonary hemorrhage, or a collagen vascular disease.

  b. The **physical examination** should be used to search for evidence of other conditions that are either associated with restrictive lung disease (eg, collagen vascular diseases) or might mimic IPF (eg, congestive heart failure [CHF]). While classic findings in IPF include Velcro rales and finger clubbing, these features are not required for the diagnosis.

  c. **Pulmonary function studies** play an essential role in the approach to the patient for whom IPF is a diagnostic consideration. Full pulmonary function studies, including spirometry, static lung volumes, and DLCO, should be obtained. In the majority of cases, these studies will indicate whether the patient's breathlessness may be a consequence of a restrictive ventilatory defect. A normal study or a study demonstrating an obstructive ventilatory defect would virtually exclude the diagnosis of IPF. Pulmonary function tests showing a mixed restrictive/obstructive abnormality suggest either two independent processes, such as IPF in a patient with preexisting chronic obstructive pulmonary disease (COPD), or processes that involve both the alveolar space and the airways, such as sarcoidosis. A reduced DLCO in the face of relatively normal lung volumes may occur in early interstitial disease but also should suggest the possibility of pulmonary vascular disease, especially thromboembolic disease or anemia. In selected individuals with significant dyspnea and relatively normal resting pulmonary function studies, cardiopulmonary exercise testing may prove extremely helpful in delineating the nature of the physiologic impairment and may suggest the diagnosis of IPF (see E. above).

d. **Radiographic studies play an essential role** in the assessment of the patient who may have IPF. **Standard posteroanterior and lateral chest radiographs should be obtained at the initial evaluation.** These studies typically reveal the presence of **bilateral nodulolinear infiltrates** that may be patchy and heterogeneous or diffuse throughout both lung fields with a lower lobe predominance (2–4,6). In a small proportion (10%) of cases, the standard chest radiograph may be entirely normal despite abnormal pulmonary physiology and unequivocal IPF by lung biopsy (10).

  i. A number of features from the chest radiograph may suggest other disease processes. Cardiomegaly with pulmonary vascular congestion suggests CHF. Hilar and mediastinal adenopathy is quite unusual in IPF and would suggest an alternative diagnosis such as sarcoidosis, infectious granulomatous disease, or tumor. Similarly, pleural involvement is not generally a feature of IPF and would lead one to consider CHF, asbestosis, collagen vascular diseases, lymphangioleiomyomatosis, or tumor. Signs of bronchiectasis on the chest radiograph would lead one to consider other diagnoses. Finally, the pattern and distribution of the infiltrates may help suggest alternative diagnoses. An infiltrate with linear, well demarcated boundaries suggests radiation exposure. Disease predominant in the upper lung zones may suggest eosinophilic granuloma or silicosis. Peripheral infiltrates with central sparing (a reverse of the typical pattern seen in pulmonary edema) is classically described in chronic eosinophilic pneumonia. Whenever possible, one should obtain old chest radiographs for assistance in defining the chronicity and progression of the disease.

  ii. In addition to standard chest radiographs, **computed tomography (CT) of the chest** may be quite useful in the evaluation of the patient with restrictive lung disease. A standard CT scan of the thorax may reveal unsuspected adenopathy or pleural disease and may better demonstrate the pattern and heterogeneity of the infiltrates. Recently, many authors have advocated **high-resolution (1-mm slices) CT (HRCT) of the thorax** (11). These scans are quite sensitive and may be used to define infiltrates in individuals with normal-appearing standard chest radiographs and to guide decisions as to the optimal sites for lung biopsy. Nonetheless, IPF can be associated with a normal-appearing HRCT scan of the chest. Although no pattern is pathognomonic for IPF, the pattern of infiltrates on these scans may suggest specific alternative diagnoses, such as lymphangioleiomyomatosis or hypersensitivity pneumonitis (Table 22-2).

Table 22-2. Lung findings on high-resolution computed tomography

Findings	Association	Characteristics
Linear shadows (irregular interlobular and interstitial thickening)	Common pattern in IPF, but may be present in many other processes including asbestosis, collagen vascular disease, radiation or drug-induced lung disease, lymphangitic carcinomatosis, and others	Honeycombing implies end-stage lung disease; common in IPF; may be seen in EG; rare in BOOP
Ground-glass opacities	Suggests alveolar filling; may be seen in IPF (DIP picture), BOOP, PAP, *P. carinii* infection, hypersensitivity pneumonitis, alveolar cell carcinoma	Distribution peripheral, with central sparing suggests chronic eosinophilic pneumonia or BOOP
Cyst formation	Thin-walled cysts suggest LAM or EG	Upper or upper and midzone predominance most common in EG, silicosis, TB, and sarcoid; unusual in IPF

BOOP = bronchiolitis obliterans organizing pneumonia; DIP = desquamative interstitial pneumonitis; EG = eosinophilic granuloma; IPF = interstitial pulmonary fibrosis; LAM = lymphangioleimyomatosis; PAP = pulmonary alveolar proteinosis; TB = tuberculosis.

     e. The results of **serologic studies** may suggest a diagnosis of pulmonary fibrosis related to collagen vascular diseases. Significant elevation in the titers of antinuclear antibodies or rheumatoid factor may direct one toward a diagnosis of interstitial lung disease associated with systemic lupus erythematosus or rheumatoid arthritis. In contrast, a significant fraction (30% to 40%) of patients with IPF may have low levels of these antibodies, likely as a consequence of generalized immunologic activation.

G. Pathologic diagnosis

    1. Open lung biopsy remains the definitive approach to making a diagnosis of IPF. Whether performed through a small thoracotomy incision or with use of a thoracoscope, surgical biopsy allows adequate tissue sampling for diagnostic purposes and is generally well tolerated, even in patients with significant lung disease. The biopsy can generally exclude other pathologic processes that mimic IPF, especially sarcoidosis, hypersensitivity pneumonitis, infection, and tumor.

       a. Several histologic patterns have been described in patients with IPF. **Usual interstitial pneumonitis (UIP)** is a patchy process with a heterogeneous mixture of normal and abnormal areas. Typical findings include interstitial fibrosis with thickening of alveolar septa and modest interstitial and intra-alveolar inflammation. Large fibrotic cysts (honeycombing) are common in advanced disease.

       b. In contrast, **desquamative interstitial pneumonitis (DIP)** often has a more uniform pattern with less fibrosis and interstitial infiltrate and a more abundant intra-alveolar mononuclear cell infiltrate (2). Although originally proposed as distinct processes, it seems more likely that UIP and DIP represent a pathologic spectrum of disease. In fact, areas typical of UIP and DIP can frequently be found within the same individual. Nonetheless, the terminology has persisted with the thought that it may be helpful for estimating prognosis and response to therapy.

2. A pathologic diagnosis by bronchoscopy and transbronchial biopsy is generally not possible because of the heterogeneous histologic pattern of IPF. The tissue specimens obtained by this technique are too small and the sampling error too great. However, bronchoscopy may be extremely useful for making other diagnoses, including sarcoidosis, infection, and tumor. Thus bronchoscopy with transbronchial biopsy should generally be done prior to open lung biopsy.

3. **Open lung biopsy** should be performed in patients with suspected IPF if the diagnosis has not been made by other techniques; the HRCT scan of the chest should be used to guide the location of the biopsy. Results of biopsy will allow the diagnosis to be made and permit a judgment of disease responsiveness to therapy. Open lung biopsy need not be done in patients with advanced lung disease of any etiology (extensive honeycombing, profound hypoxemia, hypercapnea, or cor pulmonale), since the response to therapy is likely to be low, or in those with significant comorbidities (advanced age, cardiac disease) in whom the risk of a procedure is high. Therapeutic decisions should be based solely on clinical information in these patients.

H. **Management**

1. IPF is a progressive disease without spontaneous remissions. Although the rate of disease progression may vary considerably among patients, the median survival in large series of patients with documented IPF is 3–5 years. This poor prognosis provides a strong impetus to use aggressive therapy for IPF. Unfortunately, because the etiology and pathogenesis of this disease remain poorly understood, **no specific therapy is currently available**. Since exuberant inflammation seems to be a component of the disease process, especially early in its course, most therapeutic approaches have involved the use of pharmacologic agents that suppress immune and inflammatory responses (Table 22-3) (12). Data from prospective, randomized trials are quite limited, and no large multicenter trials with extensive patient stratification have been available to guide therapeutic decisions. Complications related to therapy are very common.

    a. **Corticosteroids are the first line of therapy in IPF.** Prednisone is generally administered in doses of 60 mg/d to 1–1.5 mg/kg/d (not exceeding 100 mg/d) for 1–2 months. The dose is then reduced gradually to 0.5 mg/kg/d, with the rate and extent of further tapering determined by the patient's response. With this general approach, approximately 20% of patients will have significant improvement in physiologic abnormalities (2,4,12). Those patients who demonstrate improvement in objective measures of pulmonary function show a survival advantage (13). Some authors describe improved breathlessness without change in pulmonary function (4). An additional group of patients (20% to 30%) may show stabilization of pulmonary function and dyspnea after the initiation of steroid therapy. However, the relevance of this is difficult to assess in the absence of appropriate controls. Anecdotal reports suggest a benefit from "pulsed" intravenous corticosteroids (eg, methylprednisolone given in doses of 1

Table 22-3. Drugs proposed for the therapy of interstitial pulmonary fibrosis

Agent	Initial dose	Evidence of efficacy
Prednisone	1–1.5 mg/kg/d (<100 mg/d)	+
Cyclophosphamide	100–150 mg/d	+
Azathioprine	3 mg/kg/d (<200 mg/d)	+
Methotrexate	10–15 mg/week	0
D-penicillamine	—	0
Cyclosporine	—	0
Colchicine	0.6–1.2 mg/d	+/−

g/d for 3–4 days, followed by oral prednisone), but insufficient data are available to recommend this approach.

b. Several cytotoxic drugs have been used for therapy of IPF, either alone or in conjunction with lower doses of corticosteroids.

  i. **Cyclophosphamide** has been used most extensively. Small controlled trials have demonstrated a trend toward improved survival and improved pulmonary function in individuals who received cyclophosphamide plus prednisone (at reduced dose) compared to those who received high-dose prednisone alone (14,15). Selected individuals who have failed steroid therapy may benefit from a subsequent trial of cyclophosphamide. Cyclophosphamide is given at a dose of 100–150 mg/d, as tolerated by the patient. However, the use of this agent has been limited by major side effects (see I. below).

  ii. **Azathioprine** is another cytotoxic agent that may be helpful in IPF. Azathioprine has been used in conjunction with lower doses of corticosteroids and typically is administered at a dose of 3 mg/kg/d, not to exceed 200 mg/d. A randomized prospective trial comparing azathioprine and prednisone with prednisone alone demonstrated a trend toward prolonged survival and improved pulmonary physiology in those patients who received azathioprine (16). This drug has generally been well tolerated and may be the cytotoxic agent of choice for IPF at present.

c. Several other drugs have been suggested for the treatment of IPF, based on theoretical considerations or anecdotal reports (12). **Methotrexate**, a useful anti-inflammatory agent in rheumatoid arthritis, is well tolerated when given orally on a weekly basis and may have a role in the treatment of IPF. **Penicillamine** also is useful for treating active inflammation in rheumatoid arthritis and may act through suppression of T-cell function. **Cyclosporine** is another potent immunosuppressive agent that impairs T-cell responses and thus might be helpful in the treatment of alveolitis. However, insufficient evidence is available at present to support the use of any of these potent immunosuppressive agents in IPF, and each may cause major side effects. Finally, **colchicine** appears to have both antifibrotic and anti-inflammatory activity and is best known for its beneficial effects in the treatment of gout. A single retrospective study found this drug to have response rates similar to those described above for corticosteroids, with relatively few side effects (17).

2. **Predicting response to therapy.** A favorable response to immunosuppressant therapy (especially corticosteroids) is increased if the patient is younger or if the duration of disease prior to treatment is shorter (<12 months). A forced vital capacity (FVC) <90% of predicted may also suggest a favorable response (18,19). Patterns of infiltrates on HRCT scan of the chest are potentially of value in predicting response to therapy (20). CT scans showing ground-glass infiltrates suggest active disease that is more amenable to therapy, while linear scarring and honeycombing suggest fixed fibrotic disease that is less likely to respond (21). Similarly, a lung biopsy that shows acute inflammation with little fibrosis predicts a good response. Bronchoalveolar lavage (BAL) has been used to sample the inflammatory cells in the alveolar space in patients with IPF (6,7). Typically, increased numbers of inflammatory cells are present in the BAL fluid. A subset of individuals with increased numbers of lymphocytes in their BAL fluid has proven more likely to improve following steroid therapy. Conversely, patients with increased numbers of neutrophils or eosinophils are more likely to have refractory disease.

3. **Supportive therapy.** Patients who are hypoxemic either at rest or with exercise should receive supplemental oxygen therapy. This therapy has not been shown to prolong life; the rate of disease progression is the most important determinant of this. However, oxygen therapy may relieve symptoms, increase exercise tolerance, and slow progression to right heart failure. Similarly, pulmonary rehabilitation may help control symptoms and increase the level of ac-

tivity, although the benefits of a formal rehabilitation program are less well defined than for COPD. The physician should discuss with the IPF patient those issues related to mechanical ventilation and the aggressiveness of care at the end of life. In some instances, hospice care is appropriate.

4. **Lung transplantation** is a viable option for individuals with IPF. In general, single-lung transplantation is the procedure of choice. Patients should be considered for transplantation if they have progressive disease despite trials of therapy (steroids with or without cytotoxic agents), are not likely to survive 18–24 months, and are of an appropriate age (for most transplantation centers, <60 years). Early consideration of the possibility of transplantation is important because of the progressive nature of the disease and the long waiting period for suitable organs.

I. **Complications of therapy**

1. All of the therapies suggested for IPF have a potential for serious complications (12). Corticosteroids often are well tolerated for short periods, but the use of relatively high doses of corticosteroids for periods of months (to years) places patients at risk for a number of important complications, including very significant weight gain, alterations in mood and sleep patterns, osteopenia, hyperglycemia, myopathy, accelerated cataract formation, and opportunistic infections. Retention of salt and water by patients taking steroids may exacerbate cardiac disease and lead to worsening dyspnea or right ventricular overload. Conversely, withdrawal of steroids may result in a number of symptoms or, in rare instances, overt adrenal insufficiency.

2. **Cyclophosphamide** may induce bone marrow suppression with leukopenia or thrombocytopenia. Blood counts must be monitored closely in patients receiving cyclophosphamide, and the dose must be adjusted to maintain a total white blood cell count >3000/mm^3 with an adequate absolute neutrophil count. Hemorrhagic cystitis is a distinct complication of cyclophosphamide. To lessen the risk of this problem, cyclophosphamide should be taken early in the day along with copious fluids and frequent bladder emptying. Additional side effects of cyclophosphamide include infection, anorexia, nausea and vomiting, and azoospermia or amenorrhea. Cyclophosphamide also has occasionally been reported to induce interstitial lung disease. Finally, prolonged courses of cyclophosphamide increase the risk of late hematologic malignancy, particularly leukemia.

3. **Azathioprine** is somewhat better tolerated than cyclophosphamide but can also induce leukopenia, thrombocytopenia, or red cell aplasia. Blood counts must be monitored closely. Gastrointestinal side effects are relatively common, especially nausea and vomiting. A small proportion of patients may have mild liver function abnormalities. As with cyclophosphamide, interstitial lung disease due to azathioprine has been reported, as well as an increased risk of late malignancy.

4. The combined use of prednisone with either of these immunosuppressive drugs places the patient at significant risk of infection, especially opportunistic pneumonia. Many specialists advocate the prophylactic administration of trimethoprim/sulfamethoxazole to prevent *Pneumocystis carinii* pneumonia (PCP) in patients receiving prednisone (>20 mg/d) and full doses of cyclophosphamide. A patient with IPF on immunosuppressant therapy who presents with rapidly worsening dyspnea and a deterioration in gas exchange is a particularly difficult clinical challenge. Intercurrent infection, CHF, and progression of pulmonary fibrosis are all diagnostic possibilities. Distinguishing among these processes may be very difficult on clinical and radiographic information alone.

J. **Specialist referrals.** The care of patients who potentially have IPF requires close cooperation between the primary care physician and the pulmonologist. Patients should be promptly referred to the specialist when the diagnosis is first considered, as a thorough physiologic evaluation and consideration for fiberoptic bronchoscopy and/or open lung biopsy are essential. These procedures are best performed by individuals experienced in the care of patients with interstitial lung disease. Similarly, pathologic specimens should be reviewed by a pathologist with experience in diagnosing IPF in order to gauge inflammation and fibrosis.

II. **Bronchiolitis obliterans organizing pneumonia.** A histologic pattern of obliteration of small airways by plugs of granulation tissue (bronchiolitis obliterans) associated with extension of the organizing exudate distally into alveoli (organizing pneumonia) is found in a wide variety of pulmonary parenchymal processes, including collagen vascular diseases and inhalation injuries (Table 22-4). However, when this pathologic pattern is idiopathic and not associated with another underlying condition, the syndrome has been called either bronchiolitis obliterans organizing pneumonia (BOOP) or cryptogenic organizing pneumonitis (COP). The clinical presentation and course of this syndrome are distinctive insofar as the pathology indicates a primary airways disease that should present as chronic airflow obstruction, while the clinical syndrome more often mimics subacute pneumonitis or pulmonary fibrosis (22,23).

  A. **Clinical presentation.** BOOP typically occurs in individuals in the sixth and seventh decades, with an equal distribution among men and women. Patients most frequently present with an illness of weeks' to a few months' duration. Some patients describe a specific onset of symptoms associated with an upper respiratory infection. Dyspnea on exertion and cough are generally present. The cough is usually not productive of sputum and may be quite annoying. Systemic symptoms, including fever, weight loss, and malaise, occur in fewer than half the patients. The most common sign is rales, usually bilateral (22–24). Occasionally, patients may have a midinspiratory squeak on auscultation. Wheezing and finger clubbing are rarely present. A minority of patients have a normal examination.

  B. **Chest radiographs** in patients with BOOP reveal patchy alveolar infiltrates (22) that are usually diffuse but in rare instances may be unilateral and focal. Often the infiltrates are quite peripheral with central sparing (25).

Table 22-4. Clinical syndromes that may demonstrate a histologic pattern of obliterative bronchiolitis with organizing pneumonitis

---

Idiopathic bronchiolitis obliterans organizing pneumonia (BOOP)

Connective tissue diseases
  Rheumatoid arthritis
  Polymyositis/dermatomyositis

Hypersensitivity pneumonitis

Chronic eosinophilic pneumonia

Organizing acute infection
  Mycoplasma pneumoniae
  Legionella pneumophila
  Influenza virus
  Cytomegalovirus
  Nocardia asteroides
  Pneumocystis carinii
  Human immunodeficiency virus infection

Organizing diffuse alveolar damage following the adult respiratory distress syndrome

Organ transplantation

Vasculitis

Drug-induced lung disease

Aspiration pneumonitis

Radiation pneumonitis

Common variable immunodeficiency syndrome

Adapted from King T. Bronchiolitis. In: Schwarz M, King T, eds. *Interstitial lung disease.* St. Louis, Mo: Mosby-Year Book, 1993:463–495.

C. **Etiology and pathogenesis.** While the pathologic picture of BOOP may be found in response to a number of pulmonary insults, including toxic fume inhalation, infection, and drug reactions, none of these precipitating factors has been identified in patients with BOOP. Although precise pathologic mechanisms have not been defined, as with IPF, the basic abnormality probably involves an exuberant immunologic response. The relative importance of the obstruction of airways versus the more distal organizing pneumonia remains an open debate. The typical physiologic abnormalities found in BOOP suggest that the alveolar exudate plays a central role in the pathophysiology of this clinical entity (26).

D. **Physiology.** While bronchiolitis obliterans, a condition exclusively affecting the airways, causes an obstructive ventilatory defect, the most common ventilatory abnormality in BOOP is a mild restrictive ventilatory defect with a reduction in total lung capacity (TLC) to <80% of predicted. The FVC may be reduced to a similar extent. A small proportion of patients may have mixed obstructive/restrictive abnormalities with reductions in both FVC and FEV_1, resulting in an FEV_1/FVC ratio that is less than predicted. Patients with an obstructive defect usually have a history of cigarette smoking (22). Gas exchange is very frequently abnormal in patients with BOOP, with reductions in the DLCO to <80% of predicted and widening of the $(A-a)O_2$.

E. **Differential diagnosis.** A large number of pulmonary parenchymal processes may mimic BOOP and must be considered as diagnostic possibilities whenever the diagnosis of BOOP is entertained. These include infection, chronic eosinophilic pneumonia, hypersensitivity pneumonitis (including drug reactions), IPF, and neoplasms, especially alveolar cell carcinoma and pulmonary lymphoma (26).

F. **Diagnostic approach**
   1. The diagnosis of BOOP should be considered in the patient who presents with a subacute history of cough, breathlessness, pulmonary function studies demonstrating a restrictive ventilatory defect with impaired gas exchange, and a chest radiograph with patchy alveolar infiltrates. The results of pulmonary function studies and chest radiograph will exclude asthma or chronic bronchitis following an upper respiratory tract infection. Infectious pneumonitis is often a consideration early in the presentation of patients with BOOP, and many patients have had extensive courses of oral antibiotics prior to diagnosis. By the time the diagnosis of BOOP is considered, the duration of illness usually makes common infections less likely. Chronic infection due to fungi or mycobacteria may remain a consideration. These organisms should be sought in sputum or biopsy specimens by stain and culture. Exclusion of the known causes of BOOP is important, such as toxic fume inhalation or collagen vascular diseases, with a careful history and appropriate serologic evaluation. Patients with idiopathic BOOP do not have significant titers of antinuclear antibodies or rheumatoid factor.
   2. IPF and BOOP may share many clinical features, but there are important differences in presentation (23). BOOP frequently will present with a shorter history than IPF (>70% of patients have had symptoms for 3 months or less) and have an increased incidence of systemic symptoms. Patients with BOOP commonly have alveolar infiltrates with ground-glass opacities and air bronchograms, suggesting pneumonitis on both chest radiographs and CT scans (22,27). The typical linear and nodular infiltrates of IPF are uncommon in BOOP, and honeycombing and cyst formation are observed very rarely.
   3. Distinguishing among BOOP, chronic eosinophilic pneumonia, hypersensitivity pneumonitis, or sarcoidosis can be quite difficult on clinical grounds. Patients with BOOP do not have a history of significant exposure to antigens commonly associated with hypersensitivity pneumonitis and do not demonstrate eosinophilia. BOOP is not associated with hilar or mediastinal adenopathy, and patients lack the extrapulmonary manifestations of sarcoidosis.
   4. The **diagnosis of BOOP** can only be confirmed by the examination of lung biopsy specimens that show prominent granulation tissue obstructing bronchioles and alveolar ducts, with distal organizing pneumonia. Because features of BOOP may be found in biopsies from patients with a variety of under-

lying processes other than idiopathic BOOP, transbronchial biopsy specimens are usually insufficient to exclude these other diagnoses. However, when a transbronchial biopsy in an appropriate clinical setting demonstrates BOOP along with an absence of other disease processes, it may be appropriate to repeat fiberoptic bronchoscopy and obtain multiple specimens. We therefore recommend fiberoptic bronchoscopy with transbronchial biopsy to exclude infection, chronic eosinophilic pneumonia, sarcoid, and neoplasm. If the biopsy results are compatible with BOOP and not these other entities, therapy with steroids may be initiated (25). While such an approach may yield satisfactory results in many patients, a clinical response will not distinguish between BOOP and chronic eosinophilic pneumonia, sarcoidosis, or lymphoma. If the transbronchial biopsy is equivocal or the clinical situation unusual, we recommend open lung biopsy for a definitive diagnosis.

G. **Management.** Although a small number of patients have been described who experienced complete recovery without specific therapy, corticosteroids are the treatment of choice for idiopathic BOOP. In several series, >70% of patients have had excellent clinical response to steroids (22–24). Most of these patients had complete radiographic and physiologic improvement. In particular, those with airspace abnormalities on chest radiograph or CT scan tended to do quite well, while patients with honeycombing or interstitial infiltrates were less likely to respond. An appropriate initial therapy is prednisone, given as a single morning dose of 1 mg/kg (not to exceed 100 mg/d). With this therapy, most patients will experience significant improvement, usually over a period of weeks. Typically, patients respond somewhat more slowly than those with chronic eosinophilic pneumonia but more rapidly than patients with IPF or sarcoidosis. The steroid dose must be tapered relatively slowly; patients may experience physiologic deterioration after an initial improvement if the dose is tapered rapidly (26). Thus, after 1 month of initial therapy, the dose should be tapered over 2 months to approximately 0.5 mg/kg/d. The dose may then be tapered more slowly over the next 3–6 months. Patient symptoms, spirometry, and DLCO should be monitored closely and the dose of prednisone increased if there is evidence of deterioration. In most instances, therapy can be discontinued within 9–12 months. In the small proportion of patients who do not have significant improvement with prednisone therapy, a cytotoxic agent may be added. Little published information is available concerning the likelihood of response in these circumstances.

H. **Problems and complications of therapy.** The problems with corticosteroid therapy for BOOP are exactly those described for IPF (see I. above). Because the duration of high-dose prednisone therapy for BOOP is less than that for IPF, the therapy tends to be tolerated somewhat better in the former condition than in the latter.

I. **Specialist referral.** Patients with possible BOOP very frequently will come to the attention of a primary care physician under the guise of slowly resolving pneumonia or prolonged cough after an upper respiratory tract infection. When the presumed pneumonitis has failed to respond to therapy as expected within 6–8 weeks, the patient should then be referred to the pulmonary specialist for further diagnostic studies.

III. **Eosinophilic granuloma (EG) of the lung,** also known as primary pulmonary histiocytosis X and pulmonary Langerhans' cell granulomatosis, is a rare pulmonary disease that is part of a spectrum of diseases initially designated as histiocytosis X. Two other histiocytic diseases, Hand-Schüller-Christian disease and Letterer-Siwe disease, are aggressive conditions involving infiltration of multiple organs in adults or children. EG, the mildest form of the histiocytosis X diseases, often involves the lung alone but may also involve bone. It is characterized by a bronchocentric inflammatory reaction with poorly formed granulomas that contain proliferating Langerhans' cells, as well as lymphocytes, monocytes, and eosinophils within lung parenchyma, and often involve the alveolar walls and blood vessels (28). EG typically occurs in individuals in the third or fourth decade of life with approximately equal sex distribution.

A. **Clinical presentation**

1. The most common presenting complaints in EG are dyspnea on exertion and a nonproductive cough. However, a significant portion of patients (approximately 25%) are asymptomatic at presentation and are identified by an abnor-

mal chest radiograph (28,29). A smaller number of patients (14%) may present with chest pain and acute shortness of breath associated with a spontaneous pneumothorax. By history, at least 90% of patients have been cigarette smokers (30). This association is so strong that the diagnosis of EG must be considered with care in nonsmokers. The physical examination may be normal. Wheezes are heard only in a minority of patients. In advanced disease, patients may have signs of chronic respiratory failure and cor pulmonale. Bony lesions occur in approximately 15% of patients and are most common in the skull, ribs, or pelvis and may cause pain (29). A small number of patients may develop central diabetes insipidus.

2. The **chest radiograph** is virtually always abnormal in EG and typically reveals diffuse nodular or reticulonodular densities accompanied by small (5–10 mm) cysts. These infiltrates are often seen in the mid- and upper lung zones (29,31). The costophrenic angles often are spared. Nodules may proceed to cavitation. In more advanced cases, bullae and honeycombing may be present. The lung volume is typically normal or increased.

B. **Etiology and pathogenesis. Langerhans' cells** are normal constituents of the skin and mucosal organs, including the lung. These cells are involved in the presentation of antigen to T lymphocytes for the initiation of antigen-specific immune responses. In EG, the number of Langerhans' cells in the lung is greatly increased, with associated lymphocytes, monocytes, and eosinophils forming granulomas. This proliferation of Langerhans' cells is thought to be reactive, although the stimulus for the increase is unknown (32). The relevance of the association with cigarette smoking is unknown. Of interest, increased numbers of Langerhans' cells have been identified in the BAL fluid of healthy smokers, compared to nonsmokers.

C. **Physiology**
   1. Early in the course of EG, when the chest radiograph shows predominantly nodular densities, patients typically demonstrate a mild restrictive defect on pulmonary function studies. The TLC and FVC are reduced to <80% of predicted. As cysts and bullae are formed, air trapping develops with increases in the residual volume. Pneumothorax can occur as a consequence of local air trapping. The TLC may also become increased. In some individuals, frank airway obstruction is seen on spirometry.
   2. Abnormalities in gas transfer are quite common, with a reduction in the DLCO out of proportion to the abnormality in spirometry (28,29,33). As might be expected, the $(A-a)DO_2$ is widened, and patients may be hypoxemic, especially during exercise. In advanced disease, the $Paco_2$ may be elevated.

D. **Differential diagnosis**
   1. EG presents as an interstitial lung disease with nodular or linear and nodular infiltrates that are predominantly found in the mid- and upper lung zones. This distribution is found in conditions such as silicosis; talc-induced lung disease; sarcoidosis; chronic infectious granulomatous diseases, including fungal and mycobacterial diseases; and, rarely, metastatic disease or ankylosing spondylitis. The vast majority of patients with EG will give a history of smoking or may present with pneumothorax, diabetes insipidus, or bony lesions.
   2. Frequently, patients with EG will present with a distinctive syndrome characterized by interstitial lung disease and preserved lung volumes (by radiograph), together with airflow obstruction possibly in combination with restriction as measured by pulmonary function studies. This pattern may also be seen in lymphangioleiomyomatosis, BOOP, and sarcoidosis (Table 22-5). The presence of interstitial lung disease in a patient with a spontaneous pneumothorax should suggest EG, lymphangioleiomyomatosis, or, more rarely, IPF or PCP if the patient also has the acquired immunodeficiency syndrome.

E. **Diagnostic approach**
   1. The diagnosis of EG requires tissue confirmation. Initially, patients should undergo complete radiographic evaluation including HRCT scanning of the chest, which will reveal a mixture of nodules and thin-walled cysts (usually <10 mm in diameter). A predominance of disease will be noted in the upper and midlung zones. This appearance on CT scan should strongly suggest the

Table 22-5. Conditions associated with radiographic interstitial lung disease with physiologic studies revealing airflow obstruction or mixed obstructive/restrictive ventilatory defects

Eosinophilic granuloma of lung

Lymphangioleiomyomatosis

Sarcoidosis

Bronchiolitis obliterans with organizing pneumonia (in smokers)

Pulmonary fibrosis in an individual with preexisting chronic airflow obstruction

diagnosis of EG (27,34,35). In addition, patients should undergo complete physiologic testing including measurement of lung volumes, DLCO, and arterial blood gases.

2. A definitive diagnosis of EG generally requires pathologic study of lung tissue. An open lung biopsy is usually necessary to obtain sufficient material to observe the typical pattern of stellate lesions representing poorly formed granulomas. However, in patients with a typical clinical picture, an experienced pathologist may be able to make the diagnosis on material obtained from transbronchial biopsy (36). We therefore recommend bronchoscopy with transbronchial biopsy in most patients suspected to have EG, prior to open lung biopsy.

    a. **X bodies (or Birbeck granules) characteristic of the distinctive Langerhans' cells of EG may be identified within the lung tissue by electron microscopy** (32).

    b. **Positive staining of lung tissue with an antibody to neuropeptide, S-100, confirms the diagnosis of EG** (37).

  F. **Management**

    1. **The natural history of EG is quite variable.** All patients with EG must **stop smoking.** In individuals with asymptomatic or mildly symptomatic disease, smoking cessation alone may result in physiologic stabilization or improvement (38). In those with more severe or progressive disease, a wide variety of interventions has been advocated, including use of all of the immunosuppressant drugs used for IPF. Corticosteroids have been most commonly used. However, no controlled trials have demonstrated clear benefit from any regimen. Although occasional reports have suggested benefit from corticosteroid therapy (33), other series have shown no response (28,29). In patients with progressive disease, a trial of prednisone is probably worthwhile, but the benefit of this therapy should be monitored with physiologic measurements. The supportive measures described for IPF are appropriate for patients with EG as well. Successful lung transplantation for EG has been described.

    2. **Pleurodesis** is often necessary and beneficial in patients with recurrent pneumothorax. Painful bony lesions have responded to radiation therapy. Diabetes insipidus often is controlled by adequate free water intake, although therapy with arginine vasopressin also may be required.

  G. **Problems and complications of therapy.** The complications of therapy with immunosuppressive agents for EG are the same as those for IPF. Assessing the risk–benefit ratio of therapy is obviously problematic, given the paucity of information supporting the efficacy of any individual regimen. It should be remembered that treatment of recurrent pneumothorax by bilateral pleurectomy would preclude subsequent pneumonectomy and the possibility of future lung transplantation.

  H. **Specialist referral.** As with the other rare and complex conditions described in this chapter, the primary care physician should promptly involve the pulmonary medicine specialist in the care of patients suspected to have EG.

IV. **Lymphangioleiomyomatosis** (LAM) is a rare condition characterized by the proliferation of smooth muscle cells lining blood vessels, lymphatics, and bronchi. LAM occurs exclusively in women, almost always in the childbearing years (39,40). Histologically, LAM is indistinguishable from tuberous sclerosis, an autosomal-dominant multisystem disorder occurring equally in men and women. Tuberous sclerosis is characterized by hamartomas in skin, central nervous system, kidneys, and other organs. Pulmonary involvement is found in approximately 2% of patients with tuberous sclerosis (41).

A. Clinical presentation

1. The most frequent presenting complaint in patients with LAM is dyspnea on exertion (39,40,42). The onset of breathlessness is usually quite gradual, except in individuals with spontaneous pneumothorax, but may progress to the point of breathlessness at rest. Cough is less frequent than in the other processes discussed in this chapter; in one large series, cough was present initially in 12% of patients and sometime during the course of illness in approximately 40% (40). Occasionally, patients will present with hemoptysis, although this problem may occur in almost half the patients at some time during the illness.

2. **Pleural manifestations** of LAM are quite common. Spontaneous pneumothorax, with the abrupt onset of breathlessness and chest pain, is found in up to half the patients at presentation and in up to 80% at some point in the illness. Approximately one-quarter of patients may develop pleural effusions that are chylous in nature. A small number of patients may develop chylous ascites due to obstruction of the thoracic duct. In patients with progressive disease, the symptoms of chronic respiratory failure and cor pulmonale are found.

3. The **chest radiograph** typically demonstrates **diffuse linear and nodular infiltrates. Kerley's B lines and thin-walled cystic spaces** may be evident. The lung volumes are virtually always preserved or increased. Pneumothorax, pleural scarring, or pleural effusion may be present (39,40).

B. Etiology and pathogenesis

1. The etiology of LAM is unknown. The disease involves smooth muscle proliferation at multiple sites. The consequences of this abnormal proliferation are obstruction of lymphatics (leading to chylous effusions, Kerley's B lines, etc), airways (leading to airflow obstruction and air trapping with bleb formation and pneumothoraces), and blood vessels (resulting in hemoptysis or pulmonary hypertension) (39,40). LAM occurs in women of childbearing years or who have been exposed to estrogen, leading to the suggestion that sex hormones may be driving the abnormal smooth muscle cell proliferation. This relationship is further supported by reports of patients whose disease stabilized or improved following various hormonal interventions. However, no correlation has been found between the expression of receptors for estrogen or progesterone on the smooth muscle cells and response to therapy. Although the relationship between LAM and tuberous sclerosis remains unclear, new insights into the pathogenesis of LAM will hopefully be found when the genetic abnormality causing tuberous sclerosis is discovered.

C. Physiology

1. **Pulmonary function studies** in patients with LAM typically demonstrate an obstructive ventilatory defect, with reduction in the FEV_1 out of proportion to that of the FVC (39,43). Measurements of lung volumes generally demonstrate air trapping with an increase in residual volume. Many patients have normal or increased TLC (hyperinflation), while those who have had pleural scarring may have a reduction in TLC, consistent with a mixed obstructive/restrictive abnormality (40). The DLCO is almost always reduced. Gas transfer is often reduced out of proportion to the defect in mechanics. The $(A-a)DO_2$ is increased, and patients may have hypoxemia at rest or with exercise. Patients may develop hypercarbia and cor pulmonale.

D. Differential diagnosis

1. The diagnostic possibilities depend on the manner of presentation. If woman presents with interstitial lung disease and normal to increased lung volumes with airflow obstruction, then eosinophilic granuloma, sarcoidosis, or tuberous sclerosis would be high on the list of differential diagnostic possibilities. If dyspnea and airflow obstruction are major features of the presentation, asthma and COPD must be ruled out. If a woman presents with a pneumothorax, idiopathic spontaneous pneumothorax would also be a major consideration. A chylous pleural effusion might suggest chronic pleural inflammation due

to rheumatoid arthritis or parasitic disease or thoracic duct obstruction due to trauma or malignancy.

E. **Diagnostic approach**

1. The diagnosis of LAM is often quite difficult, because the condition is rare and usually not initially considered. In one large series, the mean time from initial presentation to diagnosis was 44 months (range, 1–219 months) (40). While the vast majority of patients are premenopausal women, there are several reports of LAM in postmenopausal women receiving estrogen therapy.

2. Following a thorough history and physical examination, the results of pulmonary function and radiographic studies can suggest the diagnosis and help exclude other, more common possibilities. In the patient with spontaneous pneumothorax, the finding of airflow obstruction with reduced DLCO or interstitial infiltrates should raise the possibility of LAM and exclude the possibility of idiopathic spontaneous pneumothorax. Similarly, a reduced DLCO and radiographic abnormalities are incompatible with asthma or chronic bronchitis. While a variety of conditions may present with interstitial infiltrates on chest radiograph that may mimic those of LAM, very few conditions (EG, sarcoidosis) combine these radiographic findings with airflow obstruction.

3. **CT scanning** can be quite helpful in the evaluation of the woman who might have LAM (42,44). LAM has a very distinctive picture of diffuse thin-walled cysts, sometimes interspersed with areas of ground-glass opacification on HRCT scans of the chest. Whether the absence of cysts on CT scan excludes the diagnosis of LAM is not yet clear. Obstruction of thoracic lymphatics with dilatation of the thoracic duct is an additional CT finding that suggests LAM.

4. **Open lung biopsy** is necessary to establish the diagnosis of LAM. However, in several cases in which there was a strong clinical suspicion of LAM and an experienced pathologist was aware of this consideration, the diagnosis has been made with specimens obtained by examination of transbronchial biopsy specimens. When transbronchial biopsy specimens do not reveal the diagnosis, open or thoracoscopic lung biopsy should be performed. Finally, as noted previously, the thoracic manifestations and pathologic appearance of tuberous sclerosis and LAM are identical. It is important for the physician to search for extrathoracic stigmata of tuberous sclerosis, when considering the diagnosis of LAM.

F. **Management**

1. The natural history of LAM is not well defined. Initial reports suggested a relentless illness that often led to death due to respiratory failure in 4–5 years (39). However, more recent evidence suggests that the disease may be less aggressive. In a relatively large series from North America, 78% of the patients were alive 9.4 years after the onset of LAM (40).

2. **The therapy of LAM is controversial.** There is no apparent benefit from immunosuppressive agents. Because estrogen may play a role in the pathogenesis of the smooth muscle proliferation, a number of hormonal manipulations designed to reduce estrogen levels have been attempted. Patients receiving estrogens should discontinue these medications.

3. The two interventions most likely to be of benefit are therapy with progesterone and surgical or pharmacologic oophorectomy. Improvement or stabilization of symptoms and physiologic abnormalities with progesterone therapy has been reported in several cases, followed by deterioration when the drug was stopped and restabilization when therapy was resumed (40). A recent meta-analysis found that >50% of evaluable cases benefited from progesterone therapy (45). However, the numbers were quite small. Patients with chylous effusions or ascites may be more responsive to this therapy.

   a. We suggest observation of asymptomatic individuals along with frequent physiologic monitoring. In women with significant symptoms or with progressive impairment, **medroxyprogesterone**, 400–800 mg, may be given intramuscularly each month. If the disease progresses or if the patient is severely impaired at presentation, pharmacologic oophorectomy (reversible) with **leuprolide or surgical oophorectomy** can be considered. This therapeutic option should be chosen only after extensive discussion with the patient and family.

   b. No information is available to suggest that tamoxifen is beneficial, and there are reports of worsening of disease with this drug, possibly attributable to its action as a mild estrogen agonist. Patients with progressive disease with LAM have successfully undergone lung transplantation.

G. Problems and complications of therapy
   1. The absence of normal estrogen may cause a number of very important side effects. Symptoms of menopause, including mood swings, hot flashes, and thinning of the vaginal mucosa, may be prominent, especially in younger women. While these symptoms may wane over time, the risks of coronary artery disease and accelerated osteoporosis are increased. Interventions to minimize these risks, such as calcium supplementation, should be considered early.

H. Specialist referral
   1. LAM is a rare condition that is often difficult to diagnose. The primary care physician should be aware of this diagnosis and refer to a pulmonary specialist those female patients who have spontaneous pneumothorax or chronic airflow obstruction with atypical presentations, including interstitial infiltrates on chest radiograph or significantly reduced DLCO. Once the diagnosis of LAM has been made, the patient will require careful joint management by the primary care physician and the pulmonary specialist.
   2. The care of patients with LAM is greatly hampered by a lack of information about the natural history of the disease and its response to therapy. No single center sees enough patients to develop these data. Accordingly, a LAM registry has been established at the National Institutes of Health.

V. Pulmonary alveolar proteinosis (PAP) is a condition in which the alveolar spaces become filled with a distinct lipid and protein mixture, but the alveolar walls are preserved. Biochemically, the mixture is composed of components of pulmonary surfactant, including surfactant phospholipids and apolipoproteins. A pathologic and clinical picture similar to PAP may be found following a variety of pulmonary insults including inhalation exposure to silica dust, *P. carinii* infection, and certain hematologic malignancies. Some authors have classified these cases as "secondary" PAP. In those instances, the natural history and therapeutic options are determined by the underlying disease. The discussion here will focus on PAP occurring in the absence of another primary disease. Typically, PAP is an illness of young or middle-aged adults, although it does occur at the extremes of age. In most series, males predominate by approximately 2:1.

A. Clinical presentation
   1. Patients typically present with a subacute illness, with progressive dyspnea on exertion as the hallmark (46–48). Eventually, they may complain of breathlessness with minimal exertion or at rest. Cough is frequently but not always present. In some instances, the cough may be a prominent complaint, and on rare occasions the patient may describe large volumes of "gummy" sputum. Patients often experience systemic symptoms such as weight loss, malaise, and fatigue. However, fever is not a sign of PAP and, when present, should suggest an alternative diagnosis or the possibility of a superimposed infection. Classically, patients with PAP have been considered to be at increased risk for infections with unusual organisms, especially *Nocardia asteroides* (49). Other reports have suggested an increased risk of infection with mycobacteria, especially *Mycobacterium avium-intracellulare* complex (50).
   2. **Examination of the chest** may reveal inspiratory rales or bronchovesicular breath sounds. However, normal breath sounds can commonly be heard on examination. Cyanosis and clubbing of the fingers may be present.
   3. The **chest radiograph** reveals bilateral ground-glass or nodular infiltrates with acinar shadows, indicating alveolar filling. These infiltrates may be patchy and are often most prominent in the perihilar region and may be suggestive of cardiogenic pulmonary edema. Hilar or mediastinal adenopathy and pleural effusions are not features of PAP.

B. Etiology and pathogenesis
   1. PAP is due to the abnormal accumulation of excessive quantities of pulmonary

surfactant within the alveolar space, blocking the diffusion of gas. Recent evidence has suggested an abnormality in the recycling or processing of surfactant, so that phospholipid and protein are not cleared from the alveolar space at a normal rate. In a few instances, pulmonary fibrosis has developed in patients with preexisting PAP. Whether this represents an end-stage progression of PAP is not known.

2. The **etiology of PAP** has not been determined, although various injuries are known to produce a similar, if not identical, pathologic and physiologic picture. In most instances, no discrete precipitating event can be identified, although a significant fraction of patients with PAP may have had exposure to inorganic dusts, as evidenced by increased quantities of birefringent material in biopsy specimens (48). No current evidence suggests that PAP in humans is an immunologically mediated disease. Although a pathologic picture identical to human PAP develops in mouse models utilizing immunodeficient animals, humans with PAP appear to be immunologically intact. Decreases in the levels of granulocyte–macrophage colony-stimulating factor in the lung may be important, because such deficiencies in mice result in accumulation of surfactant lipids and protein in alveolar spaces (51).

C. **Physiology**

1. The physiologic hallmark of PAP is gas exchange abnormality. The DLCO is reduced, often quite severely. The $(A-a)O_2$ is significantly increased (>20 mm Hg), and patients frequently are hypoxemic at rest. The gas exchange abnormalities typically worsen with exertion. The Pco_2 is usually significantly reduced due to chronic hyperventilation. Abnormalities in spirometry and lung volumes are common but not universal in PAP. The FVC and TLC are often reduced, demonstrating a restrictive ventilatory defect that is not adequate to explain the impaired gas transfer (46,48).

D. **Differential diagnosis.** The differential diagnostic possibilities in patients with PAP include other processes that cause alveolar filling. These include infectious diseases such as PCP or miliary tuberculosis; inhalation injury, especially due to acute silica exposure; malignancy; and chronic diffuse pulmonary hemorrhage, as in pulmonary hemosiderosis. Amiodarone toxicity, as well as inhalation of aerosolized lipids, may present with accumulations of alveolar lipid. Chronic aspiration of mineral oil (in nose drops or as a laxative) or other oils may result in an alveolar-filling process usually more localized than PAP and with less extensive gas exchange abnormalities. Some cases of IPF with a pathologic picture of DIP may resemble PAP both radiographically and clinically. Finally, BOOP and chronic eosinophilic pneumonia may rarely resemble PAP, although the distribution in the latter condition is more often perihilar in contrast to the peripheral distribution in the former conditions.

E. **Approach to the diagnosis**

1. In most instances, the diagnosis of PAP will be suggested by the radiographic appearance of the chest in a patient with appropriate symptoms. The history and examination will help to exclude other alveolar-filling processes such as chronic CHF, inhalational lung disease, or amiodarone toxicity. The history should include the identification of risk factors for human immunodeficiency virus infection. When present, these risk factors increase the likelihood of PCP or lymphocytic interstitial pneumonitis. As noted previously, fever is not typical of PAP, except when complicated by superimposed infection, and should prompt an extensive search for such an infection or a different process (46).

2. **CT** of the chest (either standard or high-resolution) may be of some help in these patients. Adenopathy and pleural disease are not features of PAP and, when present, should suggest an alternative diagnosis. In patients with PAP, HRCT typically demonstrates an alveolar-filling process, often with visible air bronchograms. Linear interstitial shadows may also be evident. The distribution of infiltrates, both central and peripheral, is predictive of PAP rather than BOOP or chronic eosinophilic pneumonia, processes that frequently have a more peripheral distribution. However, HRCT does not provide a specific diagnosis.

3. **The diagnosis** of PAP generally is made by bronchoscopy or open lung biopsy. In most instances, bronchoscopy should be the initial diagnostic procedure

performed. In an appropriate clinical setting, bronchoalveolar lavage may provide the diagnosis and is an effective means of excluding infection with *P. carinii* or superinfection with *Nocardia*. Transbronchial biopsy is a relatively sensitive and specific means of establishing the diagnosis and should be performed in almost all cases (46). **Positive periodic acid–Schiff staining** of bronchoalveolar washings or alveolar exudate in transbronchoscopic biopsy material confirms the diagnosis. Electron micrographic analysis will reveal granular material and lamellar bodies within alveoli. When no clear diagnosis has been obtained at bronchoscopy in suspected cases of PAP, an open or thoracoscopic lung biopsy should be performed. As with any of the relatively rare conditions discussed in this chapter, it is important that the pathologist be experienced with these processes and be given clinical information that might suggest a particular diagnosis.

F. Management

1. **The natural history of PAP is variable.** Some patients may experience spontaneous remission, while others may continue with stable disease. Individuals with minimal or no symptoms may be observed closely without therapy. Therapy should be instituted when symptoms affect day-to-day activity or patients experience significant physiologic impairment.

2. Extensive experience indicates that corticosteroids and other immunosuppressive agents have no role in the treatment of PAP (48). The only clearly beneficial therapy is total lung lavage (46,47). The patient is placed under general anesthesia, and the trachea is intubated with a double-lumen endotracheal tube to allow segregation of the left and right sides of the bronchial tree. One lung is then lavaged with multiple exchanges of isotonic saline, while the patient is ventilated via the other lung. Various formulas have been used to calculate the volume for each exchange, with most based on the estimated volume of the single lung derived from the TLC. The lung is alternately filled with saline and drained, with chest percussion performed to enhance fluid recovery. The fluid recovered in the initial exchanges is cloudy due to the excess surfactant present. The lavage procedure is continued until the fluid clears. The total volume necessary varies but is typically on the order of 25–40 L. After the procedure is ended, the patient usually requires 1–2 days in hospital for recovery. Occasionally, this procedure is performed sequentially on both lungs during one hospitalization. More frequently, the two lungs are treated in separate hospitalizations a few weeks apart.

3. Patients with PAP usually have significant radiographic and clinical improvement following total lung lavage. For many patients, a single lavage of each lung is the only treatment required. Other patients may relapse over a period of months and must be treated again. The number of times an individual requires lavage is highly variable and can not be predicted from information at the time of the initial lavage. Some authors suggest that lavage may reduce the risk of superinfection (46).

G. Problems and complications of therapy

1. **Total lung lavage** is safe and effective but should only be performed in a center experienced with the procedure. The anesthesiologist plays a critical role in the management of the patient during the lavage and must be adept with the positioning of double-lumen endotracheal tubes and single-lung ventilation. Close monitoring of gas exchange and hemodynamics during the procedure is obviously critical. Careful recording of the volumes instilled and returned with each exchange during the lavage is essential. The procedure is halted if the patient is sequestering large volumes of fluid within the chest during the procedure or if there is any indication of spill of saline into the ventilated lung. Occasionally, patients may have concomitant PAP and asthma and may develop bronchospasm during lung lavage. These patients should be treated aggressively with bronchodilators and may require steroid prophylaxis for asthma prior to lung lavage.

H. Specialist referral

1. Patients suspected of having PAP should promptly be referred to a pulmonary medicine specialist for bronchoscopy and consideration for total lung lavage.

References

1. Crystal RG, Bitterman PB, Rennard SI, et al.: Interstitial lung diseases of unknown cause: disorders characterized by chronic inflammation of the lower respiratory tract (first of two parts). *N Engl J Med* 1984;310:154–166.
2. Carrington CB, Gaensler EA, Coutu RE, et al.: Natural history and treated course of usual and desquamative interstitial pneumonia. *N Engl J Med* 1978;298:801–809.
3. Crystal RG, Fulmer JD, Roberts WC, et al.: Idiopathic pulmonary fibrosis: clinical, histologic, radiographic, physiologic, scintigraphic, cytologic, and biochemical aspects. *Ann Intern Med* 1976; 85:769–788.
4. Turner-Warwick M, Burrows B, Johnson A: Cryptogenic fibrosing alveolitis: clinical features and their influence on survival. *Thorax* 1980;35:171–180.
5. King T: Idiopathic pulmonary fibrosis. In: Schwarz M, King T, eds. *Interstitial lung disease.* St Louis, Mo: Mosby-Year Book, 1993:367–403.
6. Rudd R, Haslam P, Turner-Warwick M: Cryptogenic fibrosing alveolitis: relationships of pulmonary physiology and bronchoalveolar lavage to response to treatment and prognosis. *Am Rev Respir Dis* 1981;124:1–8.
7. Watters L, Schwarz M, Cherniack R, et al.: Idiopathic pulmonary fibrosis: pretreatment bronchoalveolar lavage cellular constituents and their relationships with lung histopathology and clinical response to therapy. *Am Rev Respir Dis* 1987;135:696–704.
8. Dreisin R, Schwarz M, Theofilopoulos A, Stanford R: Circulating immune complexes in the idiopathic interstitial pneumonias. *N Engl J Med* 1978;298:353–357.
9. Marciniuk D, Gallagher C: Clinical exercise testing in interstitial lung disease. *Clin Chest Med* 1994;15:287–303.
10. Epler GR, McLoud TC, Gaensler EA, et al.: Normal chest roentgenograms in chronic diffuse infiltrative lung disease. *N Engl J Med* 1978;298:934–939.
11. Raghu G: Interstitial lung disease: a diagnostic approach. Are CT scan and lung biopsy indicated in every patient? *Am J Respir Crit Care Med* 1995;151:909–914.
12. Meier-Sydow J, Weiss S, Buhl R, et al.: Idiopathic pulmonary fibrosis: current clinical concepts and challenges in management. *Semin Respir Crit Care Med* 1994;15:77–96.
13. Turner-Warwick M, Burrows B, Johnson A: Cryptogenic fibrosing alveolitis: response to corticosteroid treatment and its effect on survival. *Thorax* 1980;35:593–599.
14. O'Donnell K, Keogh B, Cantin A, Crystall R: Pharmacologic suppression of the neutrophil component of the alveolitis in idiopathic pulmonary fibrosis. *Am Rev Respir Dis* 1987;136:288–292.
15. Johnson M, Kwan S, Snell N, et al.: Randomised controlled trial comparing prednisolone alone with cyclophosphamide and low-dose prednisolone in combination in cryptogenic fibrosing alveolitis. *Thorax* 1989;44:280–288.
16. Raghu G, Depaso W, Cain K, et al.: Azathioprine combined with prednisone in the treatment of idiopathic pulmonary fibrosis: a prospective double-blind, randomized, placebo-controlled clinical trial. *Am Rev Respir Dis* 1991;144:291–296.
17. Peters S, McDougall J, Douglas W, et al.: Colchicine in the treatment of pulmonary fibrosis. *Chest* 1993;103:101–104.
18. Schwartz D, Van Fossen D, Davis C, et al.: Determinants of progression in idiopathic pulmonary fibrosis. *Am J Respir Crit Care Med* 1994;149:444–449.
19. van Oortegem K, Wallaert B, Marquette C, et al.: Determinants of response to immunosuppressive therapy in idiopathic pulmonary fibrosis. *Eur Respir J* 1994;7:1950–1957.
20. Wells A, Hansell D, Rubens M, et al.: The predictive value of appearances on thin-section computed tomography in fibrosing alveolitis. *Am Rev Respir Dis* 1993;148:1076–1082.
21. Muller N, Ostrow D: High-resolution computed tomography of chronic interstitial lung disease. *Clin Chest Med* 1991;12:97–114.
22. Epler GR, Colby TV, McLoud TC, et al.: Bronchiolitis obliterans organizing pneumonia. *N Engl J Med* 1985;312:152–158.
23. King TE Jr, Mortenson RL: Cryptogenic organizing pneumonitis: the North American experience. *Chest* 1992;102:8S–13S.
24. Cordier JF, Loire R, Brune J: Idiopathic bronchiolitis obliterans organizing pneumonia: definition of characteristic clinical profiles in a series of 16 patients. *Chest* 1989;96:999–1004.
25. Bartter T, Irwin RS, Nash G, et al.: Idiopathic bronchiolitis obliterans organizing pneumonia with peripheral infiltrates on chest roentgenogram. *Arch Intern Med* 1989;149:273–279.

26. King T: Bronchiolitis. In: Schwarz M, King T, eds. *Interstitial lung disease*. St Louis, Mo: Mosby-Year Book, 1993:463–495.
27. Muller NL, Guerry-Force ML, Staples CA, et al.: Differential diagnosis of bronchiolitis obliterans with organizing pneumonia and usual interstitial pneumonia: clinical, functional, and radiologic findings. *Radiology* 1987;162:151–156.
28. Friedman P, Liebow A, Sokoloff J: Eosinophilic granuloma of lung: clinical aspects of primary pulmonary histiocytosis in the adult. *Medicine* 1981;60:385–396.
29. Basset F, Corrin B, Spencer H, et al.: Pulmonary histiocytosis X. *Am Rev Respir Dis* 1978;118:811–820.
30. Hance A, Cadranel J, Soler P: Pulmonary and extra pulmonary Langerhans' cell granulomatosis (histiocytosis X). *Semin Respir Med* 1988;9:349–368.
31. Lacronique J, Roth C, Battesti J-P, et al.: Chest radiological features of pulmonary histiocytosis X: a report based on 50 adult cases. *Thorax* 1982;37:104–109.
32. Marcy T, Reynolds H: Pulmonary histiocytosis X. *Lung* 1985;163:129–150.
33. Schonfeld N, Frank W, Wenig S, et al.: Clinical and radiographic features, lung function and therapeutic results in pulmonary histiocytosis X. *Respiration* 1993;60:38–44.
34. Brauner M, Grenier P, Mouelhi M, et al.: Pulmonary histiocytosis X: evaluation with high-resolution CT. *Radiology* 1989;172:255–258.
35. Moore A, Godwin J, Muller N, et al.: Pulmonary histiocytosis X: comparison of radiographic and CT findings. *Radiology* 1989;172:249–254.
36. Housini I, Tomashefski J, Cohen A, et al.: Transbronchial biopsy in patients with pulmonary eosinophilic granuloma. *Arch Pathol Lab Med* 1994;118:523–530.
37. Webber D, Tron V, Askin F, Churg A: S-100 staining in the diagnosis of eosinophilic granuloma of lung. *Am J Clin Pathol* 1985;84:447–453.
38. Von Essen S, West W, Sitorius M, Rennard S: Complete resolution of roentgenographic changes in a patient with pulmonary histiocytosis X. *Chest* 1990;98:765–767.
39. Carrington C, Cugell D, Gaensler E, et al.: Lymphangioleiomyomatosis: physiologic-pathologic-radiologic correlations. *Am Rev Respir Dis* 1977;116:977–995.
40. Taylor J, Ryu J, Colby T, Raffin T: Lymphangioleiomyomatosis: clinical course in 32 patients. *N Engl J Med* 1990;323:1254–1260.
41. Castro M, Shepherd C, Gomez M, et al.: Pulmonary tuberous sclerosis. *Chest* 1995;107:189–195.
42. Kitaichi M, Nishimura K, Itoh H, Izumi T: Pulmonary lymphangioleiomyomatosis: a report of 46 patients including a clinicopathologic study of prognostic factors. *Am J Respir Crit Care Med* 1995;151:527–533.
43. Burger C, Hyatt R, Staats B: Pulmonary mechanics in lymphangioleiomyomatosis. *Am Rev Respir Dis* 1991;143:1030–1033.
44. Sherrier R, Chiles C, Goggli V: Pulmonary lymphangioleiomyomatosis: CT findings. *AJR* 1989;153:937–940.
45. Eliasson A, Phillips Y, Tenholder M: Treatment of lymphanioleiomyomatosis: a meta-analysis. *Chest* 1989;196:1352–1355.
46. Claypool W, Rogers R, Matuschak G: Update on the clinical diagnosis, management, and pathogenesis of pulmonary alveolar proteinosis (phospholipidosis). *Chest* 1984;85:550–558.
47. Kariman K, Kylstra J, Spock A: Pulmonary alveolar proteinosis: prospective clinical experience in 23 patients for 15 years. *Lung* 1984;162:223–231.
48. Watters L: Chronic alveolar filling disease. In: Schwarz M, King T, eds. *Interstitial lung disease*. St Louis, Mo: Mosby-Year Book, 1993:309–366.
49. Larson R, Gordine R: Pulmonary alveolar proteinosis: report of six cases, review of the literature, and formulation of a new theory. *Ann Intern Med* 1965;62:292–312.
50. Witty L, Tapson V, Piantadosi C: Isolation of mycobacteria in patients with pulmonary alveolar proteinosis. *Medicine* 1994;73:103–109.
51. Dranoff G, Crawford AD, Sadelain M, et al.: The involvement of granulocyte-macrophage colony-stimulating factor in pulmonary homostasis. *Science* 1994;264:713–716.

23

Congenital Lung Disease

Daniel M.Goodenberger

Perturbations at various times during the embryonic and early development of the lung can result in specific abnormalities. The first section of this chapter considers abnormalities of lung structural development. The latter half of the chapter reviews lung involvement in genetic systemic diseases. Primarily pediatric abnormalities will not be considered.

I. **Pulmonary agenesis**
   A. **Incidence and etiology.** A relatively rare disorder, pulmonary agenesis results in total unilateral absence of lung tissue. Males and females are affected equally. The cause is unknown, and only 164 total cases had been reported by 1968 (1). The disturbance presumably occurs early in fetal life, and possible genetic influences are unknown.
   B. **Signs and symptoms.** Although an increased number of respiratory infections may occur during the first year of life, affected individuals are usually asymptomatic, unless there is an associated cardiac defect (1,2). Associated anomalies include vascular maldevelopment, notably patent ductus arteriosus and persistent left superior vena cava; cardiac defects, including atrial septal defects, patent foramen ovale, and ventricular septal defect; gastrointestinal, including imperforate anus, tracheoesophageal fistula, and Meckel's diverticulum); and skeletal and genitourinary abnormalities.
   C. **Differential diagnosis.** The plain chest radiographic features of this diagnosis include a marked mediastinal shift to the smaller affected side and variable aeration of the hemithorax caused by herniation across the midline of the contralateral lung. The differential diagnosis includes the following:
      1. Atelectasis.
      2. Prior pneumonectomy.
      3. Old tuberculosis with fibrothorax (2).
      4. Severe postinfectious bronchiectasis/lung destruction.
   D. **Radiologic approach to diagnosis.** The diagnosis is suggested by the chest x-ray findings and the absence of relevant symptoms or previous thoracic surgery (Fig. 23-1). As may be seen with other diagnoses, the remaining lung is not hyperlucent and undergoes true hyperplasia during the period between birth and 8 years of age. The diagnosis can be confirmed by computed tomography (CT) scan, which reveals complete absence of lung tissue, bronchi, and pulmonary artery, with a shrunken hemithorax.
   E. **Management.** Individuals discovered in adulthood need no treatment. The examining physician should be alert to the possible presence of associated cardiac or gastrointestinal defects that may also remain relatively asymptomatic until adulthood, such as atrial septal defect. Individuals present during infancy because the severity of the associated defects determines the course and prognosis.

II. **Bronchial atresia**
   A. **Incidence and etiology.** The exact incidence is unknown. The male-to-female ratio is 2:1. Atresia of a bronchus is usually segmental and most often involves the apicoposterior segment of the left upper lobe (3,4). The developmental mechanism resulting in atresia is unknown, but a vascular insult is often postulated (5).
   B. **Signs and symptoms.** Atresia of the bronchus is most often diagnosed in the second decade and frequently presents as an incidental radiographic abnormality in an asymptomatic young man (4,5) (Fig. 23-2). When present, symptoms are nonspe-

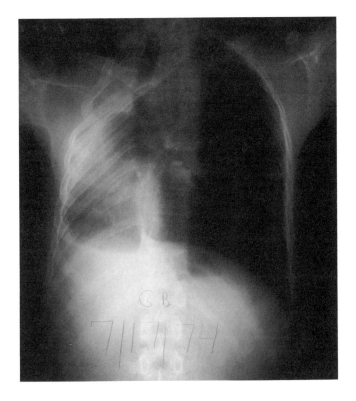

Fig. 23-1. Pulmonary agenesis in a 17-year-old male.

cific and include cough, dyspnea, and recurrent infections. These symptoms are often unrelated to the underlying lesion but prompt the chest x-ray that results in the discovery of bronchial atresia (6).

C. **Physiology.** Bronchial atresia interrupts the segmental bronchus, leaving blind pouches in the proximal and distal remnants. This results in accumulation of mucus in the bronchus distal to the interruption and accounts for the characteristic radiographic finding of a perihilar mucocele. Since the atresia is at the segmental level, collateral ventilation of the obstructed segment via the pores of Kohn and/or the bronchoalveolar channels of Lambert results in regional overinflation (7). This phenomenon results in radiographic hyperlucency that is sometimes referred to as emphysema, although alveolar destruction does not occur and is better termed *segmental overinflation*.

D. **Differential diagnosis.** Lung cancer, particularly small cell lung cancer, may sometimes simulate a mucocele (8), as will an inspissated foreign body. Mucoid impaction associated with allergic bronchopulmonary aspergillosis (ABPA) or an inspissated foreign body may also be confused with mucoceles.

E. **Diagnostic approach.** The chest x-ray will typically reveal a perihilar mass due to the mucocele. Visible branching and a detectable distal hyperlucency may be present. The young age range makes lung cancer less likely, and the usual absence of asthma mitigates against ABPA. In the event that asthma coexists, a negative skin test, negative *Aspergillus* precipitins, and normal IgE antibody levels rule out ABPA.

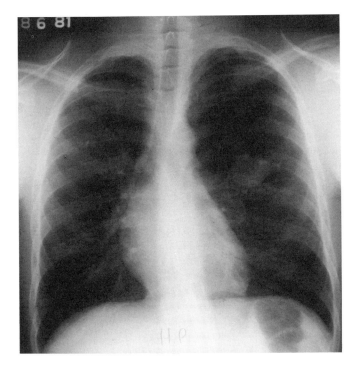

Fig. 23-2. Left upper lobe bronchial atresia and mucocele in a 17-year-old male.

Occult foreign body aspiration is rare in adults. A CT scan is generally diagnostic, showing a branching mucocele and distal localized hyperlucency (5,9).

F. **Management.** No therapy is indicated in the absence of symptoms. In the event that radiographic features are atypical, fiberoptic bronchoscopy will rule out foreign body or lung tumor.

III. **Scimitar syndrome** (hypogenetic lung syndrome, congenital venolobar syndrome)

A. **Incidence and etiology.** This anomaly occurs in 1–3 per 100,000 live births (10). The male-to-female ratio is 2:3 to 1:2 (11,12). The etiology and pathogenesis of this developmental defect are unknown.

B. **Pathophysiology**

1. The anomaly virtually always occurs on the right side. The affected lung is usually hypoplastic (58%) with an abnormal bronchial distribution to two lobes, a hypoplastic pulmonary artery, and often a systemic arterial supply via a large anomalous artery from the upper abdominal or lower thoracic aorta (11–13). An anomalous pulmonary vein descending in the major fissure in a sweeping curve resembling a scimitar drains all or part of the right lung to the inferior vena cava, connecting just below the diaphragm. This constitutes a left-to-right extracardiac shunt.

2. An infantile form exists either with multiple anomalies and an "incidental" scimitar or with associated pulmonary hypertension related to a large systemic arterial supply.

C. **Signs and symptoms.** In one large series, over two-thirds of individuals had mild symptoms that were recalled, elicited in retrospect (11). The most common symptoms of fatigue and dyspnea are particularly likely with a shunt fraction >50% (12). There may be a tendency toward increased respiratory infections. Presentation in infancy has a bad prognosis because of either early pulmonary hypertension or associated cardiac anomalies that may include hypoplastic left heart, atrial septal defect, and others. The adult form is milder, and 82% of cases are associated with a left-to-right shunt fraction <50%. Pulmonary artery pressures are normal in 77% of affected individuals and are only mildly elevated in the remainder (10). The physiology and clinical consequences of shunt are similar to those of a small atrial septal defect.

D. **Differential diagnosis.** The scimitar phenomenon is often obvious on chest x-ray, in which case the diagnosis is easy to make (11). If the scimitar is obscured by the right heart border shifted ipsilaterally (14), the differential diagnosis is that of a small hemithorax with a clear lung would include pulmonary artery agenesis and a hypogenetic lung without partial anomalous pulmonary venous return.

E. **Approach to diagnosis.** The abnormal chest x-ray may include the scimitar sign and will generally show a small right lung with diminished vascularity and a rightward mediastinal shift (11,12,15,16). CT performed with contrast is often definitive, showing the abnormal venous drainage and hypoplastic lung. Magnetic resonance (MR) angiography or right heart catheterization with pulmonary angiogram may be necessary to document the point of insertion of the anomalous vein (17).

F. **Management**
   1. Operative management for the adult form is usually unnecessary. In one large series, 93% of 85 adult patients managed medically had good results with no mortality, as compared to 33% of 37 treated surgically with an 11% mortality (10). Lung resection may be reasonable in those rare patients with recurrent infections or severe hemoptysis. Reimplantation of the anomalous vein has been recommended for large (>50%) left-to-right shunts, but this is uncommon.
   2. The operation may be technically difficult. The systemic supplying artery is easily ligated, but reimplanting the anomalous pulmonary vein in the left atrium is often technically challenging because the vein may be too short. Surgical innovations have included right atrial implantation with construction of a right-to-left atrial conduit. Chronically infected lung should be resected at a later date.

G. **Complications of therapy.** Complications include thrombosis of the reimplanted vein.

H. **Specialist referral.** Diagnosis of this disorder should prompt referral to a specialist in cardiovascular diseases or cardiothoracic surgery.

IV. **Horseshoe lung**
   A. **Incidence and etiology.** Horseshoe lung refers to a condition with variable degrees of fusion of the two lungs behind the heart, usually involving the posteroinferior lung segments. The fusion may be complete, with a continuous pleura, or may occur as an isthmus with two pleural layers or simply as posterior lung herniation with four pleural layers. This isthmus is supplied by bronchi and vessels from the right lung (18). The incidence of horseshoe lung is very low. The majority of cases (80%) are associated with the **scimitar syndrome** (18); in these cases, the right lung is often hypogenetic.

   B. The **presentation** is similar to that of the scimitar syndrome. When occurring in isolation, horseshoe lung is usually an incidental finding on CT scan. No specific therapy is required.

V. **Pulmonary arteriovenous malformations**
   A. **Incidence and etiology.** Pulmonary arteriovenous malformations (PAVMs) are abnormal connections of the pulmonary arterial circulation to the pulmonary venous circulation, with no intervening capillary bed. The majority of PAVMs consist of a saccular dilatation with a single feeding arterial vessel and a single draining vein. About 20% are more complex, with two or more of either or both types of vessels. They appear to develop between precapillary arterioles and venules, with intervening epithelial dysplasia. A variable percentage occur in isolation, with no apparent associated disease. The remainder are related to hereditary hemorrhagic telangiectasia (HHT) (also known as Osler-Weber-Rendu disease) (Figs. 23-3 and 23-4). The

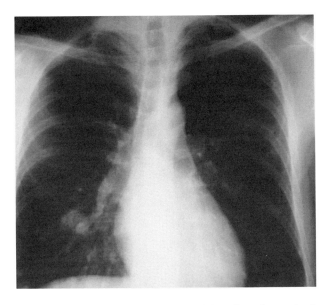

Fig. 23-3. PA chest radiograph in a 42-year-old man with hereditary hemorrhagic telangiectasia, clubbing, cyanosis, and prior strokes.

percentage of cases related to HHT varies markedly, from 36 to 88%, depending on the investigator and whether the lesions are found in symptomatic patients or by screening. One-third have more than one PAVM; the presence of multiple PAVMs is more common in HHT. The incidence of sporadic PAVMs is unknown. The reported prevalence of HHT is 1–2 per 100,000, with up to 50% having PAVMs.

B. **Genetics.** The genetics of sporadic PAVM is unknown. HHT is an autosomal-dominant disease; to date, three separate gene loci producing the syndrome have been identified on chromosomes 3, 9, and 12. The gene products of the first two sites appear to be receptors for transforming growth factor β (TGF-β); the gene product of the last, which appears to be unassociated with PAVMs, is unknown.

C. **Signs and symptoms.** PAVMs are rare in childhood. The mean age at detection in most series is late in the fourth decade, although one-quarter present before age 21 years. The most common symptom is dyspnea on exertion. Other symptoms include hemoptysis, platypnea, and orthodeoxia. In the subgroup with HHT, nosebleeds are very frequent, with gastrointestinal and genitourinary bleeding less common. Many individuals found by screening of HHT families have few or no pulmonary symptoms. The principal complications of PAVM are neurologic and due to paradoxical embolism or brain abscess, either of which may be the initial symptom. Hemothorax may also occur, particularly in association with pregnancy.

D. **Pathophysiology.** Severe intrapulmonary right-to-left shunts may result in hypoxemia and cyanosis. Long-standing shunts may result in clubbing, which may resolve after treatment. Paradoxical embolization may occur, and problems with bacterial filtering predisposes to brain abscess in a fashion similar to patients with cyanotic congenital heart disease.

E. **Differential diagnosis** depends on presentation. A differential diagnosis of presentations with which PAVM may be confused is presented in Table 23-1.

F. The **diagnostic approach** is similar to that for a lung nodule and begins with a CT scan of the chest with contrast enhancement. This will likely reveal the feeding artery and draining vein that are characteristic of and very specific for the diagnosis. The

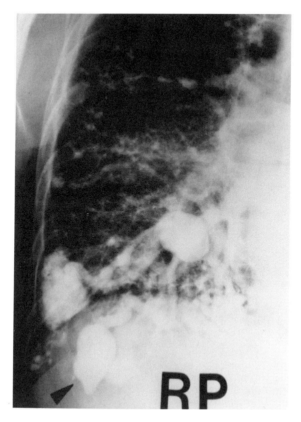

Fig. 23-4. Right lower lobe bronchogram in a 42-year-old man with hereditary hemorrhagic telangiectasia, clubbing, cyanosis, and prior strokes.

Table 23-1.

Pulmonary nodule	Hypoxemia	Hemoptysis	CVA	Brain Abscess
Malignant tumor	Cardiac shunt	Lung tumor	Cardiac embolus	Intracardiac shunt
Benign tumor	Parenchymal lung	Bronchitis	Endocarditis	Bronchiectasis
Granuloma	disease:	Bronchiectasis	Extracranial	Endocarditis
	Emphysema	Vasculitis	vascular	Suppurative
Pulmonary infarct	Interstitial lung	Lung abscess	occlusive	upper airway
	disease		disease	disease
	Pulmonary vascular		Vasculitis	
	disease			

evaluation of hypoxemia resistant to oxygen administration or an embolic cerebrovascular accident should include agitated saline contrast echocardiography. The delayed (three to five cardiac cycles) appearance of microcavitations is highly sensitive and specific for intrapulmonary shunt. Evaluation of a brain abscess should also include this modality. Evaluation of hemoptysis will include bronchoscopy, which will likely be nondiagnostic.

1. The relatives of an individual with HHT and a PAVM should be screened using contrast echocardiography to identify individuals at risk for central nervous system complications. Chest x-ray, supine and erect arterial blood gases, and arterial blood gases while breathing room air and 100% oxygen are not sufficiently accurate to identify a shunt.

G. Management. The patient should be referred to a center with experience in management of this syndrome. The treatment of choice is therapeutic embolization using coil emboli, a highly effective procedure. Resection is rarely necessary and should be reserved for large PAVMs that are technically impossible to embolize. Those with known PAVMs should be given prophylactic antibiotics using the American Heart Association protocols for endocarditis prophylaxis prior to elective procedures. Embolization may result in pleurisy, which is self-limited and treated symptomatically.

VI. Bronchogenic cyst

A. Incidence and etiology. The exact incidence is unclear. The male-to-female ratio is 4:3. Bronchogenic cysts result from anomalous supernumerary budding of the ventral (tracheal) diverticulum of the foregut. Two-thirds of bronchogenic cysts are mediastinal and paratracheal, and originate during the sixth week of gestation. The other one-third are located in the lung, usually the lower lobes, implying a later event. Rarely, the cyst is located subcutaneously, usually in the neck, abdomen, or base of the tongue (19). The cysts are usually unilocular, are lined by ciliated columnar epithelium, and have a fibrous wall containing cartilage, smooth muscle, elastic tissue, and mucous glands (20,21).

B. Signs and symptoms. Bronchogenic cysts uncommonly present with wheezing, stridor, or cyanotic spells due to airway compression in the neonatal period. More frequently, the presentation is in adulthood with recurrent infections, wheezing, cough, or as an asymptomatic lesion incidentally found on chest x-ray. Rarely, malignant degeneration to rhabdomyosarcoma, leiomyosarcoma, or anaplastic carcinoma can occur. Other unusual presentations include obstructive lobar overinflation (19), adult airway obstruction, and pneumothorax (22).

C. Pathophysiology. Many of the symptoms are due to secondary infection of the cyst. Infection and inflammation may result in communication with the tracheobronchial tree. This can occasionally result in a ball-valve effect with air trapping and enlargement, resulting in compressive symptoms, including dysphagia and wheezing.

D. Differential diagnosis. For mediastinal cysts, the differential diagnosis includes mediastinal tumors, lymphoma, esophageal duplication cysts, and other cystic lesions, including hygroma, pericardial cyst, and neuroenteric cyst. Intraparenchymal cysts have a differential diagnosis that includes acquired cystic lesions of the lung, such as lung abscess; tuberculosis with cavitation; bronchiectasis; and pneumatocele. Other developmental anomalies may be considered, including small type I cystic adenomatoid malformations and intralobar sequestrations.

E. Diagnostic approach. The chest x-ray may reveal a mediastinal or pulmonary parenchymal mass (Fig. 23-5). When infected and in communication with the tracheobronchial tree, an air–fluid level may be seen. Typically, the lesion is sharply circumscribed, solitary, and round or oval. In the mediastinum, the most frequent location is the right paratracheal area, which is easily visible on plain chest x-ray. When it is located subcarinally, it may not be seen on chest x-ray, and a CT scan will be required. If located in the lung parenchyma, it will present as a noncalcified round/oval density, usually in the lower lobe, with well defined borders and normal lung surrounding it, unless associated with pneumonia. In patients with normal chest x-rays, the evaluation of symptoms due to airway compression will most often cause a physician to obtain a chest CT and make the diagnosis. The density of the cyst tends to be uniform and can range from water (0–20 Hounsfield units) to high density (89–99 Hounsfield

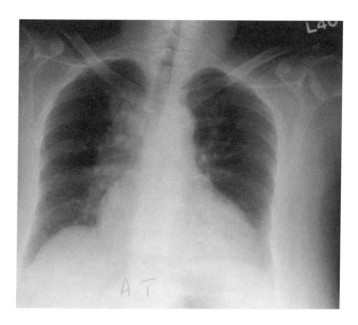

Fig. 23-5. Right paratracheal bronchogenic cyst in a 68-year-old man.

units). The higher densities are often due to calcium, blood, high protein content, or anthracotic pigment (19,23). MR imaging of the chest may be useful, as the lesion typically has a high signal intensity on T2-weighted images, approximately equal to cerebrospinal fluid. In the prenatal period, the cyst may be found on routine prenatal ultrasound. In general, this does not require any action during the pre- or postnatal period.

F. **Management**
   1. The literature generally advocates resection upon discovery, because asymptomatic cysts that are not excised may require later excision for infection or other symptoms. Some series have found more postoperative complications in this latter situation, which is used to further the argument that all bronchogenic cysts should be resected (24). An additional concern is the rare complication of malignant degeneration. However, other authors argue that surgical therapy is not necessary in asymptomatic adults (21,23,25). Infections should be treated with antibiotics appropriate for the likely organisms.
   2. If surgical removal is elected, the tendency in recent years has been the use of minimally invasive surgical techniques. Endoscopic unroofing of the cyst by mediastinoscopy with or without doxycycline sclerosis may be adequate (25, 26). An intrapulmonary bronchogenic cyst may, on occasion, be resected via thoracoscopy (27).

G. **Specialist referral.** Upon discovery, referral should be made to a physician specializing in pulmonary diseases or thoracic surgery.

VII. **Neurenteric cysts**
   A. **Incidence and etiology.** The exact incidence is unknown, but neurenteric cysts are rare. Male and female distribution is approximately equal. Neurenteric cysts result from incomplete separation of the foregut from the notochord in the third week of gestation (28). Cysts are typically lined with mucus-secreting columnar epithelium, with gastric mucosa present in up to 60%. Ninety percent of these lesions are

in the posterior mediastinum, with two-thirds above the carina and two-thirds on the right (28).

B. Signs and symptoms. These lesions may present similarly to standard bronchogenic cysts, with dyspnea, stridor, and persistent cough. However, unlike simple broncho-genic cysts, >50% will have central nervous system symptoms, including back pain, gait disturbance, and neurologic deficits. Moreover, coexistent mediastinal and/or in-traspinal lesions will be present in 25% to 75%.

C. Differential diagnosis. In general, the differential diagnosis is the same as that for posterior mediastinal lesions and includes other neurologic tumors. On occasion, lymphoma or paraspinal infection may present with a posterior mass.

D. Diagnostic approaches. Some of these lesions may come to light because of neu-rologic and/or respiratory symptoms. Plain chest x-ray may reveal a posterior medi-astinal mass. Subsequent CT scan of the chest may outline associated vertebral anomalies, including a "tunnel" through the vertebral body. MR imaging is best for evaluation of both the cyst and the spine. The finding of an associated nonenhanc-ing intraspinal cyst essentially confirms the diagnosis. In doubtful cases, a tech-netium Tc 99m scan will reveal increased activity in approximately 60% due to the presence of gastric mucosa.

E. Management. The standard treatment of these lesions is excision.

F. Specialist referral. Patients with these lesions should be referred to a thoracic and/ or neurologic surgeon.

VIII. Pulmonary sequestration

A. Etiology and pathogenesis. Sequestrations have been thought to result from ab-normal caudal accessory budding of the foregut. Dissociation from the tracheo-bronchial tree results in retention of the embryonic systemic arterial blood supply (20). Pulmonary sequestrations are divided into two types: extralobar and intra-lobar (Table 23-2).

1. Extralobar sequestrations are congenital lesions and account for 25% of se-questrations. They are completely contained within a separate pleural envelope, usually subpulmonic, and contain cysts with bronchial epithelium, cartilage, and elastic and nonelastic arteries (28). They may also be found within or below the diaphragm. In 80% of cases, the arterial blood supply is from the thoracic or abdominal aorta; in 15%, the blood supply is from the gastric artery or another systemic artery. In the remaining 5%, the pulmonary artery is the source of blood supply (29). The venous drainage is via the azygos, hemiazygos, or portal veins in 96% of cases (30).

Table 23-2.

Distinguishing features	Extralobar	Intralobar
Location	Above, below, or within the diaphragm	Usually posterior basillar lower lobe
Laterality	Left in 90%	Left in 60%
Pleural envelope	Separate	Not separate
Age at diagnosis	<1 year: 60%	>20 years: 50%
Neonatal presentation	Often	Never
Sex	Male to female: 4 : 1	Male = female
Foregut communication	Occasional	Rare
Associated anomalies	15% to 40%	Uncommon
Caliber of anomalous artery	Usually small	Usually large
Venous drainage	Azygous, hemiazygous, or portal	Usually pulmonary vein
Complications	Rarely infected	Frequent infections
Occurrence	Rare	Frequent

2. **Intralobar sequestrations** are of uncertain origin. The majority of lesions are thought to be acquired rather than congenital (31). Although representing 75% of total sequestrations, they are rarely found in infants and are rare in neonatal autopsy series (6,32). Some cases appear to be congenital, a hypothesis supported by connection to the esophagus and early presentation with infection (20). On examination, the lesion is cystic (containing mucus or pus) and lined with ciliated columnar or squamous epithelium. The walls contain smooth muscle, cartilage, and mucous glands. There are no clear anatomic planes of cleavage, and the lesion does not have a separate pleural envelope (28). The majority of lesions are supplied by an aberrant artery from the thoracic or abdominal aorta. Drainage is usually by the pulmonary vein.

B. **Incidence.** The exact incidence of these lesions is unknown. As mentioned, approximately 75% of diagnosed cases are intralobar, with 25% extralobar. The male-to-female ratio for extralobar sequestrations is 4:1; no sex differentiation is seen with intralobar sequestrations.

C. **Genetics.** The contribution of genetic abnormalities to either syndrome is unknown.

D. **Pathophysiology.** Because of the systemic arterial supply, extralobar sequestrations may occasionally present with neonatal high-output cardiac failure.
   1. In large extralobar sequestrations occurring *in utero*, the fetus may have hydrops and resultant pulmonary hypoplasia, presumably due to interference with swallowing of amniotic fluid (20).
   2. Patients with intralobar sequestrations may develop recurrent infections, perhaps due to a preexisting airway connection.

E. **Clinical presentation**
   1. **Extralobar sequestrations** are often asymptomatic. As noted above, they may present with neonatal high-output failure and occasionally with infection. Of those found in childhood, about 60% are diagnosed within the first 6 months of life, usually as a result of respiratory distress, cyanosis, or feeding difficulties. *In utero*, ultrasound may reveal polyhydramnios and hydrops fetalis. On occasion, the lesion may undergo spontaneous hemorrhage. In 50% to 65% of neonates with extralobar sequestration, there will be associated congenital anomalies (29), most often congenital diaphragmatic hernia, and congenital cystic adenomatoid malformation type II may be found in 15% to 25%. Occasionally, an individual will reach adulthood before diagnosis. The oldest known reported patient was 81 years old (33,34).
   2. **Intralobar sequestrations** diagnosed in early adulthood usually present with recurrent infections, hemoptysis, or pleural effusions (28). More than 50% are diagnosed after the age of 20 years.

F. **Differential diagnosis.** The differential in the pre- and neonatal population includes congenital cystic adenomatoid malformation, bronchogenic cyst, and congenital diaphragmatic hernia. In adults, intralobar sequestration may be confused with a variety of acquired cystic lesions of the lung, including lung abscess, bronchiectasis, cavitary tumor, and recurrent pneumonia, as well as with other congenital lesions such as an infected bronchogenic cyst.

G. **Diagnostic approach**
   1. Prenatal ultrasound may detect **extralobar sequestration**, usually a solid and highly echogenic mass that may have a detectable systemic feeding vessel and may be associated with hydrops, polyhydramnios, and mediastinal shift. The 35% of patients who have fetal hydrops are always stillborn or suffer neonatal death unless treated with fetal surgery. Postnatally, the chest x-ray typically shows a well defined lesion most often (>80% of cases) in the left lower lobe in the posterior costophrenic angle adjacent to the lower esophagus (29). The sharp margination is due to the pleural envelope. Conversely, a diaphragmatic hump or a paravertebral mass may be seen (28). Ultrasound may detect the systemic feeding artery (20,29,35). Scintigraphy, not frequently used, will reveal perfusion of the lesion in the systemic but not the pulmonary phase. CT can be diagnostic but may fail to show the feeding vessel, and MR imaging may be more useful (20,29). Aortography, although definitive, is used less fre-

quently because of the excellent results achieved by digital subtraction angiography, which is now the imaging procedure of choice (29).

2. **Intralobar sequestrations** are typically found in the posterior basilar segment of a lower lobe and on the left in 60% of cases. These lesions tend to be poorly marginated, homogenous opacities on chest x-ray, although air–fluid levels or air bronchograms may infrequently be seen (28,36). Bronchography, rarely performed, shows no bronchial connection to the lesion in the absence of an air–fluid level. CT scan typically shows normal bronchial arterial bundles draped around the mass, but it may or may not show the feeding vessel, depending on its origin and angle of penetration. MR imaging with MR angiography is the current procedure of choice for imaging (28,37,38).

   H. **Management.** The treatment of choice for symptomatic extralobar sequestrations is resection. Intralobar sequestrations typically present with symptoms, and resection, usually by lobectomy, is also the procedure of choice.

   I. **Specialist referral** should be made to a thoracic surgeon.

IX. **Congenital lobar overexpansion (congenital lobar emphysema)**

   A. **Etiology and pathogenesis.** Lobar overexpansion is the correct descriptive term, as emphysema is not present; that is, there is no destruction of alveolar septa (20). There are two types of overexpanded lobes.

     1. **Overexpanded normal lobe** may be due to bronchial obstruction that is either extrinsic (mediastinal or hilar compression by a bronchogenic cyst or anomalous vessel) or intrinsic (bronchial cartilage deficiency, mucosal flap, or intramural fibrosis) (20). No identifiable cause is found in about half of cases. The most common identified cause is a congenital deficiency of bronchial cartilage that can result in air trapping. A proportion of the remainder may be caused by enlarged vessels due to congenital left-to-right shunts (21,39). Overexpansion is most often found in the left upper lobe (42%), the right middle lobe (35%), and the right upper lobe (21%) (39).

     2. **Polyalveolar lobe** is the other type of overexpanded lobe, showing an increased number of normally expanded and normally sized alveoli.

   B. **Incidence.** The exact incidence is unknown, but the disorder may occur more frequently in whites (39). The male-to-female ratio is approximately 2:1 (40).

   C. **Pathophysiology.** The deficiency of cartilage or other cause of bronchiole obstruction results in progressive air trapping. In turn, this causes respiratory distress through compression of the remaining lung tissue and decreases in cardiac venous return and output.

   D. **Signs and symptoms.** Approximately half of affected individuals have symptoms in the first few days of life, and nearly all are symptomatic by age 4 months. The lesion is very rarely found in adults. Approximately one-eighth present as an acute emergency with respiratory compromise due to a space-occupying mass within the pleural envelope. This is manifested as neonatal respiratory distress (20,40). The usual course, however, is one of persistent and progressive respiratory distress that is frequently intermittent and provoked by excitement, crying, and feeding, and is manifested as dyspnea, tachypnea, wheezing, cough, and cyanosis (21,40). Associated cardiac anomalies are found in 14% of affected individuals; ventricular septal defect and patent ductus arteriosus are the most frequent. Other associations include cleft palate, pectus excavatum, pyloric stenosis, accessory digits, hiatal hernia, and unilateral absence of a kidney.

   E. **Differential diagnosis.** In the infant, the differential diagnosis includes pneumothorax, congenital cystic adenomatoid malformation, and congenital diaphragmatic hernia. In older children, the differential diagnosis should include aspirated foreign body, which rarely occurs before age 6 months, and a mucus plug (21). For the child presenting at an older age, the differential diagnosis includes Swyer-James syndrome. The same diagnosis must be considered in the rare adult who presents with this abnormality.

   F. **Diagnostic evaluation.** In the prenatal period, ultrasound may be diagnostic, although the lesion may also be confused with a type III congenital cystic adenomatoid malformation (41). In the neonate, a chest x-ray reveals an opacified lobe that is slow to drain and fill with air. This lobe, usually upper and left more frequently than right, may eventually become hyperexpanded with a contralateral mediastinal shift and compression of the normal lung (40). In contradistinction to a pneumothorax or a type I congenital cystic adenomatoid malformation, markings are visible in the affected lobe. Fluid drainage does not occur as quickly as might be expected in congenital diaphragmatic hernia, and, if necessary, a barium swallow will quickly differentiate these. CT scan shows lobar overexpansion and a contralateral mediastinal shift and is often diagnostic. CT scan will rule out compression of the bronchus by a subcarinal or perihilar bronchogenic cyst or large vessel. Fluoroscopy shows hyperinflation persisting during expiration, with mediastinal shift worsening during expiration. The normal lung is compressed, in contradistinction to Swyer-James syndrome, in which the normal lung is not compressed. Ventilation–perfusion (V/Q) scan documents both ventilation and perfusion, and MR imaging with MR angiography can rule out a vascular ring causing compression.

G. **Management.** It was believed that lobectomy was required in almost all individuals to relieve respiratory distress and allow long-term lung growth. However, more recent series with long-term follow-up demonstrate good results when patients are managed nonoperatively (39,41). Surgery should be recommended for those with severe or progressive respiratory distress that does not respond to medical management (39). Serial V/Q scans may be used to follow progression of both the hyper–inflated and the compressed lobes. Mortality associated with operation is in the range of 7%, related primarily to either congenital heart disease or hypoxic brain damage. Most individuals remain asymptomatic after resection, even when compensatory lung growth cannot be documented.

H. **Specialist referral.** Patients should be referred to appropriate specialists, such as a pediatric thoracic surgeon for children or a pulmonologist or thoracic surgeon for adults.

X. **Ciliary dyskinesia syndromes**

  A. **Etiology and pathogenesis**

    1. Cilia are ubiquitous throughout the body, present in the airways, sinuses, eustachian tubes, ventricles of the brain, oviducts, and vas deferens. In addition, sperm flagella function essentially as cilia and have similar ultrastructure. Cilia contain nine sets of peripheral microtubule doublets, with dynein arms attached to the A subunits of these doublets. In addition, the outer doublets are attached by radial spokes to two central microtubules. The interaction and activation of these proteins result in the movement of cilia in a coordinated fashion to promote cephalad movement in the case of respiratory epithelium. Each dynein arm is a globular protein with ATPase activity, establishing temporary cross-linkage between adjacent microtubules to cause movement.

    2. In 1975, abnormalities of cilia were recognized to result in a series of respiratory infectious complications. The normal frequency of ciliary beating is approximately 12 Hz. In the various ciliary dyskinesia syndromes, beat frequency is reduced by 40% to 69%, and the waveform is dyskinetic. In the majority of patients, this abnormal ciliary function is due to absence of the dynein arms (65% to 80%) (42,43). However, at least 20 variants of abnormal ultrastructure have been documented (43), including supernumerary central microtubules, absent radial spokes, and frank ciliary absence. Recurrent infections may be promoted by an associated abnormal motility of white blood cells as well (43,44). Interpretation of ciliary abnormalities must be undertaken with caution, as they may be found in a variety of other situations, including influenza virus infection and chronic bronchitis, among others (45). This abnormal motility also occurs in the sperm flagella, resulting in male infertility.

  B. **Incidence.** The reported incidence of ciliary dysmotility ranges from 1 in 15,000 to 1 in 68,000 (43,46). There is no sex preference.

  C. **Genetics.** The genetics of these syndromes are unclear, but some variants have been reported to be autosomal recessive (43).

  D. **Pathophysiology.** Ciliary abnormalities result in reduced mucus clearance, which promotes bacterial colonization and subsequent infection of the airways and sinuses. The abnormal function of sperm flagella is responsible for male infertility.

E. **Clinical presentation**
   1. These syndromes present as recurrent sinobronchial infections, bronchiectasis, reductions in the sense of smell, and male sterility (42). Recurrent otitis may lead to hearing loss, and progressive bronchiectasis and hypoxemia may lead to cor pulmonale (43). Infections of the upper and lower respiratory tract begin in infancy or early childhood. Nasal polyps become progressively more common with age, ranging from a 10% incidence in children to 75% in adults. The most common infecting organisms are *Haemophilus influenzae*, *Streptococcus pneumoniae*, and *Neisseria meninigitidis*. Clubbing may also be seen. Other associations include esophageal dysfunction, congenital heart disease, and scoliosis (47,48).
   2. Approximately 50% of affected individuals have situs inversus viscerum. This association suggests that under ordinary circumstances normal microtubule function during development is responsible for the appropriate orientation of the viscera within the body and that abnormal ciliary function may allow the internal orientation of organs to occur by chance (42,44).
   3. Infertility is not universal and should not be considered a necessary criterion for the diagnosis of the ciliary dysmotility syndromes. Up to 16% of affected males may have the ability to father children (49).
F. **Differential diagnosis.** In those cases with situs inversus viscerum, as well as recurrent respiratory tract infections and bronchiectasis, the diagnosis will be obvious. However, the same syndrome without situs inversus has a broader differential diagnosis. As noted above, infertility is not necessary for the diagnosis, because women and a minority of men may be fertile. Bronchiectasis tends to be panlobar, suggesting a primary host defense defect such as cystic fibrosis, humoral immunodeficiency, Young's syndrome, cartilage abnormalities, or, rarely α_1-antitrypsin deficiency. Although the distribution of bronchiectasis is usually different, the differential should also include allergic bronchopulmonary aspergillosis (ABPA).
G. **Diagnostic evaluation**
   1. Patients will ordinarily undergo evaluation because of recurrent respiratory infections, and a chest x-ray often reveals bronchiectasis and hyperinflation. Plain radiographs or CT scans of the sinuses reveal evidence of sinusitis, and high-resolution CT of the chest confirms bronchiectasis involving multiple lobes. Cystic fibrosis may be ruled out by sweat chloride determinations and, if these are borderline, genetic testing. The picture may be confused by sputum cultures showing *Pseudomonas*, but in contrast to cystic fibrosis, the *Pseudomonas* species are not mucoid (43). Ciliary dysmotility syndromes may be differentiated from ABPA by bronchiectasis that is not central, the absence of immediate and delayed skin test hypersensitivity to *Aspergillus*, normal IgE levels, and absent *Aspergillus* precipitins. α_1-Antitrypsin deficiency is ruled out by a normal α_1-globulin level on serum protein electrophoresis and by specific testing. Hypogammaglobulinemia (common variable immunodeficiency) may be ruled out by measurement of quantitative immunoglobulins.
   2. A screening test for ciliary dysfunction may be done using saccharin. In this test, a 1-mm bead is placed 1 cm from the anterior nares on the inferior turbinate, with the head tilted forward 15°. The patient is instructed not to sniff, cough, or sneeze and is not allowed to eat or drink for the duration of the test. The normal time period for saccharin to be tasted is 15–19 minutes. An abnormal test is one that takes >30 minutes, and the test is terminated at 60 minutes.
   3. Direct electron microscopy of cilia is rarely done. Samples may be obtained by brushing the nose, and it is possible to observe ciliary motion under a microscope. Some authorities recommend biopsies from two sites, both the nose and the carina, to obtain ultrastructural studies (50). Unfortunately, as noted above, nonspecific ciliary abnormalities may frequently be seen in the setting of acute or chronic infection.
H. **Management.** The treatment is similar to that for bronchiectasis of any cause and includes physical therapy with postural drainage, bronchodilator administration, and antibiotics for acute infectious flares. Sinusitis should be treated in the stan-

dard fashion, and severe chronic recurrent infections may benefit from endoscopic sinus surgery (51). At present, alpha-dornase is of uncertain benefit (50).

I. **Specialist referral.** Patients who have ciliary dysmotility and recurrent infectious complications should be referred to a chest physician.

XI. **Young's syndrome**

  A. **Etiology and pathogenesis.** Young's syndrome is the combination of chronic infectious sinobronchial disease and azoospermia due to bilateral obstruction of the epididymides at the level of the caput epididymis. The pathophysiology is not clearly understood. Individuals with this syndrome have impaired mucociliary clearance and a normal sweat test. Evaluation of ciliary ultrastructure may show disorientation of the distal ciliary ultrastructure, likely due to chronic infection and abnormal mucus. Impaired mucociliary clearance results in recurrent sinusitis and bronchitis, ultimately producing bronchiectasis.

  B. **Genetics.** On occasion, the F508 allele may be detected (52). However, unlike congenital absence of the vasa deferentia, Young's syndrome is not likely related to cystic fibrosis (53). The genetic transmission is unknown but may be autosomal recessive.

  C. **Clinical presentation** is similar to the ciliary dyskinesia syndromes, with recurrent sinobronchial infections, bronchiectasis, and male infertility. However, evaluation of the ejaculate reveals the absence of sperm rather than sperm with immotile or dysfunctional flagella (54).

  D. **Differential diagnosis** is also similar to that for ciliary dyskinesia syndrome and includes common variable hypogammaglobulinemia, cystic fibrosis, and α_1-antitrypsin deficiency.

  E. **Diagnostic approach.** Evaluation of the sinuses reveals sinusitis, and chest radiography reveals bronchiectasis. Cystic fibrosis may be ruled out by a normal sweat chloride test, and immunoglobulin deficiency may be ruled out by measurement of quantitative immunoglobulins. Ciliary dyskinesia syndrome may be ruled out by examination of ciliary ultrastructure and the male ejaculate.

  F. **Management** is similar to that for bronchiectasis of any cause, including bronchodilators, physical therapy, and antibiotics for acute exacerbations.

XII. **Congenital bronchiectasis**

  A. **Etiology and pathogenesis.** In addition to the disorders discussed in the two previous sections, bronchiectasis may be associated with several other congenital abnormalities. **Williams-Campbell syndrome** is an intrinsic disorder of cartilage with a deficiency or defect of cartilage in the fourth to sixth order bronchi that results in hyperinflation, dynamic respiratory collapse, and cystic bronchiectasis. **In Mounier-Kuhn syndrome,** tracheobronchomegaly is present and the clinical history is notable for recurrent infections. The trachea (from 20 to >31 mm) and bronchi (from 16 to >24 mm) are greatly dilated in association with a weakness of cartilage, causing dynamic airway collapse, poor mucociliary clearance, and recurrent respiratory infections, leading to bronchiectasis. Other diseases leading to chronic suppuration and bronchiectasis include Bruton's hypogammaglobulinemia, common variable immunodeficiency with hypogammaglobulinemia, yellow-nail syndrome, cystic fibrosis, α_1-antitrypsin deficiency, and selective IgG subclass deficiency. Deficiencies of IgG2, IgG3, and IgG4 all may result in severe recurrent sinopulmonary infections. Absent IgG2 and IgG3 have been associated with impaired antibody responses to bacterial polysaccharide antigens. It is unclear whether IgA deficiency, a disorder that occurs very frequently, is a specific cause of recurrent sinopulmonary infections and bronchiectasis or whether this is due to an association between IgA deficiency and selective IgG subclass deficiency.

  B. **Incidence.** These disorders are rare.

  C. **Genetics.** Bruton's hypogammaglobulinemia is an X-linked recessive disorder. Common variable immunodeficiency is thought to be autosomal recessive and occurs with approximately equal incidence in men and women. IgA deficiency occurs in 1 in 500 whites, with a slight male predominance, and appears to be autosomal dominant with incomplete penetrance. Mounier-Kuhn syndrome may be autosomal recessive. The genetics of the Williams-Campbell syndrome and the yellow-nail syndrome are unknown. Cystic fibrosis and α_1-antitrypsin deficiency are autosomal recessive.

    D. The **pathophysiology** of each of these entities relates to impaired mucociliary clearance (Mounier-Kuhn, Williams-Campbell, and cystic fibrosis) or to abnormal immune response (common variable immunodeficiency, Bruton's hypogammaglobulinemia, yellow-nail syndrome, and selective immunoglobulin subclass deficiency).

    E. **Signs and symptoms** consist of recurrent respiratory infections, which may culminate in obstructive pulmonary disease due to bronchiectasis.

    F. **Differential diagnosis** is similar to other causes of diffuse bronchiectasis as described above.

    G. **Diagnostic approach.** Immunoglobulin deficiencies are diagnosed by measurement of quantitative immunoglobulins. If suspicion of humoral deficiency remains despite a normal total IgG, immunoglobulin subclasses should be measured. Cystic fibrosis is diagnosed by sweat chloride test and genetic testing, α_1-antitrypsin deficiency by measurement of α_1-globulin, and Williams-Campbell syndrome and Mounier-Kuhn syndrome by a combination of radiologic techniques (CT with measurements of the diameter of the trachea and bronchi), bronchoscopy with direct observation, and perhaps biopsy.

    H. **Management.** Bronchiectasis should be treated as outlined above. IgG should be replaced in those with immunoglobulin deficiency. Unfortunately, IgA replacement therapy is not currently possible.

XIII. **Neurofibromatosis**

    A. **Incidence and etiology.** The incidence of this disorder is 1 in 3000. This genetic disorder is associated with dysplasia of the ectoderm and mesoderm and results in subcutaneous neurofibromata and skin discolorations (café au lait spots). The same genetic defect may result in central nervous system gliomas and meningiomas, peripheral nervous system schwannomas, and other tumors such as pheochromocytoma and angiosarcoma. The disorder is autosomal dominant, although about one-half of cases have no prior family history and are presumed to arise through spontaneous mutations.

    B. **Clinical presentation**

        1. Approximately 7% of patients with neurofibromatosis have interstitial lung disease (53). Most individuals who have lung disease present between ages 35 and 60 years, with virtually none before age 28. The patients may be dyspneic, with interstitial infiltrates in the lung bases and thin-walled bullae in the upper lobes (53). Other clinical manifestations include recurrent pneumothorax and, rarely, hemothorax due to a bleeding schwannoma (55). The histology of the interstitial fibrosis is similar to that of idiopathic pulmonary fibrosis (56).

        2. Overall, the thorax is involved in about 15% of patients with neurofibromatosis. In addition to lung abnormalities, there may be mediastinal and vagal neuromas and rib notching due to intercostal neuromas.

    C. **Differential diagnosis** includes those diseases that cause interstitial infiltrates in a basilar distribution. These include idiopathic pulmonary fibrosis, asbestosis, bronchiectasis, sarcoidosis, and connective tissue diseases.

    D. **Diagnostic approach.** There is usually very little confusion with other diagnostic possibilities. The clinical diagnosis of neurofibromatosis in association with typical interstitial infiltrates makes lung biopsy unnecessary. Intercostal neuromas may result in rib notching, raising the possibility of other etiologies of rib notching if the radiologist is unaware of the underlying diagnosis. In the same circumstance, subcutaneous neurofibromas may be mistaken for parenchymal pulmonary nodules.

    E. **Management.** No effective treatment is available for the interstitial lung disease of neurofibromatosis. Pneumothorax is treated with pleural drainage and pleurodesis when necessary. Resection of apical bullae may occasionally be necessary to achieve permanent reexpansion. Oxygen administration is necessary for patients who are hypoxemic and severely dyspneic.

XIV. **Porphyria**

    A. **Etiology and pathogenesis.** The most common acute-attack porphyrias include acute intermittent porphyria, variegate porphyria, and hereditary coproporphyria. In each of these genetic disorders, an enzyme defect results in the accumulation of neurotoxic metabolic products. Examination of affected peripheral nerves reveals demyelination and axonal degeneration. Demyelination in the central nervous system may also be seen, with chromatolysis in anterior horn cells. The nerve injury is responsible for the clinical manifestations.

B. The **incidence** is not precisely known, in part due to the variable penetrance of the disorders under discussion.

C. **Genetics.** All of the major acute-attack porphyrias are autosomal dominant in transmission. Acute intermittent porphyria, the most common of the acute-attack porphyrias, results from a deficiency of porphobilinogen (PBG) deaminase, a protein coded at chromosome 11q23. Variegate porphyria results from a deficiency of protoporphyrinogen oxidase, a protein whose gene is located on chromosome 14. This occurs most commonly in South African whites but may be seen in other populations. The least common of the three is hereditary coproporphyria, which results from deficiency of coproporphyrinogen oxidase, a protein whose gene is located on chromosome 9.

D. **Pathophysiology.** The nerve injury to both sensory and motor nerves results in severe pain, as well as motor dysfunction. Ultimately, motor nerve paralysis may result in respiratory failure.

E. **Signs and symptoms.** Acute attacks are characterized by varying combinations of abdominal pain, constipation, vomiting, urinary retention, tachycardia, hypertension, paresthesias, and weakness. When severe, the paralysis may ascend, progressing to quadriplegia and respiratory failure (57). With bulbar paralysis and cranial nerve involvement, the mortality is 60% to 90% (58). Central nervous system involvement may produce psychiatric symptoms and the syndrome of inappropriate antidiuretic hormone secretion. Seizures may also occur. When bulbar musculature is involved, aspiration pneumonia may result.

1. The disease is characterized by the 5 *P*s: onset after puberty, psychiatric abnormalities, photosensitivity (in variegate porphyria, associated with blisters, scars, and hypertrichosis), pain, and polyneuropathy.

2. Acute attacks are associated with the 4 *M*s: medicines, menses, malnutrition, and medical illnesses (especially infections). Each of these has in common the induction of aminolevulinic acid (ALA) synthetase. This increases the production of porphyrin precursors and toxic metabolites that may reaccumulate as a consequence of the reduced amounts of the affected enzymes, which under ordinary circumstances are adequate to metabolize the porphyrin precursors.

3. Many commonly used medicines may cause the syndrome. Essentially, all antihistamines, tricyclic antidepressants, benzodiazepines, barbiturates, and most calcium channel blockers may induce ALA synthetase. Other common medicines include amiodarone, captopril, carbamazepine, cephalosporins, tetracyclines, and macrolides. Alcohol, furosemide, and thiazide diuretics may also be responsible for enzyme induction, as may metoclopramide, oral contraceptives, rifampin, and valproic acid. Those caring for individuals with acute-attack porphyrias must scrutinize medication lists very carefully before prescribing any drug.

F. **Differential diagnosis** of respiratory failure due to acute porphyria includes a variety of neurologic syndromes. Ascending motor paralysis may be seen with acute infectious polyneuropathy (Guillain-Barré syndrome), and tick paralysis. Other acute syndromes of severe diffuse weakness include the periodic paralyses. Severe lead intoxication may be associated with abdominal pain and motor neuropathies but not ordinarily with diffuse involvement and respiratory failure.

G. **Diagnostic approach.** The combination of acute severe abdominal pain and progressive paralysis culminating in respiratory failure should raise the consideration of acute-attack porphyria. Diagnosis may be confirmed by appropriate tests. In acute intermittent porphyria, ALA PBG will be elevated in the serum and PBG in the urine. Diagnosis can be confirmed by measurement of erythrocyte PBG deaminase. Variegate porphyria can cause elevation of ALA and PBG during acute attacks but will also be associated with increased amounts of protoporphyrinogen in the feces and coproporphyrinogen in the feces and urine. Variegate porphyria causes increased amounts of ALA and PBG in the urine with acute attacks but also is characterized by elevated stool coproporphyrinogen greatly out of proportion to protoporphyrin.

H. **Management.** For those individuals developing respiratory failure, mechanical ventilation is mandatory (58) and may prove life saving. Once the diagnosis is made, all possible precipitating drugs should be avoided, and the patient should receive large amounts of carbohydrate, in the range of 400–500 g of glucose daily. Pain should be treated with morphine or meperidine. Administration of hematin, given in dosages of 1–4 mg/kg IV q12–24h, decreases hepatic ALA synthetase. Improvement may be expected in 2–7 days. When attacks are predictably caused by the onset of menses, hematin should be used prophylactically. Once the diagnosis has been made in an individual, family members should be screened.

XV. **Sickle cell disease**

A. **Incidence and etiology.** The incidence of the homozygous disease state is 1 in 625 African-American newborns. This genetic disease is caused by a mutation in the beta-globin gene that makes hemoglobin more susceptible to gelation. When polymerization occurs, the red cell is deformed into a sickle shape, resulting in capillary occlusion, which accounts for the majority of the clinical symptoms. Transmission is autosomal recessive.

B. **Pathophysiology.** Sickling may be precipitated by a variety of stimuli, including infection, dehydration, and hypoxemia. Sickling results in occlusion of small vessels and causes infarction of the spleen, bone, and lung. Lung lesions appear to be caused most often by *in situ* thrombosis. Even in the asymptomatic state, there is often an increased alveolar-arterial oxygen gradient [(A-a)O$_2$)], a decreased diffusing capacity for carbon monoxide, a decreased capillary blood volume, and an increased pulmonary vascular resistance with diminished lung volumes. Bone marrow emboli may occur, as suggested both by the correlation of sickle cell lung disease with aseptic necrosis (59) and by autopsy findings that show alveolar wall necrosis, focal parenchymal scars, and necrotic bone marrow emboli in 13% of fatal cases (60).

C. **Signs and symptoms.** The most common pulmonary presentation is the acute chest syndrome (ACS). Typically, fever, chest pain, leukocytosis, an increased (A-a)O$_2$, and a chest x-ray with new infiltrates are present. This syndrome accounts for 14% of adult sickle cell admissions and 10% of those in childhood.

1. Acute episodes may be associated with pneumococcal and *Haemophilus* pulmonary infections, but vascular occlusive crises are more common. Currently, approximately 12% of episodes of ACS are due to bacterial pneumonia (3% due to pneumococci), 8% due to viral pneumonia, 16% due to mycoplasma pneumonia, and 64% of undetermined origin (61). The lower frequency of pneumonia in ACS compared to 25 years ago may be due to pneumococcal immunization and penicillin prophylaxis. Those individuals who have bacterial pneumonia tend to be sicker, febrile for a longer period of time, hospitalized longer, have more pleural effusions, and require larger numbers of transfusions.

2. Recurrence of ACS may result in chronic lung disease. The average age of onset of identifiable chronic disease is slightly <24 years, with diagnosis around age 25. Severe chronic sickle cell lung disease is usually present by age 33. Risks for severe sickle cell lung disease include the number of episodes of ACS, of hospitalizations, of all sickle crises, and of episodes of ACS with sickle crisis. It is also correlated with aseptic necrosis of bone (59). Sickle cell lung disease is a significant cause of mortality for adults with sickle cell disease.

D. **Differential diagnosis** of ACS includes acute infectious pneumonia, thrombosis *in situ*, and bone marrow embolization syndrome. Given the ease of diagnosis of the underlying disease in adults, the diagnosis is usually made without difficulty. However, because cocaine use can present with pulmonary infiltrates and hypoxemia, those individuals who have been known to use drugs should be screened for cocaine metabolites.

E. **Management.** For mild episodes of ACS, oxygen, intravenous fluids, and pain medicines are appropriate. For severe episodes accompanied by fever, treatment should include antibiotics appropriate for common community-acquired pneumonias, particularly those due to encapsulated organisms, as the patient is at increased risk for fatal bacteremia due to the functionally asplenic state. When the disease is life threatening with severe abnormalities of gas exchange, exchange transfusion is indicated to reduce hemoglobin S to <30% of total hemoglobin. Anticoagulation is not indicated. For those who have had recurrent severe episodes, hydroxyurea administration to raise the concentration of hemoglobin F and decrease the mean corpuscular concentration of hemoglobin S may be indicated.

F. Specialist referral. Patients with recurrent ACS should be seen by a hematologist with experience in management of the disease. For those with significant sickle cell lung disease, management of the lung disease is best handled by a chest physician.

XVI. Ehlers-Danlos syndrome

A. Etiology and pathogenesis. Eleven types of Ehlers-Danlos syndrome have been identified, presumably representing different genetic abnormalities. The common abnormality is thought to involve type 1 or type 3 collagen, but the defect has not been identified. Moreover, Ehlers-Danlos type 10 is thought perhaps to be due to an abnormality of fibronectin. Autosomal-dominant and X-linked recessive modes of transmission have been described (62). In general, the pathogenesis of the disease is related to tissue with inadequate strength.

B. Clinical presentation. The India rubber men of side show fame were probably individuals with Ehlers-Danlos syndrome. This syndrome is characterized by hypermobile joints, hyperelastic skin, and a variety of morphologic manifestations due to weak connective tissue. These include aortic dissection, spontaneous bowel perforation, cutaneous blood vessel rupture, and, in some subtypes, a bleeding tendency. Affected individuals are fragile and bruisable and may have thin, so-called "cigarette paper" scars. Other associations include diaphragmatic hernia and gastrointestinal diverticula. The major pulmonary manifestation is pneumothorax due to subpleural bullae that rupture into the pleural space. Histologic examination reveals multiple bullae and nodular areas with fragmented elastin and emphysema (62,63).

C. Differential diagnosis. The characteristic body habitus in association with pneumothorax makes other diagnoses unlikely.

D. Management. Pneumothorax should be treated with reexpansion by tube thoracostomy. Thoracoscopic resection of bullae should be considered for patients with persistent leak or recurrence.

XVII. Marfan syndrome

A. Incidence and etiology. The incidence of this abnormality is approximately 1 in 20,000 births. This genetic disease is caused by a mutation in the gene for fibrillin, a large glycoprotein that is a component of elastin-associated microfibrils in the extracellular matrix. Genetic transmission is autosomal dominant. The gene product is produced on chromosome 15 q15-q21.

B. Clinical presentation

1. The characteristic body habitus of the patient with Marfan syndrome includes arachnodactyly, an arm span greater than height, pectus excavatum, hyperextensible joints, ectopia lentis, and aortic abnormalities including progressive aortic root enlargement, resultant aortic insufficiency, and eventual aortic dissection. The patient may also have mitral valve prolapse, and some individuals have kyphoscoliosis.

2. Typical pulmonary presentation involves a combination of recurrent pneumothorax, upper lobe fibrosis, and occasional bronchiectasis. Pneumothorax occurs at a rate of 4% to 11% in individuals >12 years of age. Pneumothorax is frequently recurrent and bilateral and associated with apical blebs. Bullae may occur in 5% of patients and pulmonary fibrosis in 4% (64). Other respiratory manifestations include recurrent respiratory infections, bronchiectasis, and, rarely, aspergilloma (65).

C. Diagnosis. The body habitus abnormalities and the aortic disease overshadow the pulmonary disease. When pulmonary disease is present, the cause is usually obvious because of the underlying genetic disease, and no significant differential diagnosis is required.

D. Management. Affected individuals should be instructed to avoid cigarette smoking in order to prevent additional small-airways disease, air trapping, and bullae expansion, as well as decreasing the risk of pneumothorax. For the same reason, individuals with Marfan syndrome should be instructed to avoid scuba diving because of the potential for bullae expansion and pneumothorax during the ascent. In those who have had pneumothoraces, the treatment is no different from that for other causes of pneumothorax. However, consideration should be given to resection of bullae to prevent recurrence, with consideration of definitive treatment at the first occurrence (66).

References

1. Maltz DL, Nadas AS: Agenesis of the lung: presentation of eight new cases and review of the literature. *Pediatrics* 1968;42:175–188.
2. Soulen RL, Cohen RV: Plain film recognition of pulmonary agenesis in the adult. *Chest* 1971;60:185–187.
3. Mori M, Kidogawa H, Moritaka T, et al.: Bronchial atresia: report of a case and review of the literature. *Jpn J Surg* 1993;23:449–454.
4. Jederlinic PJ, Sicilian LS, Baigelman W, Gaensler EA: Congenital bronchial atresia. *Medicine* 1986; 65:73–83.
5. Meng RL, Jensik RJ, Faber LP, et al.: Bronchial atresia. *Ann Thorac Surg* 1978;25:184–192.
6. Smith RA: A theory of the origin of intralobar sequestration of the lung. *Thorax* 1956;11:10–24.
7. Haller JA, Tepas JJ, White JJ, et al.: The natural history of bronchial atresia. *J Thorac Cardiovasc Surg* 1980;79:868–872.
8. Swensen SJ, Aughenbaugh GL, Brown LR: Chest case of the day. *AJR* 1993;160:1318–1322.
9. Talner LB, Gmelich JT, Liebow AA, Greenspan RH: The syndrome of bronchial mucocele and regional hyperinflation of the lung. *Am J Roentgenol Radium Ther Nucl Med* 1970;110:675–686.
10. Dupuis C, Charaf LAC, Breviere GM, et al.: The "adult" form of the scimitar syndrome. *Am J Cardiol* 1992;70:502–507.
11. Kiely B, Filler J, Stone S, Doyle EF: Syndrome of anomalous venous drainage of the right lung to the inferior vena cava: a review of 67 reported cases and three new cases in children. *Am J Cardiol* 1967;20:102–116.
12. Foreman SG, Rosa U: The scimitar syndrome. *South Med J* 1991;84:489–493.
13. Ellis K: Developmental abnormalities in the systemic blood supply to the lungs. *AJR* 1991;156:669–679.
14. Mathey J, Galen JJ, Logeais Y, et al.: Anomalous pulmonary venous return into inferior vena cava and associated bronchovascular anomalies (the scimitar syndrome): report of three cases and review of the literature. *Thorax* 1968;23:398–407.
15. Woodring JH, Howard TA, Kanga JF: Congenital pulmonary venolobar syndrome revisited. *RadioGraphics* 1994;14:349–369.
16. Roehm JDF, Jue KL, Amplatz K: Radiographic features of the scimitar syndrome. *Radiology* 1966; 86:856–859.
17. Sener RN, Tugran C, Savas R, Alper H: CT findings in scimitar syndrome. *AJR* 1993;160:1361.
18. Dupuis C, Remy J, Remy-Jardin M, et al.: The "horseshoe" lung: six new cases. *Pediatr Pulmonol* 1994;17:124–130.
19. Ribet ME, Copin MC, Gosselin B: Bronchogenic cysts of the mediastinum. *J Thorac Cardiovasc Surg* 1995;109:1003–1010.
20. Hernanz-Schulman M: Cysts and cyst-like lesions of the lung. *Radiol Clin North Am* 1993;31:631–649.
21. Nuchtern JG, Harberg FJ: Congenital lung cysts. *Semin Pediatr Surg* 1994;3:233–243.
22. Matzinger MA, Matzinger FR, Sachs HJ: Intrapulmonary bronchogenic cyst: spontaneous pneumothorax as the presenting symptom. *AJR* 1992;158:987–988.
23. Suen HC, Mathisen DJ, Grillo HC, et al.: Surgical management and radiological characteristics of bronchogenic cysts. *Ann Thorac Surg* 1993;55:476–481.
24. Patel SR, Meeker DP, Biscotti CV, et al.: Presentation and management of bronchogenic cysts in the adult. *Chest* 1994;106:79–85.
25. Urschel JD, Horan TA: Mediastinoscopic treatment of mediastinal cysts. *Ann Thorac Surg* 1994; 58:1698–1701.
26. Dab Z, Malfroot A, van de Velde A, Deneyer M: Endoscopic unroofing of a bronchogenic cyst. *Pediatr Pulmonol* 1994;18:46–50.
27. Hazelrigg SR, Landreneau RJ, Mack MJ, Acuff TE: Thoracoscopic resection of mediastinal cysts. *Ann Thorac Surg* 1993;56:659–660.

28. Haddon MT, Bowen A: Bronchopulmonary and neurogenic forms of foregut anomalies: imaging for diagnosis and management. *Radiol Clin North Am* 1991;29:241–254.
29. Rosado-de-Christenson ML, Frazier AA, Stocker JT, Templeton PA: Extralobar sequestration: radiologic-pathologic correlation. *RadioGraphics* 1993;13:425–441.
30. Savic B, Birtel FJ, Thelen W, et al.: Lung sequestration: report of seven cases and review of 540 published cases. *Thorax* 1979;34:96–101.
31. Simopoulos AP, Rosenblum DJ, Mazumdar H, Kiely B: Intralobar bronchopulmonary sequestration in children: diagnosis by intrathoracic aortography. *J Dis Child* 1959;97:796–804.
32. Stocker JT, Kagan-Hallett K: Extralobar pulmonary sequestration: analysis of 15 cases. *Am J Clin Pathol* 1979;72:917–925.
33. Katlic MR, Nardell KM, Reiff DA: Extralobar pulmonary sequestration in the elderly. *J Am Geriatr Soc* 1994;42:213–214.
34. Sugio K, Kaneko S, Yokoyama H, et al.: Pulmonary sequestration in older child and in adults. *Int Surg* 1992;77:102–107.
35. White J, Chan Y, Neuberger S, Wilson T: Prenatal sonographic detection of intra-abdominal extralobar pulmonary sequestration: report of 3 cases and literature review. *Prenat Diagn* 1994;14:653–658.
36. Felson B: The many faces of pulmonary sequestration. *Semin Roentgenol* 1972;7:3–16.
37. Donovan CB, Edelman RR, Vrachliotis TG, et al.: Bronchopulmonary sequestration with MR angiographic evaluation: a case report. *Angiology* 1993;45:339–344.
38. Doyle AJ: Demonstration of blood supply to pulmonary sequestration by MR angiography. *AJR* 1992;158:989–990.
39. Stigers KB, Woodring JH, Kanga JF: The clinical and imaging spectrum of findings in patients with congenital lobar emphysema. *Pediatr Pulmonol* 1992;14:160–170.
40. Murray GF: Congenital lobar emphysema. *Surg Gynecol Obstet* 1967;124:611–625.
41. Richards DS, Langham MR, Dolson LH: Antenatal presentation of a child with congenital lobar emphysema. *J Ultrasound Med* 1992;11:165–168.
42. Armengot M, Juan G, Barona R, et al.: Immotile cilia syndrome: nasal mucociliary function and nasal ciliary abnormalities. *Rhinology* 1994;32:109–111.
43. LeMauviel L: Primary ciliary dyskinesia. *West J Med* 1991;155:280–283.
44. Losa M, Ghalfi D, Haf E, et al.: Kartagener syndrome: an uncommon cause of neonatal respiratory distress? *Eur J Pediatr* 1995;154:236–238.
45. Lurie M, Rennert G, Goldenberg S, et al.: Ciliary ultrastructure in primary ciliary dyskinesia and other chronic respiratory conditions: the relevance of microtubular abnormalities. *Ultrastruct Pathol* 1992;16:547–553.
46. Kinney TB, DeLuca SA: Kartagener's syndrome. *AFP* 1991;44:133–134.
47. Engesaeth VG, Warner JO, Bush A: New associations of primary ciliary dyskinesia syndrome. *Pediatr Pulmonol* 1993;16:9–12.
48. DeIongh RU, Rutland J: Ciliary defects in healthy subjects, bronchiectasis, and primary ciliary dyskinesia. *Am J Respir Crit Care Med* 1995;151:1559–1567.
49. Munro NC, Currie DC, Lindsay KS, et al.: Fertility in men with primary ciliary dyskinesia presenting with respiratory infection. *Thorax* 1994;49:684–687.
50. Schidlow DV: Primary ciliary dyskinesia (the immotile cilia syndrome). *Ann Allergy* 1994;73:457–469.
51. Hicks LM, Mansfield PB: Esophageal atresia and tracheoesophageal fistula. *J Thorac Cardiovasc Surg* 1981;81:358–363.
52. Hirsh A, Williams C, Williamson B: Young's syndrome and cystic fibrosis mutation DF508. *Lancet* 1993;342:118.
53. Burkhalter JL, Morans JU, McCay MB: Diffuse interstitial lung disease in neurofibromatosis. *South Med J* 1986;79:944–946.
54. LeLannau D, Jezequel P, Blayan M, et al.: Obstructive azoospermia with agenesis of vas deferens or with bronchiectasia (Young's syndrome): a genetic approach. *Hum Reprod* 1995;10:338–341.
55. Larrieu AJ, Hashimoto SA, Allen P: Spontaneous massive haemothorax in von Recklinghausen's disease. *Thorax* 1982;37:151–152.
56. Webb WR, Goodman PC: Fibrosing alveolitis in patients with neurofibromatosis. *Radiology* 1977;122:289–293.
57. Becker DM, Kramer S: The neurologic manifestations of porphyria: a review. *Medicine* 1977;56:411–423.

58. Doll SG, Bower AG, Affeldt JE: Acute intermittent porphyria with respiratory paralysis. *JAMA* 1958;168:1973–1976.
59. Powers D, Weidman JA, Odom-Maryon T, et al.: Sickle cell chronic lung disease: prior morbidity and the risk of respiratory failure. *Medicine* 1988;67:66–76.
60. Haupt HM, Moore GW, Bauer TW, Hutchins GM: The lung in sickle cell disease. *Chest* 1982;81: 332–337.
61. Sprinkle RH, Cole T, Smith S, Buchanan GR: Acute chest syndrome in children with sickle cell disease: a retrospective analysis of 100 hospitalized cases. *Am J Pediatr Hematol Oncol* 1986;8: 105–110.
62. Smit, J, Alberts C, Balk AG: Pneumothorax in the Ehlers-Danlos syndrome: consequence or coincidence. *Scand J Respir Dis* 1978;59:239–242.
63. Robitaille GA: Ehlers-Danlos syndrome and recurrent hemoptysis. *Ann Intern Med* 1964;61: 716–720.
64. Pyeritz RE: Connective tissue in the lung: lessons from the Marfan syndrome (editorial). *Ann Intern Med* 1985;103:289–290.
65. Wood JR, Bellamy D, Citron KM: Pulmonary disease in patients with Marfan syndrome. *Thorax* 1984;39:780–784.
66. Hall JR, Pyeritz RE, Dudgeon DL, Haller JA: Pneumothorax in the Marfan syndrome: prevalence and therapy. *Ann Thorac Surg* 1984;37:500–504.

24

Lung Abscess and Empyema

Brian B. Bloom and Ronald H. Goldstein

Lung abscess refers to a localized area of necrosis and suppuration within the lung parenchyma. Empyema refers to a collection of pus within the pleural space. Both conditions share risk factors, bacteriology, and clinical presentations and will therefore be discussed together in this chapter.

I. **Lung abscess** usually forms as a complication of a bacterial pneumonitis. **A single lung abscess**, or a simple abscess, is a discrete area of infiltration with a necrotic center. This infection is classically caused by aspiration of mixed aerobic and anaerobic oral flora and presents as an indolent process. **Multiple lung abscesses** can develop as a complication of necrotizing pneumonias, resulting from rapidly destructive processes caused by aspiration of large volumes of gastric contents or by virulent aerobic organisms: *Staphylococcus aureus*, *Klebsiella*, and other gram-negative species. Other causes of cavitary lung infections include pneumonitis from fungi and mycobacteria, hematogenous seeding of the lung with pyogenic bacteria, and postobstructive pneumonias.

A. **Simple lung abscess**

1. **Signs and symptoms**

   a. Patients with an anaerobic lung abscess usually have a history of factors that predispose to aspiration: alcoholism, stroke, seizure disorder, esophageal disease, or impaired consciousness. Patients often have poor oral hygiene; lung abscess is rare in edentulous patients. Patients with an abnormal bronchial tree due to obstruction, neoplasm, or bronchiectasis are also at increased risk (1,2). Infection is caused by aspiration of oral flora containing multiple organisms to produce an indolent necrotizing infection (1).

   b. Patients with a simple lung abscess often present subacutely with prolonged constitutional symptoms, weight loss, anemia, putrid sputum, and leukocytosis. Fever and cough develop insidiously, and symptoms may have been present for several weeks (1,2).

2. **Etiology and bacteriology**

   a. Most cases of lung abscess are caused by aspiration of oral anaerobes into the lung. These organisms produce an indolent pneumonitis resulting in cavity formation. Most abscesses are found in areas of the lung at risk for aspiration: the posterior segment of an upper lobe or the superior segment of a lower lobe. However, atypical locations may occur depending on the position of the patient during the aspiration.

   b. Virtually all patients with simple lung abscesses have anaerobes, usually multiple isolates (more than three species per patient), and many in combination with aerobes found in sputum. The most common organisms include *Fusobacterium nucleatum*, *Bacteroides melaninogenicus*, and peptostreptococci. Common aerobic organisms include several species of microaerophilic and aerobic streptococci (1,2).

3. **Diagnosis**

   a. The differential diagnosis of simple lung abscess (indolent primary bacterial infection with anaerobes or mixed flora) is listed in Table 24-1.

Table 24-1. Differential diagnosis of simple lung abscess

Fulminant necrotizing pneumonia (aerobic bacteria)

Tuberculosis

Fungi

Cancer with central necrosis

Wegener's granulomatosis and related vasculitides

Infection of existing cavities (bullae, postsurgical, post-tuberculosis)

Postobstructive pneumonitis (cancer, foreign body)

Septic emboli

Empyema

Sequestration

?s/p infarction

?s/p bronchiectasis

---

   b. **Posteroanterior (PA) and lateral view chest radiographs** should be obtained in any patient with a suspected lung abscess.

      i. Classically, a simple lung abscess will appear as an infiltrate with a central cavity partially filled with fluid, creating an air–fluid level. Abscesses may not always contain air–fluid levels and conversely may be found in other conditions (empyema, necrotizing bronchogenic carcinoma). Anaerobic abscesses following an aspiration are usually found in dependent segments of the lung.

     ii. **When the abscess cavity is located adjacent to the chest wall, differentiation from an empyema may be difficult.** Unlike empyemas that tend to extend inward from the chest wall, forming an obtuse angle, abscesses tend to grow outward from the parenchyma, forming an acute angle. This rule is not always true; in one study, 14% of empyemas formed acute angles with the chest wall (3). Unlike empyemas, abscesses do not cross fissure lines. In addition, air–fluid levels will appear similar on both PA and lateral chest radiographic views in a fairly round abscess, but they usually appear compressed in one of the views in empyema (3,4). Associated lung consolidation is frequently found in both disorders.

    iii. **The finding of lung abscess in association with atelectasis, mass, or foreign body suggests a postobstructive process.** Septic emboli appear as multiple round cavities with surrounding infiltrate. These occur more commonly in the lower lobes because of greater perfusion to these areas. Infected bullae are characterized by the development of an air–fluid level in a preexisting bulla with minimal inflammation of the adjacent parenchyma. An old chest film available for comparison is of prime importance in making this diagnosis.

   c. **Computed tomography (CT) of the chest can clearly confirm the diagnosis of lung abscess if any question remains after evaluation of the plain films.** CT performed with intravenous contrast is particularly useful in distinguishing between pleural and parenchymal processes (see pleural empyema below). CT can also help distinguish an infected bulla from an abscess, because the walls of the cavity of a bulla will usually be thinner than an abscess. Tobacco users with a lung abscess should undergo CT scanning for evidence of necrotizing bronchogenic carcinoma as the etiology of the cavity. The suggestive findings on CT include a thick and irregular wall, distorted or compressed pulmonary vessels, and bronchi in proximity to the cavity wall (3,4). A lesion or foreign body obstructing a bronchus may also be seen on CT.

    d. The mixed flora of lung abscesses will often be demonstrated by **Gram's stain of expectorated sputum,** which will reveal many polymorphonuclear leukocytes, necrotic debris, and the presence of multiple bacterial species. Although sputum Gram's stain analysis is neither sensitive nor specific, a finding of large numbers of a single bacterial species in a good quality specimen suggests the diagnosis of necrotizing pneumonitis caused by an aerobic bacterial species rather than simple lung abscess. **The presence of clumps of elastin fibers on a potassium hydroxide wet prep strongly supports the diagnosis of a necrotizing pulmonary process** (5). **Acid-fast smears and mycobacterial cultures** should be performed in patients at risk for mycobacterial infections.

    e. Bronchoscopy is not required in the evaluation of lung abscess but should be performed if airway obstruction is the suspected cause of the abscess (6). A history suggestive of foreign body aspiration should prompt bronchoscopy. Similarly, a lung abscess in a smoker without other risk factors for aspiration should prompt a search for an endobronchial malignancy. Location of an abscess in an nondependent segment of lung or the absence of an infiltrate surrounding the abscess also raises the clinical suspicion of cancer. **An obstructive lesion such as a foreign body or a malignancy should also be considered if the abscess fails to completely resolve with antibiotic therapy** (6,7).

      i. Bronchoscopy may also be indicated to obtain material for culture if an atypical organism (nontuberculous mycobacteria, fungi) is suspected and adequate sputum is not otherwise available (7).

      ii. A diagnostic bronchoscopy is usually well tolerated and is not risky in these patients; however, **therapeutic endobronchial drainage of an abscess can produce a rapid, sudden flow of purulent material to otherwise uninvolved lung and cause an acute impairment of gas exchange and spread of infection**. The risks of this procedure can be reduced by performing bronchoscopy through an endotracheal tube; this permits insertion of a large suction catheter in the case of large quantities of secretions or spillage. Therapeutic endobronchial drainage of a lung abscess is generally not recommended because of a high risk of spillage. **If exogenous drainage is thought to be required, radiographically guided transthoracic catheter placement is safer than endobronchial manipulations through a fiberoptic bronchoscope** (7).

    f. Blood cultures will usually be positive in cases caused by hematologic seeding of the lung. Blood cultures may also identify the causative organism(s) in primary pulmonary processes.

    g. Any pleural fluid should be sampled via thoracentesis and aerobically and anaerobically cultured.

4. Management

    a. Prolonged antibiotic therapy is the preferred clinical management for simple lung abscess. Virtually no cases require surgical drainage, since infectious debris may be spontaneously mobilized via the bronchopulmonary tree and pulmonary lymphatics (1).

    b. In Bartlett and colleagues' series (1), most of the anaerobes isolated were sensitive to penicillin. However, four cases grew *Bacteroides fragilis,* and several of the aerobic or facultative copathogens were penicillin resistant. Two subsequent reports have shown frequent treatment failure with penicillin alone due to resistant bacteroides (8,9). **We therefore recommend clindamycin (600 mg q8h) as first-line therapy. Addition of a second antibiotic to cover gram-negative organisms should be considered in the critically ill, as well as patients who fail to respond to initial therapy. Penicillin (10–15 million U/d) in combination with metronidazole (1–2 g/d) is also an effective regimen.** Abscesses can also be caused by infection with atypical organisms such as fungi or mycobacteria.

    i. Patients should initially be treated with intravenous antibiotics. Once the patient is afebrile and asymptomatic and the abscess has stabilized radiographically, an equivalent oral regimen (clindamycin 300 mg q6h or penicillin VK 500–750 mg QID) may be instituted (2). In a typical clinical course, fever, anorexia, and sputum odor will resolve in the first week of therapy. However, massive sputum production may persist for weeks. Postural drainage may be a useful adjunct to therapy as long as the risk of large volume spillage from the abscess is low.

    ii. Length of antibiotic therapy is determined empirically. A total of at least 6 weeks of antibiotics is recommended for most cases. Antibiotics should be continued until radiographic infiltrates have completely cleared or evolved into a small, stable residual lesion. Very large or otherwise complicated abscesses may need additional treatment.

  c. During the course of treatment, **serial radiographs** should be obtained to follow abscess size, as well as whenever clinical changes occur suggestive of complications (intrabronchial spread of infection, pleural involvement). Radiographic infiltrates may progress during the first several days of successful treatment (as in other pulmonary infections). Cavity closure occurs slowly; the temporal rate of improvement is inversely proportional to the size of the cavity, with an average time to resolution of 65 days in one study (10). In general the prognosis is good, and the vast majority of patients are cured. Follow-up radiographs are indicated both to verify resolution and to rule out occult carcinoma.

5. Problems and complications of therapy

  a. In the preantibiotic era, amyloidosis and brain abscess were the most common complications of simple lung abscess.

  b. Parapneumonic effusions, empyema, and bronchopulmonary fistulas are now the most common complications of simple lung abscess. Abscesses and parapneumonic effusions often coexist. Empyemas require tube thoracostomy drainage. Bronchopulmonary fistulas may form in highly necrotic areas of lung.

  c. **Large cavities** (>6 cm) with air–fluid levels may abruptly drain and spill infected or necrotic material into the tracheobronchial tree, causing rapid clinical deterioration and asphyxiation. Extensive pneumonitis may appear in individuals who survive the initial event. Percutaneous needle aspiration of very large bulging cavities, with transthoracic placement of a pigtail catheter, or alternatively abscess resection should be considered to prevent this complication.

6. Treatment failure

  a. A **mechanically obstructed bronchus** may prevent rapid response to antibiotics by inhibiting drainage of pus. **Patients who do not respond to antibiotic therapy should undergo diagnostic bronchoscopy to rule out obstruction.** Obstructions may be divided into intrinsic, as caused by a bronchogenic carcinoma, or extrinsic, as caused by consolidated lung or swollen airway mucosa. Specific therapies will depend on the etiology of the obstruction. Surgery or radiotherapy may be required in the case of a carcinoma, whereas inhaled bronchodilators and steroids, together with postural drainage, may suffice in the case of pure inflammatory causes.

  b. A small percentage of patients will not respond to conservative medical therapy in the absence of obstruction. Patients who do not show radiographic improvement, have persistent sepsis, or develop bronchopulmonary fistula or significant hemoptysis are candidates for **percutaneous catheter drainage** or pulmonary resection.

    i. Catheters can be placed percutaneously into the abscess with CT, sonographic, or fluoroscopic guidance. After confirmation of catheter position, the abscess cavity should be aspirated and irrigated with saline, and then placed at suction drainage at -20 cm H_2O. The catheter should be irrigated twice daily to maintain patency and should be kept in place until clinical resolution occurs (11). This regimen was found to prevent surgery in 84% of patients (12), with a mean time to abscess resolution of 10–15 days and marked clinical improvement within 48 hours of drainage. Complications include pneumothorax, bronchopleural fistula, empyema, and hemorrhage (11).

B. **Postobstructive abscess** is difficult to treat and often persists unless the obstruction is removed.

    1. In some series, the incidence of bronchogenic carcinoma presenting with lung abscess ranges from 8% to 18% (6). Obstructing malignancies can be resected or irradiated. In nonoperable individuals, endobronchial debulking via rigid bronchoscopy using laser photocoagulation, brachytherapy, endobronchial stents, or a combination of these modalities may be helpful in relieving obstruction as palliative interventions. Antibiotics should be continued for a full 6-week course, if the patient improves after treatment of the obstruction. If a bronchus obstructed by malignancy cannot be reopened, very long-term antibiotic therapy may eventually sterilize the abscess or at least allow the patient to survive with low-grade infection.

C. **Necrotizing pneumonia**

    1. Infection by large numbers of virulent organisms may result in a fulminant, rapidly progressive, necrotizing pneumonia with the abrupt onset of cough, productive sputum, high fever, and leukocytosis, as well as radiographic evidence of an extensive pneumonia with multiple air–fluid levels (pneumonic abscesses). Organisms responsible for this infection include *Klebsiella pneumoniae*, *Pseudomonas aeruginosa*, *S. aureus*, β-hemolytic streptococci, pneumococci, *Nocardia*, *Pseudomonas pseudomallei*, and *Legionella* species.

    2. **Necrotizing pneumonia** should initially be managed with broad-spectrum antibiotics, followed by a regimen based on blood and sputum culture results. Ventilatory and hemodynamic support is often required in these critically ill patients.

D. **Infected bullae** are not associated with necrosis of tissue and therefore are not true abscesses. Infection of a preexisting bulla usually presents as a mild, subacute illness, and the chest x-ray usually shows an air–fluid level in a preexisting emphysematous bulla and minimal infiltrate in the surrounding parenchyma. Oral aerobes and anaerobes are the likely pathogens. Patients with infected bullae usually respond to antibiotics that cover oral flora (penicillin) and to postural drainage. Response is usually prompt, and invasive procedures are rarely required.

E. **Septic emboli** are caused by hematologic seeding of the lung by pyogenic bacteria that results in multiple round cavitary infiltrates. Cavities are found more frequently in dependent lung zones (proportional to degree of vascular flow). Usually the primary infective source is obvious (cardiac valve, vascular prosthesis). The most common organisms are *S. aureus*, *Staphylococcus epidermidis*, and *Candida* species. Antibiotic treatment is frequently prolonged, and the primary source may require surgical removal.

II. **Pleural empyema.** Management of empyema is difficult due to the progressive, changing nature of the infected pleural space and the myriad therapeutic options for drainage. The treatment plan must be tailored to each patient after consultation with experienced thoracic surgeons, radiologists, and pulmonologists. The most common errors in management of empyema are due to delays in both diagnosis and institution of effective drainage (13–15).

A. **Signs and symptoms.** The clinical presentation depends on whether the underlying infection is caused by aerobic or anaerobic bacteria.

    1. **Empyemas complicating aerobic pneumonia** usually present with symptoms due to the pneumonia (acute febrile illness, cough, sputum, pleurisy, dyspnea, and leukocytosis). In immunocompromised patients, a more indolent presentation may occur. The length of time that the patient has symptoms before seeking medical attention correlates with the likelihood that a parapneumonic effusion has developed and that the effusion is complicated (16). While most pneumonias will respond to antibiotic therapy alone, empyemas require drainage. Without drainage, the patient will have persistent fever, weight loss, and malaise. Persistent infection can result in the development of a pleurocutaneous fistula. Even when the pleural space is eventually sterilized with parenteral antibiotics, a loss of residual lung function due to a pleural peel and trapped lung often results in significant morbidity. However, slow resolution of the pleural thickening occurs with improvement in lung function in a majority of cases of empyema (17,18).

2. **Empyemas complicating infections caused by anaerobes and mixed infections** are due to the same risk factors as those described above for simple lung abscesses. Not surprisingly, the two conditions frequently coexist. Two factors are of great importance in predisposing a patient to aspiration of oral anaerobes. The first is the presence of poorly maintained dentition; edentulous patients rarely develop anaerobic lung infections. The second is impairment of normal upper airway defenses due to mechanical dysfunction of the larynx or, more commonly, to neurologic dysfunction secondary to central nervous system injury or intoxication (2,15,19,20). Compared with aerobic infections, anaerobic infections often present with a subacute illness with prolonged symptoms of a week or longer, together with weight loss, anemia, putrid sputum production, and leukocytosis (1). Chronic empyema may rarely cause back pain and pleurocutaneous fistula with drainage of pus.

B. The causes of empyema are listed in Table 24-2, and the differential diagnosis includes entities listed in Table 24-3.

C. **Classification of empyemas**
   1. **Uncomplicated parapneumonic effusions** occur in the setting of pneumonia. Pleural fluid is seen on the chest x-rays in 20% to 40% of bacterial pneumonias, and the determination of which require drainage is critical. The earliest pleural response to infection is a low-viscosity exudate without loculation. At this stage, antibiotic therapy of the underlying process will usually result in resolution of the effusion. By definition, an effusion that resolves on antibiotic therapy alone is an uncomplicated effusion. Biochemical characteristics of an uncomplicated effusion are consistent with an exudate and include a low

Table 24-2. Etiology of empyema

Direct extension from bacterial pneumonia or lung abscess

Direct extension from other primary site (pharynx, esophagus, mediastinum, subdiaphragm)

Penetrating chest trauma

Hematogenous infection of the pleural space

Nonbacterial infections (*M. tuberculosis*, fungus)

Iatrogenic (following thoracotomy, thoracentesis)

Table 24-3. Differential diagnosis of empyema

Pulmonary embolism

Acute pancreatitis

Dressler's syndrome

Connective tissue diseases (lupus pleuritis, rheumatoid pleurisy)

Esophageal rupture with effusion

Malignancy

Drug hypersensitivity reactions

white blood cell (WBC) count, a low lactate acid dehydrogenase (LDH) level, a normal glucose level, and a normal pH (4,7,14,21).

2. **Complicated parapneumonic effusions** occur when bacterial invasion of the pleural space occurs. At this time, neutrophils migrate into the pleural fluid and a fibrin matrix begins to form on the visceral and parietal pleura. This fibrin matrix can produce an inelastic pleural peel and loculations, thereby trapping the adjacent lung. Although the peel and loculations may prevent the extension of empyema, drainage of the pleural space is quite difficult. The goal of early therapy is to rapidly sterilize and drain the pleural space before loculation of the fluid and entrapment of the lung occur. Untreated loculations increase the risk that infected fluid may drain spontaneously into the lung (bronchopleural fistula), through the chest wall (pleurocutaneous fistula), or both (broncho-pleurocutaneous fistula) (4,14,16,21). Loculations suspected of being infected may require multiple CT-guided transthoracic aspirations for diagnosis and therapy. The long-term outcome of patients who survive severe pleural disease is variable. In most cases, the pleural thickening slowly resolves with corresponding restoration of underlying lung function (17).

3. **True empyema generally is defined as pus in the pleural space.** However, usage varies and empyema may refer to any complicated parapnuemonic effusion that contains pus, demonstrable pathogens, or chemical characteristics predictive of a complicated course.

D. **Bacteriology of empyema**

1. The bacteriology of empyema varies with the site of primary infection and with host factors. The parenchyma is the most common primary site of infection. In patients at risk for aspiration, oral flora are responsible for pneumonitis and subsequent empyema. Organisms mirror those found in lung abscesses. Common anaerobes include *F. nucleatum, B. melaninogenicus,* and peptostreptococci. Aerobes include several species of microaerophilic and aerobic streptococci.

2. In patients without the risk for aspiration, aerobic gram-positive species (*S. aureus, Streptococcus pneumoniae,* and *Streptococcus pyogenes*) can cause empyema as a complication of pneumonia. Enteric gram-negative rods are often responsible for parapneumonic empyemas in patients with chronic illness or nosocomial infections acquired in nursing homes, hospital wards, and particularly intensive care units (2,19,20).

3. Different infecting organisms have varying propensities to induce pleural disease. *S. pneumoniae* is still responsible for most bacterial pneumonias. Although parapneumonic effusions are common, only a small percentage (4%) will have positive cultures (16). *S. aureus* pneumonia often causes pleural effusions, with 20% positive on culture (16). *S. pyogenes* pneumonia, while uncommon, is often associated with empyema and pleural effusion, with a high rate of complication. (16). A third of the anaerobic lung infections in Bartlett and coworkers' series (1) were associated with empyema. *Escherichia coli* and *Pseudomonas* species account for over half of gram-negative organisms cultured from pleural fluid. These infections are often due to nosocomial pneumonias and frequently require drainage procedures (16). Half of cases of *Haemophilus influenzae* pneumonia are associated with parapneumonic effusions, with one-third progressing to empyema (16). *K. pneumoniae* and *Proteus* species infections usually do not cause pleural effusions (16). *Rhodococcus equi* pneumonia occurs in immunocompromised patients and is frequently complicated by empyema. *Actinomyces* and *Nocardia* species are rare causes of empyema. Tuberculous pleural effusions, though technically empyemas, do not require surgical drainage and respond well to antibiotic therapy (see chapter 8).

4. Empyemas that originate from sources other than the pulmonary parenchyma will demonstrate flora appropriate to the primary infection. Infections from subdiaphragmatic sources are typically due to common enteric organisms (and also rarely to amebae). Hematogenous seeding of the pleura can occur from staphylococci, although usually there is parenchymal involvement. Esophageal perfo-

ration allows oral flora to enter the mediastinum and often the pleural space. Iatrogenic and traumatic violation of the pleural space can result in pleural infections with skin flora.

E. **Diagnostic evaluation**

1. **Plain chest radiographs (PA and lateral views) should be obtained in any patient with a new clinical diagnosis of pneumonia or in any patient not responding as expected to antibiotic therapy.** Free-flowing pleural fluid can be demonstrated by plain films. More complicated fluid collections (loculated pleural fluid, intraparencymal collections) may require more extensive imaging.

   a. If the posterior costophrenic angle is obliterated on the lateral chest radiograph, decubitus films should be obtained to estimate the amount of pleural fluid. **If the thickness of the pleural fluid on the decubitus film is >10 mm, a sufficient volume of free-flowing fluid is present to warrant biochemical and bacteriologic evaluation to rule out a complicated effusion** (4,16).

      i. When pleural fluid is loculated (not free-flowing), it may be difficult to distinguish between intraparenchymal and pleural processes. Several radiographic findings will help distinguish between the two. Loculated pleural collections tend to extend inward from the chest wall, forming an obtuse angle between the chest wall and the fluid collection. Abscesses tend to grow outward and form an acute angle with the chest wall.

      ii. These findings are neither sensitive nor specific. Air can develop in empyemas either from gas-producing organisms introduced during thoracentesis or, more commonly, due to bronchopleural fistulas. Both empyemas and abscesses may develop air–fluid levels; however, an air–fluid level will appear similar on both PA and lateral films in a fairly round abscess, while a pleural-based collection usually will appear compressed in one of the views. Lastly, empyemas cross fissure lines, while abscesses do not (3,4,15).

   b. A **diagnostic thoracentesis** should be performed promptly because delay in instituting proper pleural drainage in patients with complicated effusions substantially increases morbidity (22).

2. **Chest CT scans should be done to confirm the diagnosis, delineate the anatomy, and determine the extent of parenchymal versus pleural disease.** In most cases, CT scans will readily define the anatomy.

   a. CT findings consistent with empyema include the **split-pleura sign:** separation of uniformly thickened visceral pleura from parietal pleura (seen in 68% of all empyemas and in a higher percentage of scans employing intravenous contrast material, and never seen in lung abscess) and compression of uninvolved lung revealed by distorted and bowed bronchi and/or pulmonary vessels around the periphery of the empyema. In lung abscess, bronchi and pulmonary vessels terminate abruptly at the advancing wall of an abscess and are not compressed or distorted.

   b. Other helpful distinguishing radiographic features relate to wall characteristics. At least part of the wall of almost all empyemas is thin, smooth, and uniform, whereas lung abscesses have walls that are thick and irregular (3,4).

3. **Pleural ultrasound** is most useful in guiding diagnostic thoracentesis and therapeutic drainage procedures. The presence of internal echoes or septations in the pleural space increases the likelihood that a parapneumonic fluid collection is an empyema. If used to guide therapeutic or diagnostic thoracentesis, the procedure should be performed with continuous ultrasound guidance. **Marking the prospective needle site on the patient's skin in the radiology department and then sending the patient back to his or her room for the thoracentesis is not recommended because the relationship between the skin and the underlying pleural fluid may be dependent on position** (16).

4. **Thoracentesis** is required to assess the biochemical and bacteriologic properties of pleural fluid. Based on these results, a parapneumonic effusion can be classified as uncomplicated (not requiring tube drainage) or complicated (includes empyemas and requires drainage).

   a. Thoracentesis is a low-risk procedure if pleural fluid is free-flowing and layers >1 cm in a decubitus view. Depending on the experience and level of expertise of the physician and the degree of difficulty of a given case (ie, small volume or loculations), some thoracenteses are more safely performed under ultrasound guidance. If the effusion is loculated, large locules should be sampled under ultrasonic guidance, because the character of the pleural fluid may vary from one locule to another. When multiple locules are present, the fluid contained within each locule is considered to be a complicated effusion (thereby requiring drainage) unless proven otherwise by sampling each locule separately under ultrasound guidance. As this is usually either impractical or impossible, large loculated effusions require surgical drainage.

   b. Approximately 30–50 mL of pleural fluid are adequate for diagnostic evaluation. Pleural fluid must be collected anaerobically and placed on ice. The sample should be grossly inspected for color, turbidity, and odor and aliquots sent for determination of pH, LDH, glucose, total protein, amylase, cell count with differential, Gram's stain, and culture (aerobic and anaerobic). Feculent odor is strongly suggestive of anaerobic infection. If there is clinical suspicion, samples should also be cultured for fungi, mycobacteria, and unusual organisms such as *Actinomyces* and *Nocardia* (4,16).

   c. Empyema may be diagnosed if the fluid reveals gross pus (thick purulent fluid) or thin fluid with organisms on the Gram's stain. Thick purulent material on visual examination is sufficient to determine the presence of an empyema and the need for tube drainage; such thick material should not be sent for pH determination, as it may damage the analyzer (16).

5. The biochemical characteristics that distinguish a parapneumonic effusion requiring drainage (complicated effusion) from one that is likely to resolve without drainage (uncomplicated) are unclear. The present consensus guidelines are listed in Table 24-4 (14,16). These recommendations do not apply to nonparapneumonic (asbestos-related, neoplastic, rheumatoid, etc) or tuberculous effusions.

   a. Of these parameters, pH and glucose have the highest diagnostic accuracy. The clinical presentation and clinical suspicion of empyema should modify interpretation of these values. A recent meta-analysis of studies of parapneumonic effusions (21) suggests that pH values <7.21–7.29 indicate the need for tube drainage, if the clinical situation is compatible.

   b. Biochemically equivocal effusions may be followed with serial thoracenteses until the clinical fate of the effusion becomes clear.

F. **Management**

   "It is sad to think of the number of lives which are sacrificed annually by the failure to recognize that empyema should be treated as an ordinary abscess, by free incision. The operation dates from the time of Hippocrates and is by no means serious. A majority of the cases get well, providing that free

Table 24-4. Biochemical characteristics of effusions

Characteristic	Uncomplicated	Complicated
pH	>7.2	<7.0
Glucose	—	<40 mg/dL
Lactate dehydrogenase	<1000 IU/L	

drainage is obtained, and it makes no difference practically what measures are followed so long as this indication is met."
William Osler, MD 1892 (23)

1. Treatment of empyema requires antibiotic therapy directed to the primary site and to the organism causing infection, together with drainage of the pleural space. The approach to the first two of these goals is straightforward; however, the selection of a method of drainage is a source of much debate and considerable confusion.

   a. The choice of antibiotics should be directed by the results of the Gram's stain and culture of the empyema fluid. Until these results are available, empiric coverage should be selected based on the known frequency of infecting organisms in a given patient population, community, and hospital. The propensity of various organisms to invade the pleura may be somewhat helpful in selecting empiric coverage (see Section II.D). Patients thought to have aspiration pneumonitis as the etiology of an empyema should be treated with clindamycin or penicillin and metronidazole to cover anaerobes. Empiric coverage of empyemas occurring as complications of surgical procedures should include vancomycin to treat staphylococci. Empyema occurring in a hospitalized or nursing home patient should be treated empirically with a broad-spectrum antibiotic, including adequate coverage for nosocomial gram-negative rods (ie, a third-generation cephalosporin or penicillinase-resistant synthetic penicillins). Antibiotic levels in the pleural fluid will be comparable to those in serum. Standard systemic doses should be given (16).

   b. The primary origin of infection must be treated. In most cases, this will be an underlying pneumonitis that will be treated with antibiotics as outlined above. When pneumonia and empyema are associated with bronchial obstruction, the obstruction should be relieved, if possible (as above with postobstructive lung abscess). Lung distal to a bronchial obstruction may not reexpand after drainage of effusion if the obstruction persists. If empyema is the result of direct extension from another primary site or of hematogenous seeding, the primary infectious focus must be eradicated.

2. **Drainage**

   a. Rapid and complete drainage of empyemas leads to quicker clinical resolution and earlier hospital discharge. In the case of a highly organized empyema, the clinician is often faced with balancing the morbidity of more extensive drainage procedures against the high frequency of failure of minimally invasive drainage procedures. The drainage procedure selected is based on the quantity and quality of the fluid, the presence of a pleural peel or loculations, the ability of the patient to tolerate surgery, and local experience and expertise. Consultation with a pulmonologist, thoracic surgeon, and radiologist is recommended. After drainage is initiated, frequent radiologic and clinical reassessment is required to determine whether further procedures are needed. If initial drainage is inadequate, further interventions should be undertaken without delay (13).

   b. **A single therapeutic thoracentesis** may be adequate to drain a small-volume, nonloculated parapneumonic empyema that is thin and caused by an easily treated organism such as *S. pneumoniae*. This type of empyema may also be treated by serial needle drainage procedures (13,15).

   c. **Closed chest thoracostomy** is the most commonly used initial drainage procedure indicated for removal of turbid fluid. Success rates vary, but tube thoracostomy is adequate for most (up to 80%) cases of parapneumonic empyema (24–26). Failure is more likely in cases with multiple loculations or a thick pleural peel (22), in immunocompromised patients, and in postoperative empyema (25). In cases in which tube thoracostomy is likely to be inadequate, an initial operative approach has been recommended by some (25,27).

i. Large-bore straight chest tubes, usually a 28–36 French, are the preferred tubes because they are rigid and do not kink. The tube should be placed in a dependent position so that the empyema will drain. Blunt dissection under local anesthesia is the most common method of insertion. These tubes are usually inserted blindly at the bedside and sometimes require repositioning with radiographic guidance. **An important contraindication to initiation of tube drainage is the presence of a lobar or mainstem bronchial obstruction.** Clinical suspicion of this condition should arise when a large effusion fails to cause contralateral mediastinal shift. Bronchial obstruction precludes efficient lung reexpansion after drainage, and the pleural space will not be obliterated (28). Bronchial obstruction should be relieved whenever possible; in cases of untreatable obstruction (usually due to malignancy), drainage may not be possible (16).

ii. **Chest tubes should be kept in place and on suction until the patient is improving clinically, minimal fluid remains on the chest radiograph, and drainage is <50 mL/day** (28). In one study, this required an average of 17 days (24). Before removal, the tube should be clamped for 12–24 hours to demonstrate that the lung remains expanded and that no air leak is present. A chest film should be obtained 12–24 hours after the tube is removed (28). Intravenous antibiotics should be continued for as long as the tube is in place.

iii. **Small-bore (8–14 French) tubes** may sometimes be used to drain empyemas. These tubes are placed under direct radiographic guidance (fluoroscopy, CT, or ultrasound) and are usually placed over a guidewire (Seldinger technique) or inserted with a trocar. Radiographically guided placement may reduce complications of lung laceration, diaphragmatic rupture, and damage to other thoracic and abdominal structures. These smaller tubes are flexible and more comfortable than the larger stiff ones (11,15) but may not be as effective in draining thick pus.

d. **Complicated closed drainage** may be necessary in the presence of loculations or thick pus that cannot be drained by simple tube thoracostomy. If no improvement is noted within 24 hours of chest tube placement, the proper location of the tube should be confirmed by chest CT. If the tube is properly placed, other techniques may be used to promote drainage. These techniques all have significant failure rates but may help avoid thoracotomy in selected patients (24). Minimally invasive interventions have less success in the presence of a thick-walled pleural peel that prevents reexpansion of the lung. Closed chest drainage procedures are also appropriate in patients unable or unwilling to undergo thoracotomy.

i. When several loculated areas of effusion are detected by CT scan or ultrasound, multiple small-bore (8–14 French) percutaneous catheters may be placed under radiographic guidance. The decision to place a chest tube into a loculated space depends on the size of the loculation and evidence of ongoing infection, such as persistent fever and elevated WBC.

ii. **Fibrinolytic agents** may be instilled through a chest tube and may prevent the need for open drainage in patients with loculated, complicated pleural effusions. **Streptokinase** is the most commonly used drug but should not be used if the patient has a suspected sensitivity to the agent (ie, recent streptococcal infection or streptokinase administration). The technique is performed by instilling 250,000 U in 60–100 mL of normal saline through the chest tube. The tube is then clamped for 2–4 hours and the procedure repeated daily, as needed, over several days. Most patients require two to five instillations. Pleural administration generally does not result in significant local or systemic side effects (15,29,30). **Urokinase** (100,000 U) is a more expensive alternative, administered in the same fashion to patients in whom sensitivity to streptokinase is suspected (15). This fibrinolytic technique is more likely to be helpful in the treatment of multiloculated empyemas than in the treatment of a single large locule with a pleural peel, and is more effective in the absence of thick pus (13).

iii. **Videothoracostomy** is used in selected centers in an attempt to avoid open thoracotomy. Only anecdotal information is available concerning the effectiveness of this modality (15,31).

e. **Open chest drainage via thoracotomy** may be performed with a high rate of cure and a low morbidity in any stage of empyema in selected patients. However, the number of surgically treated patients who eventually would have recovered with full function with conservative management remains unknown. Medically managed patients with large empyemas, thick pleural peels, and restrictive ventilatory deficits have been reported to recover full function over a period of months, once the infection is controlled (17,18). Unfortunately, the lack of randomized studies makes it impossible at this time to select those patients who would most benefit from operative drainage rather than conservative treatment.

   i. Patients presenting with empyema in the organizing phase (extensive loculations, pleural peel) may be suitable surgical candidates for thoracotomy for debridement and decortication, providing the underlying lung is normal. This treatment has been shown to markedly reduce the length of hospital stay in selected cases (14,28). When an underlying condition of the lung prevents full reexpansion or when extensive thoracotomy and decortication is too risky, rib resection and open drainage may be an acceptable option. Later closure may then be performed with a thoracoplasty or other procedures to obliterate residual pleural spaces (4,13,15,22,25).

   ii. **Late decortication** can also be performed after the empyema has resolved to release a trapped lung. It is usually prudent to wait several months after healing to see whether spontaneous improvement in function occurs before performing a decortication (4).

G. **Problems and complications of therapy**

1. Persistent fevers and constitutional symptoms imply continued infection, warranting a careful search for undrained pockets of fluid. CT scan should be obtained to locate persistent fluid collections; these should be drained and the fluid analyzed.

2. After tube drainage of empyema, **the lung may become trapped** and will not expand fully due to extensive pleural fibrosis. Some surgeons believe that any residual pleural space should be obliterated to prevent recurrent pleural space infections. Rib resection and open drainage, thoracoplasty, or thoracotomy and filling of the cavity either with extrathoracic muscle or omental flap have been advocated. We suggest a more conservative approach of waiting several months for signs of improvement before considering surgery.

3. **Bronchopleural fistulas** are usually associated with pneumonias and are due to purulent empyema material draining into bronchi that are ineffectively cleared. Bronchopleural fistulas usually present with the production of large amounts of sputum, and the clearance is often positional. Primary management includes treatment of the infection and drainage of the pleural cavity (15). Prolonged tube drainage is often needed. In the setting of fibrothorax or postpneumonectomy, closed drainage alone is unlikely to be successful. Persistent fistulas may require bronchoscopic plugging of the culprit bronchus with blood clot or fibrin glue, and closure via thoracotomy may be necessary (15).

4. Untreated empyema may erode though the chest wall, creating a **pleurocutaneous fistula**. Spread to the mediastinum and abdomen has been reported (23). Surgical drainage is required.

5. **Postpneumonectomy/postlobectomy empyemas** are difficult to treat and

are frequently associated with bronchopleural fistulas. Bronchoscopy should be performed to evaluate the integrity of the bronchial stump. Although there are case reports of successful management by closed chest tube drainage with pleural irrigation, many patients require surgical intervention. Open drainage via rib resection may be necessary. The open pleural cavity may be irrigated with antibiotic solutions. If infection resolves and granulation begins, primary closure can then be performed (15,25).

References

1. Bartlett JG, Gorbach SL, Tally FP, Finegold SM: Bacteriology and treatment of primary lung abscess. *Am Rev Respir Dis* 1974;109:510–518.
2. Bartlett JG: Anaerobic bacterial infections of the lung and pleural space. *Clin Infect Dis* 1993; 16(supp 4):S248–S255.
3. Stark DD, Federle MP, Goodman PC et al.: Differentiating lung abscess and empyema: radiography and computed tomography. *AJR* 1983;141:163–167.
4. Sahn SA: State of the art: the pleura. *Am Rev Respir Dis* 1988;138:184–234.
5. Schlaes DM, Lederman MM, Chmielewski R, et al.: Sputum elastin fibers and the diagnosis of necrotizing pneumonia. *Chest* 1984;85:763–766.
6. Sosenko A, Glassroth J: Fiberoptic bronchoscopy in the evaluation of lung abscesses. *Chest* 1985; 87:489–494.
7. Byrd RB: When to use bronchoscopy in patients with lung abscess. *J Respir Dis* 1995;16:603.
8. Levison ME, Mangura CT, Lorber B, et al.: Clindamycin compared with penicillin for the treatment of anaerobic lung abscess. *Ann Intern Med* 1983;98:466–471.
9. Gudiol F, Manresa F, Pallares R, et al.: Clindamycin vs. penicillin for anaerobic lung infections: high rate of penicillin failures associated with penicillin-resistant *Bacteroides melaninogenicus*. *Arch Intern Med* 1990;150:2525–2529.
10. Landau, MJ, Christensen EE, Bynum LJ, Goodman C: Anaerobic pleural and pulmonary infections. *AJR* 1980;134:233–240.
11. Klein JS, Schultz S, Heffner JE: Interventional radiology of the chest: image-guided percutaneous drainage of the pleural effusions, lung abscess, and pneumothorax. *AJR* 1995;164:581–588.
12. van Sonnenberg E, D'Agostino HB, Casola G, et al.: Lung abscess: CT-guided drainage. *Radiology* 1991;178:347–351.
13. LeMense GP, Strange C, Sahn SA: Empyema thoracis: therapeutic management and outcome. *Chest* 1995;107:1532–1537.
14. Light RW: *Pleural diseases*, 3rd ed. Baltimore: Williams & Wilkins, 1995.
15. Molinary E, Colice GL: Managing bacterial empyema. *Clin Pulm Med* 1994;1:279–288.
16. Light RW, Girard WM, Jenkinson SG, George RB: Parapneumonia effusions *Am J Med* 1980; 69:507–512.
17. Sahn SA, Antony VB, Good JT Jr: Decortication is rarely necessary following empyema. *Clin Res* 1981;29:88A.
18. Neff CC, van Sonnenberg E, Lawson DW, Patton AS: CT follow-up of empyemas: pleural peels resolve after percutaneous catheter drainage. *Radiology* 1990;176:195–197.
19. Bartlett JG, Gorbach SL, Thadepalli H, Finegold SM: Bacteriology of empyema. *Lancet* 1974;1: 338–340.
20. Brook I, Frazier EH: Aerobic and anaerobic microbiology of empyema: a retrospective review in two military hospitals. *Chest* 1993;103:1502–1507.
21. Heffner JE, Brown LK, Barbieri C, DeLeo JM: Pleural fluid chemical analysis in parapneumonic effusions: a meta-analysis. *Am J Respir Crit Care Med* 1995;151:1700–1708.
22. Ashbaugh DG: Empyema thoracis: factors influencing morbidity and mortality. *Chest* 1991;99: 1162–1165.
23. Osler W: *The principles and practice of medicine.* New York: Appleton, 1892:563–571.
24. Alfageme I, Munoz F, Pena N, Umbra S: Empyema of the thorax in adults. *Chest* 1993;103:839–843.
25. Lemmer JH, Botham MJ, Orringer MB: Modern management of adult thoracic empyema. *J Thorac Cardiovasc Surg* 1985;90:849–855.

26. Varkey B, Rose HD, Kutty CPK, Politis J: Empyema thoracis during a ten-year period. *Arch Intern Med* 1981;141:1771–1776.
27. Mayo P, McElvein RB: Early thoracotomy for pyogenic empyema. *Ann Thorac Surg* 1966;2:649–655.
28. Miller KS, Sahn SA: Chest tubes. *Chest* 1987;91:258–264.
29. Henke CA, Leatherman JW: Intrapleurally administered streptokinase in the treatment of acute loculated nonpurulent parapneumonic effusions. *Am Rev Respir Dis* 1992;145:680–684.
30. Taylor RFH, Rubens MB, Pearson MC, Barnes NC: Intrapleural streptokinase in the management of empyema. *Thorax* 1994;49:856–859.
31. Ridley PD, Braimbridge MV: Thoracoscopic debridement and pleural irrigation in the management of empyema thoracis. *Ann Thorac Surg* 1991;51:461–464.

25   Drug-Induced Pulmonary Disease

Geoffery L. Chupp and Jeffrey S. Berman

The power of modern medicine is due in part to the extensive array of drugs that physicians have at their disposal to treat patients. Along with the benefits that derive from the use of these drugs are toxicities that may be severe or fatal. Although any organ may be adversely affected by a given medication, pulmonary toxicities are among the most severe. Drugs should always be considered in the differential diagnosis, since the clinical presentation of toxicity may closely parallel many common lung diseases. This chapter will describe the most common and most severe drug-induced lung diseases and offer the clinician a basic approach to diagnosis and treatment. In an effort to simplify the approach, this chapter will discuss only those drugs known to cause specific lung reactions that are not anaphylactic in nature. When a drug is known to cause more than one type of reaction, the more common presentation will be covered in detail. More detail on the subject of drug-induced lung disease may be found in several excellent reviews (1–6) from which the tables in this chapter have been compiled.

I. **Drugs causing interstitial pneumonitis/fibrosis.** This reaction is the most common form of drug-induced lung toxicity. Diagnosis and treatment may be difficult, as cessation of the drug may be life threatening; conversely, the lung damage caused by the drug may be irreversible. Table 25-1 includes a list of the most common drugs associated with this syndrome.

   A. **Clinical manifestations.** Most patients present with a slowly progressive clinical course indistinguishable from idiopathic pulmonary fibrosis. The first symptoms are usually nonspecific and include nonproductive cough, mild dyspnea on exertion, fatigue, malaise, and, rarely, weight loss. Symptoms may progress insidiously over weeks to months. Lung auscultation may reveal rales that are bibasilar and end-expiratory early in the disease and become more diffuse and heard throughout the respiratory cycle as the disease progresses. Rarely, patients present with the acute onset of symptoms that develop over hours to days (7).

   B. **Radiographic studies** are the mainstay of diagnosis in evaluating drug-induced interstitial pneumonitis. Standard chest radiography most commonly reveals bilateral interstitial infiltrates with the variable presence of Kerley's B lines. Pleural effusions are rarely seen. In the unusual case with a normal chest radiograph, high-resolution computed tomography (HRCT) may confirm interstitial infiltration.

   C. **Pulmonary function** abnormalities are nonspecific and are consistent with restrictive ventilatory physiology. A reduced diffusion capacity for carbon monoxide (DLCO) may be the earliest abnormality detected. Periodic pulmonary function tests are now performed in patients receiving agents known to cause interstitial pneumonitis in the hope that early recognition can help to limit toxic effects. While intuitively correct, no evidence currently supports this approach. Of note, a reduced DLCO may be caused by many etiologies and is not predictive of fibrosis.

   D. **Diagnosis** is difficult given the nonspecific clinical and histologic findings and should be based on the clinical picture. **Bronchoalveolar lavage** cytology may reveal the presence of neutrophils, lymphocytes, and eosinophils (8). **Lung biopsy** may show the classic changes of pulmonary drug toxicity with bizarre-shaped type II pneumocytes, septal thickening, and areas of interstitial fibrosis. Because these findings are nonspecific, **open lung biopsy should be reserved for those patients in whom the diagnosis is unclear and infectious etiologies need to be excluded.**

Table 25-1. Drugs causing interstitial pneumonitis/fibrosis

Chemotherapeutic agents	Nitrosoureas
	Carmustine (BCNU)
Cytotoxic antibiotics	Semustine (methyl CCNU)
Bleomycin	Lomustine (CCNU)
Mitomycin	Chlorozotocin
Mitomycin with vinca alkaloids	**Other agents**
Pepleomycin	
Neocarzinostatin (zinostatin)	Nitrofurantoin
Alkylating agents	Sulfasalazine
Busulfan	Amiodarone
Cyclophosphamide	Tocainide
Chlorambucil	Flecainide
Melphalan	Gold
Antimetabolites	Penicillamine
Methotrexate	
Azathioprine	
6-Mercaptopurine	

BCNU = bischloroethynitrosourea; CCNU = chloroethylcyclohexylnitrosourea.

E. **Management** of toxicity should begin with the pulmonary evaluation of patients prior to treatment with an agent known to cause interstitial fibrosis. In most cases, the immediate withdrawal of the suspected drug and supportive care are all that are required for full recovery. Corticosteroids may be useful in patients with more acute presentations.

F. **Specific etiologies: chemotherapeutic agents** (cytotoxic drugs). These drugs act by irreversibly damaging rapidly dividing neoplastic cells. The mechanisms by which these drugs cause lung fibrosis is not known.

   1. **Bleomycin, mitomycin, pepleomycin,** and **neocarzinostatin** are cytotoxic antibiotics used as chemotherapeutic agents and known to cause interstitial pneumonitis.

      a. **Bleomycin** was first isolated from *Streptomyces verticillus* by Umezawa (reviewed in 9) and is used primarily in the treatment of lymphomas, squamous cell carcinomas, and testicular tumors (10). It acts by causing DNA strand scission via production of oxygen free radicals, resulting in impaired RNA and protein synthesis. Studies have reported the **incidence** of interstitial fibrosis from bleomycin at 3% to 40%, although most reviews indicate a rate of 5% to 15% (2). **Risk factors** for the development of interstitial fibrosis from bleomycin include age >70 years, cumulative dose >400 U, concomitant chest radiotherapy, supplemental oxygen therapy, renal insufficiency, administration by bolus injection, and concomitant use of other chemotherapeutic agents such as doxorubicin, cyclophosphamide, and vincristine. Withdrawal of corticosteroids may potentiate bleomycin toxicity, although no direct evidence supports this. The **prognosis** for patients afflicted with bleomycin toxicity is generally considered to be good. Mortality related to lung toxicity is 1% to 2%. Over 80% of patients with mild toxicity completely recover, although the median time to chest-radiographic resolution is 9 months (11).

      b. **Mitomycin** has been reported to cause pulmonary toxicity in over 30 cases. The mechanism of pulmonary toxicity from mitomycin is similar to that of the alkylating agents (busulfan, cyclophosphamide). Two studies have estimated the **incidence** of pulmonary toxicity related to mitomycin to be 3% (12) and 12% (13). **Risk factors** for the development of pulmonary disease from mitomycin are not well established. Mitomycin in combination with or taken in close proximity to **vinca alkaloid** therapy is believed to be associated with a higher likelihood of pulmonary toxicity and an acute form of the disease (14). Most patients, however, present with the insidious onset of shortness of breath, and a chest radiograph reveals interstitial infiltrates. Pleural effusion from mitomycin therapy has been reported more frequently (15). Recognition of symptoms and prompt cessation of therapy may improve the chance of recovery; otherwise, the mortality may be as high as 50% (16). The use of **corticosteroids** has been reported to result in dramatic recovery and therefore is recommended (1).

    c. There is one report of interstitial pneumonitis from **neocarzinostatin** after an accidental overdose. The clinical course was identical to that of bleomycin toxicity. Circulating antineocarzinostatin antibodies were identified postmortem, suggesting an immune-mediated mechanism (17).

    d. **Pepleomycin** has also been linked to irreversible progressive pulmonary fibrosis despite corticosteroids in 6% of patients receiving the drug in one study (18).

2. **Cyclophosphamide, busulfan, chlorambucil,** and **melphalan** are alkylating agents that cross-link DNA strands and block cellular replication.

    a. **Cyclophosphamide** is used in the treatment of many autoimmune and malignant diseases, including lung cancer and Wegener's granulomatosis. The **incidence** of pulmonary toxicity related to cyclophosphamide is estimated to be <1%, although clusters of cases have occurred (12). The **risk** of developing toxicity from cyclophosphamide is thought to increase with cumulative dose, concomitant oxygen therapy, and radiation; however, no definite links for risk have been established (4). **Clinical presentation** is variable. Although most patients present within weeks of initiating therapy, patients have presented years after therapy has been discontinued (19). No unique symptoms are associated with cyclophosphamide except that >50% patients develop fever. **Prognosis** from lung toxicity from cyclophosphamide is poor, with a mortality as high as 50% (20). Therefore, **management** of patients requires prompt discontinuation of therapy. Although no studies have clearly demonstrated the efficacy of corticosteroids, anecdotal reports suggesting their efficacy have led some authors to advocate their use (1,21).

    b. **Busulfan** was the first agent associated with pulmonary toxicity in 1961 (22). Busulfan is used primarily in the treatment of myeloproliferative disorders such as chronic myelogenous leukemia. The **incidence** of clinically relevant pulmonary toxicity is 4% (1,23); however, in an autopsy series of 14 patients treated with busulfan, 46% revealed pulmonary damage that was not clinically apparent at the time of death (24). The major **risk factor** for developing busulfan toxicity is **duration of therapy**. The average duration of therapy prior to the development of pulmonary toxicity is 3–4 years, with a range of 6 weeks to 10 years (25). Similarly, total cumulative dose appears to be important, and toxicity nearly always develops during the course of therapy. Scattered reports have suggested that risk is increased with concomitant radiotherapy or chemotherapy. Patients usually present with the insidious onset of shortness of breath, cough, and weight loss. **Radiographic studies** show the typical symmetric lower lung zone reticular pattern. However, airspace disease with air bronchograms can occur more commonly than with other agents (1). Pleural effusions are rare but have been reported. Lung volumes and DLCO are decreased. Prospective studies have shown that monitoring pulmonary function during therapy does not reduce the likelihood or improve the prognosis of busulfan toxicity (26,27). While sputum and bronchoalveolar lavage fluid may contain atypical mononuclear cells, the diagnosis usually requires open lung biopsy to exclude other diseases. Management requires discontinuation of therapy. Despite the limited evidence on the efficacy of corticosteroids, their use is recommended because the mean survival after development of pulmonary disease is only 5 months.

    c. **Chlorambucil** is an alkylating agent used in the treatment of hematologic malignancies such as chronic lymphocytic leukemia. Pulmonary toxicity from chlorambucil is rare. The 10 cases that have been reported involved patients being treated for 6 months to 3 years, and all but one had a clinical course consistent with pulmonary fibrosis. Anorexia is a predominant symptom. Half of these patients died after the development of pulmonary failure (1).

  d. **Melphalan** is a nitrogen mustard derivative used in the treatment of multiple myeloma. In an autopsy study, pulmonary fibrosis was found in 5 of 10 patients treated with melphalan (28). The clinical course is more typical of that associated with cytotoxic antibiotic use, with symptoms developing weeks to months after the initiation of therapy. Therapy should be discontinued and corticosteroid therapy initiated as soon as toxicity is suspected, as only two of the seven reported patients survived (1).

 3. **Nitrosoureas,** a class of chemotherapeutic agents that carbamoylate and alkylate DNA, are used in the treatment of malignancies such as intracranial tumors, melanoma, lymphoma, and gastric cancer.

  a. **Carmustine** (bischloroethylnitrosourea [BCNU]) was the first nitrosurea used clinically. Retrospective analysis suggests that 20% to 30% of patients treated with BCNU develop pulmonary toxicity (29). This risk is directly proportional to the cumulative dose, as patients who survive longer and received higher doses have a higher risk of pulmonary toxicity (4). A history of preexisting lung disease and tobacco use also increased the risk of pulmonary toxicity developing. Patients present with the typical symptoms of dyspnea over weeks to months, although rapid progression of respiratory failure over days leading to death has been reported (30). A unique feature of pulmonary toxicity from BCNU is that lung biopsy may show fibrosis in the absence of an inflammatory cellular infiltrate. Most patients reported were receiving corticosteroids for intracranial lesions, so the benefit of these agents was impossible to determine. The mortality from BCNU pulmonary toxicity is unknown, but estimates range from 15% to 90% (1).

  b. **Lomustine** (chloroethylcyclohexylnitrosourea [CCNU]), **semustine** (methyl-CCNU), and **chlorozotocin** are other nitrosoureas linked to pulmonary fibrosis in isolated cases (31–33).

 4. **Antimetabolites. Methotrexate** is most commonly associated with hypersensitivity-like reactions resulting in granulomatous pneumonitis, skin eruptions, and eosinophilia, but it can also cause interstitial pneumonitis and fibrosis (34). It is extensively discussed in section II (see below). **Azathioprine** and its metabolite **6-mercaptopurine** are widely used to suppress rejection in organ-transplant patients and have been rarely associated with interstitial pneumonitis, even given its widespread use (35). Interstitial pneumonitis develops and may progress to fibrosis.

G. **Specific etiologies: noncytotoxic drugs**
 1. **Antiarrhythmic agents**
  a. **Amiodarone** is an antiarrhythmic agent widely used in the treatment of refractory supraventricular and ventricular tachycardias (36). Chemically, it is an iodinated aromatic compound that resembles thyroxine. The large volume of *in vivo* distribution is due to extensive tissue binding, and amiodarone has an elimination half-life of approximately 30 days. The **incidence** of all pulmonary reactions related to amiodarone is 0% to 27% (37). The only clear **risk factor** for toxicity is being on a maintenance dose of the drug. In the United States, the daily maintenance dose of amiodarone is ≥400 mg, and the incidence of toxicity is higher than in European countries, where the daily dose is 200–400 mg (38). Patients have usually been treated for at least 5 months before pulmonary toxicity develops, although toxicity has been reported as early as 1 month and as long as 9 years after the initiation of therapy. The **clinical presentation** is insidious and not unique. **Radiographic studies** classically show reticular infiltrates, and because of the iodine in the amiodarone, the infiltrate may be slightly radiopaque. **CT** scan of the liver can show increased Hounsfield units typical of amiodarone deposition in the liver (5). **Bron-**

choalveolar lavage fluid may show foamy macrophages containing intracytoplasmic lamellar inclusions believed to be phospholipid accumulation. This finding is not specific, and these cells may be found in patients on amiodarone without pulmonary toxicity (39). **Management** requires stopping therapy and consideration of the use of corticosteroids in patients with life-threatening toxicity or in those who must be maintained on amiodarone therapy. If a decision is made to treat with corticosteroids, prednisone (40–60 mg/d) should be given for 6 weeks and then tapered to 20 mg/d. Therapy can then be tapered slowly over 4–months (5). In patients who must remain on amiodarone despite pulmonary toxicity, prednisone 10 mg every other day has been used successfully to alleviate symptoms (40). The **prognosis** for patients with pulmonary toxicity from amiodarone is favorable. Discontinuing therapy usually results in complete resolution of abnormalities, although this can take months. **Mortality** from amiodarone pulmonary toxicity is thought to be <30% (41).

    b. **Tocainide** is an oral antiarrhythmic used in the treatment of refractory ventricular arrhythmias. Interstitial pneumonitis has been described in over 40 cases, beginning 3 weeks to 4 months after the initiation of therapy with tocainide (42). **Flecainide** has been linked to one case of interstitial lymphocytic pneumonitis (43).

2. **Anti-inflammatory agents**

    a. **Penicillamine** is a hydrolyzed derivative of penicillin that chelates copper, mercury, zinc, and lead. It is used in a variety of clinical settings, including lead poisoning, Wilson's disease, and cystinuria. Penicillamine also possesses anti-inflammatory properties and has been used in rheumatoid arthritis, scleroderma, and primary biliary cirrhosis. Penicillamine is most commonly associated with a Goodpasture's-like syndrome of pulmonary hemorrhage (44,45), drug-induced systemic lupus erythematosus (46), bronchiolitis obliterans (47,48), and, rarely, with interstitial pneumonitis/fibrosis (49).

    b. Chrysotherapy with **gold salts** used in the treatment of inflammatory arthritis has been associated with interstitial pneumonitis/fibrosis. The **incidence** of pulmonary toxicity is <1% and may be more common in patients receiving sodium aurothiomalate rather than aurothioglucose (5). Symptoms develop insidiously weeks to months after therapy is initiated and may include fever and rash (50). **Radiographic studies** of the chest show diffuse interstitial infiltrates. **Bronchoalveolar lavage** cells are often enriched with lymphocytes, and histologically the lung shows an interstitial lymphocytic infiltrate, fibrosis, and type II pneumocyte hyperplasia. Cessation of therapy results in normal or improved pulmonary function in a majority of cases within weeks to months. The role of **corticosteroids** is not clear, as most patients improve regardless of their use and therefore should be reserved for patients with severe toxicity or respiratory failure.

3. **Antibiotics**

    a. **Nitrofurantoin** is an antibiotic used in the treatment of urinary tract infections that is associated with both acute hypersensitivity pneumonitis and chronic interstitial pneumonitis/fibrosis. The majority of reactions are acute, while the chronic form of toxicity accounts for only about 5% of toxic reactions. Toxicity afflicts women more commonly than men. The chronic form of toxicity can occur after months to years of therapy, and patients present with chronic progressive dyspnea and a nonproductive cough. Fever, eosinophilia, and other systemic manifestations are uncommon in this form of the disease. Chest x-ray reveals diffuse interstitial infiltrates, sometimes associated with pleural effusions. Pulmonary function testing reveals restrictive physiology. Histologic findings are indistinguishable from idiopathic pulmonary fibrosis, although an eosinophilic infiltrate may be present. The efficacy of corticosteroids in the chronic form of nitrofurantoin toxicity is not proven. An acceptable approach to management is cessation of therapy and close monitoring for 2–4 months with chest x-rays and pulmonary function studies. If no improvement occurs, a trial of corticosteroids is warranted (5). Prognosis is favorable, with a mortality of 10% for patients with chronic nitrofurantoin toxicity (51).

  b. The sulfonamide antibiotic **sulfasalazine** used in the treatment of inflammatory bowel disease has been linked to hypersensitivity pneumonitis, bronchiolitis obliterans, and, in two cases, to interstitial pneumonitis/fibrosis (52,53).

II. Drugs associated with hypersensitivity lung reactions. Hypersensitivity pneumonitis or extrinsic allergic alveolitis is a clinical syndrome associated with the inhalation of organic dusts. While this term has also been used to describe pulmonary hypersensitivity reactions related to therapeutic drugs, these reactions are both pathophysiologically and clinically distinct from the syndrome associated with toxic drug reactions. For the purposes of this discussion the term *hypersensitivity lung reaction* will be used to describe lung drug hypersensitivities. Table 25-2 lists the drugs that will be discussed in this section.

  A. Clinical manifestations. Patients afflicted with hypersensitivity lung reactions typically present with dyspnea, nonproductive cough, and occasionally pleuritic chest pain hours to days after beginning therapy; symptoms are not dose related. Unlike interstitial pneumonitis/fibrosis–related toxicity, patients with hypersensitivity reactions also have prominent systemic complaints including fever and chills, myalgia, and headaches. Physical examination suggests a systemic reaction, as most patients will have fever and a diffuse rash. Localized or diffuse rales are heard on lung auscultation, and findings compatible with pleural effusion may be present.

  B. Laboratory studies are also suggestive of systemic hypersensitivity. Eosinophilia is found in up to 40% of cases, and elevated transaminases suggesting hepatitis have been reported.

  C. Chest radiographs are always abnormal and most commonly reveal diffuse alveolar infiltrates compatible with the systemic nature of the reaction. Unlike interstitial pneumonitis/fibrosis reactions, pleural effusions may be present, as noted above. HRCT scan is useful in imaging abnormalities when patients present with normal chest radiographs.

  D. Pulmonary function tests reveal restrictive physiology and reduced diffusion capacity for carbon monoxide, as expected.

Table 25-2. Drugs associated with hypersensitivity lung reactions

Cytotoxic agents	Neuromuscular/anticonvulsant agents
Bleomycin	Dantrolene
Procarbazine	Mephenesin carbamate
Paclitaxel	Phenytoin
Immunosuppressive agents	Carbamazepine
Methotrexate	**Anti-inflammatory agents**
Gold salts	Naproxen
Antibiotics	Beclomethasone (inhaled)
	Cromolyn (inhaled)
Nitrofurantoin	**Psychiatric medications**
Antituberculous: isoniazid, para-aminosalicylic acid	Chlorpromazine
β-Lactams: penicillin, ampicillin, cephalosporins	Imipramine
	Desipramine
Sulfonamides: sulfasalazine, sulfadimethoxine	Methylphenidate
Tetracyclines: tetracycline, minocycline	Febarbamate
Illicit drugs	**Cardiovascular agents**
Cocaine (section VII)	Captopril
Hypoglycemic agents	Hydralazine
	Mecamylamine
Chlorpropamide	
Tolazamide	

E. Diagnosis is usually straightforward, given the rapid onset of symptoms and a history of a new medication. Of note, patients may have received the medication in the past without difficulty. Transbronchial or open lung biopsy is rarely required because discontinuance of the suspected agent usually results in rapid clinical improvement. Lung biopsy should be reserved for patients who either fail to improve or worsen after cessation of the suspected agent. The biopsy generally shows interstitial and airway eosinophilia, edema, and little fibrosis.

F. Management and prognosis. Identifying and discontinuing the drug believed to be causing toxicity will nearly always result in resolution of infiltrates within a few weeks. Corticosteroids are generally thought to hasten resolution and should be reserved for patients who fail to improve after the culprit drug is stopped. The **prognosis** for patients with hypersensitivity lung reactions is favorable. Virtually all patients recover completely, and <10% show residual chest-radiographic abnormalities.

G. Specific etiologies

1. **Cytotoxic agents.** Most of these agents are associated with interstitial pneumonitis/fibrosis; however, **bleomycin** and **procarbazine** have been linked to several cases of hypersensitivity reactions (54,55).

2. **Paclitaxel (taxol)** is a chemotherapeutic agent used in palliative and adjuvant chemotherapy on non-small cell carcinoma of the lung and other solid tumors (81). Reactions associated with the lung include an acute hypersensitivity reaction with flushing, urticaria, hypotension, and dyspnea with bronchospasm which occurs shortly after administration of the drug. This reaction has been attributed to an anaphylactoid response to the polyoxyethylated castor oil vehicle and has decreased in incidence (<1%) with routine pretreatment with dexamethasone, benadryl, and H2 blockers (81,82).

   Pulmonary infiltrates following paclitaxel administration have been reported (83). Infiltrates may develop usually 2 days to 2 weeks following administration of the drug at doses of 200 to 300 mg/m^2. The pathogenesis of these infiltrates is unknown. The short time course suggests a hypersensitivity reaction, eosinophilia has not been reported. Treatment with corticosteroids was found to be helpful in several studies, while other cases resolved spontaneously. The frequency of these reactions, dose dependence, and case fatality are not known.

3. **Antimetabolites. Methotrexate** is a folic acid analogue that inhibits cellular reproduction by causing an intracellular deficiency of folate coenzymes. Used extensively in the treatment of both malignancies and autoimmune disorders, including leukemias, psoriasis, carcinomas, and sarcoidosis, methotrexate has been recognized as a cause of pulmonary disease since 1969 (1,5). Although pulmonary reactions from methotrexate can take many forms (see I.F.4), hypersensitivity is the most common reaction. The drug can be given orally, intravenously, intramuscularly, or intrathecally; pulmonary toxicity has been linked to all routes of administration. The **incidence** of pulmonary toxicity from methotrexate is estimated at 7.6% of patients on therapy. No specific **risk factors** have been identified for the development of pulmonary toxicity, although patients who receive the drug weekly or daily appear to be at increased risk. Patients usually present in the typical fashion described above. Prognosis is excellent with discontinuation of the drug, and mortality is reported to be <1%. The role of **corticosteroids** remains unclear and should be reserved for patients who fail to improve after the cessation of therapy or suffer respiratory failure.

4. **Antibiotics**

   a. Acute **nitrofurantoin** toxicity is one of the most common toxic pulmonary reactions and is the prototypical hypersensitivity reaction. Women develop toxicity more frequently (although this may be related to the common use of nitrofurantoin for urinary tract infections); <1% of patients receiving the drug develop the acute reaction. Risk of toxicity does not appear to be dose related. Symptoms typically begin hours to days after initiation of therapy and include dyspnea, cough, fever, and pleuritic chest pain. Eosinophilia and an elevated erythrocyte sedimentation rate are common laboratory findings. Chest radiographs most commonly show bibasilar, diffuse infiltrates and sometimes pleural effusion (30%). Treatment of acute nitrofurantoin toxicity requires only stopping the drug. There is no role for the use of corticosteroids. Prognosis is excellent, as most patients fully recover and mortality is <1%.

b. Several **sulfonamides** (oral and vaginal preparations) are associated with pulmonary hypersensitivity reactions (55), and the antibiotic **sulfasalazine** is the most common of these. Sulfasalazine, metabolized to sulfapyridine and 5-aminosalicylic acid, is poorly absorbed through the gastrointestinal tract and is used primarily in the treatment of inflammatory bowel disease. A previous history of sulfonamide or salicylate allergy may identify patients at risk for the development of toxicity (56).

c. There are rare reports of β-lactam antibiotics [**penicillin** (57), **ampicillin** (58), **cephalosporins** (59)], tetracyclines [**tetracycline** (60), **minocycline** (5)], and antituberculous drugs [**isoniazid** (61) and **para-aminosalicylic acid** (62)] causing pulmonary hypersensitivity reactions.

5. **Cardiovascular agents.** In contrast to the antiarrhythmic agents known to cause interstitial pneumonitis/fibrosis, the agents linked to hypersensitivity pulmonary reactions are primarily antihypertensive agents. Reports of hypersensitivity lung reactions have involved **captopril** (63), the original angiotensin II–converting enzyme (ACE) inhibitor well known to cause cough; the vasodilating agent **hydralazine** (64), which may cause a lupus-like reaction affecting the lung; and **mecamylamine** (65), an early ganglionic blocking agent.

6. **Neuromuscular and anticonvulsant agents.** Diphenylhydantoin (66) (phenytoin) and **carbamazepine** (2) are two drugs commonly used in the treatment of seizure disorders. Both have caused hypersensitivity lung reactions. Phenytoin has also been suggested to cause chronic interstitial pneumonitis/fibrosis, but this has not been substantiated. **Mephenesin carbamate** (2), the oldest muscle relaxant, and **dantrolene** (7), a long-acting skeletal muscle relaxant structurally similar to nitrofurantoin and used in the treatment of spastic neurologic disorders such as neuroleptic malignant syndrome, have been reported to cause pulmonary hypersensitivity reactions in isolated cases.

7. **Anti-inflammatory agents. Naproxen** has been linked to at least four cases of pulmonary hypersensitivity. All patients developed acute fatigue, cough, fever, peripheral eosinophilia, and alveolar infiltrates. Symptoms resolved rapidly after the drug was discontinued (67). Isolated cases of inhaled **beclomethasone dipropionate** (68) and **cromolyn** (69) causing pulmonary hypersensitivity reactions have been reported. **Gold salts** usually associated with interstitial pneumonitis (see I.G.2) have also been linked to several hypersensitivity lung reactions (2).

8. **Psychiatric medications.** The tricyclic antidepressants **imipramine, trimipramine,** and **desipramine** are associated with the acute development of pulmonary infiltrates and eosinophilia (4). Pulmonary hypersensitivity has also been reported with **methylphenidate** (70), **chlorpromazine**, and **febarbamate** (71) use.

9. **Hypoglycemic agents.** The sulfonylureas **chlorpropamide** and **tolazamide** have been reported to cause pulmonary hypersensitivity in isolated cases.

III. **Drugs associated with noncardiogenic pulmonary edema/adult respiratory distress syndrome (ARDS).** Therapeutic and toxic doses of many drugs are associated with noncardiogenic pulmonary edema. Drug-induced ARDS is clinically indistinguishable from the initial presentation of ARDS due to other causes but differs at later stages of the reaction. Patients suffering from drug-induced ARDS have an excellent prognosis with a rapid resolution of the pulmonary edema after the drug is discontinued, whereas patients with ARDS due to other causes often develop pulmonary fibrosis. For the purposes of this discussion, the term *noncardiogenic pulmonary edema* will also be used to describe drug-related ARDS.

A. **Clinical manifestations.** Individuals typically present within hours of beginning the drug with the acute onset (minutes to hours) of severe dyspnea. Most cases are seen in the setting of drug overdose by oral, topical, intravenous or intrathecal administration. **Chest radiograph** shows a classic pulmonary edema pattern with diffuse perihilar alveolar infiltrates. **Laboratory studies** are usually not revealing. **Prognosis** for patients suffering from drug-induced pulmonary edema is excellent, as the etiology is usually rapidly recognized and the drug stopped. Nevertheless, some patients develop full-blown ARDS and subsequent pulmonary fibrosis. Table 25-3 provides a list of agents associated with the development of noncardiogenic pulmonary edema.

B. Specific agents

1. **Chemotherapeutic agents.** With the exception of intrathecal **methotrexate** and **cytosine arabinoside** (cytarabine), these agents are primarily associated with pulmonary fibrosis and hypersensitivity and are discussed elsewhere in this chapter. The intrathecal administration of methotrexate has precipitated the development of pulmonary edema in several patients (1). Cytosine arabinoside has been linked to multiple cases of pulmonary edema. A recent review estimated that pulmonary edema develops in 13% to 28% of patients receiving the drug. Pathologic findings showed intra-alveolar proteinaceous fluid and minimal inflammation. Unlike most types of drug-induced pulmonary edema, the mortality in this population is reported to be 69% (6). **Oxygen** can induce ARDS in patients who have received **bleomycin** within the previous 12 months (6).

2. **Anti-inflammatory agents**
   a. In addition to its relationship to asthma and hypersensitivity, **aspirin**-induced pulmonary edema can occur after overdose or with chronic use when the serum salicylate level is >40 mg/dL. It occurs more commonly in smokers and in elderly patients taking salicylates for rheumatic conditions. Arterial blood gas analysis may reveal a respiratory alkalosis and hypoxemia, reflecting both a diffusion abnormality and the effects of aspirin on respiratory drive (72).
   b. **Colchicine** has been linked to one case of pulmonary edema occurring 18 hours after an overdose (150 mg). The patient died 42 hours later. Autopsy revealed pulmonary and interstitial edema and neutrophilic inflammation (73).

3. **Antibiotics. Amphotericin B,** both liposomal and in conjunction with granulocyte transfusions, has been associated with pulmonary edema (6). **Nitrofurantoin** (discussed in detail I.G.3 and II.G.3) may cause pulmonary edema. Unlike cases of fibrosis or hypersensitivity, affected patients have usually

Table 25-3. Drugs associated with noncardiogenic pulmonary edema

Chemotherapeutic agents	Narcotics
Bleomycin/O_2	Heroin
Mitomycin	Methadone
Cyclophosphamide	Propoxyphene
Cytosine arabinoside (cytarabine)	Codeine
Intrathecal methotrexate	Naloxone
Antibiotics	**Psychiatric drugs**
Nitrofurantoin	Neuroleptic malignant syndrome
Amphotericin B	Haloperidol
Immunologic therapy	Tricyclic antidepressants
	Chlordiazepoxide
Interleukin-2	Ethchlorvynol
Tumor necrosis factor	**Anti-inflammatory agents**
Sclerotherapy agents	Aspirin
Morrhuate sodium	Colchicine
Sodium tetradecyl sulfate	**Other**
Ethanolamine oleate	
Tocolytic agents	Protamine
	Hydrochlorothiazide
Terbutaline	Lidocaine (oralpharyngeal topical)
Ritodrine	Low-molecular-weight dextran
Isoxsuprine	Amiodarone

received nitrofurantoin previously, and dyspnea and diffuse infiltrates develop rapidly within 24 hours of initiating therapy (2).

4. **Tocolytic agents.** These drugs are widely used in the prevention of premature labor and assert their action via stimulation of β-adrenergic receptors. Tocolytic-induced pulmonary edema is associated with many agents including, terbutaline, albuterol, and ritodrine. The incidence varies from 0.5% to 5% and increases with concomitant corticosteroid administration, fluid overload, anemia, and twin gestation. The usual clinical scenario is an unsuccessful trial of a tocolytic, which is then discontinued, and a corticosteroid is given to improve fetal lung maturation. Treatment is supportive and includes oxygen therapy and diuresis (74).

5. **Opiates** have been known to cause noncardiogenic pulmonary edema since Osler's description in 1880 (4). Although all opiates probably can cause pulmonary edema, drugs clearly associated with this reaction include **codeine, methadone, propoxyphene, naloxone,** and **heroin.** Pulmonary edema develops minutes to hours after an intravenous overdose of the drug by bolus injection. Reactions have been reported after normal oral doses as well. Patients often present to emergency departments in coma with pink frothy oral and nasal secretions and require intubation. The resolution of pulmonary effects of opiates occurs in 24–48 hours and is complete in nearly all patients.

6. **Esophageal sclerotherapy agents.** The endoscopic treatment of esophageal varices now includes injection of sclerosing agents into varices. The most commonly used agents are **morrhuate sodium, sodium tetradecyl sulfate,** and **ethanolamine oleate.** Up to 20 mL of sclerosing agent may be injected into the varices, leading to fibrosis and resolution of the lesions. Some of this material may enter the venous system and travel to the lung. A recent review suggested that up to 85% of chest x-rays are abnormal after sclerotic procedures but clinically significant pulmonary edema develops in only 1% of patients (75).

7. **Immunologic therapy. Interleukin-2** and **tumor necrosis factor** are cytokines used to boost the host immune response against malignancies such as melanoma and renal cell carcinoma. Many patients receiving these agents develop pulmonary edema within hours to days. This effect does not appear to be dose related and usually resolves rapidly (6).

8. **Psychiatric medications.** Many agents used in the treatment of psychiatric diseases are associated with the **neuroleptic malignant syndrome.** Patients with this syndrome can develop noncardiogenic pulmonary edema. About one-third of patients with **tricyclic antidepressant** overdose develop pulmonary complications, of which approximately half are noncardiogenic pulmonary edema. **Chlordiazepoxide, haloperidol,** and **ethchlorvynol** have been reported to cause noncardiogenic pulmonary edema in isolated cases.

9. **Other drugs** (hydrochlorothiazide, nebulized lidocaine, protamine sulfate, amiodarone) have all been recognized as uncommon causes of noncardiogenic pulmonary edema (76). Mechanisms are not known.

IV. **Drugs associated with pleural disease.** This section will discuss drugs that produce isolated pleural effusion or significant pleural effusion in association with other lung reactions. In addition, drug-induced lupus will be discussed briefly since pleural disease is prominent in this syndrome.

A. **Clinical features.** Patients may be asymptomatic or present with the typical symptoms of pleural effusion including shortness of breath and pleuritic chest pain. Although information on the characteristics of the pleural fluid is limited, most drug-related effusions are exudative.

B. **Etiologies**

1. **Methysergide** (once commonly used to treat vascular headaches) and **bromocriptine** are chemically similar and can cause pleural effusion. Patients present with typical symptoms after months to years of therapy. Pleuritic chest pain is uncommon. Pleural thickening and small effusions are the usual findings on chest x-ray. The limited data that exist show that bromocriptine effusions contain exclusively lymphocytes (>90%). The effusion usually resolves with discontinuation of therapy.

2. **Tocolytic agents and chemotherapeutic agents** may cause pleural effusion

in association with their primary toxic pulmonary effects. **Methotrexate** may cause pleural effusion in the absence of parenchymal disease.

3. **Dantrolene** is chemically similar to nitrofurantoin and is primarily associated with exudative pleural or pericardial disease. Patients with pleural disease experience typical symptoms and may have fever. Effusions are unilateral and occur after months to years of therapy. Pleural fluid analysis is reported to show an exudative, eosinophilic effusion. Patients improve rapidly with discontinuation of therapy, although resolution of the effusion may take months.

4. **Antibiotics. Nitrofurantoin** is discussed in detail in previous sections (see I.G.3 and II.G.3). Up to 20% of patients with acute nitrofurantoin toxicity may have pleural effusions, and isolated pleural disease can occur in 3% of these patients. Patients present within a month of starting therapy with dyspnea, cough, and fever. Most patients have peripheral eosinophilia, and limited data suggest an eosinophilic effusion as well.

5. **Esophageal variceal sclerotherapy agents** can be associated with pleural effusion. Reports suggest that from 0% to 50% of patients have asymptomatic pleural effusions shortly after injection of varices with one of these agents. Effusions are more likely when large volumes of sclerosing agent are used (77).

6. **Interleukin-2** therapy is well known to cause pulmonary reactions, including isolated pleural effusion in approximately 25% of patients. Effusions develop within hours to days of therapy and resolve spontaneously.

7. **Amiodarone** has been rarely reported to cause isolated pleural disease.

8. **Drug-induced systemic lupus erythematosus** (SLE) has been reported in association with over 40 drugs, but only those listed in Table 25-4 are commonly seen in clinical practice.

   a. Patients present months to years after initiating drug therapy with fever, arthralgia, rash, and pleurisy. As opposed to patients with idiopathic SLE, >50% of patients with drug-induced SLE have exudative pleural effusions, and renal disease is rare. Chest x-ray findings include bilateral interstitial infiltrates and pleural effusion. Cardiomegaly may be seen if pericardial effusion is also present.

   b. The antinuclear antibody assay is positive in all patients with drug-induced SLE, and the double-stranded DNA test is negative. Pleural fluid analysis reveals an exudate with a normal glucose. Withdrawal of the offending agent usually results in resolution of symptoms, although corticosteroids may hasten improvement in more severe cases (2,5).

V. **Drugs associated with cough and bronchospasm** (78). The evaluation of the patient with recent onset asthma or cough must include a careful drug history with emphasis on the agents associated with these symptoms. Even known asthmatics can develop worsening bronchospasm as a reaction to a prescribed inhaler. Table 25-5 includes a list of the agents commonly associated with these symptoms. It is important to note that many of these drugs affect individuals with underlying airways disease, such as asthma or chronic obstructive pulmonary disease (COPD), and rarely cause symptoms in normal individuals. The mechanisms by which many of these drugs induce bronchospasm and cough are complex and not completely understood.

A. **Cardiovascular agents**

1. **β-Blockers** are the classic agents associated with the induction of bronchospasm. This reaction occurs primarily in patients with underlying airways disease such as asthma or COPD and rarely in normal individuals. Although β_1-selective agents were developed in part to minimize the potential of bronchospastic side effects, all β-blockers should be considered potentially hazardous in high-risk patients, and therefore alternative agents should be considered (6).

2. **ACE inhibitors** cause cough in as many as 25% of patients. Patients describe a chronic, persistent dry cough that begins days to months to a year after the initiation of therapy. The cough then resolves within weeks of discontinuing the drug. Any ACE inhibitor can cause cough, and cross-reactivity between agents producing this side effect is common.

B. **Anti-inflammatory agents. Aspirin,** along with other nonsteroidal anti-inflammatory drugs leads to bronchospasm in susceptible individuals. Aspirin-induced broncho-

Table 25-4. Drugs associated with pleural disease

Drug-induced lupus	Chemotherapeutic agents
Procainamide	Methotrexate
Hydralazine	**Antibiotics**
Isoniazid	
Penicillamine	Nitrofurantoin (acute)
Hydantoins	**Other drugs**
Esophageal sclerotherapy agents	Amiodarone
Morrhuate sodium	Bromocriptine
Sodium tetradecyl sulfate	Dantrolene
Ethanolamine oleate	Methysergide
	Interleukin-2

spasm is reported to affect approximately 0.3% of normal adults, up to 20% of asthmatics, and as many as 80% of asthmatics with nasal polyps. Women in the third or fourth decade of life are most frequently susceptible. The usual symptoms begin with rhinitis and coryza followed by bronchospasm.

    C. **Inhaled agents.** Any drug administered by nebulization or metered-dose inhaler can induce bronchospasm by the irritant effects of propellants, solutions, and medications on the airways. **Beclomethasone** is the only inhaled steroid that has been reported to induce bronchospasm. Aerosolized **pentamidine** is well known to cause bronchospasm that may be prevented by premedicating with albuterol.

    D. **Chemotherapeutic agents.** The combination of **vinblastine** and **mitomycin C** in chemotherapy regimens has been linked to the induction of bronchospasm.

    E. **Other agents** linked to bronchospasm are listed in Table 25-5.

VI. **Unusual pulmonary drug reactions.** The previous sections have outlined the most common drug reactions that a physician will encounter in clinical practice. As might be expected, other unique pulmonary reactions have been described less frequently. This section will only briefly describe these syndromes to familiarize the physician.

    A. **Bronchiolitis obliterans with organizing pneumonia (BOOP)** is a clinical syndrome characterized by fever, cough, and flu-like symptoms that may continue for weeks. Chest x-ray shows bilateral patchy ground-glass densities in 81% of cases. Diagnosis requires biopsy that reveals bronchiolitis and organizing pneumonia. BOOP is associated with viral infections, bone marrow transplantation, or connective tissue disorders, or it may be idiopathic. BOOP is also associated with a number of medications listed in Table 25-6. As with idiopathic BOOP, drug-induced BOOP usually responds to corticosteroid therapy (6).

    B. **Granulomatous reactions** mimicking sarcoidosis or tuberculosis have been de-

Table 25-5. Drugs associated with cough and bronchospasm

Cardiovascular agents	Inhaled agents
Angiotensin-converting enzyme inhibitors	Pentamidine
β-Blockers	Beclomethasone
Propafenone	Propellants used in metered-dose inhalers
Dipyridamole	**Other agents**
Anti-inflammatory agents	Contrast media
Aspirin	Cholinesterase inhibitors
Hydrocortisone	Interleukin-2
Acetaminophen	Cocaine (section VII)
Nonsteroidal anti-inflammatory drugs	Neuromuscular blocking agents
Chemotherapeutic agents	Ophthalmologic agents (timolol eye drops)
Vinblastine/mitomycin	Protamine
Paclitaxel	

scribed after therapy with **methotrexate,** especially when administered with **nitrofurantoin,** or **nitrosoureas.** Pulmonary granulomatous reactions are classically associated with **talc** exposure either by intravenous injection of crushed tablets or inhalation in conjunction with cocaine (6).

C. **Pulmonary veno-occlusive disease (PVOD)** is a rare cause of pulmonary hypertension that affects primarily infants, children, and young adults. Clinically indistinguishable from other forms of pulmonary hypertension, PVOD is histologically unique and shows intimal thickening of veins and *in situ* thrombosis. PVOD has also been described as a complication of bone marrow transplantation and in association with chemotherapeutic agents such as bleomycin and BCNU. Treatment with anticoagulation, corticosteroids, or azathioprine has resulted in variable success rates (5).

D. **Pulmonary hypertension** has been reported in association with use of the weight loss drug **Dexfenfluramine** (84). The risk of developing pulmonary hypertension is increased over 20-fold in persons using the drug for more than 3 months and rises with time, though the onset of symptoms has been observed within weeks after beginning the drug. The characteristics of the illness appear to be identical with that of Primary Pulmonary Hypertension (PPH); onset of exertional dyspnea despite weight loss should trigger suspicion of the development of PPH. Treatment and prognosis are identical to that for PPH.

E. **Pneumothorax** has been most commonly associated with **bleomycin** therapy; **BCNU** was associated with pneumothorax in 30% of patients in one series (77).

VII. **Cocaine.** Cocaine is one of the most widely used illicit drugs that is highly addictive. Because of the availability of cheap crack cocaine, cocaine is now used by all socioeconomic classes. Insufflation, injection, and smoking of the drug can all result in pulmonary complications (Table 25–7) (79). Noncardiogenic pulmonary edema is probably the most common pulmonary reaction associated with cocaine use and has been described with all routes of administration. Particulate embolization resulting in pulmonary infarction and talc granulomatosis usually results from chronic intravenous use of cocaine. Diffuse alveolar hemorrhage is a common autopsy finding in cocaine users who die suddenly and has been associated with massive hemoptysis in free-base users (80). Cocaine is also well known to cause pneumomediastinum, pneumothorax, and pneumopericardium.

Table 25-6. Unusual pulmonary drug reactions

Bronchiolitis obliterans with organizing pneumonia (BOOP)	**Pulmonary veno-occlusive disease**
	Bleomycin
Gold	Mitomycin C
Penicillamine	Carmustine
Sulfasalazine	Etoposide
Bleomycin	Cyclophosphamide
Amiodarone	**Pulmonary hypertension**
Methotrexate	
Mitomycin C	Dexfenfluramine
Cyclophosphamide	**Pneumothorax**
Cocaine (section VII)	
Alveolar proteinosis	Bleomycin
	Carmustine
Busulfan	Cocaine (section VII)
Granulomatous pulmonary reactions	
Methotrexate with nitrofurantoin	
Talc	
Nitrosoureas	

Table 25-7. Pulmonary reactions associated with cocaine use

Noncardiogenic pulmonary edema	Alveolar hemorrhage
Diffuse alveolar damage	Hypersensitivity lung reaction
Pulmonary infarction	Bronchiolitis obliterans with organizing pneumonia
Talc granulomatosis	Barotrauma
Bronchospasm	

References

1. Cooper JA, White DA, Matthay RA: Drug-induced pulmonary disease, part I: cytotoxic drugs. *Am Rev Respir Dis* 1986;133:321–340.
2. Cooper JAD, White DA, Matthay RA: Drug-induced pulmonary disease. *Am Rev Respir Dis* 1986; 133:488–505.
3. Cooper JAD, ed Drug-induced pulmonary disease. *Clin Chest Med* 1990;11(1).
4. Fraser RG, Pare JAP, Pare PD, et al.: Drug- and poison-induced pulmonary disease. In: Fraser RG, Pare JAP, Pare PD, et al., eds. *Diagnosis of diseases of the chest.* Philadelphia: WB Saunders, 1991:2417–2479.
5. Rosenow EC III: Drug-induced pulmonary disease. In: Murray JF, Nadel JA, ed. *Textbook of respiratory medicine.* Philadelphia: WB Saunders, 1994:2117–2144.
6. Rosenow EC, Myers JL, Swensen SJ, Pisani RJ: Drug-induced pulmonary disease: an update. *Chest* 1992;102:239–250.
7. Cooper JA jr, Matthay RA: Drug-induced pulmonary disease. *Dis Monthly* 1987;33:61–120.
8. Akoun GM, Cadranel JL, Rosenow EC, et al.: Bronchoalveolar lavage cell data in drug-induced pneumonitis. *Allergy Immunol* 1991;23:245–252.
9. Jules-Elysee K, White DA: Bleomycin-induced pulmonary toxicity. *Clin Chest Med* 1990;11:1–20.
10. Yagoda A, Mukherji B, Young C, et al.: Bleomycin, an antitumor antibiotic: clinical experience in 274 patients. *Ann Intern Med* 1972;77:861–870.
11. Van Barneveld PWC, Sleijfer D, Van Der Mark THW, et al.: Natural course of bleomycin-induced pneumonitis: a follow-up study. *Am Rev Respir Dis* 1987;135:48–51.
12. Gunstream SR, Seidenfeld JJ, Sobonya RE, McMahon LJ: Mitomycin-associated lung disease. *Cancer Treat Rep* 1983;67:301–304.
13. Orwoll ES, Kiessling P, Patterson R: Interstitial pneumonia from mitomycin. *Ann Intern Med* 1978;89:352–355.
14. Luedke D, McLaughlin TT, Daughaday C, et al.: Mitomycin C and vindesine associated pulmonary toxicity with variable clinical expression. *Cancer* 1985;55:542–545.
15. Ozols RF, Hogan WM, Ostchega Y, Young RC: MVP (mitomycin, vinblastine and progesterone): a second-line regimen in ovarian cancer with a high incidence of pulmonary toxicity. *Cancer Treat Rep* 1983;67:721–722.
16. Andrews AT, Bowman HS, Patel S, Anderson WM: Mitomycin and interstitial pneumonitis. *Ann Intern Med* 1979;90:127.
17. Selzer SE, Griffin T, D'Orsi C, et al.: Pulmonary toxicity associated with neocarzinostatin therapy. *Cancer Treat Rep* 1978;62:1271.
18. Shinkai T, Saijo N, Tominaga K, et al.: Pulmonary toxicity induced by pepleomycin, 3-[(S)-1-phenylethylaminol propylamino-bleomycin]. *Jpn J Clin Oncol* 1983;13:395.
19. Abel Karim FW, Ayash RE, Allam C, Salem PA: Pulmonary fibrosis after prolonged treatment with low-dose cyclophosphamide: a case report. *Oncology* 1983;40:174–176.
20. Twohig KJ, Matthay RA: Pulmonary effects of cytotoxic agents other than bleomycin. *Clin Chest Med* 1990;11:31–54.
21. Spector JI, Zimbler H, Ross JS: Cyclophosphamide and interstitial pneumonitis. *JAMA* 1980;243:1133.
22. Oliner H, Schwartz R, Rubio F, Dameshek W: Interstitial pulmonary fibrosis following busulfan therapy. *Am J Med* 1961;31:134–139.
23. Burns WA, Macfarland W, Matthews MJ: Busulfan-induced pulmonary disease: a case report and review of the literature. *Am Rev Respir Dis* 1970;101:408–413.
24. Heard BE, Cooke RA: Busulfan lung. *Thorax* 1968;23:187–193.

25. Ginsberg SJ, Comis RL: The pulmonary toxicity of antineoplastic agents. *Semin Oncol* 1982;9: 34–51.
26. Littler WA, Ogilvie C: Lung function in patients receiving busulfan. *BMJ* 1970;4:530–532.
27. Comhaire F, Van Hove W, Van Ganse W, Van Der Straeten M: Busulfan and the lungs: absence of lung function disturbance in patients treated with busulfan. *Scand J Respir Dis* 1972;53:265–273.
28. Taetle R, Dickman PS, Feldman PS, et al.: Pulmonary histopathologic changes associated with melphalan therapy. *Cancer* 1978;2:1245.
29. Aronin PA, Mahaley MS, Rudnick SA, et al.: Predication of BCNU toxicity in patients with malignant gliomas: an assessment of risk factors. *N Engl J Med* 1980;303:183–188.
30. Pattern GA, Billi JE, Rotman HH: Rapidly progressive, fatal pulmonary fibrosis induced by carmustine. *JAMA* 1980;244:687–688.
31. Cordonnier C, Vernant J-P, Mital P, et al.: Pulmonary fibrosis subsequent to high doses of CCNU for chronic leukemia. *Cancer* 1983;51:1814–1818.
32. Lee W, Moore RP, Wampler GL: Interstitial pulmonary fibrosis as a complication of prolonged methyl-CCNU therapy. *Cancer Treat Rep* 1978;62:1355–1358.
33. Ahlgren JD, Smith FP, Kerwin DM, et al.: Pulmonary disease as a complication of chlorozotocin chemotherapy. *Cancer Treat Rep* 1981;65:223–229.
34. Sostman HD, Matthay RA, Putman CE: Methotrexate-induced pneumonitis. *Medicine* 1976;55: 371–388.
35. Sostman HD, Matthay RA, Putman CE: Cytotoxic drug-induced lung disease. *Am J Med* 1977;62: 608–615.
36. Mason JW: Amiodarone. *New Engl J Med* 1987;316:455–466.
37. Kennedy JI: Clinical aspects of amiodarone pulmonary toxicity. *Clin Chest Med* 1990;11:119–138.
38. Rakita L, Sobol SM, Mostow N, Vrobel T: Amiodarone pulmonary toxicity. *Am Heart J* 1983;106: 906–916.
39. Liu FL, Cohen RD, Downar E, et al.: Amiodarone pulmonary toxicity: functional and ultrastructural evaluation. *Thorax* 1986;41:100–105.
40. Zaher C, Hamer A, Peter T, et al.: Low-dose steroid therapy for prophylaxis of amiodarone-induced pulmonary infiltrates. *New Engl J Med* 1983;308:779.
41. Kennedy JI, Meyers JL, Plumb VJ, et al.: Amiodarone pulmonary toxicity: clinical, radiographic, and pathologic correlations. *Arch Intern Med* 1987;147:50–55.
42. Feinberg L, Travis WD, Ferrans V, et al.: Pulmonary toxicity associated with tocainide. *Am Rev Respir Dis* 1990;141:505–508.
43. Akoun GM, Cadranel JL, Israel-Biet D, et al.: Flecainide-associated pneumonitis. *Lancet* 1991; 337:49.
44. Sternlieb I, Bennett B, Scheinberg IH: D-penicillamine-induced Goodpasture's syndrome in Wilson's disease. *Ann Intern Med* 1975;82:673–676.
45. Matloff DS, Kaplan MM: D-penicillamine-induced Goodpasture's syndrome in primary biliary cirrhosis: successful treatment with plasmapheresis and immunosuppressives. *Gastroenterology* 1980;78:1046–1049.
46. Chalmers A, Thompson D, Stein HB, et al.: Systemic lupus erythematosus during penicillamine therapy for rheumatoid arthritis. *Ann Intern Med* 1982;97:659–663.
47. Epler GR, Snider GL, Gansler EA, et al.: Bronchiolitis and bronchitis in connective tissue disease: a possible relationship to the use of penicillamine. *JAMA* 1979;242:528–532.
48. Murphy KC, Atkins CJ, Offer RC, et al.: Obliterative bronchiolitis in two rheumatoid arthritis patients treated with penicillamine. *Arthritis Rheum* 1981;24:557–560.
49. Camus P, Degat OR, Justrabo E, Jeanin L: D-penicillamine-induced severe pneumonitis. *Chest* 1982;81:376–378.
50. Morley TF, Komansky HJ, Adelizzi RA, Giudice JC: Pulmonary gold toxicity. *Eur J Respir Dis* 1984;65:627–632.
51. Holmberg L, Boman G: Pulmonary reactions to nitrofurantoin: 447 cases reported to the Swedish Adverse Reaction Committee 1966–1976. *Eur J Respir Dis* 1981;62:180–189.
52. Williams T, Eidus L, Thomas P: Fibrosing alveolitis, bronchiolitis obliterans, and sulfasalazine therapy. *Chest* 1982;81:766–768.
53. Davies D, MacFarlane A: Fibrosing alveolitis and treatment with sulphasalazine. *Gut* 1974;15: 185–188.
54. Jonesse J, Moore M, Blank N, Castellino RA. Hypersensitivity to procarbazine (Matulane) manifested by fever and pleuropulmonary reactions. *Cancer* 1972;29:498–500.

55. Feinman L: Drug-induced lung disease: pulmonary eosinophilia and sulphonamides. *Proc R Soc Med* 1975;68:440–441.
56. Averbuch M, Halpern Z, Hallak A, et al.: Sulfasalazine pneumonitis. *Am J Gastroenterol* 1985; 80:343–345.
57. Geller M, Kriz RJ, Zimmerman SW, et al.: Penicillin-associated pulmonary hypersensitivity reaction and interstitial nephritis. *Ann Allergy* 1976;37:183.
58. Poe RH, Condemi JJ, Weinstein SS, Schuster RJ: Adult respiratory distress syndrome related to ampicillin sensitivity. *Chest* 1980;77:449–451.
59. Dreis DF, Winterbauer RH, Van Norman GA, et al.: Cephalosporin-induced interstitial pneumonitis. *Chest* 1984;86:138.
60. Ho D, Tashkin DP, Bein ME, Sharma O: Pulmonary infiltrates with eosinophilia associated with tetracycline. *Chest* 1979;76:33–36.
61. Demeter SL, Ahmad M, Tomashefski JF: Drug-induced pulmonary disease I: patterns of response. *Cleve Clin Q* 1979;46:89–99.
62. Wold DE, Zahn DW: Allergic (Loeffler's) pneumonitis occurring during antituberculous chemotherapy: report of three cases. *Am Rev Tuberculosis* 1956;74:445.
63. Schatz PL, Mesologites D, Hyun J, et al.: Captopril-induced hypersensitivity lung disease: an immune-complex-mediated phenomenon. *Chest* 1989;95:685–687.
64. Bedrossian CWM: Pathology of drug-induced lung diseases. *Semin Respir Med* 1982;4:98–105.
65. Rokseth R, Strostein O: Pulmonary complications during mecamylamine therapy. *Acta Med Scand* 1960;167:23–27.
66. Mahatma M, Haponik EF, Nelson S, et al.: Phenytoin-induced acute respiratory failure with pulmonary eosinophilia. *Am J Med* 1989;87:93–94.
67. Nader DA, Schillaci RF: Pulmonary infiltrates associated with naproxen. *JAMA* 1984;251:65.
68. Mollura JL, Bernstein RA, Fine SR, Vevania J: Pulmonary eosinophilia in a patient receiving beclomethasone dipropionate aerosol. *Ann Allergy* 1979;42:326–328.
69. Burgher LW, Kass I, Schenken JR: Pulmonary allergic granulomatosis: a possible drug reaction in a patient receiving cromolyn sodium. *Chest* 1974;66:84–86.
70. Wolf J, Fein A, Fehrenbacher L: Eosinophilic syndrome with methylphenidate abuse. *Ann Intern Med* 1978;89:224–225.
71. Gali JM, Vilanova JL, Mayos M, et al.: Febarbamate-induced pulmonary eosinophilia: a case report. *Respiration* 1986;49:231–234.
72. Heffner JE, Sahn SA: Salicylate-induced pulmonary edema: clinical features and prognosis. *Ann Intern Med* 1981;91:405–409.
73. Hill RN, Spragg RG, Wedel MK, Moser KM: Adult respiratory distress syndrome associated with colchicine intoxication. *Ann Intern Med* 1975;83:523–524.
74. Pisani RJ, Rosenow EC III: Pulmonary edema associated with tocolytic therapy. *Ann Intern Med* 1989;110:714–718.
75. Zeller FA, Cannon CR, Prakash UBS: Thoracic manifestations after variceal sclerotherapy. *Mayo Clin Proc* 1991;66:727–732.
76. Howard JJ, Mohsenifar Z, Simmons SM: Adult respiratory distress syndrome following administration of lidocaine. *Chest* 1982;81:644–645.
77. Durant JR, Norgard MJ, Murad TM, et al.: Pulmonary toxicity associated with bischloroethylnitrosourea (BCNU). *Ann Intern Med* 1979;90:191–194.
78. Meeker DP, Wiedemann HP: Drug-induced bronchospasm. *Clin Chest Med* 1990;11:163–175.
79. Haim DY, Lippmann ML, Goldberg SK, Walkenstein MD: The pulmonary complications of crack cocaine: a comprehensive review. *Chest* 1995;107:233–240.
80. Murray R, Smealek J, Golle M, Albin R: Pulmonary vascular abnormalities in cocaine users. *Am Rev Respir Dis* 1988;137:459.
81. Rowinsky EK, Donehower RC. Paclitaxel (taxol). *NEJM* 1995;332:1004–1014.
82. Weiss RB, Donehower RC, Wiernik PH, et al. Hypersensitivity reactions from taxol. *J Clin Oncol* 1990;8:1263–1268.
83. Ramanathan RK, Reddy VV, Holbert JM, Belani CP. Pulmonary infiltrates following administration of paclitaxel. *Chest* 1996;110:289–92.
84. Voelkel NF, Clarke WR, Higenbottam T. Obesity, dexfenfluramine, and pulmonary hypertension. *Am J Resp Crit Care Med* 1996;155:786–788.

26

HIV-Related Respiratory Problems

Randall P. Wagner and Harrison W. Farber

Respiratory illnesses in persons infected with the human immunodeficiency virus (HIV) provide practitioners with some of the most interesting diagnostic and therapeutic challenges in medicine. Although HIV-related pulmonary neoplastic and immunologic disorders are increasingly recognized, the vast majority of pulmonary complications of HIV are infectious (1–3). These infections are the natural consequence of the extended period of profound immunosuppression caused by HIV infection. The degree of immunosuppression, reflected by the CD4 lymphocyte count, is critical in understanding the pulmonary consequences of HIV infection (4). Further, a careful social, occupational, and travel history are vital in establishing a sensible differential diagnosis. Algorithms for the evaluation of pulmonary disorders and lists of differential diagnoses based on radiographic findings are located in the final section of this chapter.

I. **Bacterial pneumonia.** Community-acquired pneumonia (CAP) occurs frequently in patients with HIV infection and is more common than Pneumocystis carinii pneumonia (PCP) (3).
   A. **Presenting signs and symptoms**
      1. In patients with normal or near normal numbers of CD4 lymphocytes, the presenting signs and symptoms are indistinguishable from those seen in the seronegative population. Fever, cough, and sputum production predominate.
      2. The chest radiograph usually demonstrates a focal infiltrate. As immunosuppression proceeds, the onset of pneumonia occurs more rapidly, and multilobar disease is more likely, with unusual radiographic appearances and bacteremia (2,5).
   B. **Etiologies**
      1. Streptococcus pneumoniae is the most common bacterial cause of pneumonia in the HIV-infected patient regardless of CD4 lymphocyte count. Staphylococcus aureus, an uncommon cause of CAP in the seronegative population, is also more common in the HIV-infected, as are Haemophilus influenzae, Pseudomonas aeruginosa, Klebsiella pneumoniae, and Escherichia coli (6,7). Pneumonia due to Legionella species and Chlamydia pneumoniae has been reported, but the extent to which excess cases have emerged is still unclear (2,8). Among less common organisms, Nocardia asteroides, Rhodococcus equi, and Salmonella species are reported with increasing frequency in the HIV-infected population. Several studies have demonstrated that injection drug use and smoking increase the risk for bacterial pneumonia in this population (3,8).
         a. **S. pneumoniae.** Pneumococcal pneumonia is the most common cause of bacterial pneumonia in patients with HIV infection, with >50% having positive blood cultures (5). In light of the recent emergence of penicillin-resistant strains of pneumococcus, a cephalosporin or macrolide antibiotic should be used until sensitivities are known.
         b. **S. aureus.** This organism is a frequent cause of CAP in HIV-infected patients, with an even greater risk in injection drug users (8). Although pneumatoceles are frequently seen in immunocompetent patients with S. aureus pneumonia, this radiographic finding is much less common in HIV-infected patients.

c. **_H. influenzae._** Because of its well known virulence, the increased incidence of _H. influenzae_ as a causative agent in the immunocompromised population is not surprising. Emerging evidence suggests that _H. influenzae_ is of particular concern in patients who smoke, as is the case in the immunocompetent population.

d. **_P. aeruginosa_ and _K. pneumoniae._** Isolation of _P. aeruginosa_ from the respiratory tract of HIV-infected patients is now a frequent occurrence. Although some patients have a syndrome of recurrent bronchitis and airway colonization reminiscent of patients with cystic fibrosis, community-acquired _Pseudomonas_ pneumonia is described in virtually every survey of bacterial pneumonia associated with the acquired immunodeficiency syndrome (AIDS) (5–10). The radiographic appearance is quite variable, with cavitation occurring in 50% of cases in one series (11). The rate of bacteremia is significant, and empyema has also been reported (10). AIDS patients with gram-negative bacteremia should receive two antibiotics directed against _Pseudomonas_, until the organism has been identified and sensitivities determined. Although _Klebsiella_ species have typically been associated with alcoholism, HIV-infected patients appear to be at an even greater risk for pneumonia caused by this organism.

e. **_N. asteroides._** The diagnosis of nocardial pulmonary infection in AIDS is complicated by the diversity of its radiologic presentation: alveolar infiltrates (>60%), reticulonodular patterns (>25%), cavitation (>20%), pleural effusion (15%), and hilar adenopathy (10%) (12). Diagnosis requires the demonstration in respiratory secretions of branching, beaded, filamentous, gram-positive organisms that are weakly positive with acid-fast bacilli stains, or growth of the organism on selective media. Because the radiographic and clinical appearance of _Nocardia_ can be confused with reactivation of tuberculosis, the diagnosis is frequently made by bronchoscopy. The choice of antibiotics should be guided by sensitivities, although a sulfonamide or ampicillin with or without a β-lactamase inhibitor is a good initial choice. At least 6 months of therapy is required; >50% of patients relapse unless chronic suppressive therapy is used.

f. **_R. equi._** Frequent exposure to farm animals or their habitats is nearly universal in patients with _R. equi_ pneumonia. Cough, fever, fatigue, and pleuritic chest pain are nearly universal. Chest radiographs typically show dense consolidation with cavity formation; pleural effusion is common. Cultures of blood and/or respiratory secretions are frequently positive, but bronchoscopy with biopsy and/or thoracentesis may be required (13). Initial treatment should include a sulfonamide or ampicillin with or without a β-lactamase inhibitor; vancomycin should be considered in hospitalized patients. Therapy is individualized and based on culture and sensitivity results; surgical resection of an abscess is occasionally required. The optimal duration of treatment is unknown, but lifelong suppressive therapy may be necessary (13).

g. **_Salmonella_ species.** Although traditionally recognized as a cause of empyema, the nontyphoidal _Salmonella_ species are now recognized as a cause of necrotizing, cavitating pneumonia in patients with AIDS (14). Bacteremia is common, and a history of salmonella bacteremia can occasionally be obtained. Initial therapy should include a fluoroquinolone such as ciprofloxacin, since resistance to both ampicillin and sulfonamide is common.

2. **Hospital-acquired infections** (nosocomial pneumonia) are more common in HIV-infected patients than seronegative persons. Frequent hospitalization and impaired local and systemic immune function magnify the risk of pulmonary infection with _S. aureus P. aeruginosa_, and enteric gram-negative organisms (8).

C. **Differential diagnosis.** Bacterial pneumonia should be considered if the radiograph demonstrates focal airspace consolidation, diffuse reticulonodular densities, pleural effusion, or nodular and/or cavitary infiltrates (Table 26-1).

Table 26-1. Differential diagnosis of chest x-ray (CXR) patterns in the HIV-infected patient

CXR pattern	Bacterial agent	Fungal and mycobacterial agents	Other infectious agents	Noninfectious causes
Diffuse reticulonodular infiltrate	Nocardia asteroides	Histoplasmosis Coccidioidomycosis Aspergillosis Mycobacterium kansasii	Toxoplasmosis Strongyloidosis (overwhelming)	Lymphoma Lymphoid interstitial pneumonitis
Diffuse interstitial infiltrate		Mycobacterium tuberculosis Histoplasmosis Cryptococcal pneumonia Bronchial aspergillosis	Pneumocystis carinii Toxoplasmosis Varicella-zoster virus Cytomegalovirus	Lymphoma Lymphoid interstitial pneumonitis Nonspecific interstitial pneumonitis Kaposi's sarcoma
Alveolar infiltrates	N. asteroides	Histoplasmosis	Strongyloidosis (overwhelming) P. carinii	Kaposi's sarcoma
Focal airspace consolidation	All etiologies Rhodococcus equii (dense consolidation)	M. tuberculosis Cryptococcal pneumonia Histoplasmosis Coccidioidomycosis	P. carinii	Bronchogenic carcinoma
Lymphadenopathy	N. asteroides	M. tuberculosis Histoplasmosis Coccidioidomycosis Cryptococcal pneumonia		Lymphoma Kaposi's sarcoma
Nodules/nodular densities	All etiologies	Coccidioidomycosis Cryptococcal pneumonia	P. carinii	Lymphoma
Cavitation	Pseudomonas aeruginosa N. asteroides R. equii Salmonella sp.	M. tuberculosis M. kansasii (thin-walled) Coccidioidomycosis (thin-walled) Cryptococcal pneumonia Histoplasmosis (rare, reported)	P. carinii Lymphoma (rare, reported)	Kaposi's sarcoma (poorly defined nodularities)

Pleural effusion	All etiologies, most common: *P aeruginosa* *N. asteroides* *R. equii* *Streptococcus pneumoniae*	Cryptococcal pneumonia Histoplasmosis (reported) Coccidioidomycosis (reported)	Kaposi's sarcoma	Nonspecific interstitial pneumonitis Pulmonary hypertension
Normal	Bronchitis	*M. tuberculosis* Aspergillosis (tracheobronchial) Histoplasmosis *Mycobacterium avium-intracellulare* complex	*P. carinii* Associated with diarrhea: Microsporidiosis Cryptosporidiosis Strongyloidosis	

D. Initial management. Hospitalized patients with suspected bacterial pneumonia should receive empiric broad-spectrum antibiotics. Because *Legionella* species are more common in certain areas, some institutions will need to add macrolide antibiotics to the regimen. Sputum Gram's stains should be used to identify agents that may require additional coverage. For example, gram-positive cocci on sputum Gram's stain should lead to regimens with heightened coverage for *S. aureus*, whereas the presence of gram-negative rods should lead to regimens with coverage for *Pseudomonas* and *Klebsiella*. Recovery of organisms by culture from sputum, blood, and bronchoalveolar lavage (BAL) fluid is common and is the only rationale for the use of more limited-spectrum antibiotics.

E. Problems and complications of therapy. Pneumonia in the HIV-infected individual tends to recur, necessitating protracted courses of oral antibiotics. Some organisms, such as *N. asteroides*, *R. equi*, and *Salmonella* species may require lifelong suppressive therapy.

II. Bronchitis and bronchiectasis. Bronchitis is the most common respiratory illness in HIV-infected persons, especially those who smoke (3). Patients typically present with persistent sputum production and coarse rales following recurrent lower respiratory infections.

A. Presenting signs and symptoms. In addition to cough productive of purulent sputum, HIV-infected patients frequently complain of dyspnea. Persistent wheezing is common in patients with *Aspergillus* tracheobronchitis.(15)

B. Etiologies. Bronchitis is typically caused by the same agents that cause HIV-associated bacterial pneumonia. *S. pneumoniae*, *H. influenzae*, and *P. aeruginosa* predominate, but *S. aureus* and *Streptococcus viridans* are also important causes of bronchitis (9). Intestinal parasites of the order Microsporida and the genus *Cryptosporidium* can infest the tracheobronchial tree and cause a severe cough that is usually only modestly productive. The respiratory syndromes associated with aspergillosis, microsporidiosis, and cryptosporidiosis are discussed later in this chapter.

C. Differential diagnosis. The differential diagnosis of fever, cough, dyspnea, and a normal chest radiograph in HIV-infected patients should include PCP, disseminated histoplasmosis, disseminated *Mycobacterium avium-intracellulare* infection, and aspergillus tracheobronchitis. For patients with diarrheal disease, microsporidiosis and cryptosporidiosis should also be considered. Usually, bronchitis is diagnosed on clinical grounds: fever, productive cough, normal chest radiograph, and normal arterial blood gases. A sputum culture to help guide therapy is quite useful. Patients with fever, dyspnea, and a normal chest radiograph may require bronchoscopy, which usually reveals beefy-red airway mucosa with purulent secretions (9).

D. Management. Oral antibiotics, guided by culture and sensitivities when possible, are usually sufficient: empiric therapy with trimethoprim/sulfamethoxazole, a macrolide, or second-generation cephalosporin is generally acceptable. Treatment of *P. aeruginosa* infection is best guided by culture and sensitivities. The treatment of bronchiectasis should include postural drainage and chest percussion, as well as an extended course of antibiotics.

E. Problems and complications of therapy. As in most infections in the HIV-infected patient, recurrence is common. Although response to appropriate antibiotics is usually prompt, a considerable delay may be seen when the etiologic agent is *P. aeruginosa* (9).

III. *Pneumocystis carinii* pneumonia. Seroepidemiologic studies suggest that *P. carinii* has a global distribution and that exposure occurs early in life. PCP is the most common AIDS-related opportunistic infection in the United States, occurring in 70% of HIV-infected individuals. Infection is believed to be by inhalation, but neither the environmental reservoir nor the infective form of this organism has yet been discovered (2).

A. Presenting signs and symptoms

1. The clinical features of PCP are nonspecific but usually include fever, dyspnea, malaise, and a nonproductive cough; chills, chest pain, and sputum pro-

duction may also occur. Physical examination is notable for fever and tachypnea; auscultation of the lungs may be normal (2).

2. The **chest x-ray** frequently shows diffuse, bilateral interstitial infiltrates, although bilateral alveolar infiltrates, cavitary lesions, focal infiltrates, and nodular densities have also been described (see Table 26-1) (2,16). Apical infiltrates have become more common, and the chest x-ray is normal in a minority of cases. Pleura-based blebs and cystic lesions are common and particularly well demonstrated on high-resolution computed tomography (HRCT) of the chest (17). Intrathoracic adenopathy and/or pleural effusion are unusual and suggest another diagnosis or a copathogen (18,19).

3. **Arterial blood gas determination** usually reveals hypoxemia and an abnormal alveolar-arterial oxygen gradient (A-a)O_2 but may be normal in mild or early cases. Even with normal arterial blood gases, exercise-induced oxygen desaturation is common, the diffusing capacity for carbon monoxide (D_LCO) is diminished, and gallium scintigraphy reveals diffuse parenchymal uptake (2). Elevation of the serum lactic dehydrogenase at the time of diagnosis correlates with the severity of PCP but lacks the specificity to be useful in making the diagnosis.

B. **Differential diagnosis**

1. Table 26-1 lists the differential diagnosis of various respiratory diagnoses based on radiographic appearance. Because of the protean radiographic presentations of PCP, several diagnoses are possible with each radiographic pattern; however, intrathoracic adenopathy and/or pleural effusion are unusual and suggest another diagnosis or a copathogen.

2. Identification of the organism on methenamine silver or Giemsa staining of respiratory secretions or lung tissue is the gold standard for diagnosis. Fluorescent antibody staining of induced sputum (sensitivity 60% to 80%) is a cost-effective initial diagnostic test (2). In facilities lacking the capacity to perform induced-sputum analysis or in patients with a high clinical suspicion of PCP and a negative induced-sputum result, fiberoptic bronchoscopy with BAL remains the diagnostic mainstay. The sensitivity of multiple lobe BAL, where an area of infiltrate and upper lobe are both sampled, is approximately 95% (20). Although transbronchial biopsy improves the yield in the initial episode of PCP in patients receiving aerosolized pentamidine prophylaxis, multiple lobe BAL is likely equally sensitive.

C. **Management.** The various regimens for the treatment of PCP are listed in Table 26-2. All regimens are 21 days in length. Empiric therapy can be initiated without affecting the ability to establish a definitive diagnosis.

1. **Trimethoprim/sulfamethoxazole** (TMP/SMX), given intravenously or orally, is the drug of choice (21). Intravenous (IV) administration offers no clear advantage for patients with normal gastrointestinal function, since absorption is complete and excellent serum drug levels are achievable when the drug is taken by mouth. HIV-infected patients treated with TMP/SMX have an unusually high incidence of adverse effects, including fever, rash, leukopenia, thrombocytopenia, hyperkalemia, and renal dysfunction (2,21,22). If there is no clinical response after 5–7 days or if drug toxicity develops, pentamidine is used as an alternative agent.

2. **Pentamidine isethionate** is nearly as effective as TMP/SMX in a dose of 3–4 mg/kg/d IV; however, severe hypotension can result if it is administered too rapidly. Intramuscular administration can lead to sterile abscesses and should not be used. Neutropenia, renal impairment, and hepatic dysfunction are frequent complications (2,21). Hypoglycemia is common, and glucose intolerance or frank diabetes mellitus may occur following completion of therapy. Combination therapy with TMP/SMX and pentamidine offers no additional benefit and should be avoided because of cumulative toxicity.

   a. **Aerosolized pentamidine** has been used as treatment of mild-to-moderate PCP. Because aerosolized pentamidine is not as effective as the systemic regimens, it should be reserved for patients with mild disease who cannot tolerate other forms of therapy (23).

Table 26-2. Drugs used for the treatment of acute *Pneumocystis carinii* pneumonia (PCP)

Agents with accepted therapeutic efficacy	Dose	Comments
Trimethoprim/ sulfamethoxazole (TMP/SMX)	TMP 15–20 mg/kg/d, SMX 75–100 mg/kg/d IV or PO	Fixed combination; avoid doses >960 mg/d TMP; administer in three divided doses
Pentamidine	4 mg/kg/d, IV	Infuse over 1–2 h to prevent hypotension
Trimethoprim plus dapsone	TMP 15–20 mg/kg/d, PO, dapsone 100 mg/d PO	Investigational but readily available
Atovaquone	750 mg TID PO	Administer with food; less effective and less toxic than TMP/SMX; use in patients with mild to moderate PCP who cannot tolerate TMP/SMX
Primaquine plus clindamycin	Primaquine 15–30 mg base PO, clindamycin 600 mg q6h to 900 mg q8h IV or 300–450 mg q6h PO	Investigational but readily available
Trimetrexate	45 mg/m²/d IV	Use with leucovorin 20 mg/m² QID PO or IV
Prednisone	40 mg BID PO for 5 days, followed by 20 mg BID for 5 days, then 20 mg/d until the end of anti-	Begin adjunctive corticosteroid therapy at the onset of anti-PCP therapy (effective within 72 h of the start of therapy); use in
patients	microbial therapy	with a Pao$_2$ <70 mm Hg or an (A-a)O$_2$ >35 mm Hg

Adapted from Lane HC, moderator. Recent advances in the management of AIDS-related opportunistic infections. *Ann Intern Med* 1994;120:945–955.

3. **Dapsone and trimethoprim** given in combination is a highly effective oral regimen for the treatment of mild-to-moderate PCP; glucose-6-phosphate dehydrogenase deficiency is a contraindication to the use of this regimen (22). Side effects have been milder than with TMP/SMX but are of a similar nature. Methemoglobinemia has been detected but is rarely of clinical significance.

4. **Clindamycin** given **IV or orally in combination with oral primaquine** is also acceptable for mild-to-moderate PCP. All three of these regimens are probably equivalent for the treatment of mild-to-moderate PCP (22).

5. **Atovaquone,** an oral hydroxynaphthoquinone, is a well tolerated but less efficacious alternative for patients with dose-limiting side effects to the above regimens (24).

6. **Trimetrexate,** an analogue of methotrexate, is probably as effective as dapsone/trimethoprim or clindamycin/primaquine. While its use has been limited by the lack of an oral preparation, the expense of the required adjuvant therapy with leucovorin (folinic acid), and the high early-relapse rates, trimetrexate is nonetheless a reasonable alternative for patients intolerant to other regimens. It should be considered in patients with severe PCP who have failed or are intolerant of TMP/SMX and pentamidine(23).

7. **Adjuvant systemic corticosteroids** are now standard of care in patients with PCP and respiratory compromise. Prednisone 40 mg, or its equivalent, twice daily (BID) for 5 days followed by 20 mg BID for 5 days and 20 mg daily for an additional 11 days is now recommended for patients with moderate-to-

severe PCP [room-air Pao$_2$ <70 Torr or (A-a)O$_2$ >35] (25). Currently, no data are available to justify the use of steroids in mild PCP, in children, or as rescue therapy.
   D. **Problems and complications of therapy.** Despite early recognition and aggressive therapy, PCP still carries a 10% to 20% mortality per episode. Clinical response of PCP to antimicrobial therapy usually becomes evident between the second and sixth day of treatment (2,22). If no improvement is noted by the seventh day, the diagnosis of PCP should be confirmed (if therapy was empiric), or a second diagnosis should be considered (7). Concurrent bacterial pneumonia, often difficult to diagnosis, is a frequent cause for poor response to therapy. Patients treated initially with TMP/SMX have a survival rate >80%. Patients who are started on TMP/SMX but switched to pentamidine have lower survival rates; the rate is 70% if pentamidine is used because of TMP/SMX toxicity and 30% in patients who have no clinical response to TMP/SMX (2). Subsequent episodes of PCP, the need for assisted mechanical ventilation, and concurrent bacterial pneumonia are associated with a poorer prognosis. Pneumothorax, a common complication of PCP in patients with recurrent disease and/or those receiving aerosolized pentamidine PCP prophylaxis, will be discussed latter in this chapter.
   E. **Secondary prophylaxis** should begin immediately after the completion of therapy because of the high incidence of relapse. (26)
IV. *Mycobacterium tuberculosis.* The rise in the incidence of tuberculosis (TB) in the United States, which began in 1986, was partially due to cases occurring in the HIV-infected population (see chapter 8).
   A. **Presenting signs and symptoms**
      1. The signs and symptoms of TB in HIV-infected persons vary significantly depending on the state of immunosuppression (27). Presenting symptoms include cough, fever, weight loss, and night sweats (2). Extrapulmonary disease is common, and symptoms related to liver, bone marrow, central nervous system, or lymphatic involvement may predominate.
      2. **Chest x-rays** frequently do not reveal cavities, apical scarring, or pleural effusion and may be normal in up to 10% of patients (2). The most common abnormalities in the severely immunocompromised are diffuse or miliary infiltrates, focal infiltrates, and mediastinal or hilar adenopathy (see Table 26-1); patients with milder degrees of immunosuppression have radiographic findings more typical of TB (27,28). The wide variety of clinical and radiographic findings makes the diagnosis of TB problematic in those with AIDS.
   B. **Management.** All HIV-infected patients with suspected mycobacterial disease should receive a treatment regimen effective against *M. tuberculosis*, as untreated TB is both fatal and transmissible. Pending culture results, initial therapy should consist of isoniazid 300 mg/d, rifampin 600 mg/d, pyrazinamide 25 mg/kg/d, and ethambutol 15 mg/kg/d (29). Therapy should be adjusted once culture results are available and continued for 9–12 months for isoniazid-sensitive organisms and 18 months for isoniazid-resistant organisms (Table 26-3). The key to success in the treatment of TB is adherence of the patient to the prescribed regimen (29). Directly observed therapy is strongly recommended, since the margin of safety in treating HIV-infected patients is reduced.
   C. **Problems and complications of therapy.** Outbreaks of **multidrug-resistant TB** have been reported in health care facilities in Miami and New York City. Nosocomial transmission of multidrug-resistant TB has had the greatest impact in patients with advanced HIV disease and, despite the use of multidrug regimens, has been uniformly fatal in this population.
V. *Mycobacterium avium-intracellulare* **complex (MAC)** infection most often occurs in patients with advanced immunosuppression (CD4 lymphocytes <100 cells/mm^3).
   A. **Presenting signs and symptoms.** HIV-infected patients with MAC infection present with fever, weight loss, night sweats, and anemia. MAC infection is generally disseminated even in its early stages. The lungs are frequently colonized and are often the initial site from which the organism is identified (2). Most of the clinical manifestations are extrapulmonary, and pulmonary involvement does not alter prognosis.

Table 26-3. Mycobacterial pathogens in HIV-infected persons

Mycobacterium species	Treatment
M. tuberculosis†	**Sensitive strains:** PPD* positive: isoniazid 5 mg/kg/d (max. 300 mg/d) plus pyridoxine 25 mg/d for 6–12 mo Active disease: 9–12 mo regimen (for $6 mo after culture conversion): isoniazid 5 mg/kg/d (max. 300 mg/d), rifampin 10 mg/kg/d (max. 600 mg/d), pyrazinamide 25 mg/kg/d (max. 2 g/d), and ethambutol 15 mg/kg (max. 2.5 g/d). Adjust therapy based on culture sensitivity **Likely exposure to multidrug-resistant strains:** PPD positive: efficacy data lacking; regimens such as 6–12 mo of isoniazid plus rifampin plus ethambutol, ethambutol plus rifampin, ethambutol plus ciprofloxacin, or pyrazinamide plus rifampin have been proposed. Active disease: no clinically effective regimen yet established; institute directly observed therapy with a multidrug regimen usually including second-line agents, preferably including two or more drugs to which the organism has *in vitro* sensitivity. One alternative approach is to use ethambutol 15 mg/kg/d, ciprofloxacin 750 mg BID, rifampin 10 mg/kg and amikacin 7.5 mg/kg BID. Consider surgery if localized disease
M. bovis†	No consensus regimen established; sensitivity testing of isolates recommended as a guide to antimycobacterial drug selection
M. avium-intracellulare complex	Multidrug regimens recommended, usually ethambutol plus one or both of the following drugs (based on symptomatology; *in vitro* sensitivities do not correlate well with *in vivo* drug activity); clarithromycin 500–1000 mg BID or azithromycin 500–1000 mg/d; ciprofloxacin 750 mg BID or ofloxacin 400 mg BID; amikacin 7.5–10.0 mg/kg/d IV; or rifampin 10 mg/kg/d (max. 600 mg/d)

Other atypical mycobacteria

Photochromogens (Runyon group I): *M. kansasii*†, *M. simiae*†, *M. asiaticum*†, *M. marinum*

Scotochromogens (Runyon group II): *M. gordonae*†, *M. scrofulaceum*†, *M. flavescens*†, *M. szulgai*†

Nonchromogens (Runyon group III) other than *M. avium-intracellulare* complex: *M. xenopi*†, *M. malmoense*†, *M. triviale*, *M. terrae*, *M. ulcerans*, *M. gastri*

Rapid growers (Runyon group IV): *M. fortuitum*†, *M. chelonei*†, *M. smegmatis*.

No consensus regimens established with many species; testing of isolates recommended as the best guide to appropriate antimycobacterial drug selections; for example, *M. kansasii*: isoniazid 5 mg/kg/d (max. 300 mg/d), rifampin 10 mg/kg/d (max. 600 mg/d), ethambutol 15 g/d (max. 2.5 g/d) for 15–18 mo

---

†Organisms that have been identified as causing infection in HIV-infected persons.

*PPD: purified protein derivative tuberculin test.

Adapted from Lane HC, moderator. Recent advances in the management of AIDS-related opportunistic infections. *Ann Intern Med* 1994;120:945–955.

      B. Management. Current recommended therapy includes ethambutol and clarithromycin or azithromycin; in patients who are very symptomatic from MAC infection, a third agent, such as ciprofloxacin or short-term amikacin, may be added (30). Recommendations for therapy are outlined in Table 26-3.

      C. Problems and complications of therapy. Drug interactions are common when both macrolide and rifampin compounds are used in the treatment of MAC, especially when azole antifungal agents are also prescribed.

  VI. *Mycobacterium kansasii* is the second most common AIDS-associated nontuberculous mycobacterial infection. In contrast to MAC infection, the lungs are the major focus of disease; dissemination is reported in those with severe immunosuppression.

      A. Presenting signs and symptoms

          1. Patients usually present with fever, cough, and dyspnea.

          2. The **chest x-ray** frequently shows thin-walled cavities, reticulonodular infiltrates, and many features reminiscent of the abnormalities associated with TB (31).

      B. Management. Regimens containing isoniazid, rifampin, and ethambutol are generally effective and may provide bacteriologic cure (23). Further recommendations are outlined in Table 26-3.

  VII. **Other nontuberculous mycobacteria.** Several species of atypical mycobacteria have been isolated from the respiratory tract of patients with AIDS. Because all these organisms have different environmental reservoirs, there may be significant regional differences in their frequencies. In contrast to the situation of the immunocompetent patient, in whom isolation of these organisms is frequently required for therapy, a decision to begin therapy in HIV-positive individuals should be made based on symptoms and the chest radiograph. Many patients with atypical mycobacterial infections have symptoms or radiographic abnormalities that resolve with appropriate therapy. Recommendations are outlined in Table 26-3.

  VIII. **Cytomegalovirus (CMV) pneumonitis.** Disseminated CMV infection commonly occurs in patients with advanced HIV disease, and the virus is typically recovered from BAL fluid during the disseminated stage of disease.

      A. Presenting signs and symptoms. Clinical manifestations include chorioretinitis, encephalitis, esophagitis, hepatitis, colitis, adrenalitis, and pneumonitis (2). Pulmonary symptoms and signs, as well as chest x-ray findings of diffuse interstitial infiltrates, are not specific. Definitive diagnosis requires demonstration of characteristic intranuclear inclusions on histologic examination of lung parenchyma obtained by fiberoptic bronchoscopy and transbronchial biopsy (2). CMV pneumonitis is often associated with other pulmonary infections, such as PCP (32).

      B. Management. The implication of finding CMV in the lungs of HIV-infected patients is still controversial. Therapy should be instituted for CMV pneumonitis when histologic demonstration of pulmonary parenchymal infection has occurred and no other pathogen has been identified (2). Therapy should include either ganciclovir or foscarnet (23). There appears to be no relationship between pulmonary CMV and survival in patients with a first episode of PCP (32). Evidence of pulmonary involvement should prompt a careful ophthalmologic examination, since therapy for CMV chorioretinitis has been shown to prevent blindness. Like most of the opportunistic infections associated with AIDS, lifelong prophylaxis is required to sustain a disease-free state (26).

  IX. **Herpesvirus infections** are an infrequent cause of pneumonia in patients with HIV disease (2).

      A. Herpes simplex pneumonitis should only be considered when there is histologic evidence of pulmonary infection and no other pathogen is isolated (2). Because oral herpes simplex infection is common, isolation of the virus from respiratory tract specimens is not unusual.

      B. Varicella-zoster virus (VZV) pneumonia is generally less difficult to diagnose; patients present with diffuse, bilateral infiltrates on chest x-ray in the setting of widely disseminated VZV infection. Acyclovir is the drug of choice for both herpes simplex and VZV pneumonitis; foscarnet can be used to treat resistant organisms.

C. **Human herpesvirus 6** (HHV-6) has recently been reported as a cause of fatal pneumonitis in severely immunocompromised patients (33). Although foscarnet and ganciclovir are effective against HHV-6, their role in pneumonitis has yet to be evaluated.

X. **Cryptococcal pneumonia.** *Cryptococcus* species are yeasts ubiquitous in the environment and global in distribution. The route of infection of cryptococcal disease is almost always through inhalation of infectious particles (2).

A. **Presenting signs and symptoms**
   1. Cryptococcal disease is usually confined to patients with CD4 lymphocyte counts <200 cells/mm^3. The infection generally presents as meningitis, with a history of recent pneumonia in the majority of patients and a concomitant pneumonitis in as many as 30% of cases.
   2. The **chest x-ray** usually demonstrates a focal or diffuse interstitial infiltrate, mass-like lesions, nodules, cavitary lesions, adenopathy, and/or pleural effusion (16,19,34). Disseminated cryptococcosis can also present as a sepsis syndrome characterized by a respiratory alkalosis, tachycardia, hypotension, and oliguria without an obvious respiratory or central nervous system focus.

B. **Differential diagnosis.** Cryptococcal pneumonitis should be considered in the differential diagnosis of interstitial infiltrates, mass lesions, cavitary lesions, miliary disease, intrathoracic adenopathy, and pleural effusion (see Table 26-1). A positive serum cryptococcal antigen or a rising antigen titer in an AIDS patient with a history of cryptococcal meningitis should prompt therapy. BAL fluid is usually culture or smear positive when *Cryptococcus* is the cause of an AIDS-related pneumonia; blood cultures may also be positive (34).

C. **Management.** Because cryptococcosis is life threatening in patients with AIDS, the threshold to treat should be low. Cryptococcal pneumonitis, like meningitis, is treated with either fluconazole or amphotericin B (Table 26-4). For a more complete discussion, see chapter 9.

D. **Problems and complications of therapy.** Identification of this organism in sputum or BAL specimens should prompt a lumbar puncture to rule out meningeal involvement. Lifelong prophylaxis is required to sustain a disease-free state in AIDS patients (26).

XI. **Histoplasmosis** is a common AIDS-related opportunistic infection in endemic areas, such as the valleys of the Ohio and Mississippi Rivers, Haiti, Puerto Rico, and Central and South America (2). Current or previous residence in any endemic area imparts a lifelong risk of reactivation for patients with AIDS. (For a more complete discussion, see chapter 9.)

Table 26-4. Fungal pathogens in HIV-infected persons

Candida	Itraconazole 100–400 mg/d or amphotericin B 0.5–1.0 mg/kg/d depending on symptomatology
Cryptococcus	Primary infection: amphotericin B 0.5–1.0 mg/kg/d depending on symptomatology; combination therapy with flucytosine 100 mg/kg/d in HIV-infected patients is controversial
	Chronic maintenance therapy: fluconazole 200 mg/d or amphotericin B 1.0 mg/kg/wk. Fluconazole is the preferred regimen
Histoplasma	Primary infection: itraconazole 200 mg BID or amphotericin B 500 mg before switching to itraconazole
	Chronic maintenance therapy: itraconazole 200 mg BID
Coccidioides	Amphotericin B 0.5–1.0 mg/kg/d
Aspergillus	Amphotericin B 0.5–1.0 mg/kg/d. Role of itraconazole is not yet clear

Adapted from Lane HC, moderator. Recent advances in the management of AIDS-related opportunistic infections. *Ann Intern Med* 1994;120:945–955.

A. Presenting signs and symptoms

1. Patients typically present with fever, weight loss, and adenopathy. Although cough and/or shortness of breath are reported in about 60% of cases, pulmonary symptoms are generally not the chief complaint.

2. **Chest radiographs** showing focal infiltrates and hilar adenopathy, the hallmarks of histoplasmosis in the immunocompetent host, occur in <10% of all cases. Bilateral infiltrates predominate, described as interstitial, reticulonodular, or alveolar. Cavitation and pleural effusion are unusual but have been reported. Normal radiographs are reported in about 40% of AIDS patients with disseminated histoplasmosis (28,34).

B. Differential diagnosis. Histoplasmosis should be considered as the primary diagnosis in patients with a present or past history of residence in endemic areas and with a characteristic radiograph (see Table 26-1). Stains of BAL fluid have a sensitivity of 70%, while cultures are 90% sensitive in AIDS-related pulmonary histoplasmosis. Blood cultures and bone marrow biopsy are most likely to yield the organisms in patients with disseminated disease. Detection of *Histoplasma capsulatum* antigen in urine, serum, cerebrospinal fluid, and BAL fluid is a sensitive (80% to 95%) test for diagnosis and should be obtained in HIV-positive patients with appropriate travel and/or residency histories (34).

C. Management. Amphotericin B or itraconazole are the treatments of choice (see Table 26-4).

D. Problems and complication of therapy. Lifelong suppressive therapy is necessary (26).

XII. Coccidioidomycosis. Individuals with HIV infection residing in the southwestern United States are at considerable risk for the development of coccidioidomycosis. While most cases outside the endemic area result from reactivation of latent disease, the majority of disease results from recent infection in patients with CD4 counts <250 cells/mm^3 (34).

A. Presenting signs and symptoms

1. Patients are typically febrile and dyspneic.

2. The **chest x-ray** is abnormal in approximately 70% of cases, with diffuse reticulonodular infiltrates or focal infiltrates with hilar adenopathy and pleural effusion. Nodules and cavitary lesions typical of coccidioidomycosis in the seronegative population are also seen (16). The degree of respiratory distress roughly parallels the extent of pulmonary infiltrates on the chest radiograph.

B. Differential diagnosis. Coccidioidomycosis should be considered in the differential diagnosis of pulmonary nodules, focal or diffuse infiltrates, pleural effusion, or thin-walled cavities in patients with a recent or past history of residence in an endemic area. Cytologic examination of transbronchial biopsies is typically diagnostic when diffuse reticulonodular infiltrates are present. The organism may be cultured from lymph nodes, blood, urine, and skin, as well as pulmonary specimens; colony formation occurs in 3–5 days, but the characteristic arthrospore formation may require an additional 48 hours of culture. Despite severe immunosuppression, tube precipitin or complement-fixing antibodies are present in >90% of cases and should be considered diagnostic (2,34).

C. Management. Amphotericin B is the drug of choice for patients with diffuse disease (see Table 26-4) (34).

D. Problems and complications of therapy. Patients with a diffuse nodular pattern on chest x-ray have a poor prognosis, with 50% mortality within 1 month of diagnosis despite aggressive therapy with amphotericin B. Lifelong suppressive therapy with itraconazole, ketoconazole, fluconazole, or amphotericin B is required (26).

XIII. Aspergillosis. Pulmonary infection with *Aspergillus* species can occur as either an invasive parenchymal process or an obstructive bronchial disease. Invasive aspergillosis usually occurs in the later stages of AIDS and often in patients with a history of neutropenic episodes, broad-spectrum antibiotics, or corticosteroid therapy (2,34). Bronchial disease with or without bronchial obstruction, mucosal ulceration, or pseudomembrane formation may afflict patients without risk factors for invasive aspergillosis who have early-stage AIDS (15).

A. **Presenting signs and symptoms**
1. The clinical picture consists of cough and fever; many patients have chest pain.
2. The **chest radiograph** in invasive aspergillosis usually demonstrates unilateral or bilateral reticulonodular infiltrates with cavities or pleura-based lesions. Diffuse interstitial infiltrates are less common (16). Patients with bronchial disease may have chest radiographs that reveal diffuse interstitial infiltrates or may be normal (34).
B. **Differential diagnosis.** Demonstration of tissue invasion or microscopic identification of fungal elements in bronchial pseudomembrane is required for diagnosis. Aspergilli are frequently identified and cultured from respiratory secretions; this is not sufficient evidence to begin therapy.
C. **Management.** Despite aggressive therapy with amphotericin B, median survival is about 3 months for patients with invasive aspergillosis. Itraconazole may be useful in patients who cannot tolerate amphotericin (see Table 26-4).

XIV. *Candida* **species.** Although cultures obtained at bronchoscopy frequently grow *Candida* species, the diagnosis of pulmonary candidiasis rests on the demonstration of fungal forms invading the lung parenchyma. Pulmonary candidiasis is exceedingly uncommon (34) and rarely occurs except in gravely ill patients with disseminated candidiasis. Patients may respond to treatment with amphotericin B, ketoconazole, or fluconazole, but mortality remains high (see Table 26-4).

XV. **Toxoplasmosis.** Although occurring in only 1% to 3 % of AIDS patients in the United States, toxoplasmosis is much more common in Spain, Haiti, France, and other endemic areas.
A. **Presenting signs and symptoms.** Pneumonitis may occur alone or as a complication of central nervous system disease. Actual pneumonitis is infrequent, whereas necrotizing encephalitis with multiple ring-enhancing lesions on CT scan is the most common presentation (35). The chest x-ray generally shows bilateral nodular or interstitial infiltrates or irregular consolidation. The demonstration of the parasite on Wright's or Giemsa staining of biopsy material is required for diagnosis (35).
B. **Management.** Treatment with sulfadiazine and pyrimethamine is generally effective, but lifelong suppressive therapy is required (see Table 26-2) (23,26).

XVI. **Pulmonary cryptosporidiosis, microsporidiosis, and strongyloidosis.** The intestinal parasites of the genuses *Strongyloides* and *Cryptosporidium* and the order Microsporida may cause pulmonary symptoms in patients, in addition to diarrhea from gastrointestinal infestation (36–38).
A. **Presenting signs and symptoms**
1. While dyspnea is typical of HIV-related pulmonary strongyloidosis, patients with respiratory cryptosporidiosis or microsporidiosis complain of unremitting cough.
2. The **chest radiograph** is frequently normal, but overwhelming strongyloidosis has been reported to cause diffuse nodular or alveolar infiltrates. Diagnosis is made by the identification of the parasites from respiratory secretions or BAL fluid.
B. **Management.** Thiabendazole or ivermectin should be used as therapy for *Strongyloides* infection (38). Albendazole has been found effective against some but not all of the microsporidians. No effective therapy exists for disseminated cryptosporidiosis, and patients usually succumb to overwhelming gastrointestinal infestation (37).

XVII. **Kaposi's sarcoma** (KS) in the HIV-infected patient usually presents as a multicentric disease involving the skin and oral mucosa. Internal organ involvement is common; 30% of patients with KS have symptomatic lung involvement, accounting for 1% to 10% of the pulmonary complications of AIDS (2,3,39).
A. **Presenting signs and symptoms**
1. While nonspecific systemic symptoms such as fever and weight loss predominate, some patients complain of wheezing, hemoptysis, pleuritic chest pain, or stridor. Physical examination is usually not revealing, although stridor suggests bulky lesions of the upper airway.

2. **Chest x-ray** findings include bilateral interstitial and/or alveolar infiltrates, often with poorly defined nodularity and accompanying pleural effusion (see Table 26-1) (16,19,39). Pulmonary KS usually occurs in the setting of disseminated disease, although isolated pulmonary involvement has been reported.

B. **Differential diagnosis.** Definitive diagnosis of pulmonary KS usually requires open lung biopsy. However, visualization of the typical macular or plaque-like cherry-red lesions of KS in the trachea or endobronchial tree during bronchoscopy is considered adequate in patients with established disease. Endobronchial biopsy, transbronchial biopsy, or bronchial brushing with cytology is generally not diagnostic (2). Pleural biopsy occasionally provides useful specimens. HRCT scans in patients with oral lesions are highly suggestive, even for patients without identifiable lesions on bronchoscopy (39).

C. **Management.** Therapy for pulmonary KS is palliative and consists of radiation, combination chemotherapy, and/or interferon alfa.

XVIII. **Lymphoma.** The incidence of both Hodgkin's and non-Hodgkin's lymphomas is increased in HIV infection. HIV-associated non-Hodgkin's lymphoma usually has a highly malignant histology, with widespread and/or extranodal distribution at the time of presentation (2,40).

A. **Presenting signs and symptoms**
   1. Patients with lymphoma in the lungs or mediastinum usually present with systemic symptoms such as weight loss, fever, anorexia, or peripheral adenopathy. Pulmonary or mediastinal involvement is usually discovered radiographically during evaluation for another illness.
   2. The **chest radiograph** may demonstrate mediastinal or hilar enlargement, interstitial or nodular infiltrates, or solitary masses/nodules in the pulmonary parenchyma (2,41). Pleural thickening, pleural effusion, and cavitation of the parenchymal masses have all been reported (see Table 26-1) (16).

B. **Differential diagnosis.** Transbronchial biopsy or thoracentesis rarely provide a diagnosis, and lung or pleural biopsy is generally required.

C. **Management.** In general, therapy does not produce lasting control of HIV-related lymphoma.

XIX. **Lymphoid interstitial pneumonitis** (LIP) is an immunologic disorder of unknown etiology that typically occurs in pediatric AIDS patients but has also been described in adults with AIDS. The mononuclear infiltrate of LIP is composed of CD8 lymphocytes and plasma cells. Although the antigen has not been defined, the lymphocytic infiltration is phenotypically suggestive of a response to an undefined chronic antigenic stimulation (42).

A. **Presenting signs and symptoms**
   1. Patients typically present with slowly progressive dyspnea and nonproductive cough; fever and weight loss may also be present. Physical examination often reveals adenopathy, hepatosplenomegaly, uveitis, and/or parotid gland enlargement (2). Although examination of the chest may be normal, crackles at the bases are frequently noted on auscultation (2,42).
   2. The **chest x-ray** demonstrates bilateral lower lobe interstitial or reticulonodular infiltrates occasionally with areas of alveolar filling defects. Hypergammaglobulinemia and lymphocytosis may occur (42).

B. **Differential diagnosis.** Diagnosis of LIP in adults is difficult. The clinical presentation is nonspecific, and LIP is rare and not usually considered in the initial evaluation of dyspnea. Recurrent bacterial pneumonia is strongly associated with LIP and may further hinder diagnosis. Patients with LIP may respond to treatment of pathogens recovered from sputum, and chest x-rays may improve but rarely return to normal. Histology from transbronchial or open lung biopsy shows alveolar and interstitial infiltration with lymphocytes and plasma cells (2).

C. **Management.** Therapeutic benefit has been demonstrated with corticosteroid and zidovudine therapy. Abnormalities demonstrated on chest x-ray show considerable improvement, and oxygenation may return to normal or near normal. In many cases, there is no recurrence of symptoms after discontinuation of corticosteroid treatment (42). However, in some patients, clinical and radiologic deterioration follows within days of stopping therapy, and steroids must be continued on a long-term basis.

XX. Nonspecific interstitial pneumonitis. Although this entity was initially described as a sequela of PCP, it is now clear that nonspecific interstitial pneumonitis can be seen in a number of settings (43).

    A. Presenting signs and symptoms

        1. Nonspecific symptoms such as cough and dyspnea predominate. Constitutional symptoms are usually mild when present. Arterial blood gases may be nearly normal, but a widened (A-a)O$_2$ is more common (3,43).

        2. Chest radiographs often reflect a resolving infectious process but may be normal or demonstrate an interstitial pattern indistinguishable from PCP.

    B. Differential diagnosis. The diagnosis relies on the demonstration of a mild mononuclear cell infiltrate with varying degrees of interstitial edema, fibrin deposition, alveolar cell hyperplasia, septal thickening and fibrosis, and the exclusion of another underlying process within the lung parenchyma (2,43).

    C. Management. The clinical course usually stabilizes or improves without specific therapy (2,43). Steroids may be useful in symptomatic patients but seldom need to be continued for more than a few weeks.

XXI. Bronchogenic carcinoma. Several HIV-infected patients have now developed bronchogenic carcinoma (3,44). Whether bronchogenic carcinoma can be considered a complication of HIV infection has not yet been clarified, since most affected patients have been smokers. Nonetheless, the biologic behavior of the disease in HIV-infected patients appears much more aggressive than that seen in the seronegative population (44).

    A. Presenting signs and symptoms. Cough, fever, dyspnea, and chest pain are the most common symptoms of bronchogenic carcinoma in the HIV-infected patient. These symptoms may be an indication of postobstructive pneumonia; HIV-infected patients are more likely to have an infiltrate in addition to the primary lesion than are seronegative controls (44).

    B. Management. In general, these patients should be managed in the same fashion as seronegative patients. Patients with concurrent HIV infection and bronchogenic carcinoma are much younger than seronegative patients and present at a later stage of disease. The malignancy progresses more rapidly, even controlling for stage, and few patients survive 2 months after diagnosis (44).

XXII. Pulmonary hypertension. The etiology of HIV-associated pulmonary hypertension remains unknown. Even though pulmonary hypertension occurs 10–100 times more frequently in the HIV-seropositive than in the seronegative population; it occurs in <1% of these patients.

    A. Presenting signs and symptoms

        1. The presentation of HIV-associated pulmonary hypertension is remarkably similar to that of primary pulmonary hypertension except that the disease appears to advance more rapidly. Patients may present early in the course of HIV infection, prior to occurrence of opportunistic infection. Complaints of rapidly progressive dyspnea on exertion are usual, but evaluation yields no evidence of infection or malignancy.

        2. The **chest x-ray** typically shows normal pulmonary parenchyma with right-sided cardiac enlargement and pruning of the pulmonary vasculature (45).

    B. Differential diagnosis. Echocardiography with Doppler evaluation of the tricuspid valve documenting a high gradient is suggestive, but direct measurement of the pulmonary artery pressure is required to formalize the diagnosis.

    C. Management. No current therapy has been uniformly effective for pulmonary hypertension; however, certain patients will have hemodynamic and clinical improvement with high-dose calcium channel blockers (diltiazem or nifedipine), angiotension-converting enzyme inhibitors (captopril or enalapril) or prostaglandin analogues (misoprostol or epoprostenol) (46).

XXIII. Pneumothorax. Spontaneous pneumothorax in HIV-infected patients is almost always the consequence of active infection.

    A. Etiology and pathogenesis. The insidious onset of PCP allows significant pulmonary parenchymal destruction, leading to the development of cysts, cavities, bullae, and pneumothorax (2,16,17). The risk of pneumothorax is increased in patients with recurrent PCP and in those receiving aerolosized pentamidine prophylaxis (2). Pneumothorax has also been identified in patients with active TB and necrotizing bacterial pneumonia, although much less commonly. A sample of pleural fluid is helpful for diagnosis and should be submitted for biochemical analysis, culture, and cytologic staining.

  B. Management. Treatment of pneumothorax with chest tube suction is adequate in <50% of patients; air leaks are slow to resolve and sclerotherapy and/or thoracotomy are frequently required. The use of Heimlich valves or small-bore chest tubes is a reasonable alternative and may allow earlier discharge from the hospital. Pneumothorax is highly associated with PCP infection, and PCP treatment should begin immediately in AIDS patients with spontaneous pneumothorax and continued for 21 days, unless this diagnosis is excluded or an alternative etiology is identified.

XXIV. Intrathoracic lymphadenopathy. The differential diagnosis of intrathoracic adenopathy is listed in Table 26-1. Persistent generalized lymphadenopathy is a common finding in HIV disease. However, hilar and mediastinal adenopathy are not a part of this syndrome (2,18,47). Consequently, patients with radiographic evidence of thoracic adenopathy should be evaluated carefully for infectious or neoplastic diseases. Extrathoracic lymph node biopsy will often identify the cause, but mediastinoscopy or open biopsy should be considered when no diagnosis has been made.

XXV. Lung abscesses and cavitary lesions

  A. Presenting signs and symptoms. The vast majority of patients with lung abscesses or cavitary lung lesions present with fever and cough (48). Surprisingly, the majority of lung abscesses occur in the upper lobes; the distribution of cavitary lesions is less well studied (16,48).

  B. Etiology. The differential diagnosis of cavitary lesions is presented in Table 26-1. In patients with only modest immunosuppression, TB should be the leading diagnosis, and bronchoscopy should be performed if TB cannot be excluded (16).

  C. Differential diagnosis. Because the vast majority of cavitary lesions and abscesses are caused by treatable infectious processes, every effort should be made to determine the etiologic agent involved. Examination of induced or expectorated sputum is the first step in the diagnostic process, with subsequent CT followed by BAL with or without transbronchial biopsy or percutaneous biopsy when necessary.

XXVI. Pleural effusion. Pleural effusion occurs in approximately 25% of hospitalized AIDS patients. Effusions are typically small and usually the consequence of a parenchymal infectious process.

  A. Etiology. The differential diagnosis of pleural effusion in AIDS patients is given in Table 26-1. Approximately 66% are infectious; most are parapneumonic effusions or empyemas secondary to bacterial pneumonia (19,28). Of the fungi, only *Cryptococcus neoformans* is commonly associated with pleural effusion. When acid-fast bacilli are identified or cultured from the pleural space, *M. tuberculosis* should be considered, since *M. avium-intracellulare* complex rarely causes a pleural effusion. Pleural effusion, often bilateral, can occur in up to 50% of patients with KS. In some studies, small effusions have been noted during episodes of PCP, although significant effusions are very uncommon in this entity (19).

XXVII. Diagnostic approaches

  A. Abnormal chest radiographs. HIV-infected patients should have chest radiography performed for systemic symptoms, as well as for respiratory complaints. Evaluation of a normal chest x-ray in patients with respiratory complaints is discussed in the next section.

  B. The differential diagnosis of commonly observed chest x-ray patterns is presented in Table 26-1. An algorithm useful in the evaluation of radiographic abnormalities is presented in Fig. 26-1.

   1. If the chest x-ray reveals a **focal abnormality**, an attempt should be made to identify a "routine" infection. Staining and culturing of sputum for conventional bacteria and acid-fast bacilli should be included in this evaluation.

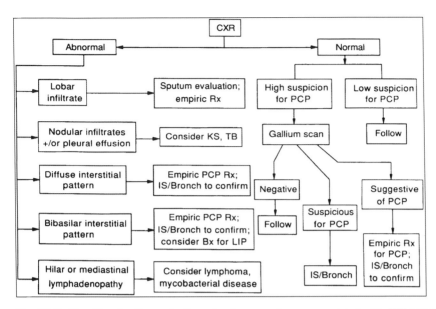

Fig. 26-1. Algorithm for the evaluation of pulmonary disease associated with HIV infection based on chest x-ray (CXR) appearance. IS/Bronch = induced sputum/bronchoscopy; Bx = biopsy; LIP = lymphoid interstitial pneumonitis; Rx = treatment; KS = Kaposi's sarcoma; TB = tuberculosis; PCP = *Pneumocystis carinii* pneumonia. (Lipman H, Witzburg RA. *HIV infection*, 3rd ed. Boston: Little, Brown, 1996).

2. If the chest x-ray shows **diffuse infiltrates,** an empiric trial of therapy for PCP is reasonable in AIDS patients with mild-to-moderate gas exchange abnormalities. In the outpatient setting, patient reliability, as well as accessibility and availability of health care, should be considered prior to initiation of empiric therapy.

3. A firm diagnosis must be pursued **for those patients not meeting the surveillance definition of AIDS** or those with more severe gas exchange abnormalities. Induced-sputum studies for *P. carinii*, acid-fast bacilli, and other pathogens should be the first step in the evaluation. In institutions lacking the capacity to perform this procedure, flexible fiberoptic bronchoscopy with BAL is appropriate. At least two lobes should be lavaged, including an upper lobe segment and an area of infiltration. A similar approach is warranted in patients whose chest x-ray abnormalities are focal, mild, or otherwise atypical of PCP after a "routine" pneumonia has been excluded.

4. If examination of induced **sputum or initial fiberoptic bronchoscopy with BAL is nondiagnostic,** fiberoptic bronchoscopy with BAL, bronchial brushings, and multiple-site directed transbronchial biopsies should be performed (49). The biopsy and BAL specimens should be processed with appropriate stains and cultures for bacterial pathogens, including *Legionella, P. carinii,* acid-fast bacilli, fungi, and cytomegalovirus. Specimens should also be evaluated by cytologic and histologic analysis.

5. An **open lung biopsy** should be performed if the transbronchial biopsy is nondiagnostic and the clinical condition is deteriorating.

6. **Observation alone is reasonable if the transbronchial biopsy is nondiagnostic** and the clinical condition is stable. Clinical response can be evalu-

ated by the $(A-a)O_2$, the D_LCO, and/or gallium scan. The diagnostic yield of repeat transbronchial biopsy appears to be low, and open lung biopsy should be considered if a firm diagnosis is required.

B. Diagnostic approach for respiratory symptoms. Patients with fever, cough, shortness of breath, or dyspnea on exertion should have chest radiography performed (1). The differential diagnosis and evaluation of commonly observed chest x-ray patterns is discussed in the previous section. If the chest x-ray is normal, one should measure the $(A-a)O_2$ and the D_LCO and obtain an additional imaging study such as gallium scanning of the lungs or HRCT of the chest. If these studies are unremarkable, pulmonary disease is highly unlikely and a cardiac evaluation should be considered. Echocardiography is probably the single best choice, since information regarding the pericardium, left ventricular function, and estimates of pulmonary artery pressures can be obtained.

References

1. Murray JF, Felton CP, Garay SM, et al.: Pulmonary complications of the acquired immunodeficiency syndrome: report of a National Heart, Lung, and Blood Institute workshop. *N Engl J Med* 1984;320:1682–1688.
2. Meduri GU, Stein DS: Pulmonary manifestations of acquired immunodeficiency syndrome. *Clin Infect Dis* 1992;14:98–113.
3. Wallace JM, Rao AV, Glassroth J, et al.: Respiratory illness in persons with human immunodeficiency virus infection. *Rev Respir Dis* 1993;148:1523–1529.
4. Masur H, Ognibene FP, Yarchoan R, et al.: CD4 counts as predictors of opportunistic pneumonias in human immunodeficiency virus (HIV) infection. *Ann Intern Med* 1989;111:223–231.
5. Magnenat J-L, Nicod LP, Auckenthaler R, Funod AF: Mode of presentation and diagnosis of bacterial pneumonia in human immunodeficiency virus-infected patients. *Am Rev Respir Dis* 1991; 144:917–922.
6. Hirschtick RE, Glassroth J, Jordan MC, et al.: Bacterial pneumonia in persons infected with the human immunodeficiency virus. *N Engl J Med* 1995;333:845–851.
7. Baughman RP, Dohn MN, Frame PT: The continuing utility of bronchoalveolar lavage to diagnose opportunistic infection in AIDS patients. *Am J Med* 1994;97:515–522.
8. Witt D, Craven D, McCabe W: Bacterial infections in adult patients with the acquired immune deficiency syndrome (AIDS) and AIDS-related complex. *Am J Med* 1987;82:900–906.
9. Verghese A, Al-Samman M, Nabhan D, et al.: Bacterial bronchitis and bronchiectasis in human immunodeficiency virus infection. *Arch Intern Med* 1994;154:2086–2091.
10. Baron AD, Hollander H: *Pseudomonas aeruginosa* bronchopulmonary infection in late human immunodeficiency virus disease. *Am Rev Respir Dis* 1993;148:992–996.
11. Schuster MG, Norris AH: Community-acquired *Pseudomonas aerguinosa* pneumonia in patients with HIV infection. *AIDS* 1994;8:1437–1441.
12. Uttamchandani RB, Daikkos GL, Reyes RR, et al.: Nocardiosis in 30 patients with advanced human immunodeficiency virus infection: clincal feature and outcome. *Clin Infect Dis* 1994;18:348–53.
13. Verville RD, Huycke MM, Greenfield RA, et al.: *Rhodococcus equi* infections of humans: 12 cases and a review of the literature. *Medicine* 1994;73:119–132.
14. Ankobiah WA, Salehi F: Salmonella lung abscess in a patient with acquired immunodeficiency syndrome. *Chest* 1991;100:591–593.
15. Kemper CA, Hostetler JS, Follansbee SE, et al.: Ulcerative and plaque-like tracheobronchitis due to infection with *Aspergillus* in patient with AIDS. *Clin Infect Dis* 1993;17:334–52.
16. Gallant JE, Ko AH: Cavitary pulmonary lesions in patients infected with human immunodeficiency virus. *Clin Infect Dis* 1996;22:671–82.
17. Kuhlman JE: Pneumocystic infection; the radiologist's perspective. *Radiology* 1996;198:623–635.
18. Stern RG, Gamsu G, Golden JA, et al.: Intrathoracic adenopathy: differential features of AIDS and diffuse lymphadenopathy syndrome. *AJR* 1984;142:689–692.
19. Joseph J, Strange C, Sahn SA: Pleural effusions in hospitalized patients with AIDS. *Ann Intern Med* 1993;118:856–859.

20. Yung RC, Weinacker AB, Steiger DJ, et al.: Upper and middle lobe bronchoalveolar lavage to diagnose *Pneumocystis carinii* pneumonia. *Am Rev Respir Dis* 1993;148:1563–1566.
21. Sattler FR, Cowan R, Nielsen DM, Ruskin J: Trimethoprim/sulfamethoxazole compared with pentamidine for treatment of *Pneumocystis carinii* pneumonia in the acquired immunodeficiency syndrome: a prospective, non-crossover study. *Ann Intern Med* 1988;109:280–287.
22. Safrin S, Finkelstein DM, Feinberg J, et al.: Comparison of three regimens for treatment of mild to moderate *Pneumocystis carinii* pneumonia in patients with AIDS: a double-blind, randomized trial of oral trimethoprim-sulfamethoxazole, dapsone-trimethoprim, and clindamycin-primaquine. *Ann Intern Med* 1996;124:792–802.
23. Lane HC, moderator: Recents advances in the management of AIDS-related opportunistic infections. *Ann Intern Med* 1994;120:945–955.
24. Dohn MN, Weinberg WG, Torres RA, et al.: Treatment of mild to moderate *Pneumocystis carinii* pneumonia with atovaquone. *Ann Intern Med* 1994;122:174–180.
25. NIH-UC Expert Panel for Corticosteroids as Adjunctive Therapy for Pneumocystis Pneumonia: Consensus statement for use of corticosteroids as adjunctive therapy for *Pneumocystis* pneumonia in AIDS. *N Engl J Med* 1990;323:1500–1504.
26. USPHS/IDSA guidelines for the prevention of opportunistic infections in persons infected with human immunodeficiency virus: a summary. *Ann Intern Med* 1996;124:349–368.
27. Jones BE, Young SMM, Antoniskis D, et al.: Relationship of the manifesttions of tuberculosis to CD4 cell counts in patients with human immunodeficiency virus infection. *Am Rev Respir Dis* 1993;148:1292–1297.
28. Cadranel JL, Chouaid C, Denis M, et al.: Causes of pleural effusion in 75 HIV-infected patients. *Chest* 1993;104:655–659.
29. American Thoracic Society: Treatment of tuberculosis and tuberculosis infection and adults and children. *Am J Respir Crit Care Med* 1994;149:1359–1374.
30. Masur H and the Public Health Service Task Force: Prophylaxis and therapy for disseminated *Mycobacterium avium* complex disease in patients with the human immunodeficiency virus. *N Engl J Med* 1993;329:898–904.
31. Witzig RS, Fazal BA, Mera RM, et al.: Clinical manifestations of implications of coinfection with *Mycobacterium kansasii* and human immunodeficiency virus type I. *Clin Infect Dis* 1995;21: 77–85.
32. Jacobson MA, Mills J, Rush J, et al.: Morbidity and mortality of patients with AIDS and first-episode *Pneumocystis carinii* pneumonia unaffected by concomitant pulmonary cytomegalovirus infection. *Am Rev Respir Dis* 1991;144:6–9.
33. Knox KK, Carrigan DR: Disseminated active HHV-6 infections in patients with AIDS. *Lancet* 1994; 343:578–580.
34. American Thoracic Society: Fungal infections in HIV-infected persons. *Am J Respir Crit Care Med* 1995;152:816–822.
35. McCabe RE, Remington JS: *Toxoplasma gondii*. In: Mandell GL, Douglas RG, Bennett JE, eds. *Principles and practices of infectious diseases*, 3rd ed. New York: Churchill Livingstone, 1989: 2093–2094.
36. Hojlyng N, Jenson BN: Respiratory cryptosporidiosis in HIV-positive patients. *Lancet* 1988;1: 590–591.
37. Molina J-M, Oksenhendler E, Beauvais B, et al.: Disseminated microsporidiosis due to *Septata intestinalis* in patients with AIDS: clinical features and response to albendazole therapy. *J Infect Dis* 1995;171:245–249.
38. Lessnau K-D, Can S, Talavera W: Disseminated *Stongyloides stercoralis* in human immunodeficiency virus-infected patients. *Chest* 1993;104:119–123.
39. Zibrak JD, Silvestri RC, Costello P, et al.: Bronchoscopic and radiologic features of Kaposi's sarcoma involving the respiratory system. *Chest* 1986;90:476–480.
40. Kaplan LD, Abrams DI, Feigal E, et al.: AIDS-associated non-Hodgkin's lymphoma in San Francisco. *JAMA* 1989;261:719–724.
41. Scheib RG, Seigal RS: Atypical Hodgkin's disease and the acquired immunodeficiency syndrome. *Ann Intern Med* 1985;102:554–557.
42. Itescu S, Winchester R: Diffuse infiltrative lymphocytosis syndrome: a disorder occurring in human immunodeficiency virus-1 infection that may present as a sicca syndrome. *Rheum Dis Clin North Am* 1992;18:683–697.
43. Ognibene FP, Masur H, Rogers P, et al.: Nonspecific interstitial pneumonitis without evidence of

Pneumocystis carinii in asymptomatic patients with human immunodeficiency virus (HIV). *Ann Intern Med* 1988;109:874–879.

44. Karp J, Profeta G, Marantz PR, Karpel JP: Lung cancer in patients with immunodeficiency syndrome. *Chest* 1993;103:410–413.

45. Coplan NL, Shimony RY, Ioachim HL, et al.: Primary pulmonary hypertension associated with human immunodeficiency viral infection. *Am J Med* 1990;89:96–99.

46. Barst RJ, Rubin LJ, Long WA, et al.: A comparison of continuous intravenous epoprostenol (prostacyclin) with conventional therapy for primary pulmonary hypertension. *N Engl J Med* 1996;334:296–301.

47. Suster B, Akerman M, Orenstein M, Wax MR: Pulmonary manifestations of AIDS; review of 106 episodes. *Radiology* 1986;161:87–93.

48. Furman AC, Jacobs J, Sepkowitz KA: Lung abscess in patients with AIDS. *Clin Infect Dis* 1996; 22:81–85.

49. Cadranal J, Gillet-Juvin K, Antoine M, et al.: Site-directed bronchoalveolar lavage and transbronchial biopsy in HIV-infected patients with pneumonia. *Am J Respir Crit Care Med* 1995; 152:1103–1106.

27

Pulmonary Manifestations of Systemic Disease

Jeffrey B. Rubins

More than any other system, the lung and respiratory tract are frequently affected by extrapulmonary diseases. Pulmonary manifestations are often the first sign of systemic disease. This chapter focuses on the more common presentations of selected systemic diseases that typically involve the respiratory system and are not covered in other chapters.

I. **Abdominal diseases**
   A. **Gastroesophageal reflux disease** (GERD) is extremely common in the United States population, with a prevalence of approximately 30%, and is the most common esophageal disease of adults associated with pulmonary disease. About 10% of patients with GERD have respiratory symptoms ranging from asthma and cough to bronchitis, bronchiectasis, and pulmonary fibrosis (1).
   1. **Clinical presentation**
      a. Approximately one-third of patients with GERD have no gastrointestinal symptoms. The majority of patients present with classical reflux symptoms or with atypical symptoms of choking, sore throat, or hoarseness.
      b. In asthmatic patients, symptoms of worsening of asthma during sleep, meals, or recumbency or with bronchodilator medications (see next section) should suggest the possibility of GERD (2). In addition, patients with adult-onset intrinsic asthma should be evaluated for this condition (2).
   2. **Relevant pathogenesis**
      a. Aspiration of gastric acid causes chemical injury to the tracheobronchial mucosa, which may trigger bronchospasm and predispose patients to chronic respiratory tract infection.
      b. Reflux of gastric acid into an inflamed esophagus may also produce reflex bronchospasm and potentiate bronchoconstriction from other triggers via a vagally mediated pathway (2).
      c. Medications that decrease lower esophageal sphincter pressure may produce or exacerbate GERD and its associated pulmonary disease
         i. Common medications include antihistamines, antiparkinsonian agents, calcium channel blockers, nitrates, and tricyclic antidepressants.
         ii. Among some asthmatics, methylxanthines and β-agonists may produce GERD and paradoxically exacerbate bronchospasm through this mechanism.
   3. **Approach to diagnosis**
      a. Although radiographic esophageal studies and endoscopy are widely available tools for diagnosis of GERD, they cannot determine whether GERD is the cause of respiratory symptoms. Ambulatory intraesophageal pH monitoring is the gold standard for determining the correlation between acid reflux and respiratory disease, but it may not be generally available. Similarly, radionuclide studies using technetium Tc 99m–labeled gastric contents are a sensitive means of detecting aspiration but are expensive and often unavailable.

b. With these considerations, a diagnostic algorithm (2) is suggested:

    i. Empiric medical treatment of patients with classic symptoms of GERD.

    ii. For other patients, ambulatory intraesophageal pH monitoring with recording of respiratory events by patient, if available.

    iii. If ambulatory intraesophageal pH monitoring is unavailable, esophagram or endoscopy of patients with atypical symptoms or inadequate response to medical therapy.

    iv. If radiographic and endoscopic studies are indeterminant in these patients or if patients with positive studies do not respond to medical treatment,

        (a) Perform radioisotope aspiration studies in patients with abnormal chest radiographs.

        (b) Perform pulmonary function testing before and after intraesophageal acid provocation in patients with normal chest radiographs.

4. Management

    a. Conventional antireflux measures, including elevating the head of the bed 4–6 inches, eliminating caffeine, and avoiding food for several hours before bed, are recommended for all patients with GERD.

    b. Drug therapy with omeprazole 20 mg/d PO is more effective than H_2-blockers for GERD, although experience with treatment of respiratory symptoms with omeprazole is limited (2). Because approximately one-third of patients require doses >20 mg/d for maximal effect, the dose should be increased to 40 mg/d if symptoms have not improved after 2 weeks. A full 12-week course of treatment is recommended before the final effect on respiratory symptoms should be assessed (2). Cisapride 10–20 mg TID may be an effective adjunctive treatment; in one study, this agent improved asthma, when combined with conventional antireflux measures (3).

    c. Surgical repair (laparoscopic fundoplication) may be the procedure of choice for severely symptomatic patients (2). Although surgery has been shown to be superior to H_2-blockers, no controlled trials have yet to compare surgery to medical therapy with the more effective agents, omeprazole and cisapride.

B. Hepatic cirrhosis. Hepatic cirrhosis is the most prevalent chronic liver disease in the United States and is associated with respiratory disease in up to 45% of affected individuals. The most significant pulmonary manifestations are arterial hypoxemia from the hepatopulmonary syndrome, pleural effusion, and pulmonary hypertension.

    1. Hypoxemia (hepatopulmonary syndrome)

        a. Clinical presentation. Most patients with cirrhosis have mild arterial hypoxemia and hemoglobin desaturation, with minimal or absent pulmonary symptoms, normal pulmonary function, and a normal chest radiograph. However, a small percentage of patients present with severe hypoxemia associated with profound dyspnea, cyanosis, and clubbing.

        i. Hypoxemia may worsen with exercise and with change from supine to standing position (orthodeoxia); it may also be associated with dyspnea from changing in position (platypnea) (4).

        ii. Digital clubbing and cutaneous spider nevi are often present. The latter are considered to be a marker of systemic vascular involvement in hepatic cirrhosis (5).

        iii. Chest radiographs may demonstrate nodular pulmonary infiltrates in the lower lung fields.

        iv. The severity of the pulmonary manifestations usually parallels the severity of the underlying liver disease.

        b. Relevant pathogenesis. Hypoxemia results from intrapulmonary vascular dilation and ineffective hypoxic pulmonary vasoconstriction producing right-to-left intrapulmonary shunting. The reversibility of arterial hypoxemia with liver transplantation in some patients (5) indicates that functional pulmonary vasodilation rather than anatomically fixed intrapulmonary shunting causes this syndrome. In addition, reversibility with liver transplantation suggests that this functional pulmonary vasodilation may be caused by increased concentrations of unknown vasodilators produced or inadequately catabolized by cirrhotic liver (5).

c. **Diagnosis**
   i. Arterial blood gases should be obtained while the patient is breathing room air and while breathing 100% oxygen in both supine and upright positions. Because any Pao_2 >100 Torr corresponds to hemoglobin saturations of 100%, oximetry does not suffice to determine arteriovenous shunt.
      (a). A Pao_2 >500 Torr while breathing 100% oxygen excludes the diagnosis of intrapulmonary shunt, while a Pao_2 <100 Torr indicates a true anatomic shunt (intracardiac or intrapulmonary).
      (b). A Pao_2 of 100–500 Torr suggests the need for further diagnostic studies to evaluate the possibility of a reversible functional intrapulmonary shunt (5,6).
   ii. Contrast-enhanced echocardiography is the preferred noninvasive procedure to document intrapulmonary shunting (5). Whereas microbubbles move immediately from the right to left heart chambers in an intracardiac shunt, the delayed appearance of microbubbles in the left heart chambers after three to six cardiac cycles supports an intrapulmonary shunt. Transesophageal echocardiography increases specificity by documenting the passage of microbubbles into the left atrium but presents undue risks in cirrhotic patients with esophageal varices.
   iii. Perfusion scanning using Tc 99m macroaggregated albumin can demonstrate right-to-left shunting by detecting passage of particles past the pulmonary capillary bed to the brain and kidney. However, perfusion scanning lacks the ability of echocardiography to distinguish between intrapulmonary and intracardiac shunts.
   iv. Pulmonary angiography excludes chronic pulmonary emboli as the cause of hypoxemia and may demonstrate large, discrete arteriovenous malformations that are best treated with embolization (5).

d. **Management**
   i. Drug therapy with either octreotide acetate (somatostatin) or indomethacin produces transient improvement in oxygenation but is of limited long-term benefit.
   ii. Percutaneous transcatheter embolization of large, discrete pulmonary arteriovenous malformations may improve refractory hypoxemia (7).
   iii. Liver transplantation should be considered for patients with hepatopulmonary syndrome who have a room-air Pao_2 >50 Torr and show a fourfold improvement in oxygenation while breathing 100% oxygen (5,6).

2. **Pleural effusion** occurs in 5% to 10% of cirrhotic patients and is termed *hepatic hydrothorax*.
   a. **Clinical presentation.** Most pleural effusions are small to moderate and asymptomatic. Occasionally, an effusion is massive and can cause dyspnea and hypoxemia. Effusions may be right-sided or bilateral and are nearly always associated with ascites.
   b. **Relevant pathogenesis.** The underlying mechanism of pleural effusion in the setting of cirrhosis is the development of anatomic diaphragmatic defects that permit one-way transfer of ascitic fluid into the pleural space due to negative pleural pressures (8,9). In some cases, ascites may not be clinically evident but can be demonstrated by computed tomography (CT) or ultrasonography.

   c. Diagnosis. Small unilateral or bilateral effusions in association with ascites do not require thoracentesis in the asymptomatic patient. For large effusions or in symptomatic patients, simultaneous thoracentesis and paracentesis are recommended. Both pleural and ascitic fluids should be transudative with similar, though not necessarily identical, chemistries (9).

   d. Management. Palliation of symptomatic effusions in cirrhotic patients is often difficult.

   i. Because negative intrapleural pressures favor the transudation of even small amounts of ascitic fluid into the pleural cavity, treatment of ascites with conventional measures of restricting dietary sodium and promoting diuresis with spironolactone and furosemide often have limited effect on pleural effusions (9).

   ii. Palliative therapeutic thoracentesis provides only temporary relief, as effusions usually reaccumulate rapidly. Simultaneous paracentesis with thoracentesis may provide somewhat longer palliation (9).

   iii. Chest tube drainage, like thoracentesis, rarely provides lasting palliation and depletes protein, electrolytes, and intravascular volume.

   iv. Pleurodesis is often ineffective due to persistent fluid reaccumulation. However, it may be successful when combined with continuous positive airway pressure to produce positive intrapleural pressures and paracentesis to decrease the amount of ascitic fluid (10).

   v. Peritoneojugular shunts are often ineffective because the pressure gradient favors transfer of fluid across the diaphragm rather than through the shunt (9).

   vi. Direct surgical repair of diaphragmatic defects appears to be the only treatment providing lasting palliation. However, surgery has increased risk due to the underlying liver disease and should be reserved for patients who are very symptomatic and refractory to other treatments (9).

3. Pulmonary hypertension is a rare complication of cirrhosis, occurring in <1% of cirrhotic patients.

   a. Clinical presentation is similar to primary pulmonary hypertension with the insidious development of exertional dyspnea often progressing to right ventricular failure and death.

   b. Relevant pathogenesis is controversial. The association of pulmonary hypertension with portal hypertension and specifically with portacaval shunt procedures (11), and its reversal with liver transplantation (12), suggest the involvement of unidentified humoral mediators that are not inactivated by the diseased liver.

   c. Diagnosis is similar to that of primary pulmonary hypertension (see chapter 17).

   d. Management. In addition to treatments used for primary pulmonary hypertension (see chapter 17), liver transplantation may produce resolution of pulmonary hypertension in some patients (12).

C. Acute pancreatitis. Pulmonary complications are among the most frequent and serious complications of acute pancreatitis and account for >50% of deaths from pancreatitis (13). The three most common types of pulmonary involvement in pancreatitis are hypoxemia with a normal chest radiograph, pleural effusion, and adult respiratory distress syndrome (ARDS).

   1. Hypoxemia with a normal chest radiograph is associated more often with pancreatitis than with any other intra-abdominal inflammatory process. Hypoxemia is usually mild, and patients are typically asymptomatic; however, profound hypoxemia occasionally occurs. The crucial clinical observation is that a normal chest radiograph does not preclude marked arterial hypoxemia in patients with acute pancreatitis. Although poorly understood, hypoxemia appears to be caused by perfusion of poorly ventilating alveolar units and is corrected with supplemental oxygen (14). Consequently, supplemental oxygen should be administered to maintain PaO_2 >70 Torr.

2. **Pleural effusion** is noted in approximately 25% of patients with active pancreatitis.
   a. **Clinical presentation**
      i. **Acute effusions** are typically asymptomatic, small to moderate in size, and left-sided. Acute effusions usually resolve spontaneously with resolution of pancreatitis and do not require specific treatment.
      ii. **Chronic effusions** are more commonly symptomatic with dyspnea, chest discomfort, and dry, nonproductive cough (15). Chronic effusions are more often large to massive left-sided effusions and require drainage. They may occur several months after the episode of pancreatitis and may pose a diagnostic puzzle when the antecedent episode of pancreatitis was not clinically evident.
   b. **Relevant pathogenesis** of acute effusion involves increased permeability of thoracic diaphragmatic lymphatics from proteolysis due to released pancreatic enzymes, increased permeability of diaphragm capillaries due to subdiaphragmatic inflammation, and movement of peripancreatic exudates through diaphragm pores or through the esophageal or aortic hiatus (16). In addition to these mechanisms, large chronic effusions can develop from pancreatic fistula formation or rupture of a pseudocyst into the left hemithorax.
   c. **Diagnosis**
      i. Thoracentesis is usually performed for acute effusion to exclude infection in the acutely ill patient with pancreatitis. Acute effusions are usually serosanguinous and exudative with amylase concentrations higher than serum levels. In contrast, chronic effusions can be bloody, serosanguinous, or purulent exudates. Amylase concentrations are highly elevated (>100,000 U/mL).
      ii. Abdominal CT scan and ultrasonography may help in the diagnosis of chronic pancreatic effusions by demonstrating pancreatic inflammation, abscess, or pseudocyst.
   d. **Management.** While acute effusions usually resolve spontaneously with supportive treatment of acute pancreatitis, chronic effusions require drainage via repeated thoracentesis or chest tube.
      i. Drainage of effusions should be supplemented by medical treatment. Patients should receive total parenteral nutrition and agents to suppress pancreatic secretion, such as cimetidine (17).
      ii. Effusions resulting from pancreatopleural fistulas require surgical management of the fistulas (17).
      iii. Chronic effusions occasionally produce restrictive pleural thickening that requires decortication.
3. **ARDS** occurs in 8% of patients with acute pancreatitis and is the most important fatal complication of this disease. The mechanisms of ARDS in pancreatitis remain unclear, but neutrophil-generated toxic oxygen products appear to play a major role (18). In addition, circulating nonpancreatic synovial-type phospholipase A_2 affecting pulmonary microvasculature, or catabolized pulmonary surfactant (19), may be involved. Although specific therapies may be developed to counter these mechanisms, management of ARDS in pancreatitis is identical to that in acute lung injury from other causes (see chapter 19).

II. **Renal diseases**
   A. **Chronic renal failure** is associated with prominent pulmonary manifestations, including pulmonary edema, pleural effusion, and pulmonary calcification.
      1. **Pulmonary edema**
         a. Pulmonary edema in chronic renal failure is usually precipitated by hypervolemia. Cardiac disease is also very common in chronic renal diseases due to associated diabetes, anemia, atherosclerotic coronary vascular disease, and possibly uremic cardiomyopathy. Additional precipitating factors in these patients include hypertension and hypoalbuminemia.

b. Uremia may also directly produce pulmonary edema in some patients by increasing alveolar capillary permeability, causing uremic pneumonitis (20), although this association remains controversial. Uremic pneumonitis is reported to progress to interstitial fibrosis in approximately 70% of untreated cases.

c. Pulmonary edema in chronic renal disease responds to dialysis, which improves infiltrates and dyspnea in oliguric patients.

2. Pleural disease

    a. As with pulmonary edema, pleural effusion in chronic renal disease is commonly transudative due to hypervolemia or congestive heart failure.

    b. In addition, **uremic pleuritis** is recognized as a common cause of pleural disease in these patients, with a prevalence estimated at 20% to 40% in autopsy studies (20).

        i. Clinical presentation. Most patients are asymptomatic, but some present with pleuritic pain and friction rubs. Pleural effusion may be large and bilateral.

        ii. Relevant pathogenesis. Although the mechanisms of uremia-induced inflammation remain unknown, the development of uremic pleuritis does not correlate with the adequacy, duration, or delay of dialysis (21).

    c. Diagnosis. Thoracentesis usually shows serosanguinous fluid that is transudative. If hemorrhage into the pleural space has occurred, the fluid becomes exudative and lymphocytic, although fluid-shifts during dialysis can dilute chemistries so that they appear transudative. Pleural biopsy may reveal nonspecific findings of chronic inflammation, organized fibrinous exudate, or granulation tissue. However, neither pleural fluid nor biopsy findings are diagnostic.

    d. Management. Uremic pleuritis usually resolves spontaneously within weeks (21). Dialysis may relieve symptoms by reducing pleural fluid but does not hasten resolution of pleuritis. Very rarely, uremic pleuritis progresses to fibrothorax requiring decortication.

3. Pulmonary calcification

    a. Clinical presentation. Pulmonary calcification is an extremely common pulmonary manifestation of chronic renal disease (22), although usually asymptomatic and undetectible by chest radiograph. When symptomatic, patients present with dyspnea and arterial hypoxemia. Chest radiographs reveal nodular infiltrates, with nodules typically <2 mm in diameter. Pulmonary function testing shows restrictive physiology.

    b. Relevant pathogenesis. Metastatic calcification along alveolar and vascular basement membranes, with associated pericalcific fibrosis, produces restrictive lung disease and radiographic infiltrates (22). Age, underlying renal disease, and duration of dialysis do not correlate with pulmonary deposition of calcium.

    c. Diagnosis

        i. The stability of chest-radiographic infiltrates over time suggests a noninfectious etiology.

        ii. Scintigraphic scanning with Tc 99m pyrophosphate that concentrates in calcium deposits in the involved lung supports the diagnosis, although the sensitivity and specificity of this test remain controversial (23,24).

        iii. When the diagnosis is in doubt and infection must be excluded, transbronchoscopic or open lung biopsy is required.

    d. Management is usually not very effective. Restriction of dietary vitamin D and calcium may prevent progression of the pulmonary disease. Renal transplantation may be beneficial but can paradoxically cause rapid progression of pulmonary calcification (25).

B. Goodpasture's syndrome is the prototypical pulmonary–renal syndrome. Whereas most systemic diseases causing pulmonary–renal syndromes are vasculitides (see chapter 28), Goodpasture's syndrome produces diffuse pulmonary hemorrhage and progressive glomerulonephritis by a unique mechanism.

1. **Clinical presentation**
   a. Goodpasture's syndrome is most common in young white men 15–30 years old, who typically present with hemoptysis and dyspnea. The diagnosis is suggested by concurrent renal dysfunction, but pulmonary symptoms precede overt renal disease by days or weeks at least half of the time (26).
   b. The chest radiograph shows bilateral airspace disease with mixed interstitial infiltrates or alveolar infiltrates similar to pulmonary edema. Very dense infiltrates may appear and resolve within days, corresponding to the onset and cessation of pulmonary hemorrhage. Occasionally, residual reticulonodular infiltrates develop from recurrent hemorrhage.
   c. Pulmonary hemorrhage produces rapidly progressive hypoxemia and iron deficiency anemia.
   d. Extrarenal involvement other than pulmonary disease is rare with Goodpasture's disease and suggests vasculitis. A pulmonary–renal syndrome in a female patient with evidence of serositis strongly suggests systemic lupus erythematosus.

2. **Relevant pathogenesis.** Goodpasture's syndrome results from circulating anti–glomerular basement membrane (AGBM) antibodies against type IV collagen located in the kidney and lung. Inflammatory responses to AGBM antibodies produce diffuse pulmonary hemorrhage and rapidly progressive glomerulonephritis (26).

3. **Diagnosis** entails distinguishing pulmonary hemorrhage from infection or pulmonary edema and differentiating Goodpasture's syndrome from other etiologies of pulmonary–renal syndrome.
   a. **Measurement of diffusing capacity for carbon monoxide** (DLCO). A rise of >30% in the DLCO over 48 hours supports the diagnosis of pulmonary hemorrhage. The hemoglobin binds carbon monoxide, resulting in an apparent increase in diffusion. In contrast, infection or edema typically decreases the DLCO (27).
   b. **CT and magnetic resonance (MR) imaging.** CT is generally superior to chest radiography in identifying localized hemorrhage. MR imaging may have increased sensitivity for diagnosing pulmonary hemorrhage by detecting parenchymal hemosiderin (26,28), although the role of this procedure in the evaluation of pulmonary hemorrhage has not been fully determined.
   c. **Bronchoscopy.** When bronchoscopy is performed to exclude infection, hemorrhage is indicated by hemosiderin-laden macrophages in bronchoalveolar lavage fluid.
   d. **Serology**
      i. Serum should be tested for circulating AGBM antibodies. The current enzyme-linked immunosorbent assay methods are more sensitive than previous methods, and a high or rising titer has a diagnostic specificity of 95% (26). However, serum titers do not always correlate with the degree of pulmonary injury, and titers may not rise despite massive pulmonary hemorrhage. (In contrast, falling antibody titers nearly always correspond to improving renal function.)
      ii. Serum should also be screened for antinuclear antibody, anti–double-stranded DNA, serum complement, and antineutrophil cytoplasmic antibody to evaluate for other causes of pulmonary–renal syndrome.
   e. **Tissue** should be obtained for immunofluorescent studies if serology results will not be available rapidly or are nondiagnostic. Immunofluorescent stains demonstrating linear deposits of AGBM antibodies along the glomerular basement membrane are diagnostic. Renal biopsy is superior to lung biopsy, as the latter is not essential to establish the diagnosis and is less likely to be diagnostic (26). If the lung is to be biopsied, open lung

biopsy is preferred to transbronchial biopsy, which frequently yields inadequate tissue and false-negative results (26).

4. **Management.** The high mortality from Goodpasture's syndrome can be reduced to approximately 50% if early treatment is begun. In a patient with pulmonary hemorrhage, histology from a renal biopsy documenting necrotizing proliferative crescentic glomerulopathy is sufficient to initiate treatment before definitive immunofluorescent stains are completed (27).

   a. Daily plasmapheresis (four exchanges every 1–3 days) is the mainstay of treatment for patients with circulating AGBM antibodies (26,29).

   b. Nonoliguric patients should receive prednisone 1–2 mg/kg/d and cyclophosphamide 2–3 mg/kg/d. Oliguric patients and those with serum creatinine >6 mg/dL respond poorly (29), and aggressive immunosuppressive therapy may not be warranted in these patients.

   c. Renal transplantation may be considered for patients not responding to medical treatment as long as circulating AGBM antibodies are no longer present (29).

III. **Connective tissue diseases**

A. **Rheumatoid arthritis** (RA) is the most common connective tissue disease, affecting 2% of people in the United States. Pulmonary disease is second only to infection as the most frequent cause of death in patients with RA. Pulmonary involvement in RA exemplifies the range of pulmonary disease associated with connective tissue diseases and has several notable features. First, pleuropulmonary involvement is more common in patients with active RA, and 80% of patients with lung disease have positive rheumatoid titers. However, pulmonary disease may precede systemic arthritis by months, presenting a diagnostic puzzle in such cases. Second, although RA typically afflicts women in their third to sixth decade, pulmonary manifestations are at least twice as common in men with RA. Third, almost half of patients with RA demonstrate abnormalities on pulmonary function testing or chest radiographs, although only 5% of patients with RA have respiratory symptoms.

Of the myriad pulmonary manifestations of RA, the most characteristic include pleural disease, necrobiotic nodules with or without associated pneumoconiosis, obstructive airways disease, interstitial disease, bronchiolitis obliterans, cricoarytenoid disease, and bronchiectasis.

1. **Pleural disease**

   a. **Clinical presentation**

      i. Pleural disease is the most common pulmonary manifestation of RA. Approximately 20% of patients have pleural effusion on chest radiographs; however, up to 75% of patients have evidence of pleural involvement at autopsy (30).

      ii. Effusions are usually small, right-sided, and asymptomatic and are typically found incidentally on chest radiographs.

      iii. Pleural disease is more common in patients with subcutaneous nodules, high rheumatoid factor titers, and active arthritis.

      iv. Effusions typically resolve over weeks with systemic treatment of RA. Occasionally, effusions can persist as chronic or recurrent disease.

   b. **Diagnosis**

      i. Thoracentesis is necessary to rule out secondary bacterial infection and malignancy.

      ii. Effusions are typically exudative, lymphocytic, and occasionally bloody. Chronic effusions may be pseudochylous due to a very high cholesterol content.

      iii. Distinguishing pleural fluid characteristics include:

         (a) **Low pleural fluid glucose** (<25 mg/dL) in >80% of rheumatoid effusions, which does not increase with intravenous glucose infusion (30).

         (b) **High lactate dehydrogenase** (often >1000 U/L).

         (c) **Positive pleural fluid rheumatoid factor,** with titers that may exceed serum levels.

(d) **Pleural RA cells**, which are macrophages containing cytoplasmic inclusions with phagocytosed immune complexes.

(e) However, none of these characteristics is sensitive or specific enough to be diagnostic for rheumatoid effusions (30).

iv. Although rarely indicated, pleural biopsy may reveal pleural rheumatoid nodules which are diagnostic.

c. **Management**

i. Most rheumatoid effusions are asymptomatic and resolve spontaneously. For symptomatic effusions, systemic steroids (prednisone 0.5–1 mg/kg/d) with repeated thoracentesis or chest tube drainage may speed resolution. Intrapleural administration of steroids does not provide additional benefit over systemic treatment and may increase the risk of secondary pleural infection (31).

ii. Rarely, pleurodesis with talc slurry may be required for palliation of recurrent effusions. Surgical decortication is rarely necessary.

2. **Pulmonary necrobiotic nodules**

a. **Clinical presentation**

i. Necrobiotic nodules are peripheral parenchymal nodules, ranging in diameter from a few millimeters up to 7 cm, that are histologically identical to subcutaneous rheumatoid nodules. Usually multiple nodules are present, and they may wax and wane with the activity of the underlying RA, progressing to cavitation in 50% to 70% of patients (31). Rarely, necrobiotic nodules precede systemic manifestations of RA.

ii. Small necrobiotic nodules are usually asymptomatic unless they cavitate, which may cause productive cough and hemoptysis. Large nodules may cause compressive symptoms. Nodules can be superinfected by bacteria or by aspergillosis, occasionally eroding into the pleura to produce bronchopleural fistula.

b. **Diagnosis**

i. Multiple nodules in patients with active RA and subcutaneous nodules do not require further evaluation and can be observed.

ii. Solitary nodules require biopsy, usually by transthoracic needle, to exclude malignancy.

iii. Because samples obtained by needle biopsy are often insufficient to establish the diagnosis of rheumatoid nodules, open lung biopsy is usually required to diagnose necrobiotic nodules in patients without systemic manifestations of RA.

c. **Management**

i. Specific therapy is not required in asymptomatic patients, as necrobiotic nodules usually resolve either spontaneously or with treatment of RA (31).

ii. Symptomatic nodules are frequently treated with systemic corticosteroids (prednisone 1 mg/kg/d). Patients on steroid therapy should be followed closely, as steroids have been reported to cause clinical deterioration in this condition (32).

3. **Caplan's syndrome** is a variant of rheumatoid necrobiotic nodules occurring in association with pneumoconiosis. Caplan first described this association in South Wales coal miners with rheumatoid disease, but exposure to iron, silicates, asbestos, or aluminum can produce a similar syndrome. For unclear reasons, this disease is uncommon in North America, and most reports come from Europe (32). Diagnosis can be made by biopsy showing the offending mineral within the necrobiotic nodule. The clinical presentation and management are identical to those discussed above for necrobiotic nodules.

4. **Interstitial lung disease (ILD)**

a. **Clinical presentation**

i. Diffuse interstitial pneumonitis or fibrosis clinically indistinguishable from idiopathic pulmonary fibrosis (IPF) occurs in <5% of patients with RA. However, ILD is the most serious pulmonary complication of RA (32). ILD usually occurs in middle-aged men with seropositive RA, and arthritis precedes lung involvement in >90% of cases. However, no correlation has been found between the severity of ILD and either the level of rheumatoid factor *or* the duration or severity of RA.

    ii. ILD presents with **clinical features similar to IPF** (see chapter 22). Rheumatoid-associated ILD is usually mild but can progress to fatal pulmonary fibrosis.

    iii. Typically, ILD presents radiographically as **bibasilar reticulonodular infiltrates** than can progress to honeycombing in late stages of disease. However, chest radiographs may be normal in 40% of patients with rheumatoid ILD. High-resolution CT (HRCT) may improve radiographic detection of ILD, but the clinical significance of CT findings in the absence of infiltrates on chest radiographs is unknown.

    iv. Pulmonary function testing shows restrictive physiology, reduced D_LCO, and arterial hypoxemia worsening with exercise.

  b. **Relevant pathogenesis** involves pulmonary inflammation directed at IgM antibodies and rheumatoid factor deposited in pulmonary arterioles and alveolar walls.

  c. **Diagnosis**

    i. When performed to exclude infection, **bronchoalveolar lavage** (BAL) shows variable patterns of inflammatory cells; either lymphocytes or neutrophils may predominate. The presence of appreciable numbers of eosinophils in BAL fluid is associated with a worse prognosis (33). However, because BAL findings do not generally influence therapy, this procedure is **not routinely indicated** for rheumatoid ILD (31).

    ii. A **lung biopsy** should be performed if presumed rheumatoid ILD persists or progresses despite appropriate treatment. HRCT can guide either transbronchoscopic or open lung biopsy to areas of ground-glass opacity, which have highest yield (31).

      (a) Rheumatoid ILD produces a wide spectrum of histologic findings that vary with the stage of disease. These include rheumatoid nodules, interstitial pneumonitis, bronchiolitis obliterans with obstructing pneumonitis, lymphoid hyperplasia, and cellular interstitial infiltrates (34). Of these, only nodules are specific for rheumatoid ILD.

      (b) **Immunofluorescent stains** may show IgM and rheumatoid factor deposits in pulmonary arterioles and alveolar walls, as well as adjacent to nodular lesions (35).

  d. **Management**

    i. **Daily high-dose steroids (prednisone 1–2 mg/kg)** may be effective if used in the early stages of disease and should be started if evidence of vasculitis or circulating immune complexes is present. Prognosis is poor in advanced interstitial disease, which is usually refractory to all therapy (36).

    ii. **Immunosuppressive treatment** with **azathioprine** should be considered for ILD that reactivates after steroid therapy is tapered or does not respond to steroids. **Cyclophosphamide** can be used in these cases, but is less efficacious and has a greater incidence of side effects. Methotrexate has not been proven effective for systemic manifestations of RA and can itself produce life-threatening pneumonitis (31).

5. **Proliferative bronchiolitis obliterans with/without organizing pneumonia (BOOP)** is more common and more responsive to therapy than is constrictive obliterative bronchiolitis (discussed below).

  a. **Clinical presentation**

    i. In contrast to most pulmonary manifestations of RA, proliferative bronchiolitis obliterans typically afflicts women 45–75 years old, usually after the onset of arthritis.

ii. Patients present with a subacute illness characterized by cough, dyspnea, rales, and wheezing that may be preceded by a flu-like illness in up to one-third of patients. Peripheral eosinophilia may be present.

iii. Chest radiographic findings are nonspecific, ranging from normal to bilateral patchy ground-glass or linear infiltrates.

iv. Pulmonary function testing shows restrictive physiology with decreased DLCO.

  b. Diagnosis. Open lung biopsy establishes the diagnosis in the appropriate clinical context and is usually done to exclude infection if illness does not respond to empiric antibiotics.

  c. Management. Corticosteroids can produce dramatic resolution of proliferative bronchiolitis and BOOP (37). However, the prognosis for recovery is generally poor in chronic cases of proliferative bronchiolitis.

6. **Constrictive obliterative bronchiolitis**
   a. **Clinical presentation.** In contrast to proliferative bronchiolitis and BOOP, patients present with acute cough and dyspnea. Furthermore, pulmonary function testing usually shows obstructive physiology with a normal D_LCO, although mixed obstructive/restrictive disease is occasionally noted.
   b. **Relevant pathogenesis.** Constrictive obliterative bronchiolitis has been associated with penicillamine and intramuscular gold treatments. An idiopathic form is also reported.
   c. **Diagnosis** usually requires open lung biopsy, although it is occasionally made with transbronchoscopic biopsy.
   d. **Management** includes aggressive treatment with pulsed intravenous methylprednisolone in conjunction with azathioprine or cyclophosphamide. However, the prognosis is generally poor despite aggressive therapy (38).

7. **Cricoarytenoid disease** is an important respiratory tract complication that occurs in up to 25% of patients with RA (39). Patients complain of throat fullness, hoarseness, stridor, or pain that radiates to the ears during speech or swallowing. By interfering with effective swallowing, rheumatoid cricoarytenoid disease increases the risk of aspiration pneumonitis. More important, progressive involvement may cause upper airway obstruction, especially during upper respiratory infection, which requires emergency tracheostomy. Mild cases may respond to treatment with steroids, whereas advanced cases may require elective arytenoid excision (39).

8. **Obstructive airways disease** is observed in up to a one-third of nonsmoking patients with RA, and the prevalence is further increased in association with smoking, secondary Sjögren's syndrome, HLA-DR4 antigen, or non-MM phenotype of α_1-antitrypsin (31). Airways disease may be caused by rheumatoid bronchiolitis, follicular bronchitis, decreased mucociliary clearance, or other unknown factors. Management includes the use of β-agonist bronchodilators and corticosteroids (31).

9. **Bronchiectasis,** as with forms of bronchiolitis, is typically found in middle-aged women with seropositive RA. Although the prevalence of rheumatoid bronchiectasis does not correlate with the severity of the underlying RA, it rarely precedes arthritis. Chest radiographs show bibasilar diffusely increased interstitial markings and focal infiltrates, and the diagnosis can be established by HRCT. Bronchiectasis may improve with administration of oral steroids.

10. **Pulmonary hypertension** is rare in RA, in contrast to other connective tissue diseases. It occasionally occurs in advanced stages of rheumatoid ILD and may improve with steroids, cytotoxic agents, and vasodilators.

11. **Apical fibrocavitary disease** occurs in <6% of patients with RA and may occur without other manifestations of RA. Its clinical presentation and manage-

ment are similar to those of apical fibrocavitary disease from ankylosing spondylitis.

B. **Systemic lupus erythematosus (SLE)** is an autoimmune disorder of unknown etiology with a marked predilection for women aged 20–40 years; it is more commonly found in African-Americans. Pulmonary involvement occurs in up to 70% of patients with SLE at some point during the course of disease. However, primary pulmonary disease from SLE must be differentiated from secondary pulmonary involvement due to infection, congestive heart failure, aspiration, and drug-induced complications. Of these, infection is the most frequent cause of pulmonary mortality and must be aggressively evaluated in the acutely ill febrile patient with pulmonary infiltrates. Primary pulmonary involvement from SLE includes pleural disease, lupus pneumonitis, and pulmonary hemorrhage.

1. **Pleural disease** is the most common form of pulmonary involvement in SLE, occurring in up to 75% of SLE patients. **All young women presenting with the new onset of pleurisy or pleural effusion should be evaluated for SLE.**

    a. **Clinical presentation**

        i. Pleuritis occurs in up to 50% of patients with pleural involvement, may flare during exacerbations, and is the initial presentation of SLE in one-third of cases. Pleuritic chest pain is usually localized to the costophrenic margins either unilaterally or bilaterally. Pleuritic pain is often accompanied by fever, dyspnea, productive cough, and a pleural friction rub.

        ii. Pleural effusions are usually small to moderate and bilateral but may be massive and unilateral.

    b. **Diagnosis**

        i. The differential diagnosis of effusions in patients with known SLE includes infection and pulmonary embolism. Bilateral effusions are unlikely to result from either of these diseases and often do not require evaluation by thoracentesis.

        ii. SLE effusions are usually clear or serosanguinous; grossly bloody fluid is uncommon. The fluid is exudative with a normal to high glucose.

        iii. Pleural total complement and components C3 and C4 are decreased or undetectible in 80% of SLE effusions. However, these findings are not diagnostic of SLE, as they also occur with RA and other connective tissue diseases. Pleural fluid antinuclear antibodies (ANA) are almost always present in SLE effusions and may exceed serum levels, but this test is also not diagnostic. The presence of LE cells in pleural fluid but not in blood is the most specific test for SLE or drug-induced SLE pleuritis; however, it lacks sensitivity.

    c. **Management.** Mild cases may respond to nonsteroidal anti-inflammatory agents. More symptomatic patients usually respond to systemic corticosteroids. Rarely, pleural sclerosis is necessary to palliate refractory effusions (40).

2. **Acute lupus pneumonitis** is a less common pulmonary manifestation of SLE, occurring in approximately 10% of cases, but it carries a high mortality.

    a. **Clinical presentation**

        i. Patients present with the acute onset of high fever, nonproductive cough, extreme dyspnea, pleuritic chest pain, and occasionally hemoptysis. Although pneumonitis may be the initial presentation of SLE, it always occurs in the setting of multiorgan disease. Physical findings can be surprisingly minimal.

        ii. Laboratory tests show leukocytosis, elevated erythrocyte sedimentation rate, hypoxemia, and respiratory alkalosis.

        iii. Chest radiographs characteristically reveal bibasilar alveolar infiltrates, occasionally accompanied by small pleural effusions. However, infiltrates can be localized to one lobe or to one side or be patchy.

    b. **Diagnosis.** Lupus pneumonitis is a diagnosis of exclusion, and patients should be aggressively evaluated to rule out infection.

    i. If sputum and blood cultures are nondiagnostic, bronchoscopy with BAL and transbronchial biopsy should be performed.

    ii. The purpose of bronchoscopy is to exclude infection, not to diagnose lupus pneumonitis. Histologic findings of interstitial pneumonia, edema, and arteriolar thrombi may be seen but are nonspecific. Immunofluorescent stains may reveal granular deposits of immunoglobulin and complement in alveolar walls, blood vessels, and interstitium, but findings are not diagnostic (41).

c. Management

    i. Empiric broad-spectrum antibiotic therapy should be initiated until infection is definitively ruled out.

    ii. Because the treatment of lupus pneumonitis has not been evaluated in controlled studies, therapeutic recommendations are derived from the accepted management of other major organ involvement in SLE (41).

       (a) Mild-to-moderate disease should be treated with prednisone 1 mg/kg/d.

       (b) Severe disease requires pulsed methylprednisolone sodium succinate 1 g/d IV for 3 days, with the addition of cyclophosphamide (2 mg/kg/d) or plasma exchange.

    iii. Although dramatic improvement can occur with steroid therapy, mortality as high as 50% is reported despite treatment (42).

3. ILD occurs in 3% of SLE patients and may follow episodes of acute lupus pneumonitis or develop insidiously.

a. Clinical presentation is similar to that for RA-associated ILD.

    i. Patients present with chronic, nonproductive cough, dyspnea on exertion, and recurrent pleuritic chest pain. Physical examination reveals dry end-inspiratory rales.

    ii. Pulmonary function testing shows restrictive physiology with reduced D_LCO.

    iii. Chest radiographs demonstrate patchy and irregular bilateral reticulonodular infiltrates that may progress to honeycombing but rarely to extensive interstitial fibrosis.

b. Diagnosis can be established by immunofluorescent staining of lung biopsy samples, which reveals patchy and lumpy deposits of IgG in alveolar walls.

c. Management, as with that for rheumatoid ILD, is generally ineffective.

4. Pulmonary hemorrhage is a rare but serious complication of SLE, with mortality rates of 50% to 90% (41). Although occurring in only 1% to 2% of patients with SLE, pulmonary hemorrhage is the cause of death in nearly 15% of patients (43).

a. Clinical presentation

    i. Patients present with the abrupt onset of fever, dyspnea, hypoxemia, and bilateral alveolar infiltrates.

    ii. Hemoptysis occurs in a minority of cases (43), and the amount of hemoptysis does not correlate with severity of hemorrhage.

    iii. An unexplained precipitous drop in hemoglobin (2–4 g/dL over 24–48 hours) without other identified source of blood loss suggests pulmonary hemorrhage.

b. Relevant pathogenesis

    i. SLE pulmonary hemorrhage can occur by immune or nonimmune mechanisms. The immune type occurs in the setting of systemic vasculitis. Granular deposits of immune complexes and complement in the alveolar septa and pulmonary blood vessels attract and activate neutrophils, which release toxins producing hemorrhage.

    ii. Nonimmune pulmonary hemorrhage in SLE is related to infections, pulmonary edema, uremia, coagulopathy, or oxygen toxicity (44).

c. Diagnosis

    i. Diagnostic considerations include establishing the presence of pulmonary hemorrhage and determining its cause. Because immune-mediated pulmonary hemorrhage is rare in SLE, the first priority, once hemorrhage is recognized, is to aggressively rule out nonimmune causes of hemorrhage, especially infection.

    ii. Measurement of DLCO may differentiate between pulmonary hemorrhage and pneumonia or pulmonary edema. DLCO is increased in hemorrhage due to the intra-alveolar blood binding increased amounts of carbon monoxide, whereas it is decreased in pneumonia and edema (41).

    iii. MR imaging has a high sensitivity for diagnosing pulmonary hemorrhage by detecting parenchymal hemosiderin. The role of MR imaging in the evaluation of this disease has not been established (28).

    iv. When BAL is performed, a bloody lavage with hemosiderin-laden macrophages supports the diagnosis of alveolar hemorrhage but is nonspecific for immune-mediated hemorrhage.

    v. Bronchoscopy with BAL and possibly transbronchoscopic biopsy are indicated to rule out infection.

    vi. If bronchoscopic studies are nondiagnostic, open lung biopsy may be required to exclude infection.

  d. Management

    i. Pulsed intravenous methylprednisolone or high-dose steroids (prednisone 1–2 mg/kg/d) should be given, especially if there is evidence of systemic vasculitis or nephritis.

    ii. Azathioprine and cyclophosphamide may also be used but are without definite evidence of efficacy in SLE pulmonary hemorrhage.

    iii. Plasmapheresis may be beneficial in some patients if circulating antibodies are demonstrated.

    iv. Despite treatment with these agents, mortality may still be >50% (41).

  5. Pulmonary thromboembolism occurs in 5% to 12% of patients with SLE. Risk factors include chronic low-grade disseminated intravascular coagulation, small-vessel angiitis, prolonged bed rest, and lupus anticoagulant. Lupus anticoagulant, found in up to 25% of patients with SLE, is an anticardiolipin antibody that interferes with phospholipid involved in prothrombin activation, thus prolonging the activated partial thromboplastin time. In contrast to this *in vitro* effect, lupus anticoagulant is associated with arterial and venous thrombosis and recurrent pulmonary emboli, which may eventually lead to pulmonary hypertension (45). Consequently, long-term anticoagulant therapy is required for such patients.

  6. Diaphragmatic and respiratory muscle dysfunction. Patients with SLE who complain of dyspnea and have no parenchymal abnormalities on chest radiographs may suffer from the shrinking lung syndrome (46), characterized by small lung fields, bilateral hemidiaphragm elevation, and basilar atelectasis. These abnormalities result from diaphragmatic muscle weakness, not from malnutrition or steroid-induced myopathy. Diaphragmatic muscle weakness may occur in the absence of peripheral muscle weakness and correlates poorly with overall disease activity. Neither steroids nor other immunosuppressive agents have been efficacious in this disease (46).

C. Progressive systemic sclerosis (PSS) is a systemic form of scleroderma that occurs more commonly in women, with a peak incidence between ages 20 and 60 years. However, as with RA, pulmonary involvement is more common in men and usually occurs after the diagnosis of PSS is established. The lungs may be secondarily involved in PSS, and patients may present with aspiration pneumonitis from esophageal disease or with spontaneous pneumothorax from rupture of subpleural blebs. Primary pulmonary disease in PSS manifests as ILD or vascular disease (47).

  1. Interstitial lung disease

    a. Clinical presentation

      i. Most patients have nonproductive cough and dyspnea on exertion. Physical examination reveals dry bibasilar rales in 50% of patients. In addition, Raynaud's phenomenon is present in 90% of patients.

      ii. Chest radiographs characteristically show bilateral, lower lobe interstitial infiltrates and occasionally reveal evidence of bronchiectasis. Pulmonary calcinosis may be apparent, especially with the CREST (calcinosis, Raynaud's phenomena, esophageal disease, sclerodactyly, telangiectasia) variant of PSS. Although pleural disease is common at autopsy, it is usually not apparent by chest radiograph. Localized alveolar infiltrates may represent bronchogenic carcinoma, which has a higher incidence in patients with PSS.

    iii. Pulmonary function testing shows restrictive physiology and a reduced DLCO. A DLCO >40% is associated with a 5-year survival of >10% (48).

  b. **Relevant pathogenesis.** ILD results from vasculitis, as well as from an active alveolitis that progresses to fibrosis, and may also be associated with bronchiolectasis and subpleural cysts. The incidence of ILD is increased in patients with serum anti-Scl-70 antibody.

  c. **Diagnosis**

    i. **Serologic tests** are nonspecific but may support a diagnosis of PSS in the proper clinical context. ANA testing is positive, usually with a speckled pattern, in 50% to 90% of patients with PSS.

    ii. BAL, when done to exclude infection, shows increased neutrophils, eosinophils, and occasionally lymphocytes. However, these findings are nonspecific, and BAL is not routinely indicated in evaluating patients, unless bronchoalveolar cell carcinoma is considered a possibility.

    iii. Gallium scan is often positive in ILD from PSS and may predict a better response to therapy.

  d. **Management.** Therapy is supportive, as the course of the disease is usually indolent and rarely is the cause of death in PSS. For severely symptomatic patients, therapy with penicillamine may be beneficial (49). Corticosteroids are typically not effective.

 2. **Vascular disease**

  a. **Clinical presentation**

    i. Pulmonary vascular disease presenting as dyspnea on exertion is more commonly associated with the CREST variant of PSS.

    ii. In advanced disease, the physical findings are consistent with right heart failure.

    iii. Pulmonary function testing reveals a DLCO <45% of predicted, which correlates with pulmonary hypertension.

  b. **Relevant pathogenesis** includes vascular obliteration with intimal proliferation, medial hypertrophy, and myxomatous changes.

  c. **Diagnosis** is usually established by biopsy.

  d. **Management.** No therapy has been shown to be effective.

D. **Polymyositis/dermatomyositis** (PM/DM) are inflammatory diseases of striated muscles caused by lymphocytic infiltration of tissues by activated T lymphocytes. PM–DM occurs with a 2:1 female predominance and a peak incidence in patients 40–60 years old. In addition to primary forms, PM–DM may be secondary to malignancy or to other connective tissue disorders. Secondary pulmonary manifestations include aspiration pneumonitis due to pharyngeal muscle dysfunction in end-stage disease, and hypoventilation and atelectasis due to respiratory muscle weakness. Primary parenchymal involvement manifests predominantly as ILD (50).

 1. **Clinical presentation**

  a. ILD occurs in 5% to 10% of patients with PM/DM. The severity of pulmonary involvement is unrelated to the degree of muscle weakness, and pulmonary disease may precede skin and muscle changes by years (51).

  b. Patients may be asymptomatic or complain of dyspnea and nonproductive cough. Physical examination reveals end-inspiratory dry rales at both lung bases.

  c. Pulmonary function testing shows restrictive physiology with decreased DLCO. Due to respiratory muscle weakness, maximal inspiratory pressures may be profoundly decreased.

   d. The chest radiograph shows basilar reticulonodular infiltrates and fibrosis that may progress to honeycombing.
   2. Diagnosis of ILD in established cases of PM/DM depends on recognition of clinical features. Lung biopsy is occasionally required to exclude other causes of ILD. Histology shows bronchiolitis obliterans, interstitial fibrosis, and infiltration with lymphocytes, monocytes, and plasma cells. Immune deposition and vasculitis are not found. Anti-Jo-1 antibody has been found in patients with PM/DM and ILD, but the diagnostic value of this test has not been studied (52).
   3. Management. Overall, 50% of patients with ILD respond to steroids. Patients with histologic evidence of cellular infiltration of lung tissue respond particularly well to treatment.
E. Mixed connective tissue disease (MCTD) is an overlap syndrome with features of SLE, PSS, and PM/DM. The distinctive MCTD serology is that of a positive ANA test with a speckled pattern and a high titer of circulating antibodies to extractible nuclear ribonucleoprotein antigen (ENA). Pleuropulmonary disease occurs in 20% to 85% of patients and presents primarily as interstitial or vascular disease, with similar manifestations as discussed above for SLE, PSS, and PM/DM. The most serious pulmonary complication is progressive pulmonary hypertension, which may remain clinically occult until fatal (53). Interstitial pneumonitis in MCTD reportedly responds to treatment with steroids. Pulmonary hypertension is refractory to all treatment.
F. Sjögren's syndrome (SS) is an autoimmune disease characterized by lymphocytic infiltration of the salivary and exocrine glands of the mucosa of the respiratory tract, conjunctiva, and the genitourinary and gastrointestinal tracts. SS frequently occurs secondary to other connective tissue disorders (RA, PSS, SLE) or to other autoimmune disorders, including Hashimoto's thyroiditis, primary hypothyroidism, primary biliary cirrhosis, and pernicious anemia. Pulmonary disease occurs in approximately 75% of patients.
   1. Clinical presentation differs for primary and secondary SS.
      a. ILD occurs in over half of patients with primary SS and extraglandular disease but in only 10% of patients with secondary SS (54). The ILD in SS is often of the lymphocytic interstitial pneumonia (LIP) variety. The clinical course of ILD in primary SS is usually less severe than that of ILD from other connective tissue diseases, and patients may often be asymptomatic and have normal chest radiographs. ILD in secondary SS is more likely to be fibrotic and cause progressive respiratory impairment.
      b. Obstructive lung disease occurs in 20% of patients with secondary SS, especially if associated with RA or HLA-DR4 antigen (54), but is rarely seen in primary SS.
      c. SS can also present as tracheal involvement, producing a desiccated trachea and bronchial mucus (xerotrachea). Patients complain of chronic nonproductive cough and are predisposed to recurrent respiratory infections.
      d. The most serious concern is the reported progression of pulmonary involvement in SS to pseudolymphoma or malignant B-cell lymphoma over 10–15 years (55). A decline in rheumatoid titer or a low IgM appears to correlate with onset of malignancy (55).
   2. Diagnosis. In the appropriate clinical setting, transbronchoscopic lung biopsy may provide adequate tissue to diagnose lung involvement. However, open lung biopsy is often required to distinguish LIP from lymphoma or lymphomatoid granulomatosis.
   3. Management. Approximately 50% of patients with ILD or LIP respond to steroids. Obstructive disease is treated with inhaled β-agonists and steroids. Xerotrachea is treated supportively.
G. Ankylosing spondylitis produces apical, usually bilateral fibrocavitary disease. Patients are usually asymptomatic, although they occasionally have productive cough and dyspnea. The clinical presentation and radiographic appearance can mimic pulmonary tuberculosis. Superinfection with *Aspergillus* complicates advanced disease. Management is supportive (56).

H. **Amyloidosis** is a systemic disease of tissue infiltration by a homogenous acellular material that is extracellular and eosinophilic. This material is composed of fibrillar proteins with a beta-pleated sheet conformation that associate with normal serum α-glycoproteins in the presence of calcium. Although a large number of widely different human proteins can produce amyloidogenic polypeptides, only those derived from immunoglobulin light chains (lambda and kappa) cause pulmonary disease. The major pulmonary manifestations are diffuse alveolar, tracheobronchial, and nodular amyloidosis.

1. **Diffuse alveolar amyloidosis**
   a. **Clinical presentation**
      i. Diffuse infiltration of alveolar septa produces progressive diffuse alveolar infiltrates, restrictive disease, and hypoxemia. Pulmonary involvement can progress to produce pulmonary hypertension.
      ii. Secondary pulmonary involvement includes obstructive sleep apnea due to infiltration of the tongue (macroglossia) and respiratory failure due to infiltration of the diaphragm.
   b. **Diagnosis**
      i. Diffuse alveolar amyloidosis produces a characteristic pattern of focal calcifications on HRCT (57).
      ii. The diagnosis of systemic amyloidosis should be made by rectal mucosal or abdominal subcutaneous fat biopsy. Transbronchial biopsy of alveolar septal or pulmonary vascular amyloidosis should be avoided because of an increased risk of bleeding.
   c. **Management.** Cytotoxic alkylating agents, colchicine, and dimethyl sulfoxide all have limited efficacy in preventing progressive pulmonary impairment.

2. **Tracheobronchial submucosal amyloidosis** typically presents with symptoms of chronic wheezing, cough, dyspnea, and hemoptysis. Endobronchial obstruction may produce atelectasis and recurrent or chronic pneumonia. Submucosal amyloidosis may calcify over time, producing tracheobronchopathia osteoplastica. Endobronchial submucosal amyloidosis may be diagnosed by bronchoscopic biopsy material stained with Congo red. Endobronchial laser surgery offers the safest and most effective treatment.

3. **Nodular parenchymal amyloidosis** presents variably as single or multiple nodules, either unilateral or bilateral, ranging in size from 1 cm to 15 cm. The nodules may grow gradually, cavitate, or calcify. Patients are typically asymptomatic, although hemoptysis may occur. Solitary nodules are usually resected when malignancy is suspected. However, resection is unnecessary if the diagnosis of amyloidosis is known and the patient is asymptomatic. Transthoracic needle biopsy should be avoided in cases of suspected nodular amyloidosis because of the increased risk of bleeding.

IV. **Endocrine and metabolic diseases**
A. **Acromegaly** is associated with increases in lung volumes and with obstructive sleep apnea.

1. **Lung volumes.** Increased lung volumes are noted in men with acromegaly. Women have normal lung volumes, suggesting an interaction between growth and sex hormones in producing this condition. Patients have a normal DLCO, indicating that the increases in lung volume result from an increase in the size of alveoli rather than in their number.

2. **Obstructive sleep apnea.** Patients with acromegaly have an increased incidence of obstructive sleep apnea (58) related to hypertrophy of the tongue, laryngeal mucosa, arytenoepiglottic and ventricular folds, and false vocal cords. Ventilatory drive is normal.

B. **Hyperthyroidism.** Dyspnea on exertion is a common complaint in patients with hyperthyroidism.

1. Dyspnea results from a combination of factors including increased carbon dioxide production from a hypermetabolic state, increased central ventilatory drive in response to increased Pco_2, and respiratory muscle weakness.

   2. Pulmonary function testing shows mildly restrictive physiology with reduced inspiratory and expiratory pressures proportional to the severity of hyperthyroidism. Resting minute ventilation and oxygen consumption during exercise are increased above predicted values.

   3. Dyspnea and abnormalities on pulmonary function testing improve with treatment of hyperthyroidism.

C. Hypothyroidism is associated with sleep apnea and pleural effusion.

   1. Sleep apnea. Hypothyroidism produces sleep apnea through effects on both ventilatory control and oropharyngeal anatomy.

   a. Chronic alveolar hypoventilation is caused by decreased carbon dioxide production from a reduced metabolic state. This in turn produces a progressive, severe impairment of ventilatory response to hypoxia, hypercapnia, and respiratory loading (59). Patients frequently are unable to wean readily from mechanical ventilation after surgery.

   b. Hypothyroidism predisposes to upper airway obstruction through deposition of mucopolysaccharide in oropharyngeal tissue and in upper airway muscles, including the genioglossus.

   2. Transudative pleural effusion and pericardial effusion occur in hypothyroidism and myxedema. Rarely, pleural effusion may be exudative.

   3. Sleep apnea and pleural disease respond well to thyroid replacement therapy.

D. Intrathoracic goiters are usually inactive, nodular, and benign thyroid tissue that present as superior and anterior mediastinal masses. Most intrathoracic goiters are asymptomatic but may occasionally produce tracheal or esophageal compression with stridor, hoarseness, or dysphagia.

   1. Tracheal compression presents insidiously either without symptoms or with a vague choking sensation that increases when lying supine. Compression usually progresses slowly but may suddenly accelerate and produce life-threatening obstruction.

   2. Diagnosis of intrathoracic goiter can usually be made by CT scan. When CT scans are indeterminant, iodohippurate sodium I 131 scans can identify functioning thyroid tissue in the mediastinum; however, scans may be negative if the thyroid tissue is nonfunctioning.

   3. Management with thyroid suppression is effective for asymptomatic goiters and for cases of mildly symptomatic tracheal or esophageal obstruction. However, patients should be followed closely. Surgical resection is required for progressive or significant tracheal compression.

E. Hyperparathyroidism may occasionally produce mild restrictive lung disease by causing neuromuscular respiratory muscle weakness. It is also associated with chest-radiographic findings of severe osteopenia, osteitis fibrosa cystica at the ends of the clavicle or in the scapula, and parathyroid adenoma appearing as a mediastinal mass. Most important, hyperparathyroidism produces metastatic pulmonary calcification that may progress to respiratory failure. The clinical presentation, diagnosis, and management are identical to those discussed above for pulmonary calcinosis under chronic renal disease.

F. Hypoparathyroidism affects the lung by hypocalcemia producing a generalized muscle weakness and mild restrictive physiology on pulmonary function testing. There are no pulmonary symptoms related to this disease.

G. Diabetes mellitus is the most common endocrine disorder. Although pulmonary causes account for nearly 10% of the mortality of diabetics, most pulmonary involvement is secondary to acute and chronic pulmonary infections, including bacterial pneumonia, tuberculosis, and pulmonary mucormycosis (60).

   1. Diabetics have an increased incidence of sleep apnea associated with diabetic neuropathy, which may explain the prevalence of unexplained sudden death in diabetics (60).

   2. Diabetes also predisposes patients to mucous plugging, presumably resulting from increased lethargy, altered vagal tone, and autonomic neuropathy (60).

   3. Diabetics often have mild reductions in DLCO on pulmonary function testing, probably from reduction in pulmonary capillary blood volume (61), and young insulin-dependent diabetics show reductions in lung volumes (62).

4. Diabetic ketoacidosis is rarely complicated by pneumomediastinum (60) and the adult respiratory distress syndrome (63).

References

1. Barish CF, Wu WC, Castell DO: Respiratory complications of gastroesophageal reflux. *Arch Intern Med* 1985;45:1882–1888.
2. Simpson WG: Gastroesophageal reflux disease and asthma: diagnosis and management. *Arch Intern Med* 1995;155:798–803.
3. Tucci F, Resti M, Fontana R, et al.: Gastroesophageal reflux and bronchial asthma: prevalence and effect of cisapride therapy. *J Pediatr Gastroenterol Nutr* 1993;17:265–270.
4. Krowka MJ, Cortese DA: Severe hypoxemia associated with liver disease: Mayo Clinic experience and the experimental use of almitrine bismesylate. *Mayo Clin Proc* 1987;62:164–173.
5. Jiva TM: Unexplained hypoxemia in liver disease: the hepatopulmonary syndrome. *J Crit Illness* 1994;9:934–947.
6. Eriksson LS, Soderman C, Ericzon BG, et al.: Normalization of ventilation/perfusion relationships after liver transplantation in patients with decompensated cirrhosis: evidence for a hepatopulmonary syndrome. *Hepatology* 1990;12:1350–1357.
7. Felt RW, Kozak BE, Rosch J, et al.: Hepatogenic pulmonary angiodysplasia treated with coil-spring embolization. *Chest* 1987;91:920–922.
8. Lieberman FL, Hidemura R, Peters RL, et al.: Pathogenesis and treatment of hydrothorax complicating cirrhosis with ascites. *Ann Intern Med* 1966;64:341–351.
9. Alberts WM, Salem AJ, Solomon DA, et al.: Hepatic hydrothorax: cause and management. *Arch Intern Med* 1991;151:2383–2388.
10. Boiteau R, Tenaillon A, Law-Koune JD, et al.: Treatment for cirrhotic hydrothorax with CPAP on mask and tetracycline pleural sclerosis. *Am Rev Respir Dis* 1990;141:A770. Abstract.
11. Robalino BD, Moodie DS: Association between primary pulmonary hypertension and portal hypertension: analysis of its pathophysiology and clinical, laboratory and hemodynamic manifestations. *J Am Coll Cardiol* 1991;17:492–498.
12. Scott V, DeWolf A, Kang Y, et al.: Reversibility of pulmonary hypertension after liver transplantation: a case report. *Transplant Proc* 1993;25:1789–1790.
13. Ettinger NA, Senior RM: The lungs and abdominal disease. In: Murray JF, Nadel JA, eds. *Textbook of respiratory medicine*. Philadelphia: WB Saunders, 1994:2416–2434.
14. Murphy D, Pack AI, Imrie CW: The mechanism of arterial hypoxia occurring in acute pancreatitis. *Q J Med* 1980;49:151–163.
15. Dewan NA, Kinney WW, O'Donohue JWJ: Chronic massive pancreatic pleural effusion. *Chest* 1984;85:497–501.
16. Light RW: Exudative pleural effusions secondary to gastrointestinal diseases. *Clin Chest Med* 1985;6:103–111.
17. Rockey DC, Cello JP: Pancreaticopleural fistula: report of 7 patients and review of the literature. *Medicine* 1990;69:332–344.
18. Guice KS, Oldham KT, Caty MG, et al.: Neutrophil-dependent, oxygen-radical mediated lung injury associated with acute pancreatitis. *Ann Surg* 1989;210:740–747.
19. Gronroos JM, Nevalainen TJ: Increased concentrations of synovial-type phospholipase A2 in serum and pulmonary and renal complications in acute pancreatitis. *Digestion* 1992;52:232–236.
20. Fairshter RD, Vaziri ND, Mirahmadi MK: Lung pathology in chronic hemodialysis patients. *Int J Artif Organs* 1982;5:97–100.
21. Berger HW, Rammohan G, Neff MS, Buhain WJ: Uremic pleural effusion. *Ann Intern Med* 1975; 82:362–364.
22. Gilman M, Nissm J, Terry P, Whelton A: Metastatic pulmonary calcification in the renal transplant recipient. *Am Rev Respir Dis* 1980;121:415–419.
23. Faubert PF, Shapiro WB, Porush JG, et al.: Pulmonary calcification in hemodialyzed patients detected by technetium-99m diphosphonate scanning. *Kidney Int* 1980;18:95–102.
24. Margolin RJ, Addison TE: Hypercalcemia and rapidly progressive respiratory failure. *Chest* 1984; 86:767–769.
25. Justrabo E, Genin R, Rifle G: Pulmonary metastatic calcification with respiratory insufficiency in patients on maintenance hemodialysis. *Thorax* 1979;34:384–388.

26. Kelly PT, Haponik EF: Goodpasture syndrome: molecular and clinical advances. *Medicine* 1994; 73:171–185.

27. Urizar RE, McGoldrick MD, Cerda J: Pulmonary-renal syndrome: its clinicopathologic approach in 1991. *N Y State J Med* 1991;91:212–221.

28. Hsu BY, Edwards DK, Tambert MA: Pulmonary hemorrhage complicating systemic lupus erythematosus: role of MR imaging in diagnosis. *AJR* 1992;158:519–520.

29. Cove-Smith JR, McLeod AA, Blamey RW, et al.: Transplantation, immunosuppression, and plasmapheresis in Goodpasture's syndrome. *Clin Nephrol* 1978;9:126–128.

30. Shiel WC Jr, Prete PE: Pleuropulmonary manifestations of rheumatoid arthritis. *Semin Arthritis Rheum* 1984;13:235–243.

31. Anaya J-M, Diethelm L, Ortiz LA, et al.: Pulmonary involvement in rheumatoid arthritis. *Semin Arthritis Rheum* 1995;24:242–254.

32. Hunninghake GW, Fauci AS: Pulmonary involvement in the collagen vascular diseases. *Am Rev Respir Dis* 1979;119:471–503.

33. Peterson M, Mouick M, Hunninghake GW: Prognostic role of eosinophils in pulmonary fibrosis. *Chest* 1987;92:51–56.

34. Yousem SA, Colby TV, Carrington CB: Lung biopsy in rheumatoid arthritis. *Am Rev Respir Dis* 1985;131:770–777.

35. DeHoratius RJ, Abruzzo JL, Williams RC: Immunofluorescent and immunologic studies of rheumatoid lung. *Arch Intern Med* 1972;129:441–446.

36. Hakala M: Poor prognosis in patients with rheumatoid arthritis hospitalized for interstitial lung fibrosis. *Chest* 1988;93:114–118.

37. Epler GR, Colby TV, McLoud TC, et al.: Bronchiolitis obliterans organizing pneumonia. *N Engl J Med* 1985;312:152–158.

38. Fort JG, Scovern H, Abruzzo JL: Intravenous cyclophosphamide and methylprednisolone for the treatment of bronchiolitis obliterans and interstitial fibrosis associated with cryotherapy. *J Rheumatol* 1988;15:850–854.

39. Dockery KM, Sismanis A, Abedi E: Rheumatoid arthritis of the larynx: the importance of early diagnosis and corticosteroid therapy. *South Med J* 1991;84:95–96.

40. Kaine JL: Refractory massive pleural effusion in systemic lupus erythematosus treated with talc poudrage. *Ann Rheum Dis* 1985;44:61–64.

41. Fessler BJ, Boumpas DT: Severe major organ involvement in systemic lupus erythematosus: diagnosis and management. *Rheum Dis Clin North Am* 1995;21:81–98.

42. Matthay RA, Schwartz MT, Petty TL, et al.: Pulmonary manifestations of systemic lupus erythematosus: review of twelve cases of acute lupus pneumonitis. *Medicine* 1974;54:397–409.

43. Abud-Mendoza C, Diaz-Jouanen E, Alarcon-Segovia D: Fatal pulmonary hemorrhage in systemic lupus erythematosus: occurrence with hemoptysis. *J Rheumatol* 1985;12:558–561.

44. Eagen JW, Memoli VA, Roberts JL, et al.: Pulmonary hemorrhage in systemic lupus erythematosus. *Medicine* 1978;57:545–560.

45. Espinoza LR, Hartmann RC: Significance of the lupus anticoagulant. *Am J Hematol* 1986; 22:331–337.

46. Hoffbrand BI, Beck ER: "Unexplained" dyspnoea and shrinking lungs in systemic lupus erythematosus. *BMJ* 1965;1:1273.

47. Owens GR, Follansbee WP: Cardiopulmonary manifestations of systemic sclerosis. *Chest* 1987; 91:118–127.

48. Peters-Golden M, Wise RA, Hochberg MC, et al.: Carbon monoxide diffusing capacity as predictor of outcome in systemic sclerosis. *Am J Med* 1984;77:1027–34.

49. Steen VD, Owens GR, Redmond C, et al.: The effect of D-penicillamine on pulmonary findings in systemic sclerosis. *Arthritis Rheum* 1985;28:882–888.

50. Dickey BF, Myers AR: Pulmonary disease in polymyositis/dermatomyositis. *Semin Arthritis Rheum* 1984;14:60–76.

51. Bohan A, Peter JB: Polymyositis and dermatomyositis. *N Engl J Med* 1975;292:344–347.

52. Bernstein RM, Morgan SH, Chapman J, et al.: Anti-Jo-1 antibody: a marker for myositis with interstitial lung disease. *BMJ* 1984;289:151–152.

53. Prakash UB: Lungs in mixed connective tissue disease. *J Thorac Imaging* 1992;7:55–61.

54. Papathanasiou MP, Constantopoulos SH, Tsampoulas C, et al.: Reappraisal of respiratory abnormalities in primary and secondary Sjögren's syndrome: a controlled study. *Chest* 1986;90:370–374.

55. Hansen LA, Prakash UB, Colby TV: Pulmonary lymphoma in Sjögren's syndrome. *Mayo Clin Proc* 1989;64:921–931.
56. Rosenow E, Stimlan CV, Muhm JR, Ferguson RH: Pleuropulmonary manifestations of ankylosing spondylitis. *Mayo Clin Proc* 1977;52:641–649.
57. Graham CM, Stern EJ, Finkbeiner WE, Webb WR: High-resolution CT appearance of diffuse alveolar septal amyloidosis. *AJR* 1992;158:265–267.
58. Hart TB, Radow KS, Blackard WG, et al.: Sleep apnea in active acromegaly. *Arch Intern Med* 1985;145:865–866.
59. Zwillich CW, Pierson DJ, Hofeldt FD, et al.: Ventilatory control in myxedema and hypothyroidism. *N Engl J Med* 1975;292:662–666.
60. Hansen LA, Prakash UB, Colby TV: Pulmonary complications in diabetes mellitus. *Mayo Clin Proc* 1989;64:791–799.
61. Sandler M, Bunn A, Stewart R: Cross-section study of pulmonary function in patients with insulin-dependent diabetes mellitus. *Am Rev Respir Dis* 1987;135:223–229.
62. Sandler M: Is the lung a "target organ" in diabetes mellitus? *Arch Intern Med* 1990;150:1385–1388.
63. Russel J, Follansbee S, Matthay MA: Adult respiratory distress syndrome complicating diabetic ketoacidosis. *West J Med* 1981;135:148–150.

28

Pulmonary Vasculitides

Jussi J. Saukkonen

The primary vasculitides affecting the lungs may be classified according to their predominant immunopathogenesis involving either (a) antineutrophil cytoplasmic autoantibodies (ANCA), (b) immune complex formation and deposition, (c) anti–glomerular basement membrane (AGBM) antibody deposition, or (d) cell-mediated processes (Table 28-1).

I. **ANCA-associated vasculitides.** In this group of diseases, neutrophils are chronically activated by autoantibodies and release cellular products that damage small and medium-sized vessels. Eosinophils and T lymphocytes may also contribute to injury.
   A. **Mechanisms of injury**
      1. **Neutrophil products.** Released lysosomal proteases and reactive oxygen species mediate tissue injury (1). The myeloperoxidase (MPO)-hydrogen peroxide-halide system is injurious to endothelial cells *in vitro* and may activate collagenase (1).
      2. **ANCA**
         a. **Target antigens.** ANCA are directed against neutrophil lysosomal constituents (1,2).
         b. **Neutrophil activation by ANCA.** Both ANCA and ANCA–target antigen complexes activate and degranulate neutrophils, releasing reactive oxygen species and antigenic, tissue-damaging lysosomal proteases. Complement activation and further neutrophil chemotaxis ensue (1–3).
         c. **Target antigen persistence.** ANCA-bound antigens escape inactivation by antiproteinases. Persistence of ANCA target antigens contributes to tissue injury and eventual granuloma formation (1–3).
   B. **ANCA disease associations.** Immunofluorescent staining of alcohol-fixed neutrophils demonstrates either **cytoplasmic (c-ANCA)** or **perinuclear (p-ANCA)** distribution of autoantibody (4).
      1. **c-ANCA are found in Wegener's granulomatosis** and are directed against epitopes of lysosomal proteinase 3 (PR3) and the cationic protein CAP57 (1,2).
      2. p-ANCA react with MPO, lactoferrin, elastase, and nuclear antigens and are associated with an array of immune disorders (Table 28-2). Whether p-ANCA play a significant pathogenetic role in these diseases is unclear (1,2).
   C. **Wegener's granulomatosis** (WG) is a clinicopathologic complex composed of necrotizing granulomatous inflammation of the respiratory tract, glomerulonephritis (GN), and systemic necrotizing vasculitis (3,5). Localized forms of WG affect the respiratory tract without renal involvement. Renal disease is eventually seen in nearly 80% of WG patients, with GN often developing within the first 2 years (6,7). Neutrophilic and granulomatous inflammation causes airway ulceration and stenosis, pneumonitis, and pulmonary nodules (6).
      1. **Presenting signs and symptoms** (5–7). Any organ system may be affected, but upper respiratory tract complaints predominate initially. Fever, weight loss, arthralgia, and myalgia are common. **Upper respiratory tract** signs include sinusitis, nasal ulceration or deformity, and epistaxis. **Lower respiratory tract** manifestations include chronic cough, hemoptysis, pleural rubs, and dyspnea with rales. Stridor and dyspnea suggest tracheal stenosis. **Cutaneous manifestations** are eventually seen in half of patients and include subcutaneous nodules, vesicles, papules, ulcers, and palpable purpura. Half of all

Table 28-1. Primary vasculitides with pulmonary manifestations

Antineutrophil cytoplasmic autoantibody associated

Wegener's granulomatosis
Microscopic polyarteritis
Polyarteritis nodosa
Churg-Strauss syndrome

Immune complex associated

Henoch-Schönlein purpura
Hypersensitivity vasculitis
Mixed cryoglobulinemia

Antibasement membrane antibody associated

Goodpasture's syndrome

Cell-mediated vasculitides

Behçet's disease
Takayasu's arteritis
Giant cell (temporal) arteritis
Necrotizing sarcoid granulomatosis

Connective tissue disease associated

Systemic lupus erythematosus
Rheumatoid arthritis

Table 28-2. p-ANCA disease associations

Microscopic polyarteritis

Necrotizing glomerulonephritis

Churg-Strauss syndrome

Polyarteritis nodosa

Rheumatoid arthritis

Systemic lupus erythematosus

Ulcerative colitis

Crohn's disease

Primary sclerosing cholangitis

p-ANCA = perinuclear antineutrophil cytoplasmic autoantibody. Kallenberg C, Leontine A, Cohen-Tervaert J. Anti-neutrophil cytoplasmic antibodies: a still growing class of autoantibodies in inflammatory disorders. *Am J Med* 1992;93:675.

patients eventually have **ocular involvement** including episcleritis, scleritis, conjunctivitis, uveitis, dacryocystitis, or retrobulbar involvement. Proptosis is a highly suggestive finding but is found in only 15% of patients. Otitis media and hearing loss may be present.

2. **Etiology and pathogenesis.** Neutrophils, initially activated by respiratory tract infectious or antigenic stimuli, are persistently activated by ANCA. Lymphocytes infiltrating the inflamed area proliferate in response to PR3, while monocytoid cells differentiate into giant cells in response to ANCA-PR3 complexes and form granulomas (1,3).

3. **Relevant physiology.** Vasculitis affects small and medium-sized arteries and veins. While lung involvement is seen in 85% of patients, only 17% actually develop chronic pulmonary insufficiency from either WG or its treatment (7).

Disability is related to chronic renal insufficiency, hearing loss, tracheal stenosis, and visual loss (7).

4. **Differential diagnosis.** Differential diagnostic possibilities include microscopic polyarteritis (MPA), Churg-Strauss syndrome, necrotizing sarcoid granulomatosis, bronchogenic carcinoma, lymphoma, tuberculosis, chronic fungal or helminthic infection, chronic bacterial sinopulmonary disease, AGBM antibody disease, and connective tissue diseases.

5. **Specific diagnosis**
   a. Clinical diagnostic criteria distinguishing WG from other vasculitides include nasal or oral inflammation, abnormal chest radiograph, microhematuria, hemoptysis, and granulomatous inflammation on biopsy (5).
   b. **Laboratory findings** distinguishing WG from other vasculitides:
      i. Hematologic findings include leukocytosis, anemia, thrombocytosis, elevated erythrocyte sedimentation rate (ESR), normal complement levels, hypergammaglobulinemia, eosinophilia, and increased C-reactive protein (5–7).
      ii. Biochemical findings include elevated creatinine and decreased creatinine clearance.
      iii. Urinalysis may reveal hematuria or red cell casts (GN).
   c. **Radiologic findings.** The chest radiograph may reveal nodular lesions, fleeting infiltrates, or pleural effusion or thickening. Solitary pulmonary nodules are seen in 20% of patients, usually in the upper lung fields. Multiple small nodules may be seen bilaterally in the mid- and lower lung fields with or without cavitation. Bilateral diffuse airspace disease may indicate alveolar hemorrhage (8).
   d. **ANCA.** Blood ANCA are detectable by indirect immunofluorescence or enzyme-linked immunosorbent assay (ELISA). In the appropriate clinical setting, detection of ANCA is a highly sensitive and specific test for active systemic WG. Nonetheless, renal biopsy is recommended even with a positive ANCA, given the extensive differential diagnosis and the morbidity associated with treatment for WG (7).
      i. **A positive c-ANCA is seen in at least 70% of active, generalized cases of WG.** In limited disease, without renal involvement, the sensitivity varies from 60% to 86%. Sensitivity in patients in remission is approximately 30% to 40%. p-ANCA have also been found in conjunction with WG or closely related MPA. Addition of a positive p-ANCA to that of c-ANCA increases the overall diagnostic sensitivity of ANCA for these two diseases to approximately 90% (2–4,9).
      ii. The specificity of c-ANCA for WG and MPA is at least 90%. Reports of positive c-ANCA findings in patients with relapsing polychondritis, human immunodeficiency virus infection, carcinoma of the lung, and Churg-Strauss syndrome are anecdotal (2–4,9).
      iii. **ANCA titer,** measured by ELISA, correlates with disease activity in some instances (10). However, these studies involved small numbers of patients, and rises in ANCA also occurred independently of disease flares (7).
   e. **Bronchoscopy** may reveal airway inflammation or stenosis (7). The diagnostic yield of transbronchoscopic biopsy is poor (approximately 7%) because it is difficult to make a specific diagnosis of WG from the small samples obtained, given the protean pathologic findings of WG (7,11).
   f. **Pathologic findings.** Open lung biopsy is diagnostic in 90% of samples (7), revealing prominent **granulomatous inflammation, parenchymal necrosis, and vasculitis**. Since these findings are also seen adjacent to foci of granulomatous infection, exclusion of mycobacterial, fungal, and helminthic infection is imperative (11).
      i. Parenchymal necrosis begins as punctate neutrophilic abscesses followed by geographic necrosis.
      ii. Classic necrotizing granulomatous vasculitis is an infrequent finding, but neutrophilic capillaritis with alveolar septal necrosis is common.

       iii. Nonspecific findings include interstitial fibrosis, endogenous lipoid pneumonia, alveolar hemorrhage, bronchiolitis obliterans with or without organizing pneumonia, and bronchocentric granulomatosis (11).

       iv. Biopsy of other sites (6,7). Multiple nasal or paranasal sinus biopsies are diagnostic in 20% to 60%. The size and number of biopsy samples influence the diagnostic yield. The diagnostic sensitivity of renal biopsy varies from 15% to 80%. Biopsy of any other sites is rarely diagnostic.

7. Management. Untreated WG was historically thought to have uniformly high morbidity and mortality, the latter due primarily to renal failure. However, a subset of patients with indolent, undiagnosed disease appears to have survived for years without therapy (6,7,12).

    a. Standard therapy in the United States consists of cyclophosphamide 2 mg/kg/d for 1 year accompanied by a corticosteroid (prednisone 1 mg/kg/d or an equivalent) for at least 4 weeks (7).

       i. Tapering. Cyclophosphamide should be reduced by 25 mg every 2–3 months as improvement allows. Prednisone should be reduced to 60-mg alternate-day therapy over 1–3 months and further tapered on an individual basis (7).

       ii. With this regimen, remission is achieved in 75% of patients, and marked improvement will be found in 91% of patients (7). The median time to remission is 12 months; 50% of these patients will experience a relapse within 3 months to 16 years after remission.

    b. Nonstandard therapy

       i. Patients with particularly aggressive disease have been initially managed with cyclophosphamide 3–5 mg/kg and prednisone 2–15 mg/kg (or the equivalent); these doses must be reduced as quickly as possible (7).

       ii. Azathioprine and corticosteroids. Azathioprine 150–200 mg/d for 1 year has been used alone and in combination with prednisone 40–60 mg/d (6,13). No prospective comparison with cyclophosphamide is available.

       iii. Methotrexate given weekly has been shown to induce remission in 69% of 29 patients, but 17% had progressive disease within 2–6 months of starting treatment. The regimen initially used a 0.3-mg/kg test dose, followed by up to 15 mg weekly for 1–2 weeks and then increased as tolerated in 2.5 mg/wk increments to a maximum dose of 25 mg/wk. Long-term follow-up of these patients is needed before conclusions can be made regarding this promising treatment (7,13).

       iv. Monthly high-dose pulsed cyclophosphamide given intravenously with daily prednisone has an unacceptable 72% relapse rate over 6–24 months (7,13).

       v. Treatment with corticosteroids alone results in a higher relapse rate and higher disease-related mortality (7). Patients with WG should not be treated with glucocorticoids alone.

       vi. Other cytotoxic agents and cyclosporin have been used but not adequately studied (6,14). Despite anecdotal reports to the contrary, trimethoprim/sulfamethoxazole does not appear to be efficacious in the treatment of WG (7,13).

    c. A significant increase in ANCA titer unaccompanied by disease activity should not be regarded as an indication for intensified treatment but as indication for close observation of the patient (14,15).

    d. Undiagnosed patients may present with rapidly progressive renal failure and a clinical picture suggestive of WG that may necessitate **empiric treatment**. Appropriate specialists should be consulted before embarking on this course.

    e. Other therapy includes management of subglottic tracheal stenosis by tracheostomy, manual dilatation, or laser resection and management of renal failure by dialysis (11%) or renal transplantation (5%) (7,16).

8. **Specialist referrals.** Diagnosis generally requires an invasive procedure and therefore necessitates a pulmonary, renal, or thoracic surgery consultation. The development of **dyspnea and stridor** suggests tracheal stenosis and requires immediate pulmonary consultation. Patients with subglottic stenosis will require a surgeon skilled in tracheal repair. Minor **hemoptysis** can herald a life-threatening event, and these patients should be seen by a pulmonologist or thoracic surgeon. An ophthalmologist should be consulted for episcleritis, scleritis, conjunctivitis, uveitis, dacryocystitis, or retrobulbar involvement. The latter two complications may require surgical intervention. Renal involvement is usually an indication for early nephrology consultation in WG. Since this disease can often progress rapidly, a renal biopsy may be indicated, and timely preparations for dialysis may be necessary. Physicians unfamiliar with the use of cytotoxic agents should refer patients for treatment to a rheumatologist or other specialist who is accustomed to prescribing and managing the toxicities of these medications.

D. **Microscopic polyarteritis** overlaps with WG and polyarteritis nodosa (PAN) clinically and pathologically and therefore has not been uniformly accepted as a distinct diagnostic entity (9,17). In contrast to WG, **granulomatous inflammation is not usually present** (17–20). Pulmonary manifestations include alveolar hemorrhage, pulmonary fibrosis, and pneumonitis (17–19).

1. **Presenting signs and symptoms** (17–20). Systemic and constitutional symptoms are common, including prodromal fever, malaise, myalgia, arthralgia, and weight loss (18,19). Palpable purpura, urticaria, nodules, or ulcers are seen in 60% of patients. Dyspnea and cough with or without hemoptysis are present in 30% of patients and usually occur with other systemic manifestations, although isolated pulmonary hemorrhage has been reported. Hypertension was found in 60% of patients in one series. Peripheral neuropathy, seizures, paralysis, ocular manifestations, and subarachnoid hemorrhage all have been reported. Abdominal pain, diarrhea, and bloody stools may also be seen.

2. **Etiology and pathogenesis.** Both c-ANCA and p-ANCA are found in conjunction with MPA, but the disease is notable for its lack of immune complex deposition (pauci-immune vasculitis) (9,21). Neutrophils and ANCA have a central role in inducing tissue injury in this condition, as in WG.

3. **Relevant physiology.** Crescentic GN may lead to renal failure, while alveolar capillaritis with recurrent hemorrhage may lead to pulmonary fibrosis (17–20).

4. **Differential diagnosis.** Wegener's granulomatosis, AGBM antibody disease, Churg-Strauss syndrome, PAN, systemic lupus erythematosus, Henoch-Schönlein purpura, and bacterial endocarditis are all in the differential.

5. **Specific approach to diagnosis**
   a. The lack of upper airway symptoms distinguishes this disease from WG and Churg-Strauss syndrome (17). Rales may signify hemorrhage or pulmonary fibrosis.
   b. Laboratory findings include anemia, leukocytosis, and an elevated ESR. Urinalysis nearly always reveals hematuria or an active sediment consistent with GN (18,19). Antibodies to PR3 (c-ANCA) are found in 46%, while antibodies to MPO (p-ANCA) are present in 50% to 60% of MPA patients (9, 21).
   c. The chest x-ray may reveal diffuse alveolar infiltrates consistent with alveolar hemorrhage (17–20). Interstitial fibrosis signifies repeated pulmonary hemorrhages.
   d. The diagnosis is established by the findings of crescentic GN, vasculitis involving skin, lung, or other tissues, and a compatible clinical picture. Pulmonary disease is usually confirmed by open lung biopsy, although transbronchial biopsy is occasionally diagnostic. The cardinal pathologic findings are **neutrophilic capillaritis, the absence of granulomas** (in contrast to WG), and the **lack of immune complex deposition** (in contrast to PAN) (17–20, 22).

6. **Management.** Untreated disease may be life threatening, and severe disease must be managed aggressively.

    a. **Cyclophosphamide** 2–3 mg/kg/d and corticosteroids (usually **prednisone** 1 mg/kg) should be used in aggressive disease (17–20). The adequacy of treatment with corticosteroids alone has not been established for mild disease.

    b. Plasma exchange to remove circulating ANCA has not been adequately studied to determine efficacy.

7. **Specialist referrals.** The importance of the timely diagnosis of MPA warrants early consultation with a nephrologist. The presence of pulmonary hemorrhage or diffuse infiltrates on chest x-ray warrants consultation with a pulmonologist or thoracic surgeon.

E. **Polyarteritis nodosa** is a systemic, necrotizing, immune-complex-mediated vasculitis involving small and medium-sized arteries, often resulting in aneurysm formation. Pulmonary involvement is exceedingly uncommon in classic PAN. The early sporadic case reports of lung involvement in PAN most likely represented variants of Churg-Strauss syndrome. However, lung involvement is common in MPA, and some cases of MPA may clinically overlap with PAN (17,23,24).

F. **Churg-Strauss syndrome** (CSS) or **allergic granulomatosis and angiitis** is a rare progressive disorder initially manifested as allergic symptoms, followed by **asthma, eosinophilia,** and finally **vasculitis** (25,26–28).

1. **Presenting signs and symptoms.** All patients have asthma and/or seasonal allergy. Fever, malaise, arthralgia, and weight loss are usually associated with the late-vasculitis phase. Wheezing and dyspnea eventually occur in >80% of patients. Dermatologic manifestations are seen in approximately 70% of patients and include nodules, erythema multiforme, petechiae, and multiple ecchymoses. Gastrointestinal manifestations (42% of patients) include abdominal pain, diarrhea, and bleeding. Cardiovascular abnormalities include hypertension (in 50%), pericarditis, endocardial fibrosis, valvular incompetence, congestive heart failure, and coronary arteritis. Mononeuritis or mononeuritis multiplex and polyneuropathy are seen in 50% of patients.

2. **Etiology and pathogenesis**

    a. CSS is an obscure, poorly understood disease. Inhaled antigen is thought to trigger the syndrome in susceptible individuals. Approximately 50% of patients are p-ANCA positive, suggesting that a component of tissue injury may be related to MPO and/or autoantibodies to MPO (1,2,9).

    b. Damage may also be induced by eosinophils circulating in large numbers and infiltrating tissues. A specific eosinophil peroxidase-halide system may cause tissue damage through the generation of reactive oxygen species (8). Myelin basic protein found in eosinophil granules is toxic to bronchial epithelium and causes ciliary stasis. Eosinophil cationic proteins induce both coagulation and fibrinolysis and are potent neurotoxins (29).

3. **Relevant physiology** (26,27). Obstructive airways disease often increases in severity over a period of years, with exacerbations occurring more frequently. In some instances, asthma symptoms abate while vasculitis becomes more prominent. The vasculitis and/or eosinophilic infiltration commonly lead to multiple organ-specific symptoms. Medium-sized arteries and veins are typically affected. As with other eosinophilic syndromes, endocardial fibrosis, valvular incompetence, and congestive heart failure may develop.

4. **Differential diagnosis.** Differential diagnostic possibilities include asthma, allergic bronchopulmonary aspergillosis (ABPA), idiopathic hypereosinophilic syndrome, chronic eosinophilic pneumonia, WG, MPA, PAN, and necrotizing sarcoid granulomatosis.

5. **Specific approach to diagnosis**

    a. Criteria necessary for diagnosis of CSS include asthma, eosinophilia >10%, neuropathy, fleeting pulmonary infiltrates, paranasal abnormalities, and the presence of extravascular eosinophils on tissue biopsy. The presence of four of the six criteria distinguish CSS from other vasculitides with a sensitivity of 85% and specificity of 99.7% (25). Of note, renal involvement is much less common than in WG, MPA, or PAN (26).

b. Asthma, sinus complaints, or paranasal tenderness are universally found in CSS (25–27). Dermatologic manifestations with neuropathy are suggestive of CSS. The percentage of eosinophils is usually at least 7.5% (25). Leukocytosis, anemia, and an elevated ESR are commonly seen. A low-titer rheumatoid factor, hypocomplementemia, mildly elevated IgE, circulating immune complexes, and hypergammaglobulinemia are sometimes found but are nonspecific (26,28). A positive immediate hypersensitivity skin test or positive serum precipitin level for *Aspergillus* supports the diagnosis of ABPA rather than CSS. A positive p-ANCA is supportive evidence for a vasculitis, but has only a 50% sensitivity and is not specific for CSS (1).

c. The presence of eosinophils in the sputum is nonspecific. Growth of *Aspergillus* from the sputum suggests ABPA rather than CSS.

d. Radiologic findings include transient pulmonary infiltrates, which may be patchy, nodular, or diffuse but rarely cavitate, unlike WG (30). In contrast, the infiltrates seen in chronic eosinophilic pneumonia are peripheral, progressive, and often recurrent (31). Pleural effusion may be present in CSS, but hilar lymphadenopathy is uncommon (30). Central bronchiectasis is not found in CSS but is a feature of ABPA. While pulmonary infiltrates occur in only 15% to 30% of patients, sinus films reveal paranasal opacification in 83% (25).

e. Skin or gastrointestinal or respiratory tract mucosa biopsies will reveal **angiitis, extravascular necrotizing granulomas, and tissue infiltration with eosinophils** (32). Granulomas have been reported in only 10% to 20% of patients (25,28).

6. **Management.** The rarity of this disease has not allowed for controlled treatment trials. The wide range in survival from 3 months to 20 years after the onset of vasculitis attests to the variable severity of the disease; most deaths from CSS itself occur within 5 years of onset (26).

a. **Most CSS patients respond rapidly to treatment with prednisone 1–1.5 mg/kg/d** (25,26). This dosage is reduced gradually according to the therapeutic response. Blood eosinophil count, ESR, and clinical parameters are used to assess response. High-dose pulsed intravenous methylprednisolone 500 mg/d for 3 days has been recommended for rapidly progressive disease (33).

b. Second-line therapy with cyclophosphamide 1–2 mg/kg/d or with azathioprine 1–3 mg/kg/d in combination with corticosteroids for 1 year results in clinical improvement (26,28,34).

c. Plasmapheresis provides no added benefit to that offered by immunosuppressive therapy (35).

d. Hypertension and congestive heart failure should be managed conventionally. Occasionally, valve replacement may be required.

7. **Specialist referrals.** Refractory asthma or hemoptysis warrants pulmonary consultation, and congestive heart failure in this setting warrants a cardiology consultation.

II. **Immune-complex-associated vasculitides.** A predominantly humoral response to antigen in this group of diseases unleashes inflammatory responses at sites of antigen–antibody complex deposition. Immune complexes activate the alternative complement cascade, with resulting neutrophil chemotaxis and activation inducing endothelial cell injury. Activation of the coagulation cascade may also result, leading to thrombosis and contributing to vessel necrosis. Biopsies often reveal **leukocytoclastic vasculitis:** neutrophil and mononuclear cell infiltration, fragments of neutrophil nuclei, and tissue edema. Multiple inflammatory mediators and cytokines are secreted locally by endothelial cells, macrophages, neutrophils, and lymphocytes (36).

A. **Henoch-Schönlein purpura** (HSP). The hallmarks of this clinicopathologic syndrome are **abdominal pain, gastrointestinal bleeding, nonthrombocytopenic**

purpura, and renal insufficiency. The disease most commonly affects children, but adult HSP has been described (37).

1. **Presenting signs and symptoms.** Lung involvement is rare and suggests more severe disease. Pulmonary manifestations include dyspnea, cough, pleuritis, and alveolar hemorrhage (38).
2. **Etiology and pathogenesis.** Many cases follow infection with β-hemolytic *Streptococci* or viruses. IgA immune complexes are demonstrable in the circulation and affected organs (36).
3. **Differential diagnostic possibilities** include hypersensitivity vasculitis, PAN, and urticarial vasculitis.
4. **Specific approach to diagnosis.** Two or more of the following are diagnostic, especially in an individual <20 years of age: palpable purpura, acute abdominal pain, and granulocytes infiltrating small vessels on biopsy (39).
5. **Management.** Mild cases of HSP are generally self-limited. More severe cases with significant lung or renal involvement may be treated with corticosteroids and cyclophosphamide, methotrexate, or azathioprine. The efficacy of plasmapheresis is unclear (36).

B. **Hypersensitivity vasculitis (HV)**
1. **Presenting signs and symptoms.** Manifestations may occur in any organ system, particularly the skin. Palpable purpura, maculopapular rash, or nodular ulceration are prominent features (40). Respiratory manifestations include dyspnea and cough related to pulmonary vasculitis and occur in up to 20% of patients. Respiratory failure, although rare, has been reported (41).
2. **Etiology and pathogenesis.** HV may be due to an exuberant immune response to antigenic food, medication, serum products, infection, or hematologic malignancies.
3. **Relevant physiology.** Pulmonary vasculitis may lead to pneumonitis.
4. **Differential diagnostic possibilities** include HSP, urticarial vasculitis, vasculitis associated with connective tissue diseases, PAN, CSS, and essential mixed cryoglobulinemia.
5. **Specific approach to diagnosis.** Antecedent exposure to medication is suggestive of HV. Renal and gastrointestinal manifestations are infrequent with HV but are seen with HSP and PAN. Blood eosinophilia is also not a feature of HV. Transient pulmonary infiltrates may be seen on the chest radiograph, but this is nonspecific. A biopsy of affected small blood vessels of the skin is the diagnostic test of choice.
6. **Management.** The disease process is generally self-limited: Removal or treatment of the suspected cause is often the only intervention required in mild cases. Failure of the syndrome to spontaneously resolve suggests on-going exposure, misdiagnosis, or the chronic form of the disease, which is rare. Chronic HV has been treated by selective elimination of foods from the diet in order to identify a potential allergen, as well as with immunosuppressive drugs (prednisone 1 mg/kg/d, cytotoxic therapy) (37).
7. **Specialist referrals.** Chronic disease should prompt referral for reevaluation and treatment by a rheumatologist.

C. **Urticarial vasculitis (UV).** This hypocomplementemic leukocytoclastic vasculitis is characterized by urticaria, angioedema, abdominal pain, uveitis, and enhanced susceptibility to tobacco-induced chronic obstructive pulmonary disease (COPD). Pulmonary vasculitis has not been demonstrated (42).
1. **Etiology and pathogenesis.** Food, drugs, infection, and autoimmune diseases have been associated with UV (37,42).
2. **Differential diagnostic possibilities** include HV, HSP, vasculitis associated with connective tissue diseases, and PAN.
3. **Specific approach.** UV is distinguished by urticarial nodules that become hyperpigmented (37).
4. **Management.** Antihistamines, corticosteroids, nonsteroidal anti-inflammatory agents, and antimalarials are used to treat UV (37,42). Conventional treatment of COPD and smoking cessation are indicated.

D. **Mixed cryoglobulinemia** (MC) is a **chronic relapsing leukocytoclastic vasculitis** occurring either as a primary disease or in association with connective tissue diseases or infections, particularly hepatitis C. Pulmonary involvement is common and includes obstructive airways disease, patchy nonspecific pneumonitis, bronchiectasis, interstitial fibrosis, and hemorrhage (43).

1. **Presenting signs and symptoms.** Purpura, arthralgia, weakness, neuropathy, and fever are common manifestations. Respiratory manifestations include cough, dyspnea, and wheezing as the most common respiratory symptoms; pleurisy and hemoptysis also occur (43).

2. **Etiology and pathogenesis.** Most cases of MC are associated with hepatitis C. Immune complexes are composed of antibodies bound to antigenic immunoglobulins (36).

3. **Differential diagnostic possibilities** include PAN, WG, MPA, and connective tissue disease-associated vasculitis.

4. **Specific approach to diagnosis.** Patients usually present in the fifth or sixth decade of life; gastrointestinal symptoms are uncommon (43). Proteinuria and an **active urinary sediment** are usually seen (36). Specific immunologic findings are usually present.

   a. Mixed cryoglobulins composed of IgG and IgM precipitate when serum is cooled to <37°C (36,43). Rheumatoid factor is frequently positive, and complement levels (CH_{50} and C4) are usually decreased. Hepatitis C serology is usually positive (36,43).

   b. Radiographic findings include interstitial infiltrates and small irregular opacities (43).

   c. Pulmonary function testing usually reveals reductions in diffusion capacity for carbon monoxide and small airways obstructive disease (43).

   d. Pathologic findings include a leukocytoclastic vasculitis with immune complex and complement deposition. Vasculitis may be identified most easily by **skin, nerve, or renal biopsy.** The latter generally reveals vasculitis with mesangiocapillary glomerulonephritis (GN) (36).

5. **Management.** Extrarenal disease is treated with steroids. Plasma exchange, or cryofiltration, can be used in addition to steroids to remove circulating immune complexes. Disease with renal involvement is treated with prednisone 1 mg/kg/d and cyclophosphamide 1–2 mg/kg/d to resolution of symptoms and signs. Trials utilizing interferon alfa are underway (36).

6. **Specialist referrals.** Biopsy of specific tissue sites will require appropriate referrals.

III. **Anti–glomerular basement membrane antibody disease** encompasses Goodpasture's syndrome (alveolar hemorrhage usually accompanied by renal failure) and rapidly progressive GN. Autoantibodies in AGBM antibody disease are directed against a component of basement membrane found largely in alveoli, renal tubules, and glomeruli (44–49).

A. **Presenting signs and symptoms.** Patients often have a flu-like prodrome. Major or minor hemoptysis generally precedes renal involvement by weeks to months. Pleuritis, dyspnea, and cough are frequent symptoms.

B. **Etiology and pathogenesis.** Components of the basement membrane are antigenic in certain individuals, particularly those with specific alleles of HLA-DR2 antigen. The autoantigen is a mutant domain of a type IV collagen molecule in the basement membrane. Circulating AGBM antibodies localize to basement membrane, especially if local inflammation exposes the antigenic domains, and activate complement, resulting in local injury. Cellular infiltration by neutrophils and macrophages follows. Relapses of the disease have been attributed to infection, fluid overload, anticoagulation, and cigarette smoking.

C. **Relevant physiology.** Diffuse alveolar hemorrhage causes hypoxemia. The extent of renal failure determines prognosis, with up to one-third of patients dying during their first hospitalization.

D. **Differential diagnostic possibilities** include idiopathic pulmonary hemosiderosis, WG, and MPA.

E. **Specific approach to diagnosis**. The vast majority of patients are men, with a median age of 21 years. Upper airway complaints are not common in Goodpasture's syndrome. Pallor, rales, or rhonchi and hepatosplenomegaly may be present. Anemia and leukocytosis may be seen. Proteinuria and gross or microscopic hematuria are present in approximately 90% of patients with Goodpasture's syndrome. Circulating AGBM antibodies are detected by a quantitative, highly sensitive radioimmunoassay or by ELISA. Until standardization of the assay is achieved, pathologic diagnosis remains the gold standard. Bilateral or occasionally unilateral alveolar infiltrates corresponding to intra-alveolar hemorrhage are noted on chest radiographs. **Immunofluorescence staining demonstrates linear IgG and C3 deposition along the basement membrane.**

F. **Management.** An accurate diagnosis must be made by measuring levels of circulating AGBM antibodies or by immunofluorescent staining of renal biopsy material as rapidly as possible to begin treatment and limit renal injury.

  1. Isolated pulmonary hemorrhage generally responds to treatment with intravenous high-dose corticosteroids (1–2 mg/kg/d) and plasma exchange. At least 1 month of high-dose therapy is necessary, with oral prednisone subsequently instituted and tapered over 3–4 months.

  2. Renal disease is generally treated with immunosuppressive agents and plasma exchange until AGBM antibodies becomes undetectible. Prednisone 1 mg/kg/d and cyclophosphamide 1–3 mg/kg/d or azathioprine 2–3 mg/kg/d are used. Renal disease does not respond to corticosteroids alone.

  3. Dialysis increases survival for patients with AGBM antibody disease, and mortality becomes related to the alveolar hemorrhage. Dialysis shunt infections can trigger alveolar hemorrhage.

  4. Renal transplantation has been performed when circulating AGBM antibodies have been consistently undetectible.

IV. **Cell-mediated vasculitides**

A. **Behçet's disease** (BD) is a chronic, relapsing systemic vasculitis with a high prevalence in the ancient Silk Route countries. Pulmonary manifestations are seen in only 5% of patients and are associated with an extremely poor prognosis (50–52).

  1. **Presenting signs and symptoms.** Recurrent oral and genital aphthous ulcers, papulopustular cutaneous lesions, neurologic complaints, and vascular occlusion are common manifestations. Dyspnea, chest pain, and hemoptysis develop 3–4 years after the onset of the disease. **Hemoptysis is the most common pulmonary manifestation** and indicates a poor prognosis, as well as rapid progression of the disease. The development of hemoptysis is associated with a 30% mortality risk, with 80% of this group dying within 2 years of the initial onset of hemoptysis.

  2. **Etiology and pathogenesis.** BD has **familial, ethnic, and genetic predispositions**, including a strong association with **HLA-B5(B51)**. Cross-reactivity between human proteins and mycobacterial and streptococcal **heat-shock proteins (HSP)** has been implicated. Humoral and cell-mediated responses to HSP are detectible in BD patients.

  3. **Relevant physiology.** Vasculitis leads to **large-vessel thrombosis and aneurysm formation**. Pulmonary embolism is rare. Hemoptysis results from small-vessel vasculitis or more commonly from the rupture of a large-vessel aneurysm into a bronchus.

  4. **Differential diagnostic possibilities** include Hughes-Stovin syndrome, systemic lupus erythematosus, syphilis, Takayasu's arteritis, and giant cell arteritis.

  5. **Specific approach to diagnosis.** Recurrent aphthous stomatitis is a criterion for the diagnosis of BD, together with two of the following: aphthous genital ulcers, uveitis, retinal vasculitis, and the skin lesions described above. Hematologic findings include anemia, leukocytosis, and an elevated ESR. IgA levels may be increased. Pleural effusion and infiltrates reflect intra-alveolar hemorrhage. Pulmonary vascular aneurysms appear as prominent hilar vessels and nodular densities and are better delineated with contrast computed tomography or pulmonary angiography.

  a. Bronchoscopy can identify the site of bleeding and may also reveal aphthous ulceration of the airways.

  b. Histopathologic examination of biopsied lung reveals vasculitis, infarcts, fibrosis, and aneurysms in affected lung tissue.

6. Management

  a. The bronchus from which hemoptysis is originating should be localized rapidly by fiberoptic or rigid bronchoscopy. Transfusions, bronchial artery embolization, lobectomy, or pneumonectomy may be required for life-threatening hemoptysis.

  b. Prednisone 1 mg/kg/d has been used to treat pulmonary vasculitis or hemoptysis but appears to be inadequate as monotherapy for BD.

  c. Immunosuppressive therapy

  i. Chlorambucil 0.1 mg/kg/d given with corticosteroids is generally effective for ocular and cerebral disease and is advocated by some clinicians for treatment of mild pulmonary involvement as well.

  ii. Cyclosporine, azathioprine, cyclophosphamide, and methotrexate have been used for BD. The efficacy of these agents for pulmonary disease is unclear.

7. Problems and complications of therapy. Anticoagulation for deep venous thrombosis should be avoided, as hemoptysis could be worsened.

8. Specialist referrals. Major hemoptysis is an indication for consultation with a pulmonologist or thoracic surgeon.

B. Takayasu's arteritis (TKA) is a granulomatous vasculitis affecting the aorta and its branches. The disease is characterized by three clinical stages: a flu-like prodrome, painful vascular inflammation with aneurysm formation, and vascular occlusion manifested by claudication, amaurosis fugax, headache, or angina. Pulmonary manifestations of TKA are uncommon despite frequent diagnostic evidence of pulmonary vasculitis (53–56).

1. Presenting signs and symptoms. Respiratory signs and symptoms include pleurisy, exertional dyspnea, pulmonary thromboembolism, and hemoptysis. Pulmonary hypertension is present in 27% of TKA patients but is rarely severe.

2. Etiology and pathogenesis. A cell-mediated response to a cross-reacting target antigen, perhaps mycobacterial, is thought to be responsible for vascular injury. Autoantibodies directed at the aorta may be detected.

3. Relevant physiology. Hypertension results from renal artery stenosis and decreased vascular elasticity. Vascular occlusion leads to most symptoms. As noted above, pulmonary hypertension is mild and rarely leads to cor pulmonale.

4. Differential diagnostic possibilities include temporal arteritis, polymyalgia rheumatica, giant cell arteritis, fibromuscular dysplasia, and Ehlers-Danlos syndrome.

5. Specific approach to diagnosis. Women are predominantly affected. Diagnostic findings include bruits, decreased pulses, anemia, elevated ESR, and demonstration of aneurysms or vascular ectasias by angiography, ultrasound, or magnetic resonance imaging. Pleural effusions and pulmonary infiltrates are uncommon. Medium- and large-vessel granulomatous arteritis is seen on biopsy specimens with transmural destruction and lymphoplasmacytic infiltration, especially involving the internal elastic lamella. Autopsy reports have shown pulmonary arteritis in 50% of TKA patients.

6. Management

  a. The majority of patients will respond to corticosteroid therapy (prednisone 1 mg/kg/d). The dosage is subsequently reduced by 5 mg each week. Long-term low-dose therapy is frequently required, and disease flares may necessitate higher doses.

  b. Cyclophosphamide 1–2 mg/kg/d is added for steroid-unresponsive disease.

  c. Vascular surgery (angioplasty) has been employed with success in patients with impending end-organ damage.

      7. Specialist referrals. Vascular symptoms (stenosis, ischemia) are indications for referral to a vascular surgeon.

   C. Giant cell (temporal) arteritis (GCA) affects large and medium-sized arteries, particularly the aorta and the external carotid artery and their branches. GCA is associated with polymyalgia rheumatica in at least 50% of patients (53,57–58).

      1. Presenting signs and symptoms. Only 4% of GCA patients present with pulmonary complaints. Pulmonary symptoms are eventually seen in 9% to 30% and include cough, hoarseness, and sore throat.

      2. Differential diagnostic possibilities include PAN, WG, HV, and TKA.

      3. Specific approach to diagnosis. The disease is characterized by jaw claudication, headache, amaurosis fugax, a diminished pulse or tenderness of the temporal artery, an ESR >100 mm/h, and granulomatous vasculitis on temporal artery biopsy. Chest radiographs rarely reveal interstitial infiltrates, pulmonary nodules, or aneurysms.

      4. Management. Prednisone 20–60 mg/d is generally effective in treating the disease. The exact dosage and length of treatment are controversial.

   D. Necrotizing sarcoid granulomatosis (see chapter 10).

 V. Connective tissue disease–associated vasculitis. Pulmonary vasculitis is relatively uncommon in patients with connective tissue diseases. Subclinical vasculitis is variably present in systemic lupus erythematosus and rheumatoid arthritis. Significant pulmonary hypertension leading to cor pulmonale is uncommon (59).

VI. Problems and complications of therapy of the vasculitides. Significant morbidity is associated with the individual and combined medications used to treat vasculitis (eg, *Pneumocystis carinii* pneumonia from cyclophosphamide and prednisone) (7).

   A. Cyclophosphamide-induced morbidity includes drug-induced pneumonitis, increased susceptibility to infections, leukopenia, ovarian failure, hemorrhagic cystitis, bladder cancer, myelodysplasia, and lymphoma. The dose of cyclophosphamide should be adjusted to keep the total leukocyte count between 3500 and 4500 cells/mm^3 (6,7).

   B. Glucocorticoid-induced morbidity, particularly with daily therapy, includes infections, diabetes mellitus, cataract development, fractures, and aseptic necrosis (6,7,13).

   C. Azathioprine-associated morbidity includes infections, bone marrow suppression, and lymphoma (6).

   D. Methotrexate-associated morbidity includes hepatic injury with or without elevations of serum transaminases, bacterial and opportunistic infections, hemorrhagic enteritis, and drug-induced pneumonitis (13,60).

References

1. Kallenberg C, Cohen-Tervaert J, van der Woude F, et al.: Autoimmunity to lysosomal enzymes: new clues to vasculitis and glomerulonephritis? *Immunol Today* 1991;12:61.
2. Kallenberg C, Leontine A, Cohen-Tervaert J: Anti-neutrophil cytoplasmic antibodies: a still growing class of autoantibodies in inflammatory disorders. *Am J Med* 1992;93:675.
3. Hoffman G: Wegener's granulomatosis. *Curr Opin Rheumatol* 1993;5:11.
4. Niles J: Value of tests for antineutrophil cytoplasmic autoantibodies in the diagnosis and treatment of vasculitis. *Curr Opin Rheumatol* 1993;5:18.
5. Leavitt R, Fauci A, Bloch D, et al.: The American College of Rheumatology 1990 criteria for the classification of Wegener's granulomatosis. *Arthritis Rheum* 1990;33:1101.
6. Anderson G, Coles E, Crane M, et al.: Wegener's granuloma: a series of 265 British cases seen between 1975 and 1985. *Q J Med* 1992;83:427.
7. Hoffman G, Kerr G, Leavitt R, et al.: Wegener granulomatosis: an analysis of 158 patients. *Ann Intern Med* 1992;116:488.
8. Staples C: Pulmonary angiitis and granulomatosis. *Radiol Clin North Am* 1991;29:973.
9. Beer D: ANCAs aweigh. *Am Rev Respir Dis* 1992;146:1128.
10. Cohen-Traevert J, Huitema M, Hene R, et al.: Prevention of relapses in Wegener's granulomatosis by treatment based on antineutrophil cytoplasmic titre. *Lancet* 1990;336:709.

11. Travis W, Hoffman G, Leavitt R, et al.: Surgical pathology of the lung in Wegener's granulomatosis: review of 87 open lung biopsies from 67 patients. *Am J Surg Pathol* 1991;15:315.
12. Andrassy K, Erb A, Koderisch J, et al.: Wegener's granulomatosis with renal involvement: patient survival and correlations between initial renal function, renal histology, therapy, and renal outcome. *Clin Nephrol* 1991;35:139.
13. Hoffman G, Leavitt R, Kerr G, et al.: The treatment of Wegener's granulomatosis with glucocorticoids and methotrexate. *Arthritis Rheum* 1992;35:1322.
14. Kerr G, Fleisher T, Hallahan C, et al.: Limited prognostic value of changes in anti-neutrophil cytoplasmic antibody titer in patients with Wegener's granulomatosis. *Arthritis Rheum* 1993;36:365.
15. De'Olivera J, Gaskin G, Dach A, et al.: Relationship between disease activity and anti-neutrophil cytoplasmic antibody concentration in long-term management of systemic vasculitis. *Am J Kidney Dis* 1995;25:380.
16. Lebovics R, Hoffman G, Leavitt R, et al.: The management of subglottic stenosis in patients with Wegener's granulomatosis. *Laryngoscope* 1992;102:1341.
17. Bosch X, Font J, Mirapeix E, et al.: Anti-myeloperoxidase autoantibody-associated necrotizing alveolar capillaritis. *Am Rev Respir Dis* 1992;146:1326.
18. Falk R, Hogan S, Carey T, et al.: Clinical course of antineutrophil cytoplasmic autoantibody-associated glomerulonephritis and systemic vasculitis. *Ann Intern Med* 1990;113:656.
19. Rodgers H, Guthrie J, Brownjohn A, et al.: Microscopic polyarteritis: clinical features and treatment. *Postgrad Med* 1989;65:515.
20. Imoto E, Lombard C, Sachs D: Pulmonary capillaritis and hemorrhage: a clue to the diagnosis of systemic necrotizing vasculitis. *Chest* 1989;96:927.
21. Hagen E, Ballieux B, van Es L, et al.: Antineutrophil cytoplasmic autoantibodies: a review of the antigens involved, the assays, and the clinical and possible pathogenetic consequences. *Blood* 1993;81:1996.
22. Savage C, Winearls C, Evans D, et al.: Microscopic polyarteritis: presentation, pathology, and prognosis. *Q J Med* 1985;56:467.
23. Lightfoot RW, Michel BA, Bloch DA, et al.: The American College of Rheumatology 1990 criteria for the classification of polyarteritis nodosa. *Arthritis Rheum* 1990;33:1088.
24. Conn D: Polyarteritis. *Rheum Dis Clin North Am* 1990;16:341.
25. Masi A, Hunder G, Lie J, et al.: The American College of Rheumatology 1990 criteria for the classification of Churg-Strauss syndrome (allergic granulomatosis and angiitis). *Arthritis Rheum* 1990;33:1094.
26. Lanham J, Elkon K, Pusey C, et al.: Systemic vasculitis with asthma and eosinophila: a clinical approach to the Churg-Strauss syndrome. *Medicine* 1984;63:65.
27. Chumbley L, Harrison E, DeRemee R: Allergic granulomatosis and angiitis (Churg-Strauss syndrome): report and analysis of 30 cases. *Mayo Clin Proc* 1977;5:477.
28. Leavitt R, Fauci A: Pulmonary vasculitis. *Am Rev Respir Dis* 1986;134:149.
29. Weller P: The immunobiology of eosinophils. *N Engl J Med* 1991;324:1110.
30. Staples C: Pulmonary angiitis and granulomatosis. *Radiol Clin North Am* 1991;29:973.
31. Jederlinic P, Sicilian L, Gaensler E: Chronic eosinophilic pneumonia: a report of 19 cases and a review of the literature. *Medicine* 1988;67:154.
32. Lie J: Illustrated histopathologic classification criteria for selected vasculitis syndromes. *Arthritis Rheum* 1990;33:1074.
33. Lanham J: Churg-Strauss syndrome. *Br J Hosp Med* 1992;47:667.
34. Guillevin L, Jarrousse B, Lok C, et al.: Long-term follow-up after treatment of polyarteritis nodosa and Churg-Strauss angiitis with comparison of steroids, plasma exchange and cyclophosphamide to steroids and plasma exchange. *J Rheumatol* 1991;18:567.
35. Guillevin L, Fain O, Lhote F, et al.: Lack of superiority of steroids plus plasma exchange to steroids alone in the treatment of polyarteritis nodosa and Churg-Strauss syndrome. *Arthritis Rheum* 1992;35:208.
36. Ambrus J: Small and medium vessel primary vasculitides. In: Rich R, ed. *Clinical immunology.* St Louis, Mo: Mosby-Yearbook, 1995.
37. Callen J: Cutaneous vasculitis and other neutrophilic dermatoses. *Curr Opin Rheumatol* 1993; 5:33.
38. Markus H, Clark J: Pulmonary hemorrhage in Henoch-Schönlein purpura. *Thorax* 1989;44:525.
39. Mills J, Michel B, Bloch D, et al.: The American College of Rheumatology 1990 criteria for the classification of Henoch-Schönlein purpura. *Arthritis Rheum* 1990;33:1114.

40. Calabrese L, Michel B, Bloch D, et al.: The American College of Rheumatology 1990 criteria for the classification of hypersensitivity vasculitis. *Arthritis Rheum* 1990;33:1108.
41. Prakash U: Vasculitides. In: Murray J, ed. *Pulmonary complications of systemic disease.* New York: Marcel Dekker, 1992.
42. Mehregan D, Hall M, Gibson L: Urticarial vasculitis: a histopathologic and clinical review of 72 cases. *J Am Acad Dermatol* 1992;26:441.
43. Bombardieri S, Paoletti P, Ferri C, et al.: Lung involvement in essential mixed cryoglobulinemia. *Am J Med* 1979;66:748.
44. Gunwar S, Bejarano P, Kalluri R, et al.: Alveolar basement membrane: molecular properties of the noncollagenous domain (hexamer) of collagen IV and its reactivity with Goodpasture autoantibodies. *Am J Respir Cell Mol Biol* 1991;5:107.
45. Briggs W, Johnson J, Wilson S, et al.: Anti-glomerular basement membrane antibody-mediated glomerulonephritis and Goodpasture's syndrome. *Medicine* 1979;58:348.
46. Savage CO, Pusey CD, Bowman C, Rees AJ, Lockwood CM: Anti-glomerular basement membrane antibody-mediated disease in the British Isles. *BMJ* 1986;292:301.
47. Hudson BG, Kalluri R, Reeders ST, et al.: Molecular characteristics of the Goodpasture autoantigen. *Kidney Int* 1993;43:135.
48. Walker R, Scheinkestel C, Becher G, et al.: Clinical and morphological aspects of the management of crescentic anti-glomerular basement membrane antibody nephritis. *Q J Med* 1985;213:75.
49. Watters L: Chronic alveolar filling disease. In: Schwartz M, King T, eds. *Interstitial lung disease.* St Louis, Mo: Mosby-Yearbook, 1993:309.
50. Allen N: Miscellaneous vasculitic syndromes including Behcet's disease and central nervous system vasculitis. *Curr Opin Rheumatol* 1993;5:51.
51. Raz I, Okon E, Chajek-Shaul T: Pulmonary manifestations in Behcet's syndrme. *Chest* 1989;95: 585.
52. O'Duffy JD: Pulmonary involvement in Behcet's disease. *Eur Respir J* 1993;6:936.
53. Hellman D: Immunopathogenesis, diagnosis, and treatment of giant cell arteritis, temporal arteritis, polymyalgia rheumatica, and Takayasu's arteritis. *Curr Opin Rheumatol* 1993;5:25.
54. Hall S, Barr W, Lie J, et al.: Takayasu arteritis: a study of 32 North American patients. *Medicine* 1985;64:89.
55. Kawai C, Ishikawa K, Kato M, et al.: "Pulmonary pulseless disease:" pulmonary involvement in so-called Takayasu's disease. *Chest* 1978;73:651.
56. Lupi EH, Sanchez GT, Howitz S: Pulmonary artery involvement in Takayasu's arteritis. *Chest* 1975;67:69.
57. Machado E, Michet C, Ballard D, et al.: Trends in incidence and clinical prestation of temporal arteritis in Olmsted County, Minnesota, 1950–1985. *Arthritis Rheum* 1988;31:745.
58. Bradley J, Pinals R, Blumenfeld H, et al.: Giant cell arteritis with pulmonary nodules. *Am J Med* 1984;77:135.
59. Lynch J, Hunninghake G: Pulmonary complications of collagen vascular disease. *Annu Rev Med* 1992;43:17.
60. Bernstein R, Spagnolo S: Interstitial lung disease. In: Spagnolo S, Witorsch P, eds. *Handbook of pulmonary drug therapy.* Boston: Little, Brown, 1994:185.

29 Occupational Lung Disease

Francis Cordova and Gerald J. Criner

I. **Introduction.** Occupational lung diseases are a heterogenous group of pulmonary disorders resulting from inhalational exposures to dusts, fumes, and chemicals occurring in the workplace. Occupational lung diseases have undoubtedly existed since antiquity; new diseases are continually emerging as novel materials, technology, and applications appear in the workplace.

A. **Definitions**

1. **Pneumoconiosis.** Derived from the term *pneumonokoniosis* (dusty lung), pneumoconiosis is defined as a nonneoplastic reaction of the lung to the inhalation of mineral or organic dusts.

2. **Threshold limit values.** Cumulative amounts of dusts considered safe to inhale over a working lifetime.

3. **Disability.** Legal term used to reflect the effects of exposure on the ability of a patient to perform an expected task.

4. **Impairment or dysfunction.** Defined by the American Thoracic Society as "a medical condition resulting from a functional abnormality that may be temporary or permanent and may preclude gainful employment" (1).

B. **Approach to diagnosis.** The diagnosis of occupational lung diseases requires a high clinical suspicion on the part of the physician. With the rapid growth of industry, many workers may be exposed to a variety of new and potentially toxic agents. A detailed clinical history, a physical examination, and a few diagnostic tests are usually sufficient to make the correct diagnosis. One essential aid in the evaluation of a suspected work-related respiratory illness is the chest radiograph. In fact, the radiographic pattern of some diseases (eg, silicosis, asbestosis, coal-worker's pneumoconiosis) is characteristic of the disorder. Depending on the specific occupational disease, additional tests—chest computed tomography (CT) scan, pulmonary function tests—may be ordered to support the clinical impression. In rare cases, a tissue diagnosis may be required.

C. **History.** A detailed occupational history is the key to the diagnosis of most work-related illnesses. Careful questioning about the specifics of employment will provide better insight into possible workplace exposure than a simple description of the job title. For example, knowledge of the total period of employment, the pattern of daily work activity, and the characteristics of exposure (ie, sandblasting in an enclosed space without protective mask) will provide important information about the extent and the magnitude of the occupational exposure. Since many occupational lung diseases have a long latency period before the onset of symptoms, job descriptions should detail the daily and actual periods of exposure. The nature of various pulmonary toxins (fumes, dusts, and chemicals) should also be obtained. Moreover, an attempt should be made to establish the temporal relationship of symptoms to the work environment. If the specific offending agents are not immediately obvious to the patient, additional information may be obtained from company data sheets, textbooks of occupational hygiene, or the *International Labor Organization (ILO) Encyclopedia of Occupational Health and Safety.* In addition to work-related exposures, a significant smoking history should not be overlooked as a possible contributing cause to a patient's respiratory symptoms.

D. **Physical examination**
  1. Early in the disease course, patients with occupational lung diseases may have a relative paucity of physical signs. Physical signs are generally not specific for any particular occupational lung disease but rather are useful aides in the determination of the severity of the underlying disease. Certain physical findings can be helpful in the diagnostic process.
  2. **Clubbing** can be seen in asbestosis but is usually not found in other types of pneumoconioses or hypersensitivity pneumonitis.
  3. **Crepitations** during late inspiration are heard in pulmonary fibrosis (asbestosis) and chronic allergic alveolitis but not in silicosis or coal-worker's pneumoconiosis.
  4. **Wheezing** temporally associated with the work environment may indicate the presence of occupational asthma, hypersensitivity pneumonitis, or the reactive airways disease syndrome.
E. **Radiologic imaging**
  1. **Plain chest radiograph.** Some occupational lung diseases, such as the pneumoconioses, may initially present without symptoms or may be initially diagnosed on the basis of a characteristic radiographic appearance. Table 29-1 lists the different radiographic patterns commonly seen in the occupational lung diseases. **Chest radiographs** are interpreted based on the standards set in 1980 by the ILO (2,3). Radiographic opacities are graded according to size, shape, location within the different lung zones, and the extent of the changes. A lesion >1 cm is by definition a large opacity. The simple pneumoconioses are further classified into categories 1, 2, and 3, and the complicated pneumoconioses into categories A, B, and C, depending on the extent of the lesions or profusion (concentration of infiltrates per unit area of the radiograph).
  2. **Chest CT Scan** is useful in the detection of early silicosis and coal-worker's pneumoconiosis, especially in patients with a near-normal chest radiograph or

Table 29-1. Predominant radiographic patterns of the various occupational lung diseases

Diffuse alveolar pattern
  Noxious gases exposure
    Silo filler's disease
    Acute nitrogen dioxide toxicity
    Sulfur dioxide
    Phosgene
    Acute cadmium poisoning
  Acute berylliosis
  Acute silicoproteinosis
Diffuse reticular, nodular, or reticulonodular pattern
  Simple silicosis
  Coal-worker's pneumoconiosis
  Asbestosis
  Talcosis
  Kaolin (China clay) pneumoconiosis
  Chronic berylliosis
Cystic or cavitary lesions
  Complicated silicosis
  Progressive massive fibrosis
Pleural effusion
  Asbestosis
Hilar and mediastinal lymph node enlargement
  Silicosis
  Chronic berylliosis

low profusion scores (4). In addition, high-resolution CT (HRCT) scans of the chest have been shown to be more sensitive in detecting and characterizing both pleural and parenchymal abnormalities in the asbestos-exposed population (5).

F.   Pulmonary function tests
   1.   Restrictive, obstructive, or mixed ventilatory disorders may be seen with occupational lung diseases. Table 29-2 lists the spirometric ventilatory defects of the different occupational lung diseases. Diseases with fixed airflow obstruction, such as emphysema and chronic byssinosis, are best evaluated with simple spirometry. In patients with variable obstruction, such as those with occupational asthma, serial peak-flow measurements conducted both at home and at work may be useful in diagnosis and management. Diseases causing pulmonary fibrosis are best evaluated by simple spirometry—forced vital capacity (FVC), forced expiratory volume in 1 second (FEV_1), and FEV_1/FVC ratio—as well as measurement of lung volumes and diffusing capacity for carbon monoxide (DLCO). Arterial blood gas examination is useful in detecting and assessing the severity of hypercapneic and hypoxemic respiratory failure in the setting of advanced occupational lung diseases. Cardiopulmonary reserve can be assessed by exercise testing and followed serially by a 6-minute walk.
   2.   Cardiopulmonary exercise testing may be helpful in selected patients to further assess the severity of impairment. Severe impairment indicates an inability to perform almost all jobs. A rating scale for the severity of impairment based on spirometry, DLCO, and maximum oxygen uptake is shown in Table 29-3. Assessment of the severity of impairment should be interpreted relative to the diagnosis. For example, patients with occupational asthma may have normal spirometry at baseline, while airflow obstruction may be provoked when exposure to sensitizing agents occurs in the workplace.

G.   Lung biopsy for tissue confirmation is often not required to confirm a diagnosis of occupational lung disease when the proper clinical setting and typical radiographic features are present. If a lung biopsy is required to rule out other disease entities or if the diagnosis is in doubt, an open lung biopsy offers a higher diagnostic yield than transbronchial lung biopsy and is the preferred procedure. Pleural biopsy in conjunction with thoracentesis is useful in ruling out tuberculosis in patients with pleural effusions and a history of asbestos exposure.

H.   Management. Since no specific therapeutic agents are indicated in the treatment of most occupational lung diseases, particularly the pneumoconioses, patient management is centered on the assessment of disability and on prognosis. In general,

---

Table 29-2. Patterns of abnormal spirometry in the various occupational lung diseases

Obstructive ventilatory defect
   Occupational asthma
   Industrial bronchitis
   Progressive massive fibrosis
   Reactive airways dysfunction syndrome
   Byssinosis
Restrictive ventilatory defect
   Silicosis
   Asbestosis
   Asbestos-associated pleural diseases
   Hypersensitivity pneumonitis
Mixed restrictive/obstructive defect
   Silicosis
   Asbestosis
   Progressive massive fibrosis

Table 29-3. American Thoracic Society rating of the severity of impairment using spirometry, diffusing capacity, and maximum oxygen uptake values

	Normal (%)	Impairment (%)		
		Mild	Moderate	Severe
FVC	≥80	60–79	51–59	≤50
FEV$_1$	≥80	60–79	41–59	≤40
FEV$_1$/FVC	≥57	60–74	41–59	≤40
DLCO	≥80	60–79	41–59	≤40
Max. oxygen uptake (mL/kg/min)		≥25	15–25	≤15

DLco = diffusing capacity for carbon monoxide; FEV$_1$ = forced expiratory volume in 1 sec; FVC = forced vital capacity.
Adapted from Official ATS Statement: evaluation of impairment/disability secondary to respiratory disorders. *Am Rev Respir Dis* 1982;126:945–951.

patients should be advised to avoid further exposure to occupational hazards. Regardless of the initial pulmonary function rating, the presence of cor pulmonale indicates severe impairment and should necessitate changing jobs. The presence of arterial hypoxemia at rest or during exercise does not by itself indicate severe impairment, unless accompanied by cor pulmonale; however, the majority of patients with arterial hypoxemia usually have impairment based on pulmonary function abnormalities. Patients with mild impairments should be able to work except in the most physically demanding jobs.

II. **Silicosis** is a chronic fibrotic lung disease resulting from the inhalation of dusts containing crystalline silicon dioxide. The clinical presentation varies depending on the duration and intensity of exposure, the nature of quartz crystals (tridymite and cristobalite) inhaled, and the presence of chronic obstructive pulmonary disease or pulmonary tuberculosis complicating the disease process. Although the incidence of silicosis is declining with improved industrial hygiene, an estimated one million workers are exposed to quartz crystals each year, and an estimated 1500 cases of silicosis could potentially be diagnosed annually (6).

   A. **Presenting signs and symptoms**

   1. In general, clinical symptoms and radiographic changes related to silicosis occur 15–20 years after the onset of exposure to silica dust. But individuals exposed to high concentrations of quartz may present soon after exposure and progress rapidly to acute, hypoxemic respiratory failure. In contrast, those exposed to low levels of quartz may be asymptomatic for long periods before presenting with mild symptoms of dyspnea on exertion or dry cough. The time from initial exposure to silica dusts to the onset of symptoms may be used to classify the three clinical patterns of silicosis: chronic, accelerated, and acute silicosis.

   2. **Chronic silicosis** is the most common form of silicosis and occurs in individuals exposed to low levels of silica over many years. Patients are usually asymptomatic early in the disease course but may later complain of cough and dyspnea on exertion. In advanced cases, progressive shortness of breath may occur with a paucity of physical findings. Finger clubbing and bibasilar crackles may be present but are uncommon.

   3. **Accelerated silicosis** is a rapidly progressive disease due to exposure to high concentrations of quartz over periods as short as 5 years. The disease is marked by progressive shortness of breath that can culminate in respiratory failure.

   4. **Acute silicosis** is caused by exposure to very high concentrations of quartz, and the duration of this exposure can be as short as a few weeks. The presenting symptoms include fever, cough, progressive dyspnea, and weight loss. Physical findings such as tachypnea, accessory muscle use, nasal flaring, and

cyanosis are indicative of severe, hypoxemic respiratory failure that is characteristic of rapidly progressive disease.

B. Etiology and pathogenesis

1. **Forms of silica.** Silicon dioxide consists of a central silica atom surrounded by four oxygen atoms in tetrahedral formation. Various spatial orientations of the oxygen atoms give rise to crystalline, microcrystalline, and amorphous polymorphs. Quartz is the most common form of crystalline silica. Cristobalite and tridymite are other crystalline forms thought to be more fibrogenic than quartz crystals. Freshly fractured quartz appears to be more fibrogenic compared to unfractured silica. Silicate crystals are silica combined with other minerals.

2. **Occupational exposures.** Quartz is the most common form of silica exposure found in the workplace. Occupations with potential exposure to high concentrations of quartz crystals are listed in Table 29-4.

3. **Pathophysiology.** *In vitro* and *in vivo* evidence has shown that the type of quartz and presence of other dust particles have important influences in modulating the lung's fibrogenic response. Inhaled quartz particles <10 μm in size are deposited in the alveoli and either engulfed by macrophages or deposited in the interstitial spaces. Phagocytosis of quartz crystals by macrophages leads to cell lysis due to lipid cell membrane peroxidation and subsequent disruption. Recent studies suggest that silicate inhalation can lead to oxidant generation via the formation of a silicato-iron complex (7). Cell lysis releases inflammatory mediators and initiates a cascade of events leading to an alteration in macrophage function, activation of humoral and cellular immunity, and eventually to the deposition of collagen that results in lung fibrosis. Although a portion of the quartz crystal may eventually drain to regional lymph nodes, some of the inhaled material remains in the lung and contributes to progressive disease even after the exposure has ceased.

C. Diagnosis

1. A history of significant exposure to free silica and typical chest x-ray findings are usually sufficient to make the diagnosis of silicosis. Tissue biopsy is generally not required in the proper clinical setting. Open lung biopsy is recommended if the diagnosis is in doubt, if a patient has atypical radiographic changes or an unusual presentation (eg, the acute form of silicoproteinosis), or if lung cancer cannot be definitely excluded. Active pulmonary tuberculosis must be ruled out with a purified protein derivative (PPD) tuberculin skin test and sputum examination with staining for acid-fast bacilli and mycobacterial culture.

2. The characteristic **chest radiograph** in silicosis shows **rounded densities** distributed predominantly in the upper lobes. Cavitation is unusual and raises the possibility of tuberculosis.

    a. Calcification of pulmonary nodules is uncommon and usually seen only in rheumatoid arthritis (Caplan's syndrome). **Egg shell calcification of**

Table 29-4. Industries with high risk for silica exposure

Mining, quarrying, and tunneling

Stone-cutting; dressing, polishing, and cleaning monumental masonry

Abrasives and abrasive blasting

Glass manufacturing

Foundry work

Pottery, porcelain, lining bricks

Boiler scaling

Vitreous enameling

Adapted from Ziskind M, Jones RN, Weill H. State of the art—silicosis. *Am Rev Respir Dis* 1976;113:643–665.

the hilar nodes is almost always pathognomonic of quartz exposure; however, rarely it may also be seen in sarcoidosis or with lymphoma after radiotherapy.

b. Coalescence of small nodular densities may lead to contraction of the upper lobes and the development of emphysematous changes in the lung bases. Pleural fibrosis is usually associated with massive parenchymal fibrosis. In accelerated silicosis, the radiographic features are similar to those of chronic silicosis, but the changes occur earlier and progress more rapidly.

c. In acute silicosis, diffuse bilateral alveolar and interstitial infiltrates are often present that are indistinguishable from pulmonary edema. Nodular densities are usually seen in acute silicosis, unless the disease is superimposed on the chronic form of the disease. The presence of pleural effusions often suggests another disease entity, such as tuberculosis, malignancy, or congestive heart failure.

3. **Chest CT scan** is more sensitive than the plain radiograph in detecting and defining silicotic nodules, especially with early conglomeration (4).

4. **Pulmonary function tests.** Changes in lung function are nonspecific in silicosis due to the frequency of concomitant exposures to other dusts, as well as the usual presence of a significant cigarette smoking history. Lung function is usually normal in simple silicosis; in advanced simple silicosis, mild reductions in $D_L CO$, lung volumes, and compliance are present (8). An obstructive pattern is frequently superimposed on an underlying restrictive ventilatory defect. In advanced cases, exercise-induced hypoxemia is usually evident. The annual decline in FEV_1 in simple silicosis is about 60 mL per year (9). With the implementation of current dust-control standards, the reported annual decline in pulmonary function is much less than previously estimated because the exposure is less (10).

D. **Differential diagnoses**

1. **Tuberculosis.** The PPD skin test and sputum examination for *Mycobacterium tuberculosis* are necessary in all individuals suspected of having silicosis. The development of cough, hemoptysis, and constitutional symptoms in patients with established silicosis should raise the suspicion of superimposed pulmonary tuberculosis. Radiographic changes such as new parenchymal densities, coalescence or rapid growth of new infiltrates, cavitation of lung nodules, or the development of pleural or pericardial effusions should all prompt investigation to exclude tuberculous infection.

2. **Lung cancer.** Lung biopsy may be necessary to rule out malignancy when the history of quartz exposure is remote or unclear or the radiographic changes are unusual (a solitary nodule, fibrotic changes confined to a single lobe, or rapidly developing silicosis).

3. **Chronic sarcoidosis** is a systemic granulomatous disease of unknown etiology presenting with bilateral hilar and right paratracheal adenopathy with parenchymal infiltrates and skin or eye lesions. Diagnosis is confirmed by transbronchial biopsy.

4. **Chronic allergic alveolitis** is a syndrome resulting from chronic low-grade inhalation of a variety of organic dusts, eventually leading to lung damage. As the disease progresses, linear and cystic changes occur in both upper lobes. The most helpful diagnostic test is the presence of precipitating antibodies against the suspected antigens.

5. **Ankylosing spondylitis** is an arthritic condition that involves the spine and sacroiliac joint and predominantly affects young males. The disease may be complicated by fibrobullous or fibrocavitary changes in both upper lobes, occasionally with the development of an aspergilloma.

6. **Eosinophilic granuloma** is a disease of unknown etiology of the group of diseases known as histiocytosis X. Many patients are asymptomatic on presentation, and the disease usually first suspected by an incidental abnormal chest radiograph. Characteristic chest-radiographic findings include symmetric nodular,

reticular, or reticulonodular infiltrates often with cystic changes, predominantly involving the upper and middle lobes. Diagnosis may be confirmed by transbronchial lung biopsy demonstrating the presence of Langerhans' cells.

E. Specific approach to each diagnostic possibility is shown in Table 29-5.

F. Management. Once simple silicosis develops, the fibrotic process of lung repair becomes irreversible. The goal of management is thus to prevent disease progression and avoid potential complications. Continued exposure in the workplace may lead to progressive disease and should be avoided.

    1. Supportive therapy. In advanced cases, treatment consists of supplemental oxygen, inhaled β-agonists and anticholinergics, theophylline if chronic airflow obstruction is present, and finally diuretics and/or inotropic drugs in the presence of cor pulmonale.

    2. No specific drugs have been proven effective in the treatment of silicosis. Recent reports have suggested that short courses of corticosteroids in simple and complicated silicosis may improve lung function (11,12). However, the long-term benefit of corticosteroid therapy in preventing disease progression or treating the late stages of silicosis is unproven.

    3. Treatment for silicotuberculosis using multiple antituberculous drugs is warranted in patients with silicosis when tuberculosis is suspected, even if clinical suspicion is low. Antituberculous chemotherapy should be initiated with four drugs (isoniazid, rifampin, pyrazinamide, and ethambutol) until sensitivities are known (13). Patients with culture-positive silicotuberculosis should be treated for at least 8 months (14,15). Tuberculin-positive patients should receive chemoprophylaxis with isoniazid for 12 months or 4 months of isoniazid plus rifampin, once active tuberculosis has been excluded.

    4. Bronchoalveolar lavage may be helpful in acute silicoproteinosis. The benefit of this therapy has not been fully documented and requires further investigation.

    5. Lung transplantation is a new treatment option that may be considered in select cases of advanced silicosis.

G. Problems and complications

    1. Tuberculosis is the major complication of silicosis. Diligent efforts should be undertaken to rule out active tuberculosis. In Third World countries during the 1960s, the incidence of active tuberculosis was 20% (16). In the same period in the United States, the incidence of tuberculosis in metal miners with silicosis was 5.3%, compared to 0.6% in those without silicosis (17). Infection with atypical mycobacteria (*M. kansasii* and *M. avium-intracellulare*) has also been reported.

Table 29-5. Approach to the differential diagnosis of silicosis

Pulmonary tuberculosis	History of exposure to tuberculosis PPD skin test Sputum AFB and mycobacterial culture
Lung cancer	Transbronchial biopsy
Chronic sarcoidosis	Skin anergy Evidence of extrapulmonary organ involvement Transbronchial biopsy
Chronic allergic alveolitis	History of exposure to organic dusts Positive for precipitating antibodies to suspected antigens
Ankylosing spondylitis	Radiographic evidence of bamboo spine deformity and sacroiliitis
Eosinophilic pneumonia	Presence of bone cyst Transbronchial biopsy showing Langerhans' cell

AFB = acid-fast bacilli stain; PPD = purified protein derivative tuberculin test.

2. **Pneumothorax** may result from the rupture of bullae in the setting of massive fibrosis and frequently occurs in accelerated and acute forms of silicosis.
3. **Collagen vascular diseases.** Rheumatoid nodules may appear in patients with silicosis. Antinuclear antibodies are found more commonly with rheumatoid arthritis and silicosis, although the clinical significance is unclear. Systemic sclerosis, rheumatoid diseases, and systemic lupus erythematosus may occur in 10% of patients with accelerated silicosis.
4. **Lung cancer.** Epidemiologic and experimental studies suggest an association between silica exposure and an increased risk of pulmonary malignancy. However, a causal relationship has not been established due to the presence of confounding variables (smoking and exposure to cocarcinogens) in most studies attempting to link silicosis and lung cancer (18).

H. **Prognosis.** Simple silicosis of profusion category 1 is not associated with increased mortality. The major causes of death are respiratory failure and other respiratory complications arising from silicosis. The predictors of mortality include age <45 years, advanced silicosis, and the occurrence of tuberculosis (19).

I. **Prevention.** The incidence of silicosis has decreased with the advent of preventive measures such as dust control, adequate ventilation, and the use of respirators. The Occupational Safety and Health Administration threshold limit for silica-containing dusts is 100 µg/m³ (20). For dusts containing cristobalite and tridymite, the threshold value is 50% less, while dusts with very low quartz contents have a threshold value of 10 mg/m³.

J. **Specialist referrals.** Consultation with appropriate specialists should be considered in the following situations:
1. The diagnosis of silicosis is not certain because of unclear or remote occupational exposure, unusual clinical presentations, or the presence of atypical radiographic patterns. A tissue diagnosis may be necessary to exclude other disease processes.
2. Lung transplantation evaluation in an individual with advanced silicosis.
3. Silicosis complicated by atypical and drug-resistant mycobacterial infection.
4. Acute silicosis precipitates acute hypoxemic respiratory failure and requires intensive care management and diagnostic tests to exclude other possibilities.

III. **Asbestos-related pulmonary disorders.** Asbestos is a collective term for fibrous mineral silicates of the serpentine and amphibole groups. These minerals are valued for their durability and fire-resistant qualities. Inhalation of asbestos fibers can lead to different pulmonary disorders, including asbestosis, lung cancer, malignant mesothelioma, asbestos pleural effusion, and pleural plaques or circumscribed pleural thickenings (21).

A. **Asbestosis** is a diffuse interstitial fibrosis of the lung parenchyma caused by exposure to asbestos fibers.
1. **Presenting signs and symptoms.** The onset is often insidious. The most common presenting complaint is shortness of breath on exertion, with eventual progression to breathlessness at rest as the disease advances. Persistent cough and sputum production are also commonly reported. Chest pain is not unusual and suggests pleural involvement. The earliest physical examination findings are bibasilar end-inspiratory crackles. Finger clubbing is seen in 15% to 20% of cases and portends a poor prognosis (22).
2. **Etiology and pathogenesis**
   a. **The toxicity of the fibers** depends on (a) physical and aerodynamic properties, (b) fiber length (long fibers are more toxic to the lung), (c) chemical properties, and (d) surface properties.
   b. **Sources of exposure.** Table 29-6 lists the sources of human asbestos exposure. The threshold limit for asbestos exposure is 0.2 fibers/cm³ (23). The risk of developing asbestos-related disease from occupancy in buildings made with asbestos-containing materials appears to be very low (24).
      ii. **Occupational exposure** is still the most common source of exposure.
      ii. **Indirect occupational exposure or bystander exposure** results from work-related exposure to an individual whose job involves direct handling of the material.

Table 29-6. Occupations at risk for asbestos exposure

Process	Products made or used
Mining	
Milling	
Handling	
Manufacture	
Textiles	Protective clothing, mailbags, padding, conveyor belts
Cement products	Sheets, pipes, roofing shingles, ventilation shafts, flower pots
Paper products	Millboard, roofing felt, flooring felt, fillers
Friction materials	Gasket, clutch plates, brake lining
Insulation products	Pipe and boiler insulation, bulkhead lining for ships
Application	
Construction	Boards and tiles, paints, joint fillers, cement products
Shipbuilding	Insulation materials (boards, mattresses, cloth) for engines, hull, decks
Automotive industry	Gaskets, brake linings, undercoating
Manufacture	
Repair	

Adapted from Becklake MR. Asbestos-related diseases of the lung and other organs: their epidemiology and complications for clinical practice. *Am Rev Respir Dis* 1976;114:187–227.

  iii. **Domestic exposure** is the consequence of fiber-laden work clothes that are laundered at home.
  iv. **Environmental exposure** refers to exposure unrelated to occupation and results from living in proximity to asbestos mines or mills that contaminate the environment.
3. **Pathophysiology and pathology.** Deposition of asbestos fibers in the alveoli results in macrophage-induced alveolitis. With sufficient dust loads, this may lead to increased oxidant and fibronectin production with cytokine release and recruitment of inflammatory cells, as well as to the eventual development of chronic interstitial lung disease. Pulmonary fibrosis associated with asbestosis tends to be most prominent in the lower lung lobes in the subpleural regions (25). Microscopic examination may reveal asbestos bodies or uncoated asbestos fibers that are considered pathognomonic for asbestos exposure (26). Asbestos bodies are asbestos fibers coated by an iron-containing protein that has a golden-yellow or brown color. Asbestos bodies can also be detected in sputum specimens dissolved in sodium hydroxide. The presence of asbestos bodies only indicates a past exposure to asbestos fibers and is not diagnostic of asbestosis or other asbestos-related diseases (27).
4. **A presumptive diagnosis of asbestosis** can be made with a suitable history of asbestos exposure and physical findings compatible with interstitial lung disease (persistent bibasilar, inspiratory crackles) coupled with typical chest x-ray findings. If the exposure was trivial and the diagnosis is uncertain, a lung biopsy (transbronchial or open lung) may clarify the nature of the underlying disease.
  a. **Chest radiographs** are useful for health surveillance of the asbestos-exposed worker. Typically, small irregular opacities are seen on chest x-ray examination between the rib shadows in the lower lung zones. As the opacities coalesce, the heart borders may become obscured. Rounded opacities due to asbestos are unusual, unless concomitant exposure to silica dusts occurs. In contrast to silicosis, hilar adenopathy is not seen in asbestosis.
  b. **Chest CT Scans** can image the early fibrotic changes of asbestosis, especially pleural fibrosis. In addition, they are helpful in characterizing localized pleuropulmonary lesions, such as rounded atelectasis, that must be differentiated from lung cancer.

    c. **Pulmonary function testing** usually reveals either restrictive or combined restrictive/obstructive ventilatory defects. The restrictive defect in asbestosis is due to decreased lung compliance. An obstructive defect is usually present at lower lung volumes due to the development of peribronchiolar fibrosis. In advanced cases, an impairment in gas exchange manifested by hypoxemia and a decreased DLCO is observed.

    d. **Bronchoalveolar lavage** may show asbestos bodies, indicating prior exposure to asbestos.

    e. **Transbronchial lung biopsy** is helpful in excluding other disorders such as lung cancer, infection, or sarcoidosis.

  5. Differential diagnosis. Diffuse interstitial pulmonary fibrosis from other causes (connective tissue disease, idiopathic pulmonary fibrosis, chronic sarcoidosis, drug-induced lung diseases, hypersensitivity pneumonitides) should be considered in the appropriate clinical setting.

  6. Specific approach to each diagnostic possibility. The presence of systemic symptoms and abnormal physical findings involving other organ systems (malar rash, joint deformities, etc) may provide a clue to the diagnosis of diffuse pulmonary fibrosis. Table 29-7 lists some of the diagnostic possibilities and the approach to each diagnosis.

  7. No treatment is effective once pulmonary fibrosis is established. The usefulness of steroids and other anti-inflammatory agents or cytotoxic agents in the presence of active alveolitis is unclear. Smoking cessation and the avoidance of further asbestos exposure is mandatory.

  8. Complications

    a. **Lung cancer.** Epidemiologic evidence suggests that the risk of developing lung cancer is increased 10-fold in individuals with asbestosis (28). The excess risk is directly related to the duration and intensity of asbestos exposure. Smoking further enhances the carcinogenicity of asbestos.

    b. **Mesothelioma.** Individuals with a history of exposure to asbestos have an increased risk for the development of malignant mesothelioma, which is thought to arise from pleural mesothelial cells. Unlike other asbestos-related lung diseases, no close temporal relationship has been found between the duration and intensity of asbestos exposure and the development of mesothelioma. The majority of patients present with an insidious onset of chest pain, dry cough, and shortness of breath. The most common radiographic finding is a large pleural effusion. Pleural plaques may also be seen on the contralateral side in one-third of cases. A diagnosis of mesothelioma often requires an open pleural biopsy and special staining to exclude adenocarcinoma.

  9. Specialist referrals. When the diagnosis is uncertain due to an unclear asbestos exposure or an atypical radiographic pattern, transbronchial or open lung biopsy may be required to rule out other disease entities. Patients with advanced asbestosis may benefit from participation in structured pulmonary rehabilitation programs to further improve functional capacity. In selected patients, lung transplantation may be considered.

B. Pleural reactions to asbestos. Asbestos exposure can lead to both benign and malignant pleural diseases. Benign pleural diseases may present as pleural plaques, pleural effusion, or diffuse pleural thickening that occasionally leads to a fibrothorax.

  1. Pleural plaques usually become radiographically apparent 20 years following the initial asbestos exposure. Only 5% of plaques are calcified, and most present as irregular shadows in the lateral thorax without clear margins on chest radiograph. In addition to occupational exposure, domestic and residential exposures have been implicated in the production of pleural plaques. As many as 50% of patients with pleural plaques have concomitant asbestos-induced parenchymal lung disease.

    a. **Presenting signs and symptoms.** Symptoms are generally not present in the absence of parenchymal lung disease. The diagnosis of pleural plaques is usually made as an incidental finding on the chest radiograph.

Table 29-7. Differential diagnoses for asbestoses and their distinguishing clinical features and diagnostic tests

Diseases	Etiology	Clinical history	Diagnostic tests
Interstitial pulmonary fibrosis	Unknown	Progressive and cough	Serum positive for rheumatoid factor, ANA, elevated gammaglobulins, Pulmonary function testing reveals restrictive lung defect with reduced diffusion capacity for carbon monoxide Chest x-ray reveals ground-glass opacities in early stages and diffuse reticular or reticulonodular changes in advanced stages
Drug-induced lung disease	Bleomycin Alkylating agents Methotrexate Nitrofurantoin	Symptoms may occur early or late during drug administration. Fever, cough, dyspnea may occur	Mild eosinophilia may be seen in methotrexate toxicity Chest x-ray may initially show alveolar filling process, gradually becoming interstitial pattern
Lymphoproliferative disorders	Immune disorder	Usually occurs in middle-aged women Presents with progressive dyspnea and cough	Associated with dysproteinemias or connective tissue disorders Chest x-ray with diffuse reticulonodular pattern Diagnosis often requires open lung biopsy
Hypersensitivity pneumonitis	Organic antigens	Acute symptoms (fever, dyspnea, cough) after acute exposure to antigens; chronic symptoms after repeated antigen challenge Occupations at risk are farmers, mushroom workers, grain and bagasse workers, pigeon breeders	Serologic confirmation of exposure
Sarcoidosis	Unknown	Other organs (skin, eyes, liver, central nervous system) may be involved Cough and dyspnea are common presenting complaints Erythema nodosum may be seen	Skin anergy Chest x-ray features include nodular and reticulonodular infiltrates with hilar adenopathy Elevated angiotensin-converting enzymes Biopsy typically shows noncaseating granuloma
Connective tissue diseases Systemic sclerosis Systemic lupus erythematosus Dermatomyositis	Autoimmune disorders	Multiple organ involvement gives rise to different symptom complexes	Presence of different autoantibodies (ANA, anti-SCL, anti-Ro, anti-La)

    b. **Pathology and pathogenesis.** On postmortem examination or open thoracotomy, pleural plaques appear as shiny, white, and slightly raised areas. Pleural plaques are most commonly found over the inferior lateral chest wall and central portion of the diaphragm, although the anterior or posterior chest walls may also be involved. Histologically, pleural plaques consist of hyaline fibrous tissue that is almost completely acellular and avascular. Calcifications are common, especially of the parietal pleura. Pleural plaques are believed to develop when short asbestos fibers are released into the pleural space via subpleural and parietal pleural lymphatics.

    c. **Diagnosis** is based on a history of asbestos exposure and the presence of bilateral localized pleural thickening of the anterolateral or diaphragmatic parietal pleura. Isolated pleural plaques are not usually associated with clinically detectible restrictive defects on pulmonary function testing. A reduction in vital capacity may be seen in patients with extensive pleural plaques.

2. **Pleural effusion.** Originally described as "asbestos pleurisy," benign asbestos pleural effusions usually occur in young men 10–15 years following an asbestos exposure.

    a. **Presenting signs and symptoms.** Shortness of breath and pleuritic chest pain are the usual presenting complaints, although some individuals may be asymptomatic. A pleural rub may occasionally be heard.

    b. **The usual pathologic finding** is chronic fibrous pleurisy with minimal cellularity.

    c. **Diagnosis** is made by exclusion. Malignancy, particularly mesothelioma, must be excluded. Since pleural fluid analysis is rarely conclusive, open pleural biopsy is often necessary to rule out other causes. In most cases, the pleural effusion clears spontaneously.

3. **Diffuse pleural thickening** often occurs after a short period of heavy asbestos exposure. While frequently preceded by a benign asbestos pleural effusion, this pleural thickening can occur in the absence of parenchymal involvement. Whether the presence of pleural fibrosis increases the future risk for mesothelioma is unclear.

    a. **Presenting signs and symptoms.** The most common complaint is dyspnea on exertion.

    b. **Pathology.** Pleural fibrosis commonly involves the visceral and parietal pleura of both lower lobes. On gross inspection, the lung is encased by a white peel. Occasionally, the pleural reaction may fold upon itself, trapping the underlying parenchyma and causing atelectasis of the trapped lung. This process leads to the development of pleuroparenchymal lesions known as **rounded atelectasis**.

    c. **The diagnosis** is initially suspected on the chest radiograph, which may show rounded atelectasis. This type of pleural thickening is distinguished from circumscribed pleural thickening by obliteration of the costophrenic angle and a loss of lung volume. Pulmonary function testing reveals a reduction in FVC and DLCO, which corrects when referenced to alveolar volume. The chest CT scan is helpful in evaluating the extent of pleural fibrosis and defining the nature of pleura-based masses such as rounded atelectasis. The pathognomonic chest CT appearance of rounded atelectasis is a peripheral lesion adjacent to broad-based pleural thickening with a "comet-tail" of bronchovascular structures radiating from the lesion to the hilum (29).

4. **Differential diagnosis** includes pleural fat pads, rib fractures, pleural calcification due to tuberculosis or hemothorax, silicosis, localized mesothelioma, metastatic disease, and lymphoma. In these conditions, the pleural thickening is unilateral and usually involves the visceral pleura.

5. **Management of asbestos-related pleural diseases.** Individuals with pleural plaques have an increased incidence of lung fibrosis and should avoid further exposure to asbestos. The role of surgery in diffuse pleural fibrosis is unclear, although pleurectomy may be effective in providing symptomatic relief from

pleuritic chest pain due to benign asbestos pleural disease (30). Smoking cessation programs should be offered to decrease the risk of lung cancer.

IV. Coal-worker's pneumoconiosis is a pulmonary disease resulting from the deposition of coal dust into the lungs. The disease may be classified by radiographic appearance as simple pneumoconiosis (lesions <1 cm in diameter) or complicated pneumoconiosis with progressive massive fibrosis (PMF) (lesions >1 cm in diameter). The severity of the disease is related to the cumulative exposure to coal mine dusts and concomitant exposure to silica. The inhalation of coal mine dust can also lead to silicosis, industrial bronchitis, and chronic airflow obstruction independent of smoking.

  A. Presenting signs and symptoms. In simple pneumoconiosis, patients usually have no symptoms. The diagnosis is made on the basis of the chest radiograph in individuals with a history of coal exposure. The presence of cough and sputum production early in the disease process is probably due to the development of chronic bronchitis from repeated dust inhalation. As the disease evolves to PMF, dyspnea on exertion becomes the predominant symptom. Occasionally, cough productive of black sputum (melanoptysis) may result from the rupture of cavitating PMF lesions into the airways. Blue-black discoloration of the skin on the hands, forearms, and face due to coal tattoo marks may indicate past coal exposure. Finger clubbing is not a feature of the disease and should prompt a search for an alternative diagnosis.

  B. Etiology. Coal is a mineral formed from dead vegetation over 250–300 million years old. Coal is graded by its carbon content to reflect its combustibility. The risk for pneumoconiosis is higher with the higher grades of coal. Anthracite is the highest-ranked coal, while bituminous and sub-bituminous types have the lowest coal contents. Exposure to coal dust with a quartz concentration >15% is associated with a high risk of developing a rapidly progressive form of pneumoconiosis that is clinically and pathologically similar to silicosis.

  C. Pathology and pathogenesis. The primary lesion in coal-worker's pneumoconiosis is the **coal macule**, distributed mainly in both upper lobes, although the lower lobes may eventually become involved. On histologic examination, the lesions consist of aggregates of dusts, dust-laden macrophages, and fibroblasts in the respiratory bronchioles and alveoli. The coal macule may eventually enlarge to form nodules that will eventually weaken the bronchioles and lead to focal emphysema. Coalescence of perivascular coal nodules leads to bulky rubbery masses, primarily located in the posterior segments of the upper lobes. This pattern has been called **progressive massive fibrosis.** As in the other pneumoconioses, the initial pathogenic mechanism involves the deposition of coal dusts in the distal airways, followed by macrophage-triggered alveolitis leading to fibrosis. The development of focal and centriacinar emphysema is thought to be due to the release of mediators by inflammatory cells, causing alveolar and epithelial cell damage. The exact cascade of events triggering PMF is speculative but believed to be influenced by the dust load and the degree of immunologic response.

  D. Diagnosis. A history of coal dust exposure and an appropriate chest-radiographic pattern are necessary to make the diagnosis of coal-worker's pneumoconiosis. The duration of exposure is usually >10 years, although radiologic changes may develop soon after exposure is terminated. PMF may also appear and progress after the exposure has ceased.

    1. The hallmark chest-radiographic finding in simple pneumoconiosis is the presence of small rounded opacities in the lung parenchyma. The upper lung zones are initially involved, and cavitation and calcification of the lesions may occur. Hilar adenopathy may be present, but eggshell calcification is unusual. Lesions of PMF are usually seen in the upper lobes. Bullae may develop as these lesions shrink toward the apices.

    2. HRCT scan of the chest usually detects the presence of nodules before they are visible on the chest radiograph (31).

    3. Pulmonary function tests. No identifiable patterns of impairment in lung function testing have been noted in simple pneumoconiosis. In more advanced diseases, such as PMF, a reduction in FVC and FEV_1 are usually seen, even after allowing for the effects of smoking (32). Residual volume may increase, reflecting air trapping due to emphysema and small-airways disease. Reductions in D_LCO and increases in dead space ventilation may also be noted.

E. **Differential diagnosis** includes pulmonary tuberculosis, nodular sarcoidosis, Wegener's granulomatosis, pulmonary amyloidosis, metastatic lung disease, primary lung cancer, and exogenous lipoid pneumonia. It is important to remember that different types of pneumoconiosis can coexist.

F. **Specific approach to each diagnostic possibility.** A complete medical history and physical examination, in addition to careful interpretation of the chest radiograph, will often establish the diagnosis of pneumoconiosis and exclude other diagnostic possibilities. When available, serial chest radiographs are extremely helpful in excluding other diseases. Patients with simple pneumoconiosis are often asymptomatic, and the presence of constitutional signs and symptoms should prompt further diagnostic investigations. Tests that may be helpful in the diagnostic evaluation are shown in Table 29-8.

G. **Management** is directed at the prevention, early diagnosis, and treatment of complications. The principles of management are the same as in silicosis. Job retraining is encouraged for younger patients with higher profusion categories to prevent the development of PMF. Patients with significant airflow obstruction or PMF should receive appropriate immunizations with influenza virus and pneumococcal vaccines.

H. **Problems and complications**
    1. **Mycobacterial infection.** Both *M. tuberculosis* and the atypical mycobacteria can complicate coal-worker's pneumoconiosis, although the incidence is much lower than in silicosis. Nevertheless, continued surveillance for and treatment of tuberculosis are of paramount importance.
    2. **Caplan's syndrome (rheumatoid pneumoconiosis)** describes the association between coal-worker's pneumoconiosis and rheumatoid arthritis. The chest radiograph typically shows rounded densities <5 cm in diameter that appear in groups over short periods of time. The lesions may cavitate, calcify, develop air–fluid levels, or even disappear entirely on occasion. The radiographic changes may precede the onset of rheumatoid arthritis by 5–10 years. There is a variable temporal association between the rheumatoid nodules found in the elbows and Achilles tendon and those that appear in the lungs in that the lung lesions may appear first.

I. **Specialist referrals.** See sections II.J. and III.A.9. on silicosis and asbestosis, respectively.

Table 29-8. Differential diagnoses of coal-worker's pneumoconiosis and diagnostic tests

Diseases	Diagnostic tests
Tuberculosis	PPD skin test Sputum for acid-fast bacilli stain and culture
Nodular sarcoidosis	Elevated angiotensin-converting enzyme level Skin anergy Noncaseating granuloma on transbronchial biopsy specimen
Wegener's granulomatosis	Positive for antinuclear cytoplasmic antibodies May have abnormal renal function studies
Metastatic disease	Tests should be guided by abnormal history or physical examinations Should include usual screening tests, eg, mammogram, stool for occult blood, flexible sigmoidoscopy, pelvic examination, etc
Pulmonary amyloidosis	Serum and urine protein and immunoelectrophoresis
Lipoid pneumonia	History of laxative abuse
Lung cancer	Sputum cytology Transbronchial lung biopsy

V. Occupational asthma. Occupational asthma is characterized by the presence of variable airflow obstruction and/or bronchial hyperresponsiveness due to exposure to airborne dusts, gases, vapors, and fumes in the workplace. The incidence of occupational asthma is estimated to be between 2% to 15% and is fast becoming the most prevalent occupational respiratory disease, even surpassing silicosis and asbestosis (33,34). Occupational asthma can be divided into allergic and nonallergic components. Allergic occupational asthma is caused by exposure to a specific sensitizing agent in the workplace and characterized by a preceding latency period before the onset of symptoms. Nonallergic occupational asthma is nonspecific bronchial hyperresponsiveness due to an exposure to irritants in the workplace without a latency period (35). Reactive airways dysfunction syndrome is a persistent asthma-like illness classically due to exposure to high levels of extremely irritating agents. This must be distinguished from preexisting asthma that is aggravated by irritants in the workplace.

A. Presenting signs and symptoms. The onset of symptoms may be immediate or may follow a prolonged latency of a few weeks to several years from the time of initial exposure. Symptoms such as dyspnea, cough, and wheezing usually improve on weekends and holidays and worsen on return to work. However, symptoms may be prolonged and persistent. if the disease is not recognized and treated early. Allergic symptoms such as rhinitis, itchy eyes, and sneezing often accompany the respiratory symptoms. Symptoms may first appear at night or late in the day after an exposure at work due to the late-phase response of asthma.

B. Etiology and pathogenesis. About 250 known agents can potentially cause occupational asthma. Isocyanates are the most common causative agents identified (36). Table 29-9 lists the agents that cause occupational asthma and workers who are at risk. Bronchial hyperresponsiveness is the characteristic feature of occupational asthma. The offending agent can directly stimulate or act as a hapten to produce IgE-specific antibodies. The specific interaction between the antigen and the IgE–

Table 29-9. Sensitizing agents implicated in occupational asthma and workers potentially exposed to them

Agents	Workers at risk
High-molecular-weight agents	
Cereals	Bakers, millers
Animal-derived allergens	Animal handlers
Enzymes	Detergents users, pharmaceutical workers, bakers
Gums	Carpet makers, pharmaceutical workers
Latex	Health professionals
Seafoods	Seafood processors
Low-molecular-weight agents	
Isocyanates	Spray painters; insulation installer; manufacturer of plastics, rubbers, and foams
Wood dusts	Forest workers, carpenters, cabinetmakers
Anhydrides	Users of plastics, epoxy resins
Amines	Shellac and lacquer handlers, solderers
Fluxes	Electronic workers
Chloramine-T	Janitors, cleaners
Dyes	Textile workers
Persulfate	Hairdressers
Formaldehyde, glutaraldehyde	Hospital staffs
Acrylate	Adhesive handlers
Drugs	Pharmaceutical workers, health professionals
Metals	Solderers, refiners

Source: Adapted from Chan-Yeung M, Malo J. Current concepts: occupational asthma. *N Engl J Med* 1995; 333:107–112.

antibody complex can then initiate the inflammatory cascade that results in bronchial edema and hyperreactivity. Pathologic changes are the same as seen in other forms of asthma.

C. **Diagnosis.** Any adult patient with new onset asthma should have a thorough review of the occupational history. The diagnosis of asthma should first be confirmed, then followed by establishment of the relationship between asthma and exposure in the workplace. The presence of a temporal relationship between asthma symptoms and the work environment is helpful but not specific for occupational asthma. Objective testing to confirm the diagnosis is often required.

   1. **Skin prick and radioallergosorbent tests** for IgE antibodies using appropriate allergens may be helpful in identifying the specific offending agent(s) (37). A positive test, however, only indicates prior sensitization and not disease causation.

   2. **Pulmonary function tests.** Because asthma is a reversible airflow limitation, normal spirometry does not exclude the diagnosis. Pulmonary function measured on a day away from work may be normal in up to 50% of patients with occupational asthma.

   3. **Bronchoprovocation testing.** This test is helpful when the symptoms are atypical, such as cough and chest tightness, and initial spirometry shows no evidence of airflow limitation. Once again, a negative study does not rule out occupational asthma, even if the patient has not been exposed for a period of time. The absence of bronchial hyperresponsiveness after the individual has worked for 2 weeks virtually rules out occupational asthma. Other indications for testing include identifying the safe dosage of antigen to be used later for specific bronchial challenge testing and documenting that the patient has recovered full function after cessation of exposure (38).

   4. **Peak expiratory flow rate monitoring** can help clarify the relationship of asthma to the work environment. This test is performed every 2 hours while awake for 2 weeks at work followed by 2 weeks at home, in conjunction with a diary of symptoms. The test is sensitive but not specific and depends heavily on patient effort and cooperation.

D. **Differential diagnosis.** Certain diseases can present with asthma-like symptoms: acute tracheobronchitis, vocal cord dysfunction (ie, factitious asthma), gastroesophageal reflux, hypersensitivity pneumonitis, and the organic toxic dust syndrome. Diseases with preexisting chronic airflow obstruction such as chronic asthma or chronic obstructive pulmonary disease may have intermittent exacerbations caused by irritant gases and fumes or may worsen because of the development of sensitivity to new antigens in the workplace.

E. **Specific approach to each diagnostic possibility.** The first step in the diagnosis of occupational asthma is to confirm the diagnosis of asthma and to exclude other diseases that may present with intermittent wheezing, as enumerated above. Special variants of asthma (Churg-Strauss syndrome, aspirin-induced asthma, bronchopulmonary aspergillosis) must also be excluded. Table 29-10 details the approach to the different diagnostic possibilities.

F. **The best treatment** for occupational asthma with a latency period is avoidance of further exposure to the offending agents. Ideally, the worker should be reassigned to a different workplace. If occupational asthma is due to toxic irritation of the airways, an emphasis should be placed on improving the workplace. The pharmacologic treatment of occupational asthma is similar to that of other types of asthma.

G. **Specialist referrals.** Once occupational asthma is suspected, early referral to a pulmonologist or allergist/immunologist is essential to establish the diagnosis. Since asthma is a common disease, a history of a temporal association between asthma symptoms and workplace exposure is usually not specific enough to diagnose occupational asthma. A complete history and physical examination, as well as a challenge with the suspected agents or spirometry in and out of the workplace, may be required to arrive at the correct diagnosis.

VI. **Toxic gases and fumes.** Acute exposures to toxic substances can lead to many different pulmonary disorders ranging from a nonspecific cough to upper airway injuries and

Table 29-10. Differential diagnoses of occupational asthma and its clinical features

Differential diagnoses	Clinical features and diagnostic tests
Diseases resembling asthma Acute tracheobronchitis	Prevalent during late fall and winter due to viral infections
Vocal cord dysfunction syndrome	More common in women, obese patients Associated with psychological disorders Stridorous wheezing due to abnormal adduction of the vocal cord during inspiration and expiration Routine spirometry including methacholine challenge are normal even during acute attacks Direct laryngoscopy may be used to document abnormal vocal cord movement during respiration
Gastroesophageal reflux disease	Symptoms worse in supine position May be associated with hoarseness Confirm by 24-h pH monitoring
Hypersensitivity pneumonitis	Due to organic dusts exposure Associated with specific occupational risks (farmers, grain workers, pigeon breeders, etc) Positive serum precipitin against specific antigens
Preexisting asthma	Symptoms aggravated at the workplace either due to acquired sensitivity to new antigens or to exposure to noxious gases and fumes
Industrial bronchitis	Exposure to irritant gases and fumes
Chronic obstructive pulmonary disease Chronic bronchitis	Chronic sputum production 3 months in a year for 2 consecutive years.
Emphysema	Fixed airflow obstruction on spirometry with decreased diffusion capacity for carbon monoxide

pulmonary edema with hypoxemic respiratory failure. Exposure to these irritant gases commonly occurs in the setting of industrial accidents. Occasionally, acute exposures of toxic inhalants can lead to reactive airways disease or bronchiolitis obliterans (33).

A. Presenting signs and symptoms. In general, exposure to an irritant gas causes immediate coughing, shortness of breath, and chest tightness. Mucosal irritation can cause conjunctivitis and sore throat. Upper airway obstruction can occur within hours of exposure, signaled by the presence of inspiratory stridor and the inability to swallow saliva or speak in full sentences. These grave signs require immediate endotracheal intubation. Physical findings may include accessory muscle use with tracheal tugging and intercostal and subcostal retractions. Coarse crackles and rhonchi may be appreciated due to sloughing of airway mucosa. Exposure to an asphyxiant gas initially causes nausea, vomiting, and shortness of breath, rapidly followed by mental confusion and obtundation. It is important to remember that cyanosis may not be seen in carbon monoxide poisoning in spite of severe tissue hypoxia.

B. Etiology and pathogenesis. Toxic-gas and -fume exposures can be divided into two major groups depending on the main pathophysiologic mechanism: local irritation of the airways or asphyxia. Table 29-11 lists the most common toxic gases and fumes and the occupations in which they are most frequently encountered. The site of action of a toxic gas depends on its chemical and physical characteristics.

    1. Solubility. Water-soluble gases are absorbed in the upper airways, where most damage is caused, while less soluble gases may cause damage throughout the entire respiratory tract.

    2. Size. Large particles (15–20 μm) are trapped in the nose and upper airway, while **smaller particles** (1–7 μm) are deposited in the distal airways and alveoli.

    3. Mechanism of injury. Irritant gases induce lung injury by either oxidative

Table 29-11. Toxic gases and fumes and their mechanism of injury

Agent	Occupations exposed	Mechanism of injury
Acrolein	Plastic, rubber, textile, resin making	Direct irritant effects on the mucosa of the eyes and respiratory tract
Acrylonitrile	Synthetic fibers, acrylic resin, rubber making	Asphyxiant
Ammonia	Fertilizer, refrigerator, explosive production	Direct action on mucosa of the eye and respiratory tract, tracheitis, pulmonary edema
Cadmium fumes	Ore smelting, alloying, welding	Acute tracheobronchitis, pulmonary edema, emphysema, renal effects
Carbon dioxide	Foundry work, mining	Asphyxiant
Carbon monoxide	Foundry work, petroleum refining, mining	Asphyxiant
Chlorine	Bleaching, disinfectant and plastic making	Direct action on mucosa of the eye and respiratory tract, tracheitis, pulmonary edema; possible chronic effects and airways obstruction
Copper fumes	Welding	Metal fume fever
Formaldehyde	Disinfectant, embalming fluid use, paper and photography industry	Direct action on mucosa of the eye and respiratory tract, dermatitis, asthma(?)
Hydrogen chloride	Refining, dye making, organic chemical synthesis	Direct action on mucosa of the eye and respiratory tract and tracheobronchitis
Hydrogen cyanide	Electroplating, fumigant work, steel industry	Asphyxiant
Hydrogen fluoride	Etching, petroleum industry, silk working	Direct action on mucosa of the eye and respiratory tract, tracheitis
Hydrogen sulfide	Natural gas making, paper pulp, sewage treatment, tannery work, oil-well prospecting	Systemic and local effects, pulmonary edema, toxic asphyxia
Manganese fumes	Foundry work, battery making, permanganate manufacture	Metal fume fever, predisposition to pneumonia, toxic to CNS
Mercury fumes	Electrolysis	Direct action on mucosa of eyes, GI tract, lung; interstitial pneumonitis; systemic effects; CNS effects
Nitrogen	Underwater work, mining	Asphyxiant
Nitrogen dioxide	Arc welding, dye and fertilizer making, farming	Irritant to respiratory tract, tracheitis, pulmonary edema, bronchiolitis obliterans
Ozone	Arc welding, air, sewage, and water treatment	Direct respiratory tract irritant
Phosgene	Chemical industry, dye and insecticide making	Direct respiratory tract irritant, pulmonary edema
Sulfur dioxide	Bleaching, ore smelting, paper manufacture, refrigeration industry	Direct action on the respiratory tract, bronchitis, pulmonary edema
Vanadium pentoxide fumes	Glass, ceramic, alloy making, chemical industry	Respiratory tract irritant, bronchitis, asthma
Zinc chloride	Dry-cell making, soldering, textile finishing	Respiratory tract irritant
Zinc oxide fumes	Welding	Metal fume fever

Adapted from Ross JA, Seaton A, Morgan WK. Toxic gases and fumes. In: Seaton A, Morgan WK, eds. *Occupational lung diseases*. Philadelphia: WB Saunders, 1995.

damage or an alteration in intracellular acid-base balance. Oxidant gases such as oxides of nitrogen, ozone, and chlorine directly disrupt the integrity of mitochondrial and cellular enzymes. Acidic and basic gases such as hydrogen chloride, sulfur dioxide, sulfuric acid, and ammonia alter the intracellular pH milieu and cause protein denaturation, increased capillary permeability, and cell death.

    C. **Relevant physiology.** The mechanisms of tissue hypoxia caused by toxic gas inhalation can vary according to the nature of the toxic gas.

        1. **Simple asphyxia** can occur by displacement of oxygen from the atmosphere and by a significant reduction in the ambient partial pressure of oxygen. This type of asphyxia usually occurs in an enclosed environment (ie, cave mining or underwater caisson). Toxic gases found in these environments include carbon dioxide, nitrogen, and methane.

        2. **A reduction in oxygen carrying capacity of the red blood cells** is typified by carbon monoxide poisoning. The high affinity of carbon monoxide for hemoglobin (250 times greater than oxygen) decreases the total oxygen-carrying capacity of the blood, and tissue hypoxia is further enhanced by the shift of the oxyhemoglobin dissociation curve to the left and increased affinity of the remaining hemoglobin for oxygen due to allosteric modification.

        3. **Inhibition of the cytochrome oxidase system** occurs by binding of cyanide to the cytochrome a-a_3 complex, blocking the final step in oxidative phosphorylation and mitochondrial oxygen utilization. This type of tissue hypoxia also occurs in acrylonitrile and hydrogen sulfide exposures.

    D. In general, **treatment of inhalational exposures** to toxic gases or fumes should include immediate removal from further exposure and cardiopulmonary resuscitation when indicated. All individuals exposed to potential toxins should be admitted to the hospital and observed for 24 hours, even if the initial injury appears to be trivial. **The signs and symptoms of upper airway obstruction due to mucosal injury may be delayed.** The onset of stridor and/or difficulty in clearing secretions are indications for endotracheal intubation. Steroids may be helpful in reducing upper airway edema. Upper airway examination should only be done under direct visualization in a location equipped for immediate intubation, as manipulation of the upper airway may precipitate complete airway obstruction. Management measures for specific toxic gas exposures are listed in Table 29-12.

Table 29-12. Specific antidotes available for toxic gas exposures

Agent	Specific treatment
Carbon monoxide	Immediate administration of 100% oxygen Hyperbaric oxygen is indicated after significant CO poisoning (pregnant patients) if it can be administered without delay Concomitant cyanide poisoning should be considered
Cyanide	Contaminated skin should be washed immediately Administer supplemental oxygen Give sodium nitrite 300 mg IV in 3–20 min followed by sodium thiosulfate 12.5 g, which may be repeated in 30 min. In severe poisoning, dicobalt edetate 600 mg IV should be given in 1–5 min; 50 mL of 50% dextrose is infused after 300 mg injection of dicobalt edetate
Hydrogen sulfide	Administration of supplemental oxygen Give sodium nitrite 300 mg IV in 3–20 min Hyperbaric oxygen may be helpful in unresponsive cases Monitor for latent pulmonary edema
Nitrogen dioxide	Corticosteroids may be helpful Exposure to nitrogen oxides may lead to methemoglobenemia, which can be treated by methylene blue 1–2 mg/kg

E. **Problems and complications.** Some patients with toxic inhalation injuries develop persistent impaired organ function even after the acute inhalational injury has resolved. Examples are described below.

   1. **Reactive airways dysfunction syndrome** is characterized by persistent wheezing, cough, and dyspnea on exertion after an episode of toxic gas inhalation (39). Persistent bronchial hyperactivity can be documented with methacholine challenge testing. The incidence of this syndrome has been estimated to be as high as 10% in patients with a prior history of acute inhalational injury.

   2. **Bronchiolitis obliterans** is an inflammatory disease characterized pathologically by plugging of terminal bronchioles and alveoli with granulation tissue. This disease entity may develop after apparent recovery from an acute inhalational injury (40).

   3. **Neurologic dysfunction.** Posthypoxic cerebral encephalopathy following carbon monoxide poisoning can develop in up to 10% of cases. Symptoms typically develop 4–6 weeks after acute poisoning and include parkinsonism, neurosis, or psychiatric disorders (41,42).

F. **Specialist Referrals.** In cases of severe carbon monoxide and cyanide poisoning, hyperbaric therapy may be life saving.

VII. **Other occupational lung diseases**

A. **Berylliosis** is a light metal with high tensile strength that is used primarily in the nuclear, aerospace, and electronic industries. Beryllium is highly toxic, and exposure can lead to either acute or chronic berylliosis (43). In addition, cutaneous exposures to beryllium can lead to papulovesicular eruptions or beryllium ulcers and granuloma formation. The first few reported cases of berylliosis were described in workers engaged in the manufacture of fluorescent light strips. Reports of berylliosis due to indirect domestic and neighborhood exposures were subsequently reported.

   1. **Acute berylliosis.** The direct irritant effects of beryllium on the skin and mucosal surfaces cause inflammation and edema. Exposure to high concentrations of beryllium can lead to chemical pneumonitis. The symptoms and signs of berylliosis are nonspecific. Chest radiographs may show patchy alveolar infiltrates, an acute miliary process, or occasionally a pulmonary edema pattern.

   2. **Chronic berylliosis** is a systemic granulomatous disease with the primary manifestation in the lung. The latency period is variable and may range from a few months to 25 years from the initial exposure. Noncaseating granulomas may be found in the lung, liver, spleen, and other tissues. The most common presenting symptom is dyspnea, which is then followed by cough, chest pain, and constitutional symptoms. Physical examination findings include bibasilar crackles, skin lesions, hepatosplenomegaly, lymphadenopathy, and sometimes finger clubbing. Pulmonary function testing may reveal an obstructive or restrictive ventilatory defect or a reduced D_LCO with normal spirometry and lung volumes. Chest radiographs usually show diffuse alveolar infiltrates and hilar adenopathy. Radiographic infiltrates have been described as granular, nodular, linear, or a mixed pattern.

   3. **Treatment** is supportive. Corticosteroids are useful in both acute and chronic berylliosis. An improvement in radiographic findings may occur after steroid therapy.

   4. **Differential diagnosis.** Berylliosis is difficult to differentiate from sarcoidosis. A Kveim test is reportedly always negative in berylliosis but has a false-negative rate of 20% in sarcoidosis (44). Diagnostic criteria for berylliosis have been proposed (45).

B. **Byssinosis** is a respiratory disease caused by exposure to cotton, flax, and hemps. The clinical presentation may range from chest tightness, shortness of breath, and cough to irreversible airflow obstruction. In addition, there is an increased prevalence of bronchitis manifested by persistent cough and sputum production. The prevalence of byssinosis is higher in smokers than nonsmokers. Pulmonary function tests reveal mild airflow obstruction with a normal total lung capacity and a mild increase in residual lung volume. The decrement in ventilatory capacity following an acute exposure is poorly correlated with the development of chronic airflow obstruction. The chest radiograph is usually normal. The diagnosis depends on a history of industrial exposure to cotton, flax, or soft hemp dusts, with typical symptoms as described earlier and a fall in FEV_1 or maximum mid–expiratory flow rate during the working day or week. Management includes avoidance of further exposure and the use of antihistamines, salbutamol (albuterol), beclomethasone, or sodium cromoglycate.

C. **Hypersensitivity pneumonitis**, also known as extrinsic allergic alveolitis, is an immunologic injury to the bronchioles and alveoli due to exposure to organic particles or gases. Both type III and type IV immunologic responses have been implicated in the pathogenesis of this disease. A variety of organic substances, listed in Table 29-13, have been implicated as causes of this disease, but the clinical manifestations are similar. The classic acute presentation of allergic alveolitis includes fever, myalgia, and general malaise that typically develop 4–8 hours after an acute exposure. Dyspnea with wheezing may occur during a severe attack, as well as fever, tachycardia, and tachypnea. Auscultation of the chest usually reveals mid- and end-inspiratory crackles. Symptoms usually peak 12 hours after exposure and may improve after 24 hours if no further exposure occurs. Subacute presentations may occur with chronic low-dose exposure to the responsible antigens. The presence of precipitating antibodies to the suspected antigen in the serum supports the diagnosis,

Table 29-13. Etiologic agents of hypersensitivity pneumonitis

Antigens	Source	Disease
Thermophilic actinomycetes		
Micropolyspora faeni	Moldy vegetable compost	Farmer's lung
		Mushroom worker's lung
Thermoactinomyces	Contaminated ventilation	Ventilation pneumonitis
vulgaris, T. viridis, T. sacharii,	system	Bagassosis
T. candidus		
Fungi		
Alternaria species	Moldy wood chips	Woodworker's disease
Aspergillus species	Moldy malt	Malt worker's lung
Cephalosporium species	Standing water	Hypersensitivity pneumonitis
Cryptostroma corticale	Wet maple bark	Maple bark stripper's disease
Penicillium caseii	Cheese mold	Cheese worker's lung
Penicillium frequentans	Cork dust	Suberosis
Pullularia species	Moldy wood	Sequoiosis
Trichosporon cutaneum	House dust	Summer type
Animal proteins		
Avian	Avian dust	Bird breeder's lung
Bovine and porcine	Pituitary snuff	Snuff taker's lung
Rat urinary	Animal urine	Laboratory technician's lung
Insect proteins		
Sitophilus granarius	Moldy grain	Miller's lung
Amebae		
Naegleria gruberi	Humidified water	Ventilation pneumonitis
Acanthamoeba castellani		
Chemicals		
Toluene diisocyanate	Plastic industry	Hypersensitivity pneumonitis
Diphenylmethane diisocyanate		
Trimelletic anhydride		
Phthalic anhydride		

Source: Adapted from Fink JN. Hypersensitivity pneumonitis. *Clin Chest Med* 1992;13:303–309.

but a negative result does not rule out the disease (46). Chest-radiographic changes include bilateral alveolar infiltrates indistinguishable from pulmonary edema or diffuse miliary mottling. Treatment is with high-dose corticosteroids, except in very mild cases that may spontaneously improve after avoidance of further exposure.

D. **Industrial bronchitis** is a distinct entity characterized by cough and sputum production due to the inhalation of dust, fumes, and gases in the workplace. Pathologically, the depth and number of mucus-secreting glands increases in the airways. The prevalence of bronchitis increases with cumulative dust exposure and can occur in the absence of pneumoconiosis. Even when age and smoking history are taken into consideration, pulmonary function tests show a mild decrease in large airway flows and occasionally a slight increase in residual volumes. It is important to remember that the contribution of cigarette smoking to bronchitis and airflow limitation is estimated to be three to five times greater than that of dust. Industrial bronchitis in the absence of either smoking or complicated pneumoconiosis does not cause sufficient respiratory impairment to prevent a patient from employment, nor does it seem to shorten life expectancy.

References

1. American Thoracic Society: Evaluation of impairment/disability secondary to respiratory disorders. *Am Rev Respir Dis* 1982;126:945–951.
2. Shipley RT: The 1980 ILO classification of radiographs of the pneumoconioses. *Radiol Clin North Am* 1992;30:1135–1145.
3. *Guidelines for the use of the ILO international classification of radiographs of pneumoconiosis. No 22.* Occupational Safety and Health Sciences, International Labour Office, 1980.
4. Begin R, Ostiguy G, Fillion R, Colman N: Computed tomography scan in the early detection of silicosis. *Am Rev Respir Dis* 1991;144:697–705.
5. Staples CA, Gamsu G, Ray CS, Webb WR: High-resolution computed tomography and lung function in asbestos-exposed workers with normal chest radiographs. *Am Rev Respir Dis* 1989;139; 1502–1508.
6. Valiante DJ, Rosenman KD: Does silicosis still occur? *JAMA* 1989;262:3003–3007.
7. Ghio AJ, Kennedy TP, Schapira RM, et al.: Hypothesis: is lung disease after silicate inhalation caused by oxidant generation? *Lancet* 1990;336:967–969.
8. Cowie RL, Hay M, Thomas RG: Association of silicosis, lung dysfunction, and emphysema in gold miners. *Thorax* 1993;48:746–749.
9. Ng TP, Tsin TW, O'Kelly FJ, et al.: A survey of the respiratory health of silica-exposed gemstone workers in Hong Kong. *Am Rev Respir Dis* 1987;135:1249–1254.
10. Graham WG, Weaver S, Ashikaga T, O'Grady RV: Longitudinal pulmonary function losses in Vermont granite workers: a re-evaluation. *Chest* 1994;106:125–130.
11. Goodman GB, Kaplan PD, Stachura I, et al.: Acute silicosis responding to corticosteroid therapy. *Chest* 1992;101:366–370.
12. Sharma SK, Pande JN, Verma K: Effect of prednisone treatment in chronic silicosis. *Am Rev Respir Dis* 1991;143:814–821.
13. American Thoracic Society: Treatment of tuberculosis and tuberculosis infection in adults and children. *Am J Respir Dis* 1994;149:1359–1374.
14. Hong Kong Chest Service/Tuberculosis Research Centre, Madras/British Medical Research Council: A controlled clinical comparison of 6 and 8 months of antituberculosis chemotherapy in the treatment of patients with silicotuberculosis in Hong Kong. *Am Rev Respir Dis* 1990;143:262–267.
15. Lin T, Suo J, Lee C, et al.: Short-course chemotherapy of pulmonary tuberculosis in pneumoconiotic patients. *Am Rev Respir Dis* 1987;136:808–810.
16. Chatgidakis CB: Silicosis in South African white gold miners: a comparative study of the disease in its different stages. *Med Proc* 1963;9:383.
17. Irwig LM, Rocks P: Lung function and respiratory symptoms in silicotic and nonsilicotic gold miners. *Am Rev Respir Dis* 1978;117:429–435.
18. Pairon JC, Brochard P, Jaurand MC, Bignon J: Silica and lung cancer: a controversial issue. *Eur Respir J* 1991;4:730–744.

19. Ng TP, Chan SL, Lee J: Predictors of mortality in silicosis. *Respir Med* 1992;86:115–119.
20. Theriault GP, Burgess WA, DiBerardinis LJ, et al.: Dust exposure in the Vermont granite sheds. *Arch Environ Health* 1974;28:12–17.
21. Becklake MR: Asbestos-related diseases of the lung and other organs: their epidemiology and implications for clinical practice. *Am Rev Respir Dis* 1976;114:187–227.
22. Coutts II, Gilson JC, Ken IH, et al.: Significances of finger clubbing in asbestosis. *Thorax* 1987; 42:117–119.
23. EPA Office of Pesticides and Toxic Substances: *Airborne asbestos levels in schools*. Environmental Protection Agency, 1983;560.
24. Gaensler EP: Asbestos exposure in buildings. *Clin Chest Med* 1995;13:231–242.
25. Davis JMG: The Pathology of asbestos-related disease. *Thorax* 1984;39:801–808.
26. DeVuyst P, Dumortier P, Moulin E, et al.: Diagnostic value of asbestos bodies in bronchoalveolar lavage fluid. *Am Rev Respir Dis* 1987;136:1219–1224.
27. Schwartz DA, Galvin JR, Burmeister LF, et al.: The clinical utility and reliability of asbestos bodies in bronchoalveolar fluid. *Am Rev Respir Dis* 1991;144:684–688.
28. Doll R: Mortality from lung cancer in asbestos workers. *Br J Ind Med* 1955;12:81–86.
29. Schneider HJ, Fulson B, Gonzales LL: Rounded atelectasis. *AJR* 1980;134:225–232.
30. Fielding DI, McKeon JL, Oliver WA, et al.: Pleurectomy for persistent pain in benign asbestos-related pleural disease. *Thorax* 1995;50:181–183.
31. Remy-Jardin M, Remy J, Farre I, Marquette CH: Computed tomographic evaluation of silicosis and coal worker's pneumoconiosis. *Radiol Clin North Am* 1992;30:1155–1174.
32. Love RG, Miller BG: Longitudinal study of lung function in coal-miners. *Thorax* 1982;37:193–197.
33. Reilly MJ, Roseman KD, Watt FC, et al.: Surveillance for occupational asthma—Michigan and New Jersey, 1988–1992. *MMWR* 1994;43:9–17.
34. Malo J: Compensation for occupational asthma in Quebec. *Chest* 1990;98:236S–239S.
35. Chan-Yeung M, Malo J: Current concepts: occupational Asthma. *N Engl J Med* 1995;333:107–112.
36. Chan-Yeung M, Lam S: State of the art—occupational asthma. *Am Rev Respir Dis* 1986;133: 686–703.
37. Grammer LC, Patterson R, Zeiss CR: Guidelines for the immunologic evaluation of occupational lung disease. *J Allergy Clin Immunol* 1989;84:805–814.
38. Cartier A, Bernstein IL, Sherwood Burge P, et al.: Guidelines for bronchoprovocation on the investigation of occupational asthma. *J Allergy Clin Immunol* 1989;84:823–829.
39. Brooks SM, Weiss MA, Bernstein IL: Reactive airways dysfunction syndrome (RADS): persistent asthma syndrome after high-level irritant exposure. *Chest* 1985;88:376–384.
40. Wright JL: Inhalational lung injury causing bronchiolitis. *Clin Chest Med* 1993;14:635–644.
41. Myers RA, Snyder SK, Emhoff TA: Subacute sequelae of carbon monoxide poisoning. *Ann Emerg Med* 1985;14:1163–1167.
42. Choi H: Delayed neurologic sequela in carbon monoxide intoxication. *Arch Neurol* 1983;40: 433–435.
43. Kriebel D, Brain JD, Sprince NL, Kazemi H: The pulmonary toxicity of beryllium. *Am Rev Respir Dis* 1988;137:464–473.
44. Klech H: Sarcoidosis: differential diagnosis. *Semin Respir Med* 1986;8:72–94.
45. Hardy H: Beryllium disease: a clinical perspective. *Environ Res* 1980;21:1–9.
46. Richerson HB, Bernstein IL, Fink JN, et al.: Guidelines for the clinical evaluation of hypersensitivity pneumonitis. *J Allergy Clin Immunol* 1989;84:839–844.

30

Pulmonary Diseases in Pregnancy

Khaled Al-Asad and Alan Fine

Pregnancy is associated with multiple physiologic and hormonal/biochemical changes that make it a unique medical situation. Most physicians feel uneasy when handling a medical problem during pregnancy due to the fear of inflicting harm to the fetus. One clear recommendation, however, is that **all pregnant patients who smoke should be explicitly advised to stop**. Our goal in this chapter is to provide basic guidelines for the management and treatment of pulmonary diseases during pregnancy. The discussion will initially focus on the major physiologic changes associated with pregnancy with an emphasis on the respiratory system. Illnesses have been arbitrarily divided into two main categories: infectious and noninfectious. Acute respiratory failure and mechanical ventilation are discussed in other chapters.

I. **General physiologic changes in pregnancy** (1–5). Pregnancy is associated with multiple physiologic changes in the mother enabling adaption to the metabolic demands of the growing fetus.
   A. **Cardiovascular.** The cardiac output increases by 40% or more from baseline values. This increase is due to increases in stroke volume and heart rate. There is an associated decrease in the systemic vascular resistance and systemic blood pressure (diastolic more than systolic). Blood pressures >100/70 mm Hg or an increase from baseline values >30 mm Hg systolic or >15 mm Hg diastolic are considered abnormal.
   B. **Blood and plasma.** There is an absolute increase in the plasma volume with a concomitant increase in red blood cell (RBC) mass. The increase in RBC mass is not as great as the increase in plasma volume, thus causing a minor anemia that may be accentuated by concomitant iron or folate deficiency.
   C. **Serum proteins.** Total protein levels may be reduced by 20%, primarily as a result of decreased albumin synthesis. The levels of most other proteins are within the normal range. The levels of coagulation factors X and XII may be increased, while the levels of factors XI, XIII and antithrombin III may be decreased.
   D. **Renal.** Plasma flow and glomerular filtration rate tend to increase without a measurable increase in glomerular pressure. A minor degree of proteinuria may occur and may worsen in the presence of renal disease or hypertension. The incidence of urinary tract infections and asymptomatic bacteriuria is significantly increased.

II. **Respiratory changes in pregnancy** (1–6)
   A. **Thoracic cavity.** The progressive enlargement of the uterus produces a mass effect, shifting the abdominal contents upward and elevating the diaphragm by as much as 4 cm. This leads to a change in the thoracic cavity shape and alteration of both vertical and transverse diameters. The earliest recognized radiographic sign of this shift is an increase in the depth of the substernal angle.
   B. **Oxygen consumption.** The basal metabolic rate is increased during pregnancy as evidenced by an increase in oxygen consumption. During labor, oxygen consumption may be further increased by 20% to 25%. When lung function is compromised due to pulmonary disease, the ability to increase oxygen consumption may be limited and may not be sufficient to support normal labor; as a consequence, fetal distress may result. Exercise testing of pregnant patients with pulmonary disease may

help predict which patients will encounter respiratory problems during labor. During graded testing, pregnant women should be able to increase oxygen consumption by 79% and increase ventilation by 65%. Failure to achieve these values may be predictive of incipient respiratory failure during labor.

   C. **Pulmonary function** (Table 30-1). Pregnant women without underlying pulmonary disease will have normal spirometry, including forced expiratory volume in 1 second (FEV_1), the ratio of FEV_1 to forced vital capacity (FEV_1/FVC), and compliance. Some minor changes in pulmonary function accompany a normal pregnancy. The vital capacity is usually unimpaired, the total lung capacity may be slightly decreased, and the expiratory reserve volume (ERV) and the residual volume (RV) may be mildly decreased, resulting in a 15% to 20% decrease in the functional residual capacity (FRC). These changes are evident by the second trimester and relate in part to the elevation of the diaphragm. The decreases in the FRC and ERV will be more pronounced in obese pregnant women and in the supine position. The observed decrease in FRC leads to a higher closing volume. The diffusing capacity for carbon monoxide is usually increased in the first trimester and will then decrease until about the 28th week of gestation. Minute ventilation is usually normal or increased in pregnancy, primarily due to an increased respiratory rate stimulated by an increased level of circulating progesterone.

   D. **Arterial blood gases.** The predominant abnormality is a compensated respiratory alkalosis (pH 7.40–7.47, $Paco_2$ 25–32 mm Hg). The Pao_2 is slightly elevated (>100 mm Hg) and remains at this level until delivery. The calculated alveolar-arterial oxygen gradient [$(A-a)O_2$] is usually increased, with slight differences noted between supine and sitting positions. An increase in the $(A-a)O_2$ >25 mm Hg should be considered abnormal.

   E. **Respiratory epithelium.** Mucosal congestion occurs secondary to engorgement of the superficial capillaries. This may involve the tracheobronchial mucosa and the nasopharynx, causing frequent nosebleeds, voice changes, and nasal congestion.

III. **Infectious disease** (5,7–10)
   A. **Viral infections.** Despite the presence of mucosal congestion, there is no increase in the incidence of viral infections of the upper respiratory tract during pregnancy. There may, however, be an increased morbidity and mortality from viral illnesses, particularly if there is lung involvement. This section will discuss the two most common viral illnesses affecting the respiratory system during pregnancy.
      1. **Influenza virus infection** is associated with increased mortality during pregnancy, as suggested by data derived from the influenza epidemic of 1957–1958. The benefit of the influenza virus vaccination is not settled; many physicians

Table 30-1. Physiologic changes during pregnancy

FEV_1	Unchanged
FEV_1/FVC	Unchanged
COMPLIANCE	Unchanged
VC	Unchanged
RV	Decreased
IRV	Increased
ERV	Decreased
FRC	Decreased
TLC	Decreased minimally
CV	High
DLCO	Increased early in pregnancy

CV = closing volume; DLCO = diffusing capacity for carbon monoxide; ERV = expiratory reserve volume; FEV_1 = forced expiratory volume in 1 sec; FRC = functional residual capacity; FVC = forced vital capacity; IRV = inspiratory reserve volume; RV = residual volume; TLC = total lung capacity; VC = vital capacity.

advise vaccination of high-risk pregnant patients afflicted by predisposing conditions (valvular heart disease, chronic lung diseases, diabetes, and chronic renal disease). Adverse effects associated with influenza virus vaccine include hypersensitivity reaction in patients allergic to eggs, febrile illness, Guillain-Barré syndrome, possible increases in plasma theophylline and warfarin levels, and a false-positive test for human immunodeficiency virus (HIV). These are no data to suggest an increase in the risk of these reactions during pregnancy.

2. **Varicella-zoster virus infection** during pregnancy is more commonly associated with lung involvement. Varicella pneumonia during pregnancy has a high mortality (40%) and is also associated with increases in fetal defects and mortality. At presentation, patients may complain of fever, cough, dyspnea, pleuritic pain, and hemoptysis. On examination, they may be tachypneic and cyanotic. The chest x-ray commonly reveals an interstitial pattern with nodular infiltrates. If there in lung involvement, treatment with acyclovir is indicated. The drug appears to be safe for both the mother and fetus. There is no consensus regarding the prophylactic use of globulin or varicella-zoster immune globulin following exposure in women without serologic evidence of previous infection. Furthermore, there are no clear recommendations regarding the use of acyclovir in cutaneous varicella without pulmonary involvement.

B. **Bacterial pneumonia** is the second most common cause of mortality in pregnant women after cardiac diseases. Upper respiratory tract infections precede pneumonia in approximately 50% of cases. Pneumonia appears to be more common in pregnant than nonpregnant women; in part, this may be attributed to the increasing incidence of HIV infection in women of childbearing age. *Streptococcus pneumoniae*, *Mycoplasma pneumoniae*, and *Haemophilus influenzae* continue to lead the list of the most common responsible pathogens. The mortality of community-acquired pneumonia in the absence of a comorbid disease is <5%.

1. **Diagnosis** is based on clinical presentation, physical examination, and chest x-ray. Other work-up should include sputum sample for Gram's stain, culture, and sensitivity and a blood test including white blood cell count and electrolytes.

2. **Treatment** of community-acquired pneumonia in pregnant patients should be initiated as quickly as possible to reduce the risk of abortion, premature delivery, and intrauterine fetal death. Initial antibiotic therapy may include a penicillin or cephalosporin. Erythromycin and other macrolides, though safe to use during pregnancy, are reserved for cases of allergy to penicillin or cephalosporins, or if atypical pneumonia is expected. Another safe choice are the quinolones. The major antibiotic to be avoided in pregnancy is tetracycline and related drugs because of their adverse effects on tooth coloration, and bone formation.

C. **Aspiration pneumonia (Mendelson's syndrome)**. During labor, the risk of aspiration is increased. Lung injury results from the low-pH gastric contents, which produce a severe chemical pneumonitis. Preventive measures should be initiated at the onset of labor: avoidance of oral intake once labor has started, use of H_2-blockers or antacids, and use of regional rather than general anesthesia. In addition to chemical pneumonitis, aspiration of gastric contents may induce bronchospasm, cough, cyanosis, dyspnea, and tachycardia. Aspiration of solid food may also lead airway compromise and suffocation. Therapy is supportive; antibiotics should be administered only if there is evidence of infection.

D. **Tuberculosis (TB)**. Pregnancy does not increase the risk of reactivation of an old tuberculous focus. Once developed, the course of TB is not affected by pregnancy. To avoid dissemination, progression, and congenital tuberculosis in the newborn, aggressive therapy should be started immediately in suspected cases of active disease. Importantly, the purified protein derivative tuberculin skin test is not affected by pregnancy and should be performed in all patients suspected of having TB. Chest x-rays are not contraindicated in pregnancy since the radiation exposure to the chest is only 50 mrad with significantly less pelvic exposures (teratogenic effects of radiation are thought to occur at doses >1 rad). Routine screening chest x-rays are not advisable, however, and should be performed only in cases of high suspicion for active TB or in patients with recent skin conversion.

1. **To diagnose** active disease, multiple adequate sputum samples should be stained and plated for culture. If necessary, ultrasonic nebulization or bronchoscopy can be used to obtain specimens.
2. **Treatment** of active TB with a pansensitive organism should begin with isoniazid, rifampin, and ethambutol for the first 2 months. In contrast to therapy in nonpregnant patients, pyrazinamide is generally not included in the initial regimen because of uncertainty regarding its effects on the fetus. After this, therapy should be continued with isoniazid and rifampin for a total duration of 6 months. With multidrug-resistant organisms, initial therapy should be tailored to the *in vitro* sensitivity of the organism. In these cases, treatment should be continued for at least 1 year. Available information indicates that isoniazid, rifampin, and ethambutol can be safely administered to a pregnant woman without danger to the fetus. Streptomycin is contraindicated because of effects on ear development.
3. **Response to therapy** should be monitored by repeated sputum smears and cultures to document clearing. In 85% of patients infected with a pansensitive organism receiving isoniazid and rifampin, sputum cultures will be negative after 2 months of therapy. If the sputum fails to clear and continues to be positive, the susceptibility pattern of the organism should be reviewed, and the compliance of the patient should be rigorously examined. In cases where the original susceptibility pattern of the organism has changed, two new drugs to which the organism is sensitive should be added to the regimen. Directly observed therapy and frequent sputum testing should be done in patients who are suspected of being noncompliant with therapy.
   E. **HIV-associated lung problems.** The number of women with HIV disease is increasing; the majority of these women are in the childbearing age. At this time, about 0.25% to 0.80% of pregnant women are seropositive for HIV. Fetal transmission rates appear to approach 40%. The most common pulmonary complication in HIV-positive pregnant women is bacterial pneumonia, which should be treated according to established protocols for community-acquired pneumonia.
      1. *Pneumocystis carinii* **pneumonia** is the most common opportunistic infection afflicting patients with low CD4 lymphocyte counts. Initial treatment is trimethoprim/sulfamethoxazole. Although sulfonamides may lead to hemolysis, placing the newborn at risk of kernicterus, most studies indicate that the use of this family of drugs is safe during pregnancy.
      2. **Kaposi's sarcoma** is common in homosexual men but has a low incidence in HIV-positive women, particularly pregnant women. This may be a result of the effect of human chorionic gonadotropin, which appears *in vitro* to accelerate sarcoma cell death by an apoptotic mechanism.
IV. **Noninfectious complications**
   A. **Dyspnea** is the most common pulmonary complaint encountered in pregnant women (11,12); 60% will complain of dyspnea, even in the absence of pulmonary or cardiac disease. The majority of patients complain of dyspnea in the first or second trimester. Dyspnea occurs mostly at rest and does not limit exercise. There is some evidence that dyspnea is more common in women with a higher baseline (nonpregnant) Pco_2. The cause is unknown.
   B. **Asthma** is the most common pulmonary disease in pregnant women with an incidence of 1% to 2% (13–17). About one-third of pregnant women will experience deterioration one or more times during pregnancy, another third will not have any exacerbation, and the remaining one-third will show some improvement. Many physicians and patients are reluctant to use medications during pregnancy; this may increase the frequency of exacerbations. There are studies suggesting that increases in the frequency of vaginal bleeding, toxemia, and hyperemesis occur in pregnant asthmatics. The risk of low-birth-weight infants is also thought to be increased. Episodes of severe asthma may be associated with maternal hypoxemia and respiratory alkalosis, leading to fetal distress.
      1. **Risk factors.** The failure of the IgE level to fall during pregnancy may be an independent risk factor for pregnancy-associated asthma exacerbations. Hy-

perventilation, exposure to fetal antigens, and mucosal congestion may be other exacerbating factors. To some extent, these factors may be counteracted by increased serum cortisol, decreased airway resistance, and increased serum cyclic AMP.

2. **Treatment of asthma** in pregnancy does not differ from its management in nonpregnant patients. Self-measured peak expiratory flow rate should be routinely recorded, and baseline spirometry should be performed during the early stages of pregnancy. Any exacerbation should be immediately reported to a physician. The severity of an exacerbation should be assessed by employing commonly practiced guidelines. Since the average $Paco_2$ during pregnancy is approximately 32 mm Hg, obtaining such a value during an acute episode suggests the possibility of impending respiratory failure. Such patients should be carefully observed and considered for admission to the MICU. The first step in management of the acutely ill patient is to identify predisposing factors, including the use of new medications, particularly nonsteroidal anti-inflammatory agents.

3. **Inhaled steroids** are the mainstay of outpatient therapy of the stable asthmatic. With these medications, there are no data indicating a detrimental effect on the fetus. In acute asthma, intravenous pulsed steroids at high doses (hydrocortisone 1–2 mg/kg/d) should be used. Prolonged use of steroids in animals has been associated with increased cleft palate, but this has not been documented in humans. Prolonged use of prednisone in pregnant women has only been rarely associated with transient adrenal suppression in the newborn. If the mother has been receiving high doses of steroids, hydrocortisone 100 mg IV q8h should be administered for 24 hours at the time of delivery.

4. **β-Agonists** may be used in the treatment of exercise-induced asthma and intermittent wheezing during pregnancy. These medications should be administered by inhalers or nebulizers. Oral and intravenous forms should be avoided. Inhaled terbutaline is a selective β_2-agonist frequently used in both pregnant and nonpregnant asthmatics. Based on animal studies, it may be safer for the fetus than albuterol or metaproterenol. Rarely, pulmonary edema in the latter part of the pregnancy has been associated with the use of β-agonists. More commonly, pulmonary edema may complicate the use of β-adrenergic tocolytic therapy. In addition, β-agonists may delay the progression of labor and lead to postpartum uterine atony. Subcutaneous injections of catecholamines during acute episodes should probably be avoided because of inhibitory effects on uterine contractions and placental blood flow.

5. **Theophylline** has been reported not to cross the placenta, but fetal serum levels of this drug have been documented. It is secreted in breast milk and may lead to infant irritability and insomnia. If used, it is advisable to monitor maternal serum levels to achieve a low therapeutic level. Importantly, theophylline may exacerbate morning sickness.

6. **Atropine or atropine-like drugs** can be used in difficult cases. No documented fetal malformations have been noted, but use of this drug can lead to fetal tachycardia.

7. **It is not advisable to initiate desensitization** during pregnancy, but if it is already in progress, the regular dosage schedule can probably be maintained. Large increases in doses should be avoided to prevent maternal anaphylaxis.

C. **Cystic fibrosis (CF)** (18). Because more patients with CF are surviving into adulthood, it is common for women with CF to be pregnant. Most pregnancies result in a good outcome and no associated deterioration in maternal lung function. A prepregnancy FEV_1 >60% of the predicted value is the single best indicator of good maternal and fetal outcome. Overall, there is an increased incidence of congestive heart failure, low maternal weight gain, and prematurity. In CF patients with pulmonary hypertension, termination of pregnancy may be indicated.

D. **Sarcoidosis** (19). The activity of sarcoidosis during pregnancy tends to reflect the activity in the prepregnant state. Most patients with sarcoidosis do well and may even improve during their pregnancy, possibly as a result of increased plasma level of corticosteroids. However, 3–6 months after delivery, disease activity may worsen. Use of steroids should be maintained in doses sufficient to control disease activity.

E. **Pulmonary embolism (PE) and deep venous thromobosis (DVT)** (20–27). The risk of DVT and PE is higher in the postpartum period than during pregnancy. DVT occurs in 2 in 1000 pregnancies, while superficial thrombophlebitis occurs in 12 in 1000 pregnancies. The incidence of PE is approximately 0.4 per 1000 pregnancies. The risk of these complications is closely related to use of estrogens, prolonged bed rest due to complications of pregnancy or delivery, assisted delivery, and cesarean section. Obesity, advanced maternal age, and increased venous stasis from compression of veins from the enlarging uterus may play additive roles. Further, the synthesis of fibrinogen and other clotting factors is increased. whereas the synthesis of certain proteins involved in the fibrinolysis are suppressed.

1. **Work-up and diagnosis** of DVT/PE is more complicated because the value of lower extremity ultrasound is not reliable (high false-positive and -negative rates). The use of radioactive iodine–labeled fibrinogen is contraindicated in pregnancy. Venography, the gold standard technique, is associated with significant pelvic irradiation and thus requires pelvic shielding, which obscures visualization of the external and common iliac veins. Ventilation–perfusion scans and pulmonary angiography can be safely performed and interpreted during pregnancy. Fetal exposure can be minimized by abdominal shielding. The approach to diagnosis of DVT in pregnancy is unsettled, but in early pregnancy Doppler ultrasound or plethysmography may be informative. The use of venography and pelvic shielding should be employed in the third trimester. To rule out PE, work-up and overall approach should proceed as in the nonpregnant state.

2. **Anticoagulation** remains the standard therapy during pregnancy. Warfarin sodium, a low-molecular-weight compund, crosses the placenta, leading to fetal hemorrhage, bony malformation (nasal hypoplasia, stippled epiphysis, and chondrodysplasia), and neurologic abnormalities. Its use during pregnancy is absolutely contraindicated. Heparin does not cross the placenta and accordingly does not affect fetal development. However, its use can lead to maternal bleeding, especially at delivery. Heparin therefore should be stopped 24 hour before an elective delivery. During nonelective deliveries, protamine sulfate can be administered to reverse the effect of heparin. Following the diagnosis of DVT or PE, intravenous heparin should be administered for 1–2 weeks to achieve a therapeutic activated partial thromboplastin time (PTT) 1.5–2.5 of the control. Heparin may then be given as a subcutaneous injection every 12 hours (Table 30-2).

3. **Monitoring therapy, use of thrombolytics, and future risks.** The PTT should be monitored 6 hours following heparin injection to ensure that it remains therapeutic. The use of thrombolytics are relatively contraindicated in pregnancy due to the hemorrhagic risks for both the mother and the fetus. Available data reveal a hemorrhagic rate of around 8%, fetal loss of 5%, and maternal mortality of almost 1.2%. Some advocate the use of thrombolytics only

Table 30-2. Management of deep venous thrombosis (DVT) and pulmonary embolism (PE)

Prophylactic	
History of previous DVT/PE	Low-dose heparin (5000 U SC BID); duration of therapy includes pregnancy and first 2 weeks of puerperium
Acute event	
First 2 weeks	Heparin IV (maintain a PTT 1.5–2.0 times control)
Following 3 months	High-dose heparin SC (maintain a PTT slightly elevated)
Remaining period	Low-dose heparin SC through first 2 weeks of puerperium

PTT = partial thromboplastin time.

with a life-threatening PE or clinical deterioration in the setting of therapeutic heparin administration. The risk of thromboembolism in subsequent pregnancies in a woman with a previous DVT or PE is high (recurrence in untreated individuals is estimated at 4% to 12%). In such cases, prophylaxis with subcutaneous heparin (5000 U q12h) is probably indicated throughout pregnancy. In the third trimester, some advocate increasing heparin dosage to achieve an PTT of 1.5 times control, particularly in patients with cardiac disease, hypercoagulable state or obesity.

F. **Amniotic fluid embolism** has a high mortality (>80%) but accounts for <10% of all pregnancy-associated deaths. It usually occurs during labor, but the syndrome has been reported in the postpartum period. Clinically, patients present with an acute onset of respiratory distress followed by adult respiratory distress syndrome, disseminated intravascular coagulation, and cardiovascular collapse. It is unclear which component of the amniotic fluid leads to this syndrome, as the fluid contains meconium, fat, lanugo hair, bile, mucin, and electrolytes. The diagnosis can be established by identifying squamous epithelium of fetal origin in the sputum. Swan-Ganz catheter–directed blood sampling of the pulmonary vein may also reveal the presence of fetal cells. Treatment is supportive. At autopsy, the lungs display evidence of pulmonary edema and amniotic fluid in the pulmonary vasculature.

G. **Venous air embolism** is an uncommon complication (1% of pregnancies) that occurs as a result of the passage of air into the venous sinuses of the uterus during labor, usually in the presence of placenta previa. As little as 100 mL of air may be sufficient to precipitate symptoms of air embolism. In severe cases, air emboli may cause mechanical obstruction of the pulmonary outflow, leading to death. In addition, platelet and fibrin aggregates leading to fibrin microthrombi can cause stroke, myocardial infarction, and retinal thrombosis. Patients present with the sudden onset of dyspnea, cough, diaphoresis, bronchospasm, chest pain, and occasionally cardiovascular collapse. Physical examination may reveal cyanosis, marble-like skin, tachycardia, and a "mill-wheel" murmur. If this diagnosis is considered, the patient should be emergently placed in the left lateral decubitus position to minimize obstruction of pulmonary outflow tract, and 100% oxygen should be administered to reduce thrombotic complications. Use of heparin therapy may be of some benefit.

H. **Primary pulmonary hypertension** is a rare disease that may present during pregnancy. Mortality may be exceedingly high (50%), particularly in the third trimester. Clinical deterioration relates to the burden of increased circulating blood volume and cardiac output. Elective abortion may be necessary for the health of the mother. If it is not performed, affected patients should be hospitalized early in pregnancy for close observation to minimize cardiac complications.

References

1. Gee JBL, Packer BS, Millen JE, Robin ED: Pulmonary mechanics during pregnancy *J Clin Invest* 1967;46:945–952.
2. Gazioglu K, Kaltreider NL, Rosen M, Yu PN: Pulmonary function during pregnancy in normal and in patients with cardiopulmonary disease. *Thorax* 1970;25:445–450.
3. Knuttgen HG, Emerson K Jr: Physiologic response to pregnancy at rest and during exercise. *J Appl Physiol* 1974;36:549–553.
4. Rubin A, Russo N, Goucher D: The effect of pregnancy upon pulmonary function in normal women. *Am J Obstet Gynecol* 1956;72:963–969.
5. Weinberger S, Weiss S, Cohen W, et al.: Pregnancy and the lung. *Am Rev Respir Dis* 1980; 121:559–581.
6. Eliasson A, Phillips Y, Stajduhar K, et al.: Oxygen consumption and ventilation during normal labor. *Chest* 1992;102:467–471.
7. American Thoracic Society: Treatment of tuberculosis and tuberculosis infection in adults and children. *Am J Respir Crit Care Med* 1994;149:1359–1374.
8. Snider D: Pregnancy and tuberculosis. *Chest* 1984;86S:10S–13S.
9. Barnes P, Barrows S: Tuberculosis in the 1990s. *Ann Intern Med* 1993;119:400–410.

10. Heubner R, Schein M, Bass J: The tuberculin skin test. *Clin Infect Dis* 1993;17:968–975.
11. Gilbert R, Auchincloss JH: Dyspnea of pregnancy: clinical and physiological observations. *Am J Med Sci* 1966;252:270–276.
12. Milne JA, Howie AD, Pack AL: Dyspnea during normal pregnancy. *Br J Obstet Gynaecol* 1978; 85:260–263.
13. Moore-Gillon J: Asthma in pregnancy. *Br J Obstet Gynaecol* 1994;101:658–660.
14. Chazotte C: Asthma in pregnancy: a review. *J Assoc Acad Minor Phys* 1994;5:107–110.
15. Gluck JC, Gluck PA: The effects of pregnancy on asthma. *Ann Allergy* 1976;37:164–168.
16. Cockcroft DW: Management of acute severe asthma. *Ann Allergy Asthma Immunol* 1995; 75:83–89.
17. Snyder RD, Snyder D: Corticosteroids for asthma during pregnancy. *Ann Allergy* 1978;41: 340–341.
18. Larsen JW: Cystic fibrosis and pregnancy. *Obstet Gynecol* 1972;39:880–883.
19. Dines DE, Banner E: Sarcoidosis and pregnancy: improvement in pulmonary function. *JAMA* 1967;200:726–727.
20. Clinton M, Neiderman M: Noninfectious respiratory disease in pregnancy. *Cleve Clin J Med* 1993; 60:233–244.
21. Leontic E: Respiratory disease in pregnancy. *Med Clin North Am* 1977;61:111–128.
22. Jaff M: Medical aspects of pregnancy. *Cleve Clin J Med* 1994;61:263–271.
23. Nelson-Piercy C, Waldron M, Moore-Gillon J: Respiratory disease in pregnancy. *Br J Hosp Med* 1994;51:398–401.
24. Moseley P, Kerstein MD: Pregnancy and thrombophlebitis. *Surg Gynecol Obstet* 1980;150:593– 599.
25. Ginsberg J, Hirsh J: Use of antithrombotic agents during pregnancy. *Chest* 1992;142:385S–389S.
26. Kramer WB, Belfort M, Saade GR, et al.: Successful urokinase treatment of massive pulmonary embolism in pregnancy. *Obstet Gynecol* 1995;86:660–662
27. Turrentine MA, Braems G, Ramirez MM: Use of thrombolytics for the treatment of thromboembolic disease during pregnancy. *Obstet Gynecol Surv* 1995;50:534–541.

31

Smoking Cessation

Kevin R. Cooper

I. Health impact of tobacco

A. Tobacco use is the most common preventable cause of death in the United States, responsible for about 1 in every 5 American deaths. Cigarette smoking is the most popular and most lethal form of tobacco use. Its attractiveness peaked in the U.S. in 1963, at which time half of all adult men and a third of adult women were smokers. By 1993, overall smoking rates had declined to 28% for men and 23% for women; however, each day another 3000 teenagers become smokers. Most recently, smoking prevalence among teenagers actually increased slightly (1,2). Tobacco exports have quadrupled since 1980. Even though U.S. consumption is declining, worldwide consumption grows about 2% each year, with the highest rates of growth in developing nations (3). The World Health Organization estimates that 10% of the 5.7 billion people now alive will die of a disease caused by tobacco.

B. Americans usually begin smoking in early adolescence. Half of all regular adult smokers began by the age of 14, and 90% by age 20. Although the vast majority of patients with smoking-induced diseases are older than 40, the initiation phase of this chronic disease is certainly in the realm of pediatrics, and finding effective ways of preventing children from smoking is the most elegant and effective public health strategy. People who drop out of school before eighth grade and those who graduate from college are the least likely to smoke; high school dropouts are the most likely. Among adults, smoking is slightly more prevalent among blacks than among whites, but blacks under age 25 have very low smoking rates, about 5% (4).

II. Diseases caused by tobacco

A. Of the 2.2 million Americans who die each year, tobacco kills about 400,000. The average American smoker begins smoking between ages 11 and 15, smokes 20–25 cigarettes a day until middle age, runs a one-in-three risk of dying from a disease caused by tobacco, and another one-in-three risk of developing a serious but not fatal tobacco-related disease. About one in three lifelong smokers escapes serious health effects.

B. About 90% of **lung cancer** results from tobacco use. Studies quoting a smaller percentage usually have failed to attribute cancer to former tobacco use among ex-smokers. When smokers are exposed to other lung carcinogens such as asbestos or radon daughters, the risk increases further. **The lifetime risk of dying from lung cancer for the average American smoker is 10%; the risk is about 50% for a smoker with asbestosis.**

1. The risk of lung cancer is clearly dose related, so that a 40-pack-year smoker (number of packs per day × number of years smoked) has about twice the risk of a smoker with 20 pack-years. A person who cuts down but does not quit reduces the risk of lung cancer. However, risk calculations are less reliable at rates <10 cigarettes a day because people tend to inhale more smoke from each cigarette when they smoke <10 a day. Low-tar cigarettes provide less carcinogen to the smoker when puffed by the mechanical devices that measure tar content, but this does not reflect actual use by the smoker, who can often receive much more tar and nicotine by wetting the cigarette filter or covering it with the lips. Smokers of filtered cigarettes and those with low tar and nico-

tine enjoy only a small reduction in risk of lung cancer compared with smokers of unfiltered cigarettes (5).

   2. **All cell types of lung cancer are caused by tobacco use.** The most common are small cell and squamous bronchogenic carcinomas. Most lung cancers unrelated to tobacco are adenocarcinomas; however, many adenocarcinomas are associated with tobacco use as well.

C. Many other types of cancer are associated with tobacco use since many organs are exposed to carcinogens absorbed from smoke. **Smoking increases the risk of cancers of the oral cavity, larynx, esophagus, stomach, pancreas, cervix, kidney, and bladder, with relative risks ranging from 2 for cancers of the pancreas, cervix, and bladder to 27 for lip and oral cavity cancers in males** (6). Recent epidemiologic studies have also found that cancers of the breast (7) and colon (8) are smoking associated.

D. **Disease of the heart and blood vessels** is the most common smoking-induced cause of death. The pathogenetic mechanisms are accelerated arteriosclerosis, reversible vasoconstriction, and enhanced platelet adhesiveness caused by smoking. About one-third of all heart attack deaths and 40% of stroke deaths are attributable to tobacco use. Myocardial infarction is five times more common among smokers than nonsmokers under age 50 (9). Aortic aneurysm is increased about fourfold in smokers compared to nonsmokers (10). Among patients requiring leg amputation for peripheral vascular disease, diabetes and cigarette smoking are the chief risk factors. Smoking-induced peripheral vascular disease is also the most common organic cause of impotence and causes premature skin wrinkles, especially in people with generous sun or other ultraviolet light exposure.

E. **About 85% of chronic bronchitis and emphysema is attributable to tobacco smoking,** and current smokers have far more episodes of hospital care for exacerbations of symptoms then do ex-smokers. Forty percent of 30-year-old men who smoke a pack a day have chronic bronchitis; by age 60, the rate is 80%. Overall, about 20% of lifelong smokers develop airflow obstruction detectable by pulmonary function tests. While α_1-antiprotease deficiency certainly increases the risk of chronic obstructive pulmonary disease (COPD), the vast majority of smokers with COPD have normal levels of this enzyme. Other susceptibility factors are not well understood.

F. **Other smoking-related conditions**
   1. **Spontaneous pneumothorax** is most common in young people with tall, thin stature. Smoking is the chief risk factor, increasing the risk of spontaneous pneumothorax more than 20-fold in men and ninefold in women (11). Small subpleural blebs and bullae are often found at surgery.
   2. **Eosinophilic granuloma,** a histiocytic proliferative condition, causes interstitial infiltrates with predominantly upper lobe involvement. Although the onset can occur at any age, even in infancy, the typical patient is a young adult, and >90% are current or former cigarette smokers (12).
   3. **Peptic ulcer disease** occurs more commonly and ulcers heal more slowly in smokers.
   4. **Osteoporosis** with abnormally low bone density and spontaneous fractures is more common in smokers.
   5. **Hypertension is not more prevalent among smokers but is more difficult to control.** Less medication is needed by smokers with hypertension when they quit smoking.

III. **Health effects of environmental tobacco smoke**
   A. Environmental tobacco smoke (ETS) contains over 4000 distinct chemicals; some are toxic and some are carcinogenic. Long-term exposure to ETS has been shown to cause lung cancer and coronary heart disease in adults (13).
   B. The epidemiologic studies of health effects of ETS on adults have usually examined risks to nonsmoking wives of male smokers (**second-hand smoke**), but studies also show comparable risks in other groups with similar exposure histories (14). Children who live in a home shared by a smoker and exposed to second-hand smoke have an increased risk of otitis media, colds, bronchitis, and pneumonia (15). The development of lung cancer later in life also appears more likely in these

children, whether or not they become smokers (16). Asthma, chronic cough, and wheezing are all more prevalent among children who live in homes shared by smokers.

C. **Female smokers experience a substantial decline in fertility and enter menopause about 2 years younger than nonsmokers. The woman who smokes while pregnant gives birth to a baby who is on average 1 pound lighter than the baby of a nonsmoking mother.** The incidence of prematurity and very low birth-weight babies is also higher among smoking mothers.

1. **Sudden infant death syndrome** is more common among infants born to women who smoked during pregnancy, as well as among infants who share a home with a smoker (17).

2. Nicotine and other components of smoke are present in the **breast milk** of nursing mothers who smoke; infants who ingest such milk take smaller volumes, gain weight more slowly, and have more vomiting, diarrhea, and restless behavior than infants of nonsmoking mothers (18). Overall, tobacco use accounts for about 10% of all infant mortality.

IV. **Pipes, cigars, and smokeless tobacco.** Pipe and cigar smoke and smokeless tobacco are more alkaline than cigarette smoke and allow more efficient absorption of nicotine by the buccal mucosa, so that contact with the mouth rather than inhalation provides the sought-after nicotine effects. Thus, pipe and cigar smokers have a greatly increased risk of cancer of the mouth, tongue, larynx and esophagus. The risk of coronary artery disease, lung cancer, and COPD are increased compared to nonsmokers, but not nearly as much as among cigarette smokers. Smokeless tobacco users risk periodontitis and tooth loss, along with oral cancers. All forms of tobacco use increase peptic ulcer risk.

V. **Benefits of quitting.** Former smokers live longer and remain healthier than current smokers. People who quit by age 50 have only half the risk of dying before age 65 as those who continue to smoke. The risk of sudden death from myocardial infarction and stroke declines almost immediately and continues to decrease with time after smoking is stopped. The risk of lung cancer begins to decrease 5–7 years after cessation, since most lung cancers have been growing for years by the time they are large enough to be seen on chest radiographs. The risk of other cancers also declines over time. Cancer risk declines exponentially, and approaches but never reaches the risk of lifelong nonsmokers, even after 25 years. Emphysema does not improve after quitting but worsens at a slower rate than with continued smoking. Cough and sputum usually resolve entirely in patients with simple chronic bronchitis but may persist in patients with obstructive lung disease.

VI. **Why people smoke**

A. Smokers are informed about the health risks and effects of smoking; when surveyed, smokers generally **overestimate** the likelihood that daily smoking will cause a serious disease. Two-thirds of smokers would like to quit and only one in four intends to continue smoking another 5 years, yet the long-term success rate of people trying to quit each year is only about 8%.

B. People smoke because it makes them feel good and because trying to do without tobacco makes them feel bad. For most smokers, pleasure is derived from biochemical effects of nicotine on the brain, primarily from effects on the locus ceruleus (enhanced vigilance and arousal) and actions in the mesolimbic dopaminergic system (feelings of reward and pleasure).

C. **Paradoxically, by controlling the dosing, an experienced smoker can use nicotine for either stimulation or relaxation. A series of brief, rapid puffs provides a feeling of enhanced alertness and ability to focus concentration, while a long inhalation, breath-hold, and slow exhalation produce calm.** When a person has been relying on a drug to cope with the daily stresses of life, fluctuations of mood, and issues of self-control by self- administering 200 doses a day of an addicting drug (25 cigarettes × 8 puffs per cigarette), quitting becomes quite difficult.

D. Most smokers take years to become expert at dosing nicotine and to incorporate it skillfully into a lifestyle. Although the first few smoking experiences produce physiologic responses of nausea and nervousness that are uniformly unpleasant, with dosing experience, the bad feelings can be avoided while the feelings of pleasure and control become more predictable. Daily cigarette consumption tends to increase gradually for the first 5 years before stabilizing. This pattern of increased use can be explained partly by pharmacologic tolerance to nicotine that requires larger doses for the same effect but also by acquired experience in the different ways that nicotine produces good feelings. For the typical beginning smoker (11–16 years old), this period of learning how to use a drug to alter mood coincides with the tumultuous period of adolescent personality development and coping with multiple life stresses.

1. **The first cigarette.** Why take that first cigarette, and why continue smoking when it initially produces nausea and cough? Sixth and seventh graders describe their reasons for smoking as trying something new, imitating a role model (especially an older sibling or other family member), rebelling from adult warnings not to smoke, gaining acceptance from peers, and projecting an image of confidence by taking on a dangerous and forbidden practice. Surprisingly, the most common reason to try cigarettes is: "I was bored, and it was something to do."

    a. Advertising projecting images of pleasure, thinness, and social success associated with smoking is a major force that focuses children's attention on smoking. About 3000 children start smoking everyday; surveys show that about 20% of high school seniors are regular smokers, and recently this figure has been increasing (4). An exception to this is African-American teenagers; only about 5% of black teens smoke, and the dominant reason is simply rejecting smoking as "not something we do...smoking is something white kids do" (19). This shunning of tobacco by black youth will have significant health benefits if the attitude persists.

2. **Children's knowledge of health risks.** One young smoker said with great insight: "We're old enough to know better, but too young to care." Kids who begin smoking are very well informed about the health effects, and most plan to quit before they get enough of a cumulative dose to become addicted. Very few plan to remain smokers for their whole lives, yet by age 17 half of all daily smokers have already tried to quit and failed. Others plan to quit someday before any serious harm results, but they believe they have plenty of time before that day comes. During middle age, feelings of invincibility fade, and the wisdom of quitting becomes more apparent.

VII. **Psychological dynamics of quitting**

A. Quitting tobacco is a highly individualized process. Most smokers fit a general model of substance abuse behavior that classifies the smoker in the **precontemplation** stage when happily enjoying the benefits of the drug. The **contemplation** stage occurs when the smoker is thinking about quitting, usually motivated by the fear of adverse health effects. This fear evolves into a plan of **action** and attempts to quit. A period of **maintained abstinence** may then begin, and is usually followed by **relapse**. The cycle may be repetitive. The period of abstinence may become long-lasting and finally permanent, resulting in an ex-smoker. **Fewer than 5% of smokers are permanently successful on their first attempt at quitting; the average smoker tries five or six times before achieving a durable abstinence.** The physician should determine where the smoker is in the abuse cycle at each contact and direct progress to the next stage.

B. Any particular stage in the smoking cycle may last from minutes to years, depending on the individual patient and the strength of motivating factors. Many people smoke until a first myocardial infarction or cancer surgery and then are able to quit for good. Others spend a decade vaguely considering a plan. Individual differences cannot be predicted.

C. Sometimes a patient will quit when advised by a physician or other health care provider. Some individuals quit when the price of a pack of cigarettes increases. Smokers who never find sufficient motivation to quit are in the minority. America has as many ex-smokers as current smokers; most smokers have the ability to overcome this addiction, if the desire is strong enough. Many patients who say they will never be able to quit eventually do but only with persistent effort, planning, and support.

VIII. **Features of the cessation process**

A. **Smokers' relationship to cigarettes.** Most ex-smokers share similar experiences and feelings. For many, smoking is an accessible and reliable source of pleasure, comfort, and self-esteem. The sense of a great loss that accompanies quitting may have the impact of a divorce or the death of a trusted friend; however, this loss can easily be recovered and is thus fundamentally different. While quitting is an achievement that brings great pride, the smoker often believes that cigarettes have made him or her a better person, and quitting signifies the end of a very satisfying period of life.

B. **Nicotine dependence.** Nicotine produces pharmacologic dependence and therefore **withdrawal produces symptoms**: restlessness, irritability, difficulty with concentration, insomnia, headache, nausea, abdominal discomfort, and diarrhea. Nicotine replacement by polacrilex gum or patch reduces withdrawal symptoms and is very helpful. However, nicotine gum and patches increase blood levels much too slowly to replace the pleasure of smoking. Quicker-acting delivery systems, such as nasal sprays, may eventually enable ex-smokers to reproduce more of the pleasure of smoking and may therefore improve success rates.

C. **Cigarette cravings** can be intense. Smokers describe intense desires for cigarettes at certain times, such as after dinner, after sex, when under stress, at social gatherings, and so on. Quitters must be taught in advance that these cravings will eventually subside, but they need to have techniques in place to deal with them. Otherwise, they may believe that cravings will continue forever unless they are satisfied.

D. **Smoking-associated behavior.** Associated behaviors are a frequent source of relapse. Smokers often light cigarettes after meals, during coffee breaks, or while on the phone but can be unaware or unconscious of smoking until the cigarettes are half gone. Planning ways to avoid or dissociate these connected behaviors improves success and may be as simple as keeping cigarettes in a briefcase instead of a pocket to interrupt habitual routines.

E. **Slips versus relapse.** Smokers should be taught to distinguish between a slip (smoking a few cigarettes) and a relapse (resumption of former smoking pattern). The tendency is often to abandon hopes of quitting after slipping with the first cigarette, because quitters believe that only perfect abstinence is acceptable. For some, the uncompromised goal of perfect abstinence is a subconscious strategy to assure failure. Slips during the first 2 weeks of cessation commonly lead to relapse; later slips usually do not lead to relapse. Follow-up contact with smokers 2–4 days into the quitting process increases success by addressing such issues as slips or proper use of nicotine replacement before bad habits are established. This early reinforcement presents an excellent opportunity for the physician to praise success or to help get the quitter back on track by explaining that instant total success is rare.

F. **Weight gain.** Smokers have less desire for sweets and other carbohydrates, a poorer sense of taste and smell, and the ready ability to substitute another oral activity for eating. The average smoker is about 7.5 pounds lighter than a matched nonsmoker. Caloric intake increases about 300 calories a day and metabolic rate decreases slightly during cessation, so weight increases about a pound a week without exercise or a decrease in caloric intake (20). The mean weight gain after quitting is 6–12 pounds a year. Nicotine replacement reduces this weight gain by about half (21). Increasing physical exercise during a cessation effort helps prevent weight gain and increases the quitter's chance of success (22). **The benefits of exercise should be emphasized to every quitter.**

IX. **Approach for primary care providers**

A. No single best way has been found to quit smoking. People vary greatly in motivation and in the general approach to difficult tasks. Some smokers seek hypnosis or organized group cessation programs, such as the American Lung Association Freedom From Smoking Program or the American Cancer Society's FreshStart. Others prefer personal counseling, acupuncture, or aversive conditioning therapy.

B. Ninety five percent of successful quitters do so on their own, but smokers often implore physicians to "do something to make me quit smoking." While the various techniques of cessation can help, all are adjuncts. Quitters must understand clearly that all these treatments will "help me quit, not make me quit." Most smokers regard their tobacco use as a habit to be addressed when they are ready; only a small minority view smoking as a disease requiring treatment from outside themselves. A patient who plans to rely completely on a technique delivered by a professional is laying the groundwork for blaming failure on someone else.

C. The National Cancer Institute has developed a quick and workable plan for primary care physicians based on four *As* (23):

Asking every patient about tobacco use.
Advising every tobacco user to stop.
Assisting the cessation effort.
Arranging follow-up.

This framework is adapted to each patient, emphasizes individual strengths and motivating factors, and utilizes the close personal relationship of the primary care setting.

D. **How to assist.** Assisting the effort consists of several elements:
1. Providing pamphlets about quitting.
2. Informing patients about the availability of books, videos, and audiotape programs.
3. Emphasizing that quitting is a very important health advance and that you are there to help no matter how hard it is or how long it takes.
4. Praising successes, even if followed by relapse.
5. Helping patients progress from one stage to the next in the cycle of substance abuse.
6. Prescribing nicotine replacement when appropriate.
7. Directing those who want hypnosis or group therapy to reputable providers.

E. Three critical elements of the approach deserve special emphasis:
1. **Addressing the subject.** The physician usually initiates discussion concerning smoking cessation. Smokers do not think of tobaccoism as a disease and often hope to avoid the topic for fear of their doctor's disapproval. The physician's attitude must therefore be understanding and helpful in order to ease the inevitable discomfort felt by the smoker when addressing the issue of cessation.
2. **Always be supportive.** After a failed attempt at quitting, patients are tempted to cover up the failure or even cancel return visits. This is a golden opportunity to be supportive by calling patients to offer encouragement and assurance that initial failures are common. Even when relapse has occurred after only several days, praise those days of abstinence as an excellent first try, and urge the patient to return to the active contemplation stage. One of the most helpful roles of the physician is to address the loss of self-esteem and guilt following a failed attempt, assure the patient that this is the usual path, and encourage making another attempt soon.
3. **Use several strategies simultaneously.** The utilization of different strategies increases the likelihood of successful cessation of smoking (24), such as starting an exercise program, using nicotine replacement, avoiding social gatherings with smokers, and beginning with a hypnosis session on the quit date. Most smokers eventually quit on their own, but with the help of careful planning, often directed by information from friends, physicians, and media sources. Providing literature to inform patients about available techniques is extremely important and a major way that physicians can help.

X. **Specific cessation methods**
A. **Published techniques**
1. The patient may ask for recommendations regarding tapering off, going cold turkey, joining a group, acupuncture, aversive conditioning, hypnosis, forced oversmoking, aerated cigarette holders, nicotine fading, or nicotine replacement. Published success rates vary from 0% to >80% and are usually not reproducible in a practice setting, since patient selection is such a strong determinant of published quit rates.
2. Specific approaches usually do not offer each patient the flexibility for individually tailored plans or the opportunity to select the best time to begin. In the office practice setting, these considerations become very important. The physician should inform the patient about the experience of others and then let the

patient select the method to be used. The more the patient participates in determining the process of quitting, the more likely is a successful outcome.
3. Setting a **specific quit date** is important. Urge the patient to select a specific quit date removed from stressful work and family occasions. A birthday or anniversary works well. When spouses both smoke, success rates for quitting are much greater when both spouses quit together rather than one spouse's trying alone.

B. **Tapering off and cold turkey techniques**
1. **Quitting cold turkey** has a greater success rate and makes available the option of using nicotine replacement. However, tapering appeals to smokers who believe that cold turkey is impossible and for whom a gradual reduction may be the only workable plan. Several variations are possible. A 25-cigarette/day smoker can promise to make 24 cigarettes last a whole day. After success is demonstrated, reduce to 23, and so on. Another method is requiring 45 minutes between cigarettes by using a timer to signal when the next cigarette can be smoked. The interval can then be gradually lengthened (25).
2. **Tapering techniques** often allow people to decrease the number of cigarettes smoked each day to half or fewer, but not quit completely. Since smoking-induced diseases are dose related, this can provide a major benefit. Emphasize the positive achievement by highlighting the health benefit and urging the patient not to backslide. Patients may proceed very slowly when being weaned from the last 5–10 cigarettes a day, and physicians should be patient, while encouraging the effort. Five years are usually necessary to learn to smoke expertly, and becoming smoke-free may likewise take a long time.

C. **Nicotine replacement** is the only Food and Drug Administration–approved pharmaceutical agent for use in smoking cessation and is indicated for people who are addicted to nicotine.
1. The **Fagerstrom addiction scale** (26) may be used to assess addiction; people who smoke >5–10 cigarettes a day are probably addicted. Adding nicotine replacement doubles the success rate of behavioral quitting methods in published studies of addicted smokers. The unpleasant feelings of nicotine withdrawal are reduced, although the pleasure obtained from smoking cigarettes is not replaced.
2. Nicotine replacement does not fit into a model of tapering cigarette consumption, and nicotine gum or patches should not be used while patients are still smoking cigarettes. Myocardial infarctions have been reported in patients who smoke while using nicotine patches, but no evidence exists that concurrent use of nicotine while smoking actually increases the risk of any other disease. Nicotine gum may also be used during pregnancy, when the risk of continued smoking appears greater than the risk of modest intake of nicotine only.
3. **Higher success rates are achieved when nicotine replacement is continued for at least 3 months.** Longer periods of time may be required for heavier smokers, and high-, medium-, and low-dose patches are available to permit gradual reduction of nicotine dose after the shift from cigarettes to patch is secure. Published results show comparable efficacy for patches and gum. Using nicotine polacrilex gum on schedule (eg, every hour while awake) works better than chewing as needed, since this strategy prevents rather than competes with the desire to smoke (27). The 4-mg dose is more effective than the 2-mg dose and should be started in patients who smoke >20 cigarettes a day. A typical dosing schedule would be one 4-mg piece every hour or in place of every 3–4 cigarettes (28). Be sure to advise quitters using nicotine polacrilex to follow the directions about avoiding acid beverages like colas and coffee before using the gum, since the acid pH of these beverages prevents buccal absorption of nicotine.
4. The larger the dose of nicotine supplied by gum or patch, the greater the success rate will be, at least at gum doses up to 4 mg and patch doses up to 22 mg. The margin of safety is considerable, since even the 21-mg transdermal patch, which produces the highest blood level of nicotine, provides only half the blood level achieved by a one-pack-a-day smoker. Combined or sequential use

of nicotine patch and gum suggests that the combination may be more effective than either agent used alone, but published experience is limited (29,30). High-dose nicotine replacement with a dose of 44 mg/d is safe and well tolerated by heavy smokers (31), but it did not increase the success rate in a group of individuals who smoked >15 cigarettes a day, when compared to treatment with a 22-mg patch (32). Two 22-mg patches may be effective for smokers of two or more packs of cigarettes a day, but this is as yet unproven.

  D. Adjunctive medications
    1. Lobeline has been used as a smoking cessation aid, but the benefit is unproven.
    2. Clonidine, tranquilizers, and antidepressants have also been used as adjuncts, but none has proved successful enough for use in a patient who does not have another valid indication for such a drug.
  E. Hypnosis has a high initial quit rate, but relapses after a few days are common. Long-term success rates of hypnosis followed by counseling or repeated hypnosis have been reported to exceed 50% (33), but success rates this high are not the rule after the typical single session of hypnosis. Since smokers taking charge of their own cessation plans is a predictor of success, patients wishing hypnosis or acupuncture should be referred to reputable providers of these techniques. However, the published evidence does not support sending all smokers to any one type of delivered program.

XI. Physicians as health advocates
  A. Physicians are primarily trained to diagnose and treat diseases, and about 15% of all medical care in the U.S. is devoted to diseases caused by tobacco. Since the misery of emphysema, lung cancer, and stroke is largely preventable and treatment for these diseases is often not very effective, many physicians believe they have a role in advocating that all people consume less tobacco. Many techniques are available, and while all are somewhat effective, none is sufficient for the successful cessation of smoking (34).
  B. The best approach to smoking-related diseases is to prevent children and adolescents from starting tobacco use. The decade from ages 10 to 20 is a critical period when virtually all people who will eventually die of tobacco use become daily smokers. Physicians should promote:
    1. Enforcement of laws that prohibit the sale of tobacco to minors.
    2. Requirement that each retailer be licensed to sell tobacco, so that the license could be suspended or revoked if the retailer ignores the ban on tobacco sales to minors.
    3. Forbidding the sale of tobacco by vending machines accessible to children.
    4. Curtailing advertising so that children are not barraged by images that associate cigarettes with grand outdoor vistas, social popularity, and slimness.
    5. Increasing tobacco taxes and devoting some of the revenue for broadcast media messages to discourage tobacco consumption.
    6. Expansion of the mandate for smoke-free public places and workplaces to include virtually all shared space.

References

1. Centers for Disease Control: Cigarette smoking among adults—United States, 1993. *MMWR* 1994; 43:925–930.
2. Centers for Disease Control: Trends in smoking initiation among adolescents and young adults—United States, 1980–1989. *MMWR* 1995;44:521–525.
3. Crofton J: Tobacco and the Third World. *Thorax* 1990;45:164–169.
4. Centers for Disease Control: Youth risk behavior surveillance—United States, 1993. *MMWR Surveill Summ* 1995;44(SS-1), March 24.
5. Coultas DB, Stidley CA, Samet JM: Cigarette yields of tar and nicotine and markers of exposure to tobacco smoke. *Am Rev Respir Dis* 1993;148:435–440.
6. Centers for Disease Control: Cigarette smoking—attributable mortality and years of potential life lost. *MMWR* 1993;42:645–649.

7. Bennicke K, Conrad C, Sabrore S, et al.: Cigarette smoking and breast cancer. *BMJ* 1995;310: 1431–1433.
8. Fielding JE: Preventing colon cancer: yet another reason not to smoke. *J Natl Cancer Inst* 1994; 86:162–164.
9. Parish S, Colloins R, Peto R, et al.: Cigarette smoking, tar yield, and non-fatal myocardial infarction: 14,000 Cases and 32,000 controls in the United Kingdom. *BMJ* 1995;311:471–477.
10. MacSweeney ST, Powell JT, Greenhalgh RM: Pathogenesis of abdominal aortic aneurysm. *Br J Surg* 1994;81:935–941.
11. Bense L: Spontaneous pneumothorax. *Chest* 1992;101:891–892.
12. Hance AJ, Basset F, Saumon G, et al.: Smoking and interstitial lung disease: the effect of cigarette smoking on the incidence of pulmonary histiocytosis X and sarcoidosis. *Ann N Y Acad Sci* 1986; 465:643–656.
13. U.S. Department of Health and Human Services (DHHS): *The health consequences of involuntary smoking. A report to the Surgeon General.* Washington, DC: DHHS, 1986; publication DHHS(CDC) 87–8398.
14. Samet JM, Marbury MC, Spengler JD: Health effects of indoor air pollution, part 1. *Am Rev Respir Dis* 1987;136:1486–1508.
15. U.S. Department of Health and Human Services: *Respiratory health effects of passive smoking: lung cancer and other disorders. The report of the U.S. Environmental Protection Agency.* 1993; NIH publication 93–3605.
16. Janerich DT, Thompson WD, Valera LR, et al.: Lung cancer and exposure to tobacco smoke in the household. *N Engl J Med* 1990;323:632–636.
17. Schoendorf KC, Kiely JL: Relationship of sudden infant death syndrome to maternal smoking during and after pregnancy. *Pediatrics* 1992;90:905–908.
18. Hopkinson JM, Schankler RJ, Fraley JK, et al.: Milk production by mothers of premature infants: influence of cigarette smoking. *Pediatrics* 1992;90:934–938.
19. McIntosh H: Black teens not smoking in great numbers. *J Natl Cancer Inst* 1995;87:564.
20. Sachs DPL, Leischow SJ: Pharmacologic approaches to smoking cessation. *Clin Chest Med* 1991; 12:769–791.
21. Gross J, Stitzer ML, Maldonado J: Nicotine replacement: effects on post-cessation weight gain. *J Consult Clin Psychol* 1989;57:87–92.
22. Derby CA, Lasater TM, Vass K, et al.: Characteristics of smokers who attempt to quit and of those who recently succeeded. *Am J Prev Med* 1994;10:327–334.
23. Glynn TJ, Manley MW: *How to help your patients stop smoking.* Washington, DC: Department of Health and Human Services; NIH publication 92–3064. Available by calling 1–800–4-CANCER.
24. Fisher EB, Haire-Joshu D, Morgan GD, et al.: Smoking and smoking cessation. *Am Rev Respir Dis* 1990;142:702–720.
25. Cinciripini PM, Lapitsky L, Seay S, et al.: The effects of smoking schedules on cessation outcome: can we improve on common methods of gradual and abrupt nicotine withdrawal? *J Consult Clin Psychol* 1995;63:388–399.
26. Fagerstrom KO: Measuring degree of physical dependence to tobacco smoking with reference to individualization of treatment. *Addict Behav* 1978;3:235–241.
27. Killen JD, Fortmann SP, Newman B, et al.: Evaluation of a treatment approach combining nicotine gum with self-guided behavioral treatments for smoking relapse prevention. *J Consult Clin Psychol* 1990;58:85–92.
28. Henningfield JE: Nicotine medications for smoking cessation. *N Engl J Med* 1995;333:1196–1203.
29. Fagerstrom KO, Schneider NG, Lunnel E: Effectiveness of nicotine patch and gum as individual versus combined treatments for tobacco withdrawal symptoms. *Psychopharmacology* 1993;111: 271–277.
30. Kornitzer M, Boutsen M, Dramaix M, et al.: Combined use of nicotine patch and gum in smoking cessation: a placebo controlled clinical trial. *Prev Med* 1995;24:41–47.
31. Dale LC, Hurt RD, Offord KP, et al.: High-dose nicotine patch therapy: percentage of replacement and smoking cessation. *JAMA* 1995;274:1353–1358.
32. Jorenby, DE, Smith SS, Fiore MC, et al.: Varying nicotine patch dose and type of smoking cessation counseling. *JAMA* 1995;274:1347–1352.
33. Schwartz JL: Methods for smoking cessation. *Clin Chest Med* 1991;12:737–753.
34. Phillips, BA: The physician as advocate: why bother? *J Respir Dis* 1993;14:848–854.

32   Sick Building Syndrome and Specific Building-Related Illnesses

David Ciccolella

Workers are exposed to a number of biologic and inorganic pollutants emitted from equipment, building materials, furnishings, or other people in the indoor work environment. Exposure to these indoor pollutants is thought to cause two general types of building-related illnesses. The first type is sick building syndrome (SBS) with nonspecific complaints and an unknown etiology. In SBS, there is generally no tissue damage that can be detected by a laboratory test or by physical examination (1). The second type is specific building-related illnesses (SBRI) with a well defined symptomatology and known etiology such as humidifier fever, hypersensitivity pneumonitis, or infectious syndromes (eg, legionnaires' disease). In SBRI, the illness is usually caused by an identifiable agent found in either the patient or the building (1); such illnesses account for only a small fraction of building-related medical problems (2).

I. **Sick building syndrome** is a poorly defined entity first described in the late 1970s. Numerous reports surfaced in the 1980s after the energy crisis stimulated the construction of tightly sealed buildings, employing recirculation of air and decreased ventilation rates to conserve energy. SBS has been discussed in the literature under several different names, including sealed building syndrome, tight building syndrome, and closed building syndrome. The impact has been enormous, and the World Health Organization estimates that 30% of newly built or remodeled buildings are sick, that is, associated with the production of symptoms characteristic of SBS in a large fraction of the workers in those buildings (3). This translates into large indirect economic costs due to lower worker productivity and increased absenteeism (3), as well as direct costs due to litigation, investigation, and building repairs. The syndrome is poorly characterized; typically, many workers within a building must be affected to label a building as sick (4).

   A. **Presenting symptoms and signs.** Symptoms are nonspecific and involve several organ systems. Predominant symptoms include lethargy (57%), mucous membrane irritation (46%) (eg, dry throat or nasal congestion without microbial cause), headache (43%), pruritic, irritated eyes, and dry skin (5,6). Other symptoms include chest tightness, dyspnea, pruritus, short-term memory problems, and poor attention span (5,6). Symptoms should be related to the work (building) environment, worsening at work, and improving rapidly outside of the workplace (3,7). Signs usually cannot be detected by physical examination, and laboratory findings are generally normal.

   B. **Etiology and pathogenesis**
      1. The cause of SBS is unknown, and multiple etiologies are most likely. The rates of building-related symptoms vary widely among buildings, suggesting a preventable cause (8). However, SBS tends to be more commonly found in newer, tightly sealed buildings with central air conditioning than in buildings with natural ventilation through open windows (5,9).
         a. The health problems of building occupants may derive from one or more adverse physical, chemical, biologic, or psychosocial factors. Excessive stimulation of basic sensory receptors (olfactory, thermal, auditory, and visual) may be causative. For example, stimulation of receptors by heat, noise, or glare may cause headaches. Symptoms may be induced by agents that af-

fect the sensory receptors only at thresholds slightly above irritant levels. Offending agents may include gases and vapors such as ozone, oxides of nitrogen, and bioaerosols (1).

2. Irritants implicated in the pathogenesis of SBS include volatile organic compounds emitted from carpeting, furniture, glues, and wall paints (4); noncombustion emissions such as formaldehyde (10); and bioaerosols such as airborne organisms, particles, or volatile compounds associated with and released from a living organism (11). Other possible contributing factors to the pathogenesis of SBS include environmental factors such as temperature, lighting, and noise (4). The correlation between sick-building symptoms and levels of measurable contaminants (formaldehyde, volatile organic compounds, ions, particulate matter) has been poor (8). Usually, in evaluation of SBS complaints, measurement of toxic contaminant levels are found to be well below the recommended standards.

3. Ventilation rates in buildings relate inconsistently to symptoms of SBS. Studies showing no change in SBS symptoms after rates were increased (8,12) have been met with controversy (13,14). The combination of slightly inadequate levels of ventilation along with a heterogenous distribution of ventilation within a building may be significant factors in producing SBS (4). Central air conditioning may contribute to the toxicity of these irritants by producing moisture that may enhance microbial growth and spread via ventilation systems, producing odoriferous and irritating air (15,16).

4. **Work stress** may be an important contributing factor to the reporting of SBS symptoms (4). Work stress or job dissatisfaction may enhance perception of a suboptimal physical environment or manifest as complaints about the physical environment.

C. **Relevant physiology** is unknown.

D. **Differential diagnostic possibilities** of SBS are broad and complex (Table 32-1); the diagnosis is one of exclusion. Included in the differential diagnosis are mass hysteria, chronic fatigue, and certain SBRIs such as humidifier fever and Pontiac fever (17). Specific symptoms may present singly and must be differentiated from other pathologic causes, such as allergic rhinoconjunctivitis and viral coryza.

E. **Specific approach to each diagnostic possibility.** SBS should be included in the differential diagnosis involving any individual with SBS core symptoms, especially if the symptoms are related to the workplace environment. Since the diagnosis of SBS is one of exclusion, the physician must ensure that an otherwise treatable illness is not missed. The evaluation of SBS begins with a comprehensive medical history, including a listing of environmental exposures at home and at work, and a physical examination (3). Since SBS typically involves more than one individual in the same environment, the clinical history should include questions about the health status of coworkers and family. Specifically, the physician should inquire about the type of symptoms and their severity, the relation of symptoms to physical changes in the building environment such as remodeling or addition of carpets, the time at which the symptoms are most intense, the work stress for the patient and

Table 32-1. Differential diagnostic considerations for the sick building syndrome

Viral coryzas

Allergic rhinoconjunctivitis

Acute/chronic sinusitis

Chronic fatigue

Specific building-related illnesses

Lower respiratory tract diseases

Mass hysteria

Medication hypersensitivity

other employees, any medication changes, and any changes in the home environment (18).

1. An assessment of both the home and work environments with specific inquiry into the temporal relationship of the patient's symptoms to time spent at home and work is required (10). Evaluation of SBS cases also requires information about the specific groups of workers affected and a detailed description of the characteristics of the work environment and the building. When patients may be sensitized to or biased about work-related symptoms by other employees, it is important to determine whether symptoms were present prior to the discovery that the building was believed to be sick.

2. Rarely is only one employee affected, and information should also be collected about other affected employees, with emphasis on job type (clerical/secretarial, technical, professional), the social relationships among affected individuals, time of onset in relation to the discovery that the building was sick, whether patients were diagnosed by a single physician or different physicians, job stress and job satisfaction, and the organization of the workers. The role of workman's compensation should also be considered.

3. Specific inquiry into the building would include questions of age, type of ventilation, and adequacy of temperature, lighting, and humidity. For exposures to known toxic substances in the workplace, the material safety data sheets required by law to be available from the employer should be requested and reviewed for each substance.

4. Previous medical records should be examined to determine whether there are any preexisting conditions that could explain the complaints. Although there are no known specific laboratory abnormalities associated with SBS, tests are required to exclude other specific diseases. These may include a chest radiograph, complete blood cell count, and other routine laboratory studies. Other tests such as pulmonary function tests, peak flow rate monitoring, plain films or computed tomography of the sinuses, nasopharyngoscopy, and selected skin testing should be based on symptoms and signs (6).

5. Further diagnostic testing is costly and of low yield and should be performed by physicians with expertise in evaluating building-related diseases, such as a physician trained in occupational/environmental medicine. Further analysis will involve environmental measurements (6) requiring consultations by epidemiologists, industrial hygienists, toxicologists, and building diagnosticians (6). A walk-through and on-site investigation to gather information from office managers and facility engineers, as well as an examination of the heating, ventilation and air-conditioning (HVAC) systems and control strategies, will almost certainly be required (1).

6. A **therapeutic trial** of workplace abstinence may be required to determine whether symptoms abate. This would be important in relating the symptoms to work and making the diagnosis (6). Symptoms should abate if caused by the SBS.

7. **Diagnostic errors** usually relate to the failure to consider past medical disorders, an inadequate differential diagnosis, and a wish to satisfy the patient (19). A specific cause is found in a minority of cases of SBS, and these have been related to poor building maintenance or heating, the presence of contaminants, institution of energy-conserving measures, and poor basic building design (1).

8. **Mass hysteria** can be confused with SBS, since symptoms are very similar to those associated with SBS. Mass hysteria is also a diagnosis of exclusion, and a thorough consideration should be given to the possibility of organic causes before a diagnosis of hysteria is made. Mass hysteria may occur when an employee or health care professional attributes an employee's illness or symptoms to a perceived toxin emitted in the workplace (3,20), initiating a chain reaction of perceived symptoms in coworkers. The employees commonly involved are women in low-level jobs who are dissatisfied with work and experiencing high levels of stress. The most common precipitants have been odors or gases (3).

F. Management
1. Since the specific cause of SBS is usually not determined in the majority of cases, interventions are frequently nonspecific (10).
    a. In general, measures include but are not limited to increasing building ventilation, eliminating or reducing an identifiable emission source, and cleaning all ventilation systems (6,10). Even if no irritant source is found after a thorough investigation of the building, increasing the amount of ventilation or improving ventilation efficiency may reduce or eliminate the problem (6).
    b. It has been recommended that the initial step in treating a sick-building population is to switch to 100% outside air, as this will eliminate the problem regardless of the type of airborne irritant (6). Unfortunately, not all individuals working in buildings considered sick have shown improvement in symptoms with this approach (6,7). The reasons are unclear but could relate to the presence of variable-point-source emissions and to pockets of poorly ventilated areas in a building with high overall ventilation rates (3).
2. In cases of identified toxins, reducing potential employee exposure by passive protection using high-filtration masks is not usually efficient or effective. Providing supportive treatment to patients is also relatively ineffective.

G. Problems and complications of therapy. There are no long-term sequelae known to occur from SBS. An important element of the diagnostic evaluation is to ensure that other causes of these nonspecific symptoms have been excluded and to reevaluate the patient if the symptoms worsen.

H. Specialist referrals. For the physician with expertise in building-related illnesses, consults to appropriate medical, epidemiologic, and industrial hygiene personnel are usually required to diagnose and treat all suspected sick-building problems (6). The physician will require the efforts of public health agencies, ventilation engineers, and building managers to manage building-related complaints (8).

II. **Specific building-related illnesses** are grouped into three types: infectious disorders, hypersensitivity diseases, and exposure-related diseases (6). The infectious type of SBRI includes bacterial, viral, and fungal infections of the upper and lower respiratory tracts (10). Hypersensitivity reactions caused by exposure to bioaerosols may produce hypersensitivity pneumonitis, humidifier fever, asthma, or rhinoconjunctivitis. Exposure-related diseases include those produced by chemical or nonbiologic toxins that can result from combustion (carbon monoxide) or noncombustion emissions (10). Noncombustion emissions, caused by formaldehyde and other volatile organic compounds emitted from carpet, particle board, cleaning products, solvents, paints, and pesticides (10) can produce eye and upper respiratory tract irritation, as well as headache, malaise, and dizziness (10). Agents that cause disease with long latency periods such as radon or asbestos fibers will not be discussed here.

A. **Infectious disorders.** There are a number of infections that have been linked to building-related problems: *Legionella* infections, Q fever, viral infections (influenza, measles, and varicella), and tuberculosis, as well as others related to specific buildings where animal products are processed.

B. *Legionella* **infections**
1. *Legionella pneumophila* is the major organism linked to building-related disease (21). The bacteria are spread principally through contaminated ventilation systems. *Legionella* infections present in two forms: a pneumonia, known as Legionnaires' disease, and a nonpneumonic, self-limited form resembling humidifier fever, known as Pontiac fever (2,22). The attack rate for the pneumonic form is usually lower than that for the nonpneumonic form (23).
2. **Presenting symptoms and signs.** The pneumonic presentation ranges from a mild illness with cough and fever to a severe illness with diffuse pulmonary infiltrates and multiorgan failure. The pneumonia has a 2–10-day incubation period. Nonspecific symptoms of fever, malaise, anorexia, myalgia, and headache occur early in the course of the illness. This is followed by the development of a mildly productive cough that may be accompanied by chest pain of either a pleuritic or nonpleuritic nature and occasionally by hemoptysis. Extrapulmonary symptoms

include watery diarrhea in 25% to 50% of patients and nausea, vomiting, and abdominal pain in 10% to 20%; infrequently, there will be a change in mental status. On physical examination, fever is present in most patients, and relative bradycardia may be found. Rates are heard on chest examination. Increased mortality is associated with age >50 years, alcoholism, diabetes mellitus, immunosuppression, chronic obstructive pulmonary disease, and smoking.

3. **Etiology and pathogenesis.** Pneumonia is caused by airborne transmission of the aerobic, gram-negative *L. pneumophila*, typically as a result of a contaminated mechanical ventilation system in a public building or hospital (2,22). Although there are >30 potential pathogenic species of the genus *Legionella*, approximately 90% of infections are caused by *L. pneumophila* serotypes 1, 4, and 6, and 80% of infections are caused by serotype 1. Oropharyngeal colonization with aspiration has not been definitively established as a mechanism of infection. Since the organisms are found in water and are ubiquitous, the disease has been reported to occur from exposures to contaminated water sources (cooling towers, hot water systems, humidifiers, and whirlpools) (22).

   a. The organism is cleared through the usual respiratory mechanisms; a higher infectivity rate is thought to occur in individuals with impaired mucociliary clearance as seen in chronic obstructive pulmonary disease, smokers, and alcoholics.

   b. Individuals with impaired cell-mediated immunity are at greater risk of infection, since phagocytosis and killing by alveolar macrophages is an important part of host defense.

4. **Relevant differential diagnostic possibilities.** Other building-related pneumonias that present as community-acquired pneumonias and produce epidemics include Q fever, tuberculosis, psittacosis, varicella (24), and anthrax (22) in the appropriate setting.

5. **Diagnosis.** Legionnaires' disease causes approximately 4% to 6% of community-acquired pneumonias (range, 1% to 27%) and 10% of hospital- and nursing home–acquired pneumonias (2,24). *Legionella* pneumonia cannot be differentiated from other pneumonias by clinical manifestations (25). Hyponatremia has been found to be more frequently associated with Legionnaires' disease than other etiologies of community-acquired pneumonia. Routine tests such as Gram's stain of secretions usually show polymorphonuclear neutrophils without a predominant organism. Gram's stain of normally sterile fluids may show faintly staining pleomorphic rods and gram-negative rods. Specialized laboratory tests that include culture, serologic antibody detection, and direct fluorescent antibody stain should document an organism that matches the organism from the contaminated source. The definitive diagnostic test (100% specific and 80% sensitive) is culture of respiratory fluids on special media (buffered-charcoal yeast extract agar). Culture will identify all species, while the other techniques only identify certain species or serotypes. Direct fluorescent antibody staining of respiratory fluids is less sensitive (50% to 70%) than culture and is now less frequently performed by hospital laboratories. Serologic diagnosis requires a fourfold rise in serotype-specific antibody titer from acute to convalescent of 1:128 or a single elevated titer of 1:128. The rapid urinary antigen test is easier to perform, since only urine is required, but tests only for *L. pneumophila* serotype 1, which does represent the major cause of infections. The test may remain positive for months after the acute infection. The diagnosis of legionnaires' disease as a cause of building-related illness should be based on the presence of an epidemic outbreak, with individuals having consistent clinical manifestations and laboratory tests indicating recent infection (22).

6. **Management.** Almost all outbreaks of Legionnaires' disease are associated with a contaminant source in the building, usually the ventilation system (22). Identification of the source and correction of the problem are necessary. The disease may be treated with erythromycin 4 g/d IV, but 2 g/d PO may be used in selected patients with mild disease. Rifampin may be added to the regimen of patients with severe disease. Immunocompetent patients should be treated for at least 10–14 days, and immunosuppressed patients should be treated longer.

7. **Problems and complications of therapy.** High doses of erythromycin may cause ototoxicity. The dosage may need to be increased in patients with advanced disease.

8. **Prevention.** The infection is theoretically preventable because the environmental reservoirs are known. The Centers for Disease Control and Prevention recommend culturing environmental sources after the diagnosis of legionnaires' disease is established. Others have advocated routine environmental culturing in hospitals (25). Colonization may be more likely in low water temperature, electric heaters, horizontal water tanks, plumbing systems, and situations where sediment and scale accumulate in tanks. Treatment of a contaminated source associated with disease outbreaks may require not only source removal but also regular biocidal treatment to prevent recurrences (22).

C. **Pontiac fever**

1. **Presenting symptoms and signs.** The disease was first noted in 1968 in Pontiac, Michigan, when 144 employees working in the county health building developed a mild flu-like illness. This self-limited disease is associated with fever, chills, headache, and myalgia that occur 12–36 hours after exposure and last approximately 2–5 days. The disease has not been fatal. Chest radiographs are typically normal.

2. **Etiology and pathogenesis.** The disease is caused by airborne transmission of *L. pneumophila* and other *Legionella* organisms.

3. **Differential diagnostic possibilities** include influenza and other upper respiratory tract viral infections, atypical pneumonia, humidifier fever, bronchitis, and SBS (17), among others.

4. **Specific approach to each diagnostic possibility.** Because the illness is nonspecific, the diagnosis is always made under epidemic conditions (24). The diagnosis of *Legionella* infection is typically made by serology (24).

5. **Management.** This is a self-limited illness. Identification and removal of the source are important to prevent the disease. Prevention is similar to that for the pneumonic form of *Legionella* infection.

6. There are no problems and complications of therapy.

III. **Hypersensitivity diseases**

A. **Humidifier fever**

1. **Presenting symptoms and signs.** Humidifier fever usually presents as a flu-like illness with fever, chills, myalgia, rigors, and malaise without significant pulmonary symptoms. The relatively mild symptoms usually begin within 4–8 hours of exposure on a Monday (or at the beginning of the work week) and progressively worsen over the work week. Symptoms improve during the weekend but recur after exposure upon return to work, hence the name "Monday miseries" (2,22,26). Interestingly, Monday worsening of symptoms has been noted in reports from Great Britain but not from the United States (22).

2. **Etiology and pathogenesis.** The illness is related to hypersensitivity pneumonitis (HP) due to organic dust exposures with biologic agents such as mold spores, microbial contamination of humidifier reservoirs, or inhaled endotoxin (2,22,26,27). Exposure to multiple pathogens (bacteria, fungi, protozoa) has been identified (2). The pathogenesis is similar to that of HP (see below).

3. **Differential diagnostic possibilities** include HP, mild influenza, organic dust toxic syndromes (28), metal fume fever, and bacterial and viral pneumonias.

4. **Specific approach to each diagnostic possibility.** The chest radiograph is usually normal in group outbreaks, but pulmonary fibrosis may be noted in rare instances. Precipitins to specific organisms may be found in the serum but may also be seen in asymptomatic individuals. Spirometry shows a restrictive pattern during the acute episode that resolves over 48–72 hours. The diagnosis is based on a consistent clinical history, time course, and the absence of other identifiable diseases. The major diagnosis to be considered is HP. Humidifier fever occurs more frequently than HP, is usually associated with a normal chest radiograph, and may be associated with mild wheezing and recurrent flu-like symptoms that resolve (2). Bronchoalveolar lavage is not helpful in distinguishing humidifier fever from HP (24). Other illnesses that may be

confused with humidifier fever are influenza, metal fume fever, grain fever, byssinosis, and Pontiac fever. Metal fume fever, grain fever, and byssinosis may be eliminated based on the history of exposure.

5. **Management.** Removal of the contaminated humidifier is the best management.

6. **Prevention.** The condition may be prevented by strict adherence to the guidelines of maintenance of building equipment, humidifier units, and HVAC systems.

B. **Hypersensitivity pneumonitis** (see chapters 11 and 29 for further information) occurs in a significant fraction of individuals complaining of sick-building symptoms and is the best documented of all building-related diseases. Clinical characteristics of the hypersensitivity pneumonitides are similar regardless of the types of inhaled dusts.

1. **Presenting symptoms and signs.** The disease may present in acute, subacute, or chronic forms. The acute form typically presents with chills, cough, dyspnea, fever, and malaise 4–6 hours following a dust exposure and may last 24 hours. Physical examination may show rales and fever. The subacute and chronic forms have a more insidious presentation with productive cough, progressive dyspnea, anorexia, and weight loss. Patients may have symptoms that begin hours after entering the building environment. The dust exposure may be variable from day to day and thus affect the presentation of symptoms and signs.

2. **Etiology and pathogenesis.** The disease may result from exposure to a wide variety of organic agents (bacteria, fungi, protozoa, actinomycetes) (29). Acute exposure to organic agents results in the production of an immunologic reaction with the development of a granulomatous and interstitial pneumonitis with lymphocytes, plasma cells, and histiocytes. A poorly maintained or damaged HVAC system allows dissemination of the organic agents through the building; water damaged furniture has also been a source (2,29).

3. **Differential diagnostic possibilities.** The acute presentation of the illness may be confused with bacterial or viral pneumonia. Interstitial pneumonitis and sarcoidosis should be considered in the chronic forms of the disease.

4. **Specific approach to each diagnostic possibility.** The diagnosis is based on the appropriate history, physical examination, and laboratory tests, including chest radiography, pulmonary function tests, and measurement of serum precipitins. Pulmonary function tests (spirometry, lung volumes, diffusion capacity for carbon monoxide) usually demonstrate a restrictive pattern. In cases in which the pattern is unclear, exercise testing can be useful. High-resolution computed tomography may be used to identify disease patterns of interstitial lung disease and are more sensitive than chest radiographs in this regard. Positive serum precipitins to the causative organisms may be helpful in establishing the diagnosis, but 50% of asymptomatic patients will also have positive precipitins. Lung biopsy may show interstitial lung disease and granulomas but is usually not required (22).

5. **Management.** In individual cases, effective management requires removal of the employee from exposure to the source. The patient with HP should not return to the environment since reexposure to antigen represents a significant risk. Corticosteroids may be beneficial in acute cases, as well as in chronic cases if pulmonary fibrosis has not yet developed (22). The discovery of a case of building-related HP should prompt closing of the building until the problem is corrected (26).

C. **Building-related asthma** (see chapters 5 and 29 for detailed information)

1. **Presenting symptoms and signs.** Building-related asthma is rarely reported. It should be considered as distinct from other causes of occupationally induced asthma because its diagnosis may have legal ramifications. New building-related asthma induced by exposure to chemicals such as toluene diisocyanate in the building environment (30) should also be distinguished from an exacerbation of preexisting asthma (31). Workers may present with typical

symptoms of cough, chest tightness, dyspnea, and wheeze that may occur soon after exposure to the building environment or hours after leaving the building. The temporal relationship of symptoms to the presence or absence from the workplace will help to establish the diagnosis (30).

2. **Etiology and pathogenesis.** New building-related cases of asthma have been related to contaminated ventilation systems (eg, toluene diisocyanate) and to contaminated humidifiers (biocidal agents) (32,33). Preexisting asthma may be worsened in buildings by exposure to irritants such as secondary smoke and odors or by the release of high concentrations of allergens such as dust mites, especially after a building has been repaired or remodeled (2).

3. **Differential diagnostic possibilities and approach.** The physician must determine whether the disease is related to the building in general (building-related asthma), to a chemical that the patient works with (occupational asthma), or to an exacerbation of preexisting disease. The clinical history, physical examination, and special tests (pulmonary function tests, methacholine challenge, bronchial provocation, and so on) may be required to diagnose the disease as asthma and then relate the exacerbations to the building environment. Establishing the diagnosis is helped when other workers are also affected. Peak flow rate monitoring may be helpful in evaluating the triggers.

4. **Management.** Depending on the causative agent, removal of the source of the agent causing disease, repair or improved maintenance of the building or equipment, or placement of the worker in another work area should help.

5. **Specialist Referrals.** Timely referral to an asthma specialist is critical. Reporting to the local public health department and subsequent investigation may be indicated.

IV. **Exposure-related diseases.** These conditions may be related to specific nonbiologic or chemical exposures in the indoor environment. A large number of chemicals may cause a broad range of symptoms that overlap those of the SBS and the SBRI. In general, chemical exposures causing building-related complaints can be identified without prolonged investigation. This section will be limited to some examples of specific chemical exposures.

A. **Formaldehyde** at significant concentrations produces irritant effects on the mucous membranes of the eyes and upper respiratory tract, as well as neuropsychologic effects. Formaldehyde is a water-soluble, volatile gas that can be found in a number of materials in buildings, such as urea-formaldehyde foam insulation (no longer used in the United States), particle board, plywood, and office furnishings (34,35). While frequently claimed to be a cause of mucous membrane irritation in sick buildings, strong scientific evidence is lacking because low levels are usually found (35).

B. **Carbon monoxide poisoning** rarely produces building-related illnesses. Symptoms of carbon monoxide poisoning can include headache, nausea, and fatigue. Poisoning may occur when building ventilation systems are near parking garages or large boiler stacks (31). The odor of other combustion products in the ventilation system may identify the source; carbon monoxide itself is odorless (35).

C. **Fiberglass** may cause office building–related pruritus through skin contact from particles sedimenting on furniture from ceiling tiles or ventilation ductwork (26,35). Workers typically have pruritus that may be associated with a fleeting rash. The pruritus resolves with showering (35). Fiberglass dust found on furniture may support the diagnosis.

D. **Excessive use of detergent and solvents** to clean carpets has caused cough, dry throat, and eye irritation with high frequency in workers in the affected areas. The diagnosis may be supported by a carpet maintenance history of excessive detergent use, reproduction of symptoms after carpet brushing, and the use of air filters to help solubilize agents in water that can then be analyzed (35).

E. **Vapor from carbonless copy paper** causes upper respiratory tract irritation and airway obstruction, as well as skin irritation from allergic contact dermatitis and contact urticaria (28,36,37).

References

1. Samet J: Environmental controls and lung disease. *Am Rev Respir Dis* 1990;142:915–939.
2. Bardana EJ Jr: Buildingq-related illness. In: EJ Bardana Jr, Montanaro A, O'Hollaren MT, eds. *Occupational asthma.* Philadelphia: Hanley and Belfus, 1992:237–254.
3. Rothman AL, Weintraub MI: The sick building syndrome and mass hysteria. *Neurol Clin* 1995; 13:405–412.
4. Hodgson M: The sick building syndrome. *Occup Med* 1995;10:167–175.
5. Burge S, Hedge A, Wilson S, et al.: Sick building syndrome: a study of 4373 office workers. *Ann Occup Hyg* 1987;31:493–504.
6. Lyles W, Greve KW, Bauer RM, et al.: Sick building syndrome. *South Med J* 1991;84:65–72.
7. Chang CC, Ruhl RA, Halpern GM, Gershwin ME: The sick building syndrome. 1. Definition and epidemiological consideration. *J Asthma* 1993;30:285–295.
8. Kreiss K: The sick building syndrome in office buildings—a breath of fresh air. *N Engl J Med* 1993;328:877–878.
9. Apter A, Bracker A, Hodgson M, et al.: Epidemiology of the sick building syndrome. *J Allergy Clin Immunol* 1994;94:277–288.
10. Lambert WE, Coultas WB: Epitomes—occupational medicine: evaluating and preventing illness associated with indoor air pollution. *West J Med* 1994;160:565–566.
11. Cecile R: Epitomes—occupational medicine: bioaerosols. *West J Med* 1994;160:566.
12. Menzies R, Tamblyn R, Farant J, et al.: The effect of varying levels of outdoor-air supply on the symptoms of sick building syndrome. *N Engl J Med* 1993;328:821–827.
13. Boatman JF: Sick building syndrome. *N Engl J Med* 1993;329:503
14. Edelman PA, Hethmon T: Sick building syndrome. *N Engl J Med* 1993;329:503.
15. Harrison J, Pickering CAC, Faragher EB, et al.: An investigation of the relationship between microbial and particulate indoor air pollution and the sick building syndrome. *Respir Med* 1992; 86:225–235.
16. Mendell MJ, Smith AH: Consistent pattern of elevated symptoms in air-conditioned office buildings: a reanalysis of epidemiologic studies. *Am J Public Health* 1990;80:1193–1199.
17. O'Mahoney M, Lakhani A, Stephens A, et al.: Legionnaires' disease and the sick building syndrome. *Epidemiol Infect* 1989;103:285–295.
18. Lees-Haley PR: When sick building complaints arise. *Occup Health Saf* 1993;62:46–47;53–54.
19. Bardana EJ Jr, Montanaro A: "Chemically sensitive" patients: avoiding the pitfalls. *J Respir Dis* 1989;10:32–45.
20. Colligan MJ, Murphy LR: Mass psychogenic illness in organizations: an overview. *J Occup Psychol* 1979;52:77–90.
21. Fraser DW, Tasi TF, Orenstein W, et al.: Legionnaires' disease: description of an epidemic of pneumonia. *N Engl J Med* 1977;297:1189–1197.
22. Seltzer JM: Building-related illnesses. *J Allergy Clin Immunol* 1994;94:351–361.
23. Kaufman AF, McDade JE, Patton CM, et al.: Pontiac fever: isolation of the etiologic agent (*Legionella pneumophila*) and demonstration of its mode of transmission. *Am J Epidemiol* 1981; 114:337–347.
24. Hodgson MJ: Clinical diagnosis and management of building-related illness and the sick-building syndrome. *Occup Med* 1989;4:593–606.
25. Yu VL: *Legionella pneumophila* (legionnaires' disease). In: Mandell GL, Bennett JE, Dolin R, eds. *Principles and practice of infectious diseases.* New York: Churchill Livingstone, 1995:2087–2097.
26. Sherin KM: Building-related illnesses and sick building syndrome. *J Fla Med Assoc* 1993;80: 472–474.
27. Rylander R, Haglind P, Lundholm M, et al.: Humidifier fever and endotoxin exposure. *Clin Allergy* 1978;8:511–516.
28. Marks JG: Allergic contact dermatitis from carbonless copy paper. *JAMA* 1981;245:2331–2332.
29. Banaszak EF, Thiede WH, Fink JN: Hypersensitivity pneumonitis due to contamination of an air conditioner. *N Engl J Med* 1970;283:217–221.
30. Carroll KB, Secombe CJP, Pepys J: Asthma due to non-occupational exposure to toluene (tolylene) di-isocyanate. *Clin Allergy* 1976;6:99–104.
31. Alberts WM: Building-related illness: what it is, what you can do. *J Respir Dis* 1994;15:899–912.

32. Burge PS, Finnigan M, Horsfield N, et al.: Occupational asthma in a factory with a contaminated humidifier. *Thorax* 1985;40:248.

33. Hoffman RE, Wood RC, Kreiss K: Building-related asthma in Denver office workers. *Am J Public Health* 1993;83:89–93.

34. Gold DR: Indoor air pollution. *Clin Chest Med* 1992;13:215–229.

35. Kreiss K: The epidemiology of building-related complaints and illness. *Occup Med* 1989;4:575–592.

36. Marks JG, Trautlein JJ, Zwillich CW, Demers LM: Contact urticaria and airway obstruction from carbonless copy paper. *JAMA* 1984;252:1038–1040.

37. Morgan MS, Camp JE: Upper respiratory irritation from controlled exposure to vapor from carbonless copy forms. *J Occup Med* 1986;28:415–419.

33

Disability Evaluation

Gary R. Epler

Primary care physicians and pulmonary clinicians trained to diagnose and treat disease are often asked to determine disability and quantify functional impairment. A framework for evaluation of these patients and a systematic plan for documentation of the findings are important. This chapter outlines a practical approach for the documentation and evaluation of signs and symptoms, exposure information, physical examination findings, radiographic results, and pulmonary function testing.

I. **Definitions** are a fundamental part of disability and impairment determination. The meanings vary among governmental agencies, medical societies, and world organizations.

A. **Impairment** is a medical term defined as a functional abnormality resulting from a medical condition (1–4). An objective, measurable loss of function is designated, with impairment either **temporary** or **permanent.** Impairment that persists after appropriate therapy without reasonable prospect of improvement is permanent. The degree of impairment varies in severity from mild to moderate (precludes some types of labor) to severe (precludes any type of gainful employment). The physician is expected to assess and rate the extent of impairment arising from pulmonary disease.

B. **Disability** is a general term used to indicate the total effect of impairment on the person's life (1–4) and implies an inability to perform expected roles or tasks within society. Disability is affected by such diverse factors as age, education, economic and social environment, and the energy requirement of the occupation. **Partial disability** is characterized by a degree of impairment that still allows some types of labor, while **total disability** designates an impairment severe enough to preclude any type of gainful employment.

C. **The rating of pulmonary impairment is determined by the physician.**

D. **The adjudication of disability** includes the rating of the pulmonary impairment but also requires consideration of nonmedical factors such as educational level, impact of the current state of society's norms, and availability of suitable work. Thus, disability is generally determined by administrative judges, judicial panels, or compensation boards. The role of the physician in determination of disability continues to evolve. Physicians may have considerable knowledge about how an impairment affects a person's life and must document such individual factors. This information can be utilized as part of the administrative process for determination of disability.

E. **The World Health Organization** has different wording of the definitions of impairment and disability, and the term *handicap* is added (5).

1. **Impairment** is defined as any loss or abnormality of physiologic or anatomic structure or function. Impairment is more inclusive than disorder in that it also covers losses. Impairment represents deviation from some norm in the individual's biomedical status. Definition of its constituents is undertaken by those qualified to judge physical functioning according to generally accepted standards.

2. **Disability** is defined as any impairment that restricts or prohibits the performance of an activity within the range considered normal for a human being. Disability is concerned with integrated activities expected to be performed by

the person, such as those represented by tasks, skills, and behaviors. Disability represents a departure from the norm in terms of performance of the individual.

3. **Handicap** is a disadvantage for a given individual, resulting from an impairment or a disability that limits or prevents the fulfillment of a role that is normal for that individual. Handicap is characterized by a discordance between the individual's performance or status and the expectations of the particular group of which the person is a member. Disadvantage accrues as a result of being unable to conform to the norms of the person's universe. Handicap is a social phenomenon, representing the social and environmental consequences for the individual stemming from the presence of impairments and disabilities.

4. **From these definitions**, it has been suggested that assessment of respiratory impairment and disability requires both rating of the loss of function and rating of exercise performance (6).

F. **The Americans with Disabilities Act defines disability** as a physical or mental impairment that substantially limits one or more of the major life activities of an individual (7).

G. **Referral sources** vary for patients or individuals requiring impairment and disability determination. Patients referred for pulmonary consultation or long-term care can often be claimants requesting disability reviews, and such determinations are based on available records. Such individuals are generally referred from governmental agencies, insurance companies, or attorneys.

H. **Questions from the referral source** may be specific or general. Some patients are referred specifically for evaluation and determination of impairment according to the Social Security standards (8). Others are referred for more general evaluations, and the issues can be complex and numerous. Three distinct but interrelated questions must be answered:

1. **What is the pulmonary diagnosis?**
2. **What is the degree of impairment?**
3. **Is the pulmonary condition related to the workplace?**

II. **Establishing the clinical data base is the first step in determination of impairment and disability.** A respiratory questionnaire is used to record the information systematically.

A. **Degree of dyspnea** is often the principal manifestation of impairment but can not be utilized as a sole criterion for determination of pulmonary impairment for several reasons. Dyspnea is a subjective finding, and individual responses to similar impairments of pulmonary function vary greatly for reasons such as difficulty of verbal expression, questions of comprehension, or preoccupation with health. Dyspnea can be coded from none (grade 0) to very severe (grade 4) (9).

1. **None, grade 0.** Not troubled with breathlessness except with strenuous exercise.
2. **Slight, grade 1.** Breathless going up one flight of stairs at a normal pace.
3. **Moderate, grade 2.** Breathless walking with other people of the same age on the level at a normal pace.
4. **Severe, grade 3.** Stopping for breath after walking on level surfaces.
5. **Very severe, grade 4.** Breathless when dressing or undressing.

B. **Other pulmonary symptoms** such as cough, sputum production, and wheezing should be characterized and quantified (9). This includes the frequency and duration of cough, the amount of sputum produced daily with the time of day and days of the week, and the persistence of cough and sputum for more than three consecutive months. The timing and duration of wheezing should also be documented. The degree to which the cough, sputum, or wheezing are limiting the person's capacity to function in daily work activities must be noted.

III. **Information concerning occupations and hazardous exposures** is helpful to both adjudicators assessing the workplace environment and physicians attempting to determine causation. A systematic method of obtaining this information is essential.

A. **Date and place of birth** is a good beginning and enables patients to begin to think about past exposure information. Then proceed to summer employment, military service, and conclude with a chronologic list of jobs beginning with the first and ending with the present.

B. **Job titles** should be listed, along with brief descriptions of associated duties with each employment. Titles such as plasterer, fire fighter, or engineer may be of little value. While titles may remain the same over time, job activities and hazardous exposures can change dramatically.

C. **The jobs and exposures of spouses and family members** may be revealing, especially for certain dust exposures such as asbestos.

D. **Exposures to pets, use of forced-air humidifiers, presence of neighborhood factories, and the nature of hobbies** should be also be noted.

E. **Questions about exposures to specific toxic fumes** should be asked. Whenever accidental exposures to fumes are found, the following should be noted:

    1. **Day of exposure.**

    2. **Duration of exposure in minutes.**

    3. **Amount of exposure.**

    4. **Distance from source of exposure.**

F. **Questions about exposures to specific hazardous dusts** should also be asked, with the following indices documented for each exposure:

    1. **Year first exposed to the agent.**

    2. **Year last exposed to the agent.**

    3. **Total years exposed to the agent.**

    4. **Estimation of exposure level.**

        a. **Level 1. Peripheral exposure**—administrative personnel.

        b. **Level 2. Indirect exposure**—electricians, welders.

        c. **Level 3. Direct exposure**—insulation workers, mixers.

G. **Amount of cigarette smoking or tobacco use** should be determined. Individuals can be classified as nonsmokers, current smokers, or ex-smokers if they have stopped for at least 1 year. The nature and type of smoking should be noted, such as filtered or nonfiltered cigarettes, the use of pipes, and the extent of cigar smoking. The age first started and age stopped, and the average number of packages of cigarettes smoked daily should be recorded.

IV. **The physical examination** should describe the patient's breathing, note the presence of finger clubbing or cyanosis, assess the quality of breath sounds including the presence of crackles or wheezes, and document any pertinent cardiac findings.

A. **The description of the patient's breathing** includes the use of accessory muscles, paradoxical movements of rib cage and abdomen, pursed lips during exhalation, the presence of labored breathing at rest, and inability to speak complete sentences.

B. **The signs of right ventricular failure** secondary to pulmonary hypertension include neck vein distention, dependent edema, hepatomegaly, exaggerated intensity of the second heart sound, and a right ventricular gallop that occurs early in diastole and increases with inspiration.

V. **Chest radiographs** should be obtained for all persons being evaluated for pulmonary impairment and disability.

A. **In diseases of chronic airflow obstruction,** the appearance of the chest radiograph may bear little relation to severity of disease. Severe obstructive airways disease may be accompanied by a normal chest radiograph. Nonetheless, the chest x-ray is part of the overall evaluation of disability and should be described in terms of lung size, presence of bullae, flattened diaphragms, increased posteroanterior diameter, and findings consistent with cor pulmonale.

B. **Interstitial diseases** require careful categorization of radiographic findings.

    1. **Type of opacities.** These include nodular (rounded) or reticulonodular. Large volumes of normal lung can be found between these nodular opacities, and thus the chest radiograph often poorly correlates with physiologic findings and pulmonary impairment, especially in early coal-worker's pneumoconiosis and sarcoidosis. Linear, irregular opacities, seen in chronic interstitial pneumonias as well as asbestosis, correlate better with pulmonary function, although the physiologic impairment can sometimes be underestimated because linear opacities generally represent fibrosis and are recognized late in the course of the disease.

2. **Severity of the process**: mild, moderate or severe. A scale of 1–3 can be utilized. For the interstitial disorders, the International Labor Organization radiographic classification for pneumoconiosis can be utilized.

VI. **Pulmonary function testing** is a very useful tool in classifying the degree of impairment. The available battery of tests is vast, and the evaluation can range from minimal testing to extensive, time-consuming, and sometimes invasive testing.

   A. **Three screening tests** can be utilized as the basis for classification of pulmonary impairment. More complex studies can be added whenever discrepancies between clinical findings and screening tests cannot be resolved. These tests should be performed by standardized techniques, and the equipment and methods of calibration must meet published standard guidelines (10–12).

   1. **The forced expired volume in 1 second (FEV$_1$)** is the single best test for the determination of impairment in subjects with airflow obstruction. Accepted throughout the world for almost 50 years, the FEV$_1$ is simple to perform, does not fatigue patients, and permits consistent patient cooperation with little difference in the results between first and subsequent trials.

   2. **The forced vital capacity (FVC)** is the most valuable screening test for volume determination, especially for the interstitial lung diseases. Performed routinely with FEV$_1$, FVC requires minimal time and effort and is both valid and reliable. The variance is small, and several regression equations for predicted normal values are available.

   3. **The single-breath diffusing capacity of carbon monoxide (Dsb)** is the single most important test for determination of severe impairment in patients with interstitial lung diseases (1). This test is noninvasive and suitable for rapid screening and requires little cooperation or effort; adequate regression equations for prediction of normal values are available.

   B. **Other pulmonary function tests** may be of little value in determination of impairment but may be useful to confirm the findings of the screening tests. The **maximal voluntary ventilation (MVV)** has become less important for determination of pulmonary impairment. This test is effort dependent, frequently elicits cough, and is time consuming and fatiguing for patients. Moreover, the FEV$_1$ correlates well with the MVV and is simpler to perform, and the results are highly reproducible. The **functional residual capacity (FRC)** and **residual volume (RV)** are sometimes helpful because they are effort-independent tests that may be useful with patients who have difficulty cooperating with pulmonary testing. The additional time and expense must be weighed against the the limited benefit. Particular tests, such as forced expiratory flow between 25% and 75% of vital capacity, the end-expiratory flow rate, and compliance measurements have no place in assessing disability and impairment.

   C. **Arterial blood oxygen** would appear to be an ideal objective test but is a poor initial screening tool because it is invasive and the results are difficult to standardize due to the effects of acute hyperventilation and altitude. More important, for chronic airflow obstruction no correlation exists between the resting arterial oxygen value and work status. In the interstitial lung diseases, the resting arterial oxygen value often underestimates the degree of impairment; however, arterial oxygenation during exercise in this situation can be utilized for classification of the degree of pulmonary impairment.

VII. **Pulmonary exercise testing** continues to be evaluated for its role in determination of pulmonary impairment and disability (6,13). Knowledge of testing methods and interpretation of exercise testing results have become increasingly important with the growing number of referrals for exercise studies.

   A. **The cycle ergometer and treadmill** are both suitable for exercise testing, although each has advantages and disadvantages. A higher oxygen consumption and heart rate can be achieved on a treadmill because a larger muscle mass is used. Arterial blood sampling and complex ventilatory studies are more easily performed while the patient is seated on a cycle ergometer. Cycling is not as universal as walking, thus elderly patients may find it easier and more comfortable to walk on a treadmill.

   B. **The type of exercise** used is determined by the reason for the testing, as well as the population being studied. For example, elderly patients generally tolerate one of the levels of the six-stage treadmill protocol suggested by Naughton, whereas most younger patients can perform a more strenuous protocol of Bruce. Another choice is between steady-state testing of 5–6 minutes at each level and studies of continuous progression of the workload for 6–12 minutes. Such incremental studies are becoming increasingly popular because of the ease and short duration of the tests.

C. **The estimated oxygen consumption (Vo_2)**, obtained indirectly by calculating power output of either the cycle ergometer or the treadmill, is too variable for disability determination and should not be used for this purpose. Only a poor correlation exists between the measured and the estimated Vo_2 at both low-level and high-level exercise. Vo_2 can be useful in specific situations such as evaluating a particular patient's progress in a rehabilitation program.

D. **An adequate level of exercise** is needed for meaningful results (6,13). Subjective findings by patients, as well as observations by testing personnel, should be carefully recorded, although these are insufficient to document an adequate or maximal test. Objective cardiac and pulmonary criteria are needed.

1. **Heart rate** is the easiest reflection of cardiac performance to quantify and should be used as a cardiac criterion for routine exercise monitoring. The heart rate correlates linearly with ventilation and Vo_2. A value of 80% of predicted (210 − age × 0.65) can be used for the minimal limit.

2. **A ventilatory** criterion can be utilized for subjects not able to attain an adequate heart rate, often because they are receiving cardiac medications. The amount of expired volume during exercise correlates best with Vo_2, and a maximal expired minute volume of 50% of predicted (FEV_1 × 35) can be used as a minimal limit.

E. **Exercise testing should be deferred** because of certain conditions listed in Table 33-1.

F. **Reasons for terminating the exercise study include:**

1. **Adequate or maximal test** criteria have been attained.

2. **The subject stops** secondary to dyspnea, muscle fatigue, or both.

3. **The physician terminates the study** for reasons noted in Table 33-2.

G. **The laboratory should be equipped to meet an emergency.** All personnel should be certified in basic life support and capable of maintaining life until the patient can be managed by the resuscitation team.

H. **Oxygen saturation obtained by oximetry** may be used to estimate the degree of impairment, but the direct arterial oxygen value from an indwelling arterial cannula is preferable. Arterial studies during exercise often add new information for patients with interstitial lung disease, especially if the DLCO is abnormal. Such studies also assess the carbon dioxide status during exercise.

I. **Pulmonary exercise testing interpretation** is a required step for classification of pulmonary impairment and disability. In healthy subjects, maximal exercise is limited by heart rate and cardiac output, and not by ventilation or pulmonary function.

Table 33-1. Indications for deferring pulmonary exercise testing

Acute illness

Congestive heart failure

Dissecting or ventricular aneurysms

Limiting neuromuscular impairment

Severe aortic stenosis

Severe pulmonary hypertension

Uncontrolled arrhythmia

Uncontrolled severe hypertension

Unstable angina pectoris

Table 33-2. Indications for terminating pulmonary exercise testing

Extreme fatigue

Intolerable leg muscle pain

Systolic blood pressure decreases with increasing workload

Systolic blood pressure does not increase with workload

An increase in diastolic pressure .20 mm Hg

Severe systolic hypertension

Three or more successive premature ventricular contractions

A major left ventricular conduction disturbance

ST-T depression or elevation of ≥ 2.0 mm associated with symptoms

Signs of insufficient peripheral circulation or cardiac output, such as pallor, cyanosis, clammy skin, nausea, or dizziness

During maximal exercise, the minute ventilation approaches only about 70% of the MVV. With increasing age, the maximum heart rate decreases along with a decrease in maximal Vo_2. In healthy subjects, the magnitude of the increase in heart rate and ventilation elicited by a certain amount of exercise depends on body size, fitness, amount of training, and hemoglobin content. Because of these multiple factors, work done is best measured by quantifying Vo_2 rather than determining the amount of external workload, another reason that estimated Vo_2 is not recommended.

1. **The Vo_2max** can estimate an individual's aerobic fitness. Healthy manual laborers can work comfortably at approximately 40% of Vo_2max. During shorter periods of time, such individuals can work without fatigue at a pace of 50% of Vo_2max.

2. **Vo_2 requirements** have been estimated for several recreational and occupational activities. Office work requires an estimated Vo_2 of 5–7 mL/kg/min, moderate labor about 15 mL/kg/min, and strenuous labor 20–30 mL/kg/min (2). The range of Vo_2 required for recreational activities include the following: golf, 7–10 mL/kg/min; tennis, 12–15 mL/kg/min; and marathon running or handball, 25–30 mL/kg/min.

3. **Determination of impairment and disability from pulmonary exercise testing is based on two concepts**: (a) jobs can be performed comfortably at 40% of Vo_2max and (b) Vo_2 values can be assigned to specific jobs. For example, if an individual can attain a Vo_2 of 35–40 mL/kg/min by treadmill testing, work requiring a Vo_2 of 10–15 mL/kg/min could easily be performed. However, if an individual can attain a Vo_2 of only 15 mL/kg/min by treadmill testing, moderate-to-heavy labor jobs could not be performed because an individual could not be expected to work at 100% of their Vo_2.

VIII. **Several approaches can be utilized for determination of pulmonary impairment and disability.**

   A. **An approach based only on history and clinical examination** is generally unsatisfactory except in situations of extreme illness.

   B. **A second approach is a functional profile generated and graded by computerized analyses** of many spirometric studies, lung volume measurements, diffusing capacity measurements, arterial blood gas measurements, and cardiopulmonary function during exercise. This approach may include traumatic, painful, and expensive tests available in only a few specialized centers. This method remains in an investigational phase of development.

   C. **A third approach utilizes only the results of exercise testing.** This theoretically gives the most practical estimate of functional capacity and the ability to perform any given amount of work in a job; however, standardization and reliability of the relationship between results and work status are critical. In addition, exercise testing is expensive and time consuming; often the same information can be obtained from the results of FEV_1 and DLCO tests.

D. A fourth, more flexible, approach is preferred. A database is compiled with the degree of dyspnea, the amount of cough and sputum, the detection of crackles or wheezes, and a description of the chest radiograph. Most important, the database includes three noninvasive screening tests: FVC to describe volume, FEV_1 to characterize flow rate, and Dsb to characterize gas exchange in the lungs. The need for pulmonary exercise testing depends on the outcome of these tests. This method is based on the concept of the amount of loss of function, detected by spirometry and Dsb, and the amount of remaining function, determined by exercise testing.

IX. Categories of the degree of pulmonary impairment are needed for the determination of disability due to lung disease. Some are based on criteria for obstructive or restrictive disease, others are based on three or four classes of impairment, and a few have only a category for the severely impaired. Most governmental agencies and medical societies now agree on the two ends of the impairment spectrum. Screening values ≥80% of predicted indicate no pulmonary impairment by physiologic testing. Severe pulmonary impairment is determined by either a vital capacity ≤50% predicted or an FEV_1 or Dsb ≤40% of predicted. Thus, persons with normal screening pulmonary function tests are not disabled by physiologic pulmonary impairment; if they indicate severe functional impairment, then pulmonary dysfunction is so severe that it precludes gainful employment; that is, the individual is totally disabled. Between these extremes of impairment there is less agreement because of the imprecise correlation between the results of pulmonary function testing and the ability of an individual to perform work. For example, individuals near the normal end of the spectrum can probably perform all types of jobs despite slightly abnormal values because of the large pulmonary functional reserve. Any work limitations are more likely due to poor conditioning or cardiac dysfunction. For individuals whose values range from 40% to 60% of predicted, the inability to perform certain types of work may be the result of pulmonary impairment (ie, partial disability).

A. The current recommended classification, shown in Table 33-3, is based on FVC, FEV_1, and Dsb. Each is categorized as normal, mildly impaired, moderately impaired, or severely impaired (3,4).

1. **Mildly impaired** is usually not correlated with diminished ability to perform most jobs.
2. **Moderately impaired individuals** with progressively lower levels of lung function have diminishing ability to meet the physical demands of many jobs.
3. **Severely impaired individuals** are unable to meet the physical demands of most jobs, including travel to work.

Table 33-3. Rating of pulmonary impairment

Test	Normal (% predicted)	Mild (% predicted)	Moderate (% predicted)	Severe (% predicted)
FVC	≥80	60–79	51–59	≤50
FEV_1	≥80	60–79	41–59	≤40
FEV_1/ FVC	≥70	60–69	41–59	≤40
DLCO	≥80*	60–79	41–59	≤40
Vo_2 max mL/kg/min)	≥25	15–25	15–25	<15

DLCO = diffusing capacity for carbon monoxide; FEV_1 = forced expiratory volume in 1 sec; FVC = forced vital capacity; Vo_2max = maximum oxygen consumption.
*AMA guidelines utilize 70% predicted or higher (American Medical Association. The respiratory system: guides to the evaluation of permanent impairment, 4th ed. Chicago: American Medical Association, 1993: 153–167.)

B. **Pulmonary exercise testing should be limited** because of the cost and amount of time involved, but it can be helpful in certain circumstances. Exercise testing may confirm an impairment category or indicate a more severe category for individuals with large discrepancies between perceived symptoms and screening tests. In addition, exercise testing can be very helpful in studying individuals with strenuous jobs. The exercise Vo_2 values that have been utilized in defining impairment categories include the following (3,4):

1. **Vo_2max >25 mL/kg/min**—virtually all types of work.
2. **Vo_2max 15–25 mL/kg/min**—desk work to light or moderate labor.
3. **Vo_2max ≤15 mL/kg/min**—no gainful employment.
4. **The 40% value of the individual's Vo_2max can also be calculated** and compared to the estimated Vo_2 requirement for the particular job. If the job Vo_2 requirement exceeds the worker's 40% Vo_2max value, then full-time employment in that particular job would probably be too difficult. This method must be applied with caution, as job-specific Vo_2 requirements are estimates and large variabilities exist in Vo_2 requirements among individuals (6,13).

C. **Although numeric limits to delineate degrees of impairment are necessary** for use as guidelines by administrative personnel, continuing refinements and clarification are needed. For example, the Social Security Administration has published tables of lower limits for actual values of the FVC and FEV_1 based only on height (ie, without regard to sex or age) (8). Thus, the Social Security tables tend to be designed for elderly persons, while values expressed as percentages of predicted may not favor older workers because the respiratory cost of a given task remains unchanged with advancing age. The use of the 95% confidence interval for normal limits or the percentage of predicted values is preferable in most circumstances because physicians charged with rating impairment should compare organ function or function of the whole person to that of comparable, healthy persons.

X. **Special considerations and other impairments are important issues.** The method noted above is helpful for patients or workers with stable chronic bronchitis or emphysema with airflow obstruction and those with pulmonary fibrosis; however, special situations, especially asthma, require modification of this system or other types of categorizing systems that permit case-by-case evaluations.

A. **Asthma is often considered a special category (2–4,8).** According to the Social Security classification, an asthmatic may be considered disabled if documented attacks of airflow obstruction require treatment in the emergency department or hospital at least once every 2 months, or an average of at least six times yearly despite optimal therapy (8).

B. **Guidelines developed by the American Thoracic Society** are related to the diagnosis of asthma and the classification of impairment by a numeric system based on FEV_1 studies and medication use (3).

1. **Diagnosis of asthma** requires appropriate symptoms of asthma and objective confirmation.

   a. **If the FEV_1/FVC is abnormal,** improvement in the postbronchodilator FEV_1 value of ≥12% or ≥200 mL is confirmatory. For those with values <12%, a confirmatory finding would be an improvement of FEV_1 of ≥20% after a course of corticosteroid therapy.

   b. **If the FEV_1/FVC is normal,** a 20% decrease in the FEV_1 after a challenge with methacholine 8 mg/mL is confirmatory.

2. **Impairment rating** utilizes the FEV_1 value after bronchodilators (Table 33-4), FEV_1 change after bronchodilator or methacholine challenge (Table 33-5), medication to maintain control of asthma (Table 33-6), and summary of these scores for impairment rating (Table 33-7).

C. **Occupational asthma** is a disease characterized by variable airflow limitation or airway hyperresponsiveness due to causes or conditions that are attributable to a particular occupational environment (3,14). Immunologic occupational asthma occurs on reexposure to an agent after a latent period of immune sensitization. Nonimmunologic occupational asthma does not induce immune sensitization. The diagnosis is established utilizing the same method as noted for asthma with the addition

Table 33-4. Postbronchodilator FEV_1

Score	FEV_1 (% predicted)
0	> lower limit of normal
1	70 to normal
2	60–69
3	50–59
4	<50

FEV_1 = forced expiratory volume in 1 sec.

Table 33-5. FEV_1 reversibility or degree of airway hyperresponsiveness

Score	FEV_1 (% change)	PC20 (mg/mL)
0	<10	>8
1	10–19	>0.5–8
2	20–29	>0.125–0.5
3	≥30	<0.125
4	—	—

FEV_1 = forced expiratory volume in 1 sec; PC20 = provocative challenge that induces a 20% decrease in FEV_1.

Table 33-6. Minimum medication need to control asthma

Score	Medication
0	No medication
1	Occasional bronchodilator
2	Daily bronchodilator or low-dose inhaled steroid (<800 μg)
3	High-dose inhaled steroid (>800 μg) or occasional course of systemic steroid (1–3/yr)
4	Plus daily systemic corticosteroid therapy

Table 33-7. Summary impairment rating classes

Impairment class	Total score
0	0
I	1–3
II	4–6
III	7–9
IV	10–11
V	Asthma not controlled by maximal treatment, FEV_1 <50% predicted with 20 mg/d prednisone

FEV_1 = forced expiratory volume in 1 sec.

of a documented 20% decrease in FEV_1 after a specific exposure. Once the diagnosis is made, these patients should be considered 100% impaired on a permanent basis for the job that caused the illness and for other jobs with exposure to the same causative agent. Assessment for long-term impairment should be performed 2 years after the removal from exposure.

D. Hypersensitivity pneumonia (allergic alveolitis) is a disease that is also related to a specific sensitizing agent, and the same principles apply as with individuals with occupational asthma.

E. Some respiratory disorders lead to impairment because of their effect on overall body function rather than their respiratory effects, such as carcinoma of the lung, pulmonary hypertension, sleep apnea syndromes, and severe chronic respiratory infections. Impairment results from weight loss, muscle weakness, fatigue, loss of mental alertness, and general debility. Such impairments need to be documented as accurately as possible in each individual case. There are individual circumstances leading to pulmonary impairments that are too numerous to mention and require case-by-case analysis. For example, an individual with bullous emphysema and mucous plugging should be disqualified from diving or aviation jobs because of risk of barotrauma.

F. Cor pulmonale indicates severe impairment regardless of the pulmonary function rating of impairment.

XI. **Causation** is a medical and legal term often used in requests for disability evaluation. The medical definition of cause and effect requires scientific proof, and the alleged positive element must be one recognized scientifically. Legal causation requires either a probability >50%, or that the event was more likely than not to be the cause.

A. **A thorough review** of the clinical and epidemiologic literature, recording of all available medical and occupational information, and objective determination of the nature of disease are essential elements to establish causation. There are four general aspects that can serve as guidelines for determination of an occupation-related disorder:
   1. **The exposure is a proven hazardous agent.**
   2. **The dose–response relationship and latency period** are appropriate for the exposure.
   3. **The clinical, physiologic, and radiographic findings are consistent** with a described occupational-related disorder.
   4. **There is not a more likely and established diagnostic explanation** as a cause of the pulmonary condition.

B. **A group of basic criteria for causation** of chronic disease can also be utilized (15):
   1. **Consistency of the association.**
   2. **Strength of the association.**
   3. **Specificity of the association.**
   4. **Temporal relationship of the association.**
   5. **Coherence of the association.**

References

1. Epler GR, Saber FA, Gaensler EA: Determination of severe impairment (disability) in interstitial lung disease. *Am Rev Respir Dis* 1980;121:647–659.
2. American Thoracic Society: Evaluation of impairment/disability secondary to respiratory disorders. *Am Rev Respir Dis* 1986;133:1205–1209.
3. American Thoracic Society: Guidelines for evaluation of impairment/disability in patients with asthma. *Am Rev Respir Dis* 1993;147:1056–1061.
4. American Medical Association: The respiratory system. In: *Guides to the evaluation of permanent impairment*, 4th ed. Chicago: American Medical Association, 1993:153–167.
5. World Health Organization: *Impairments, disabilities, and handicaps.* Geneva: World Health Organization, 1980:27–30.

6. Cotes JE: Rating respiratory disability: a report on behalf of a working group of the European Society for Clinical Respiratory Physiology. *Eur Respir J* 1990;3:1074–1077.

7. King, Ballow: *Americans with disabilities act compliance book.* Nashville, Tenn: M. Lee Smith Publishers, 1992:18–29.

8. *Disability evaluation under Social Security: handbook for physicians.* Washington, DC: U.S. Department of Health and Human Services Social Security Administration, 1994; SSA publication 64–039, ICN 468600.

9. Minett A: Questionnaire of the European community for coal and steel (ECSC) on respiratory symptoms. *Eur Respir J* 1989;2:165–177.

10. Standardization of spirometry—1994 update. *Am J Respir Crit Care Med* 1995;152:1107–1136.

11. Crapo RO: Pulmonary function testing. *N Engl J Med* 1994;331:25–30.

12. American Thoracic Society: Single breath carbon monoxide diffusing capacity. *Am Rev Respir Dis* 1987;136:1299–1307.

13. Sue DY: Exercise testing in the evaluation of impairment and disability. *Clin Chest Med* 1994; 15:369–387.

14. Chan-Yeung M, Malo J: Occupational asthma. *N Engl J Med* 1995;333:107–112.

15. Parkes WR: *Occupational lung disorders*, 3rd ed. Oxford: Butterworth, 1994:874.

34

Theophylline/Glucocorticoids

Helen M. Hollingsworth

I. **Theophylline**, or 1,3-dimethylxanthine, has been used as a bronchodilator in patients with asthma and chronic obstructive pulmonary disease for more than 60 years. Its narrow toxic-to-therapeutic window mandates close attention to dosage, serum levels, and potential drug interactions.

A. **Mechanism(s) of action.** The mechanism of action of theophylline is not well understood (1,2) and likely involves a constellation of effects including phosphodiesterase inhibition and adenosine antagonism (3).

1. Phosphodiesterase inhibitors reduce intracellular degradation of cyclic AMP, thus prolonging cyclic AMP's intracellular effects of relaxing bronchial smooth muscle and suppressing mast cell mediator secretion.

2. Theophylline is a weak, nonselective phosphodiesterase inhibitor that inhibits only 10% to 20% of phosphodiesterase activity at the usual therapeutic serum concentrations. Whether its bronchodilator activity is predominantly through this mechanism remains controversial (1,3).

3. Theophylline interferes with the action of adenosine. Adenosine is a naturally occurring purine nucleoside that has been shown to be a bronchoconstrictor in patients with asthma (3).

   a. Local adenosine concentrations increase with methacholine and allergen stimulation, presumably due to mast cell release.

   b. Theophylline selectively inhibits adenosine-induced bronchoconstriction at the usual therapeutic concentrations.

   c. Evidence against this mechanism is that certain methylxanthines that are active bronchodilators do not appear to be adenosine antagonists.

4. Additional possible mechanisms of theophylline-induced bronchodilation include (3):

   a. Inhibition of the generation of contractile prostaglandins.

   b. Modulation of intracellular calcium.

   c. Synergy between phosphodiesterase inhibitors and adenylate cyclase activators (eg, β-adrenergic agonists).

B. **Role of theophylline as a bronchodilator.** Theophylline is a less potent bronchodilator than inhaled or subcutaneously injected β_2-adrenergic agents. On the other hand, sustained-release preparations of theophylline provide a longer duration of action than inhaled β_2-adrenergic agents, with the exception of salmeterol. Theophylline may be helpful in the following situations:

1. Nocturnal bronchoconstriction in patients with asthma—because of the duration of action of the 12- and 24-hour sustained-release preparations (1).

2. For patients with moderately severe to severe chronic asthma, the addition of theophylline to the medical regimen decreases the frequency and severity of asthma symptoms. Theophylline provides an additional steroid-sparing benefit when added to a regimen of alternate-day prednisone or daily inhaled high-dose beclomethasone (1).

3. In patients with exercise-induced bronchoconstriction—although theophylline is not as effective as inhaled albuterol in terms of peak effect.

4. In the setting of acute asthma, the benefit of adding theophylline to the usual emergency department regimen of nebulized β-adrenergic agents remains con-

troversial (1,4–7). Theophylline may be beneficial in patients admitted to the hospital with status asthmaticus (1).

5.   In patients with chronic obstructive pulmonary disease (COPD), even when spirometry is not improved, theophylline therapy is associated with a decrease in dyspnea (2,8). Theophylline appears to provide additional benefit to patients with COPD who are already taking ipratropium bromide and a β-adrenergic agent (9).

6.   Patients who have difficulty using inhaled bronchodilator medication—despite education and use of chamber or spacer devices.

C.   **Evidence for anti-inflammatory activity.** Some patients with asthma experience significant deterioration when theophylline therapy is withdrawn. The extent of deterioration has appeared greater than expected, given theophylline's bronchodilating capacity, leading to speculation that theophylline may have anti-inflammatory activity or other effects (2).

1.   At moderate serum concentrations, theophylline attenuates the bronchoconstriction associated with the late allergic response (9) but does not affect the immediate phase.

2.   The increase in CD4 lymphocytes typically seen with the late-phase response is inhibited by theophylline. In patients with moderately severe asthma taking high-dose inhaled corticosteroids, withdrawal of theophylline has resulted in an increase in CD4/CD8 cells in the submucosa and an associated decrease in FEV_1 (10).

3.   Bronchial biopsy studies have shown a decrease in EG2-positive activated eosinophils immediately below the basement membrane in mild asthmatics treated with theophylline (11).

4.   However, the observation that allergen-induced increases in airway methacholine responsiveness are not inhibited by theophylline (12) argues against significant anti-inflammatory activity.

D.   **Respiratory muscle effects: force and endurance**

1.   At high serum concentrations, theophylline has a positive inotropic effect on normal diaphragm, but this effect is harder to demonstrate when concentrations are in the normal therapeutic range (2).

2.   In patients with COPD, theophylline improves the strength of the fatigued diaphragm and makes the diaphragm more resistant to fatigue. This may help asthma and COPD patients who are weaning from mechanical ventilation or are experiencing worsening airflow obstruction (2,13).

E.   **Clinical pharmacology.** The specific indications for theophylline therapy are given in the chapters on asthma (see chapter 4) and COPD (see chapters 14 and 15) and in recently published guidelines (1,8). Once the decision is made to initiate theophylline therapy, the following guidelines may be helpful:

1.   **Oral administration**

a.   12- and 24-hour release preparations have largely supplanted use of shorter-acting preparations.

b.   In adults, start with a low dose (12–16 mg/kg/d to a maximum of 300–400 mg/d); titrate upward slowly.

c.   Do not increase dose if patient experiences nausea, headache, tachycardia, or other side effects.

d.   Guide final dosage by measurement of serum levels, aiming for 5–15 µg/mL (lower levels for elderly patients with COPD, higher levels for younger patients with asthma) or 8–12 µg/mL in pregnancy. Measure a serum level about half way into dosing interval.

e.   Instruct patients to take medication at the same time each day with respect to meals.

f.   Reduce dosage by half for fever >24 hours; institution of quinolone antibiotic, oral contraceptive, clarithromycin, or erythromycin. Alert the patient to call for further dose adjustments at the first sign of drug toxicity. Azithromycin does not alter clearance of theophylline.

g.   Reduce dosage by half when maintenance therapy with phenytoin, carbamazepine, or other enzyme inducer is discontinued.

2. **Intravenous (IV) administration.** The main indication for IV therapy is inability to take oral medication or concern about absorption. Otherwise, sustained-release oral preparations provide stable blood levels and are just as effective (1,14).
   a. Aminophylline, a salt of theophylline with 80% bioavailability, is usually used for IV therapy.
   b. When patients on maintenance theophylline are admitted to hospital with exacerbations of asthma or COPD, oral theophylline can be continued, if the patient can take oral medication and the serum dose is appropriate.
   c. Patients with an adequate serum level on admission who are switched to IV therapy do not need a loading dose. If the theophylline level is subtherapeutic, a supplemental loading dose can be given: each 1 mg/kg aminophylline will increase serum concentration by 2 µg/mL.
   d. **Maintenance therapy**
      i. If the outpatient oral dose is known, 125% × theophylline dose = aminophylline dose to be given over 24 hours as a continuous infusion.
      ii. Usual maintenance dose is 3–9 mg/kg/h. Use lower doses for patients with fever, advanced age, liver disease, congestive heart failure, or concomitant interacting drugs. Higher doses are necessary for smokers and children. Levels need to be checked daily.
   e. The loading dose for patients not previously on oral therapy is 5 mg/kg lean body weight, given IV over 20–30 minutes.
F. **Adverse effects**
   1. Most common adverse effects include nausea, abdominal discomfort, vomiting, diarrhea, diuresis, headache, and jitteriness.
   2. Side effects tend to increase as the serum level increases but may be seen with low therapeutic levels (5–10 µg/mL).
   3. Although nausea and abdominal discomfort tend to predict when the serum level is too high, dangerous toxicity can be seen in patients without these symptoms (15,16). Therefore, monitoring of serum levels is extremely important when therapy is initiated or changed, and then at 6–12 month intervals.
   4. Signs and symptoms associated with toxic levels include palpitations, premature ventricular contractions, atrial tachyarrhythmias, tremors, seizures, and gastrointestinal bleeding.
G. **Drug interactions.** Because theophylline is metabolized in the liver, many medications that are similarly metabolized may alter theophylline clearance or may themselves be affected by theophylline (17–19). Whenever there is a potential drug interaction, the care provider must educate the patient regarding potential toxicity, obtain more frequent theophylline serum levels, and consider empiric reductions in theophylline dose.
   1. Drugs that decrease theophylline clearance and increase serum levels include erythromycin, clarithromycin, the quinolones (20), troleandomycin, birth control pills, cimetidine, ranitidine, allopurinol, propranolol, and calcium channel blockers.
   2. Drugs that increase theophylline clearance and reduce serum levels include phenytoin, barbiturates, and rifampin.
   3. **Other interactions**
      a. Lithium clearance is increased by theophylline.
      b. Furosemide diuresis is enhanced by theophylline.
      c. β-Adrenergic effects can be enhanced by theophylline and result in toxic synergism (eg, isoproterenol, ephedrine, albuterol).
      d. Interaction of reserpine and theophylline may result in tachycardia.
   4. Antibiotics that do not appear to interact with theophylline include amoxicillin, cefaclor, cotrimoxazole, and doxycycline.
H. **Treatment of theophylline intoxication.** Theophylline poisoning may result from inadvertent iatrogenic overdosage, patient error, or suicide attempt.

1. Serious toxicity is associated with levels >30 µg/mL. Serious adverse effects are more likely to be seen at any given blood level in patients with chronic rather than with acute intoxication (16). Serum levels correlate poorly with occurrence of life-threatening events. Metabolic disturbances are more common with acute intoxication (15).

2. Prevention of absorption is particularly important with the widespread usage of slow-release preparations.

3. Emptying the stomach is recommended only for patients who have ingested a large quantity within 1 hour of presenting to medical attention.

4. Activated charcoal, 50–100 g orally, with 70% sorbitol 75–100 mL.

5. **Supportive care**
   a. Monitor and maintain serum potassium concentration.
   b. Hemodynamic monitoring for volume repletion.
   c. Seizure is usually treated with diazepam or phenobarbital; phenytoin is not recommended (15,21). Refractory status may require general anesthesia with pentobarbital or thiopental and paralyzing agents. Prophylactic phenobarbital may be used for patients with serum levels ≥50 µg/mL, although this has not been studied in clinical trials.
   d. Cardiac arrhythmias. Treatment is recommended only for serious arrhythmias. Adenosine, verapamil and digoxin have been used for supraventricular arrhythmias; lidocaine and phenytoin for ventricular arrhythmias.
   e. Metabolic acidosis is common. Conservative treatment is advisable.

6. **Active removal** (15,22)
   a. Activated charcoal enhances theophylline clearance in patients with moderate intoxication, but should not be administered to patients with depressed pharyngeal reflexes and may not be tolerated by patients with vomiting.
   b. Charcoal hemoperfusion is indicated for serum levels (15,22):
      i. ≥80 µg/mL in acute ingestion for normal patients.
      ii. ≥60 µg/mL in chronic intoxication.
      iii. ≥40 µg/mL if patient is <6 months old, >60 years old, has significant liver or cardiac disease, or cannot tolerate activated charcoal.
   c. Hemodialysis doubles theophylline clearance and may be helpful when hemoperfusion is not available. This should be combined with oral activated charcoal.
   d. Other modalities such as peritoneal dialysis, plasmapheresis, and hemofiltration are unlikely to be beneficial (15).

II. **Glucocorticoids** (GCs) have broad anti-inflammatory activity and are effective in the treatment of a wide spectrum of pulmonary diseases including asthma, COPD, sarcoidosis, interstitial fibrosis, hypersensitivity pneumonitis, and bronchiolitis obliterans with organizing pneumonia. Unfortunately, GCs also have significant potential side effects that require careful monitoring and patient education. This section will focus on general concepts regarding the mechanisms of action, administration, and adverse effects of systemically administered GCs. A discussion of inhaled GCs can be found in the chapters on asthma and COPD (see chapters 4, 14, and 15).

A. **Mechanisms of action.** Recent research has increased our understanding of the cellular effects of GCs (23,24) and provides insight into the reasons why GCs have such widespread effects.

1. GCs, when administered orally or IV, circulate in the blood unbound or associated with cortisol-binding globulin.
2. Free GC binds with GC receptors (GR) on cells.
3. The GC-GR complex translocates into the cell nucleus and binds to DNA, resulting in either positive or negative modulation of gene transcription.
4. GCs also influence post-transcriptional events, such as RNA translation and protein synthesis and secretion (eg, altering the stability of certain cytokine messenger RNAs to change the intracellular steady-state).

B. **Anti-inflammatory effects.** GCs affect a multiplicity of cells to inhibit or suppress several steps in inflammation, including (23,24):

1. Traffic of leukocytes to sites of inflammation by decreasing the number of circulating lymphocytes.
2. Activation of leukocytes through suppression of interleukin-2 (IL-2).
3. Expression of endothelial cell surface adhesion molecules (ICAM-1 and VCAM-1) and elaboration of arachidonic acid metabolites and IL-1 and complement factors.
4. Fibroblast cytokine and prostaglandin secretion and collagen formation.
5. Secretion of proinflammatory molecules by mast cells and basophils.
6. Activation of basophils and mediator release.
7. Eosinophil accumulation at inflammatory sites and intravascular circulation.
8. Microvascular leakage of fluids and inflammatory cells.
9. Phospholipase A_2 release via the annexin family of proteins, which includes lipocortin-1.
10. IgE levels, possibly due to immunoglobulin catabolism, as well as inhibition of cytokines that promote IgE production.

C. **Clinical pharmacology.** Several different GC analogues have been developed for clinical use. These compounds differ in their absorption and distribution characteristics, GR binding, elimination rates, topical versus systemic potency, and mineralocorticoid activity. The choice of a specific analog and dose depends on the disease being treated and the severity of the disease. These disease-specific issues are reviewed in the chapters devoted to the individual diseases.

   1. **General observations about systemic GC use**
      a. **Smaller doses** administered more frequently are more effective than larger doses administered less frequently.
      b. **Topical or focal application** of GCs results in less toxicity than systemic administration and should be used when the desired clinical affect can be achieved. Airway diseases such as asthma and COPD can usually be managed with inhaled GCs, but pulmonary parenchymal diseases such as interstitial pulmonary fibrosis require systemic GCs.
      c. Most respiratory diseases that require oral GC therapy respond to a once-daily regimen. The preferred method is a single morning dose of prednisone or methylprednisolone to mimic the endogenous pattern of GC secretion, minimize insomnia, and reduce hypothalamic-pituitary-adrenal (HPA) axis suppression. For more severe disease, it may be desirable to maintain the clinical effect throughout the day. In this situation, prednisone or methylprednisolone can be prescribed in divided doses on a BID or TID schedule.
      d. As patients improve on therapy, particularly when the prednisone equivalent dose is ≤30 mg/d, attempts should be made to switch to alternate-day dosing to further reduce GC-related morbidity and enhance recovery of the HPA axis.
      e. After patients have been on systemic GC therapy for >3 weeks, the GC dose needs to be tapered to allow recovery of the HPA axis; longer durations of therapy require slower tapers.
      f. Timing of the dose of oral GCs may affect the therapeutic result (25), especially if the disease involved has a diurnal variation. For example, some patients with steroid-dependent asthma have improved control of asthma symptoms when the daily dose of GC is taken in the afternoon instead of the usual early-morning dosing. Potentially, the combination of low endogenous cortisol secretion and waning of the effect of the previous dose contributes to poor control at night, a time when asthma symptoms frequently flare.

   2. **Specific GCs available for use in the United States** (24)
      a. **Hydrocortisone** (half-life 1.9 hours) is usually used for physiologic replacement or "stress" coverage. The mineralocorticoid effects are helpful in patients who need physiologic replacement, but they are undesirable in patients requiring the medication for immunosuppression or anti-inflammatory activity.

   b.   Prednisone is a widely used oral GC that is inactive until converted in the liver to prednisolone by reduction at the 11-keto position. The relative potency is four times that of hydrocortisone.
   c.   Methylprednisolone differs from prednisolone in the presence of a methyl group in the 6α position; like prednisolone, it is active without hepatic conversion. Methylprednisolone is available both for oral and IV use, and the relative potency is five times that of hydrocortisone.
   d.   Triamcinolone is essentially devoid of mineralocorticoid activity and is available as a suspension for intramuscular (IM) use. The potency is about five times that of hydrocortisone. Patient-to-patient response is not uniform, but a single parenteral dose four to seven times the oral daily dose will control symptoms from 4 days to as long as 4 weeks. The major indication is the treatment of patients unable to adhere to a regimen of oral medication.
   e.   Dexamethasone is 20–25 times more potent than hydrocortisone and has the benefit of minimal salt retention. However, the potential morbidity is increased because the biologic half-life is even longer than prednisone or methylprednisolone.
   f.   A suspension of betamethasone sodium phosphate and betamethasone acetate is available for IM use. The onset of action of the betamethasone esters varies, so a single IM injection provides prompt as well as sustained GC therapy. Like IM triamcinolone, the daily GC effect in an individual patient is difficult to titrate. Betamethasone is generally reserved for patients who are not able to take oral GC preparations.
D.   Glucocorticoid resistance. Although GCs are the most effective antiasthma medications currently available, some patients with chronic asthma do not experience the expected improvement in asthma symptoms and pulmonary function following oral GC administration (23,26,27).
   1.   This phenomenon has been explored most fully in patients with asthma, but it likely pertains in other GC-requiring diseases.
   2.   A <30% improvement in FEV$_1$ after a total of 420 mg prednisolone given over 2 weeks is one accepted definition of corticosteroid resistance. These patients lack not only an ameliorative respiratory response but also the other clinical features of hypercorticolism. GC resistance may be familial or acquired.
   3.   Evaluation of suspected GC resistance
      a.   Determine whether the patient is adhering to the recommended dosing schedule (26,27).
      b.   Evaluate the absorption and clearance of orally administered GCs (26,28,29):
         i.   Measure peak and trough blood levels (available only in specialized laboratories).
         ii.   Measure total eosinophil levels.
         iii.   Enhanced plasma clearance of prednisolone or methylprednisolone has not been demonstrated except in the presence of medications that enhance cytochrome P-450 metabolism.
      c.   Evaluate conversion of prednisone into the biologically active prednisolone in the liver. This may be tested by having the patient take methylprednisolone at 80% of the usual prednisone dose, and repeat spirometry again after 2 weeks (26). Additionally, the total eosinophil count can be measured during the two regimens, looking at the relative eosinophilopenic responses.
      d.   Measure endogenous cortisol. Patients with familial GC resistance, a rare autosomal-dominant disorder with variable penetrance, have high circulating levels of cortisol and adrenocorticotropic hormone (corticotropin). These patients may also demonstrate excess of non-GC hormones (eg, hypertension, hirsutism, menstrual irregularities, hyperkalemia) (23,26).
      e.   Consider referral to a specialized center for evaluation of cellular response to GCs.

    4. Treatment of GC resistance in asthma depends on the exact mechanism and degree of resistance (23,26,27).

      a. Use additional conventional therapies such as theophylline, salmeterol, terbutaline, ipratropium, nedocromil or cromolyn, remembering that only the latter two have significant anti-inflammatory effects.

      b. Consider **steroid-sparing therapies**, such as methotrexate or cyclosporine.

      c. Consider **leukotriene inhibitors** (eg zileuton) **or receptor antagonists** (eg zafirlukast).

      d. Try an **alternate GC analog** such as oral methylprednisolone or triamcinolone instead of prednisone.

      e. Consider a trial of high-dose, possibly IV, GC therapy to reduce inflammation that may contribute to secondary GC resistance (23). One theory regarding GC resistance in asthma is that apparent secondary resistance to the effects of oral, low-to-moderate dose of GCs may be caused by severe, ongoing airways inflammation. A course of high-dose, IV GCs may reduce the inflammation, enabling improved control of the patient's asthma at doses that previously were ineffective (23).

E. Complications of glucocorticoid therapy. Oral GC therapy is frequently associated with side effects that tend to become more serious and more prevalent as the dose and duration of therapy increase (24).

    1. Certain adverse effects such as **insomnia, emotional lability, increased appetite, and weight gain** are characteristic of early therapy. Insomnia can be decreased by consolidating most or all of the GC dose to the early morning. Patient education and reassurance help with emotional instability, but serious problems in the face of ongoing need for GC therapy may require psychiatric help. Nutrition counseling helps to offset weight gain.

    2. HPA axis suppression is to be expected when systemic therapy lasts >3 weeks. After this time, steroid therapy needs to be tapered: the longer the duration of therapy, the slower the taper. The rate of tapering depends on the disease activity and adrenal recovery. **When the dose of prednisone has been >30 mg/d for several weeks, a decrease in the daily dose of 10 mg every 1–3 weeks is usually acceptable. With a daily dose 10–30 mg, the decreases may be 5 mg every 1–3 weeks. With a dose <10 mg/d, the incremental decreases may need to be 1–2 mg** (30). When systemic GC therapy is discontinued, a cosyntropin stimulation test may be used to determine whether the HPA axis has recovered. **Stress GC coverage should be given for 1 year after completion of systemic GC therapy. Patients on high-dose inhaled GCs should also receive stress coverage.**

    3. Elevations in serum glucose are common during GC therapy but only in patients with underlying glucose intolerance. **Educate patients about signs and symptoms of hyperglycemia.** Patients who already require oral hypoglycemics or insulin should have frequent blood glucose determinations. Patients who require insulin for diabetes control should be advised to monitor their blood glucose closely, anticipating elevated levels during GC treatment. **Insulin dose should be adjusted according to the blood glucose level.** Patients taking a short course of GCs who do not normally require insulin may transiently require insulin, if their blood glucose is persistently above 250 mg/dL. If long-term GC therapy is anticipated, consideration can be given to using an oral hypoglycemic agent. Measurement of gycosylated hemoglobin A (hemoglobin A_{1C}) may help guide this decision. **Adherence to an American Diabetes Association diet should help control blood glucose elevations. When insulin or oral hypoglycemics are used to control hyperglycemia, patients need to be warned that hypoglycemia may occur as the GC dose is tapered.**

    4. Hypertension and **acne** are seen when patients have other underlying risk factors.

    5. The risk of **peptic ulcer disease** is slightly increased but appears more related to coexistent risk factors, such as nonsteroidal anti-inflammatory therapy.

6. The relative risk of **infectious complications** of steroid therapy is about two times that of controls and varies according to the underlying disease process, as well as the duration and intensity of therapy.
   a. The most common infectious side effect is **oropharyngeal thrush**. Typically associated with inhaled steroids, oral thrush is also seen with oral steroids, particularly when accompanied by antibiotic therapy.
   b. **Patients who have never had varicella are at increased risk for generalized varicella. If exposed, these patients should receive hyperimmune immunoglobulin. Patients who present with a varicella skin rash should be treated with IV acyclovir.**
   c. The use of **prophylactic antituberculous therapy** for a previously untreated patient with a positive purified protein derivative (PPD) tuberculin skin test who requires steroid therapy is controversial. In general, prophylaxis with isoniazid is not necessary for patients who require intermittent GC bursts for asthma. On the other hand, patients requiring long-term GC therapy should receive prophylactic isoniazid, barring other contraindications.

7. Steroids cause bone loss by decreasing intestinal calcium absorption and increasing renal secretion. These changes in calcium metabolism result in lower serum calcium levels and an increase in parathyroid hormone secretion with subsequent bone resorption. In a study of patients with asthma, long-term steroid treatment resulted in trabecular, but not cortical, bone loss—a pattern consistent with osteoporosis.
   a. Prevention of **GC-induced osteoporosis** depends on adequate dietary calcium (1200–1500 mg/d) intake and weightbearing exercise (24,31–33). Whether calcitriol or calcitonin will ultimately be added to this prevention regimen is still under investigation. Sex hormones and vitamin D should only be replaced if deficient. **Bone density** measurement is important to determine whether prevention has been adequate for patients with long-term therapy, particularly if other risk factors for osteoporosis are present.
   b. **Calcitriol and bisphosphonates** are the usual agents for treatment of osteoporosis, but this therapy should be managed by a rheumatologist or endocrinologist (30). Long-term use of inhaled GCs may also be associated with osteoporosis (34). Studies of optimal preventive measures are ongoing. For the present, patients should be encouraged to ingest the recommended daily amount of calcium through diet or supplements and to engage in weightbearing exercise when feasible.

8. **Osteonecrosis** (avascular necrosis) of bone is a known complication of systemic GC therapy, although the exact mechanism is not known (24,35). While osteonecrosis is typically a complication of long-term GC therapy, it has also been described with short-term, high-dose therapy. The joints most commonly affected are the hips, knees, and shoulders. When the area involved is small, treatment can be conservative with avoidance of weightbearing and pain relief with nonsteroidal anti-inflammatory agents or other analgesics. More severe cases require bone grafting or joint replacement.

9. **Cataract** development related to GCs is usually associated with higher doses and longer duration of therapy. Intraocular pressures should be monitored in patients on chronic, systemic GC therapy because of the increased risk of glaucoma (36).

10. **Steroid-induced myopathy** is also associated with higher doses and longer duration of therapy and may be a cause of worsening exercise tolerance in the face of stable spirometry. Improvement is usually seen as steroids are tapered.

11. Chronic, systemic use of GCs in children may result in growth retardation. Studies are ongoing as to whether inhaled GCs alone have a significant effect on growth (37).

F. **Glucocorticoid drug interactions**
   1. Relatively few adverse drug interactions have been described for GCs.

2. **Phenobarbital, phenytoin, and carbamazepine** increase cytochrome P-450 activity, thereby reducing prednisolone, methylprednisolone, and dexamethasone effectiveness.
3. **Erythromycin** and ketoconazole impair prednisolone and methylprednisolone elimination. **Rifampin** decreases the effectiveness of prednisolone and methylprednisolone.
4. Cimetidine has no interaction with prednisolone, methylprednisolone, or dexamethasone, but **antacids** decrease the bioavailability of prednisolone.
5. Although not directly a drug interaction, patients receiving **insulin or oral hypoglycemic agents** for glucose intolerance will likely need dose adjustments as GC therapy is added or tapered.

References

1. National Heart Lung and Blood Institute/World Health Organization workshop report: *Global initiative for asthma*. NIH/NHLBI Publication 95–3659.
2. Jenne JW: Two new roles for theophylline in the asthmatic? *J Asthma* 1995;32:89–95.
3. Essayan DM, Lichtenstein LM: Phosphodiesterase inhibitors: yesterday, today and tomorrow. *Insights in Allergy* 1994;9:1–12.
4. Rossing TH, Fanta CH, Goldstein DH, et al.: Emergency therapy of asthma: comparison of the acute effects of parenteral and inhaled sympathomimetics and infused aminophylline. *Am Rev Respir Dis* 1980;122:365–371.
5. Fanta CH, Rossing TH, McFadden ER Jr: Treatment of acute asthma—is combination therapy with sympathomimetics and methylxanthines indicated? *Am J Med* 1986;80:5–10.
6. Wrenn K, Slovis CM, Murphy F, et al.: Aminophylline therapy for acute bronchospastic disease in the emergency room. *Ann Intern Med* 1991;115:241–247.
7. Huang D, O'Brien RG, Harman E, et al.: Does aminophylline benefit adults admitted to the hospital for an acute exacerbation of asthma? *Ann Intern Med* 1993;119:1155–1160.
8. American Thoracic Society: Standards for the diagnosis and care of patients with chronic obstructive pulmonary disease. *Am J Respir Crit Care Med* 1995;152:S77–S120.
9. Karpel JP, Kotch A, Zinny M, et al.: A comparison of inhaled ipratropium, oral theophylline plus inhaled-agonist, and the combination of all three in patients with COPD. *Chest* 1994;105:1089–1094.
10. Ward AJM, McKenniff M, Evans JM, et al.: Theophylline—an immunomodulatory role in asthma? *Am Rev Respir Dis* 1993;147:518–523.
11. Sullivan P, Bekir S, Jaffar Z, et al.: Anti-inflammatory effects of low-dose oral theophylline in atopic asthma. *Lancet* 1994;343:1006–1008.
12. Cockcroft DW, Murdock KY, Gore BP, et al.: Theophylline does not inhibit allergen-induced increase in airway responsiveness to methacholine. *J Allergy Clin Immunol* 1989;83:913–920.
13. Aubier M: Effect of theophylline on diaphragmatic and other skeletal function. *J Allergy Clin Immunol* 1986;78:787–792.
14. Jonasson S, Kjartansson G, Gislason D, et al.: Comparison of the oral and intravenous routes for treating asthma with methylprednisolone and theophylline. *Chest* 1988;94:723–726.
15. Goldberg MJ, Park GD, Berlinger WG: Treatment of theophylline intoxication. *J Allergy Clin Immunol* 1986;78:811–817.
16. Shannon M: Predictors of major toxicity after theophylline overdose. *Ann Intern Med* 1993;119:1161–1167.
17. Szefler SJ, Bender BG, Jusko WJ, et al.: Evolving role of theophylline for treatment of chronic childhood asthma. *J Pediatr* 1995;127:176–185.
18. Pashko S, Simons WR, Sena MM, Stoddard ML: Rate of exposure to theophylline-drug interactions. *Clin Ther* 1994;16:1068–1077.
19. Jonkman JHG: Therapeutic consequences of drug interactions with theophylline pharmacokinetics. *J Allergy Clin Immunol* 1985;78:736–742.
20. Niki Y, Soejima R, Kawane H, et al.: New synthetic quinolone antibacterial agents and serum concentration of theophylline. *Chest* 1987;92:663–669.
21. Gaudreault P, Guay J: Theophylline poisoning: pharmacological considerations and clinical management. *Med Toxicol* 1986;1:169.

22. Singer EP, Kolischenko A: Seizures due to theophylline overdose. *Chest* 1985;87:755–757.
23. Barnes PJ, Greening AP, Crompton GK: Glucocorticoid resistance in asthma. *Am Rev Respir Dis* 1995;152:S125–S142.
24. Boumpas DT, Chrousos GP, Wilder RL, et al.: Glucocorticoid therapy for immune-mediated diseases: basic and clinical correlates. *Ann Intern Med* 1993;119:1198–1208.
25. Beam WR, Weiner DE, Martin RJ: Timing of prednisone and alterations of airways inflammation in nocturnal asthma. *Am Rev Respir Dis* 1992;146:1524–1530.
26. Chrousos GP, Detera-Wadleigh SD, Karl M: Syndromes of glucocorticoid resistance. *Ann Intern Med* 1993;119:1113–1124.
27. Cypcar D, Busse WW: Steroid-resistant asthma. *J Allergy Clin Immunol* 1993;92:362–372.
28. Szefler SJ: Glucocorticoid therapy for asthma: clinical pharmacology. *J Allergy Clin Immunol* 1991;88:147–165.
29. Alvarez J, Surs W, Leung DYM, et al.: Steroid-resistant asthma: immunologic and pharmacologic features. *J Allergy Clin Immunol* 1992;89:714–721.
30. Larochelle GE Jr, LaRochelle AG, Ratner RE, Borenstein DG: Recovery of the hypothalamic-pituitary-adrenal (HPA) axis in patients with rheumatic diseases receiving low-dose prednisone. *Am J Med* 1993;95:258–264.
31. Lukert BP, Raisz LG: Glucocorticoid-induced osteoporosis: pathogenesis and management. *Ann Intern Med* 1990;112:352–364.
32. Meunier PJ: Is steroid-induced osteoporosis preventable? *N Engl J Med* 1993;328:1781.
33. Sambrook P, Birmingham J, Kelly P, et al.: Prevention of corticosteroid osteoporosis. *N Engl J Med* 1993;328:1747–1752.
34. Ip M, Lam K, Yam L, et al.: Decreased bone mineral density in premenopausal asthma patients receiving long-term inhaled steroids. *Chest* 1994;105:1722–1727.
35. Mankin HJ: Nontraumatic necrosis of bone (osteonecrosis). *N Engl J Med* 1992;326:1473–1479.
36. Urban RC Jr, Dreyer EB: Corticosteroid-induced glaucoma. *Int Ophthalmol Clin* 1993;33:135–139.
37. Allen DB, Mullen ML, Mullen B: A meta-analysis of the effect of oral and inhaled corticosteroids on growth. *J Allergy Clin Immunol* 1994;93:967–976.

Oxygen Therapy

Scott K. Epstein

Oxygen (O_2) is one of the most commonly prescribed therapeutic modalities for the prevention and treatment of hypoxemia. Proper use of O_2 therapy requires an understanding of the mechanisms and consequences of hypoxemia, as well as the principles of available delivery and monitoring systems.

I. Overview of hypoxemia

A. Relationship between hypoxemia and tissue hypoxia

1. Normal or expected arterial partial pressure of O_2 (Pao_2) decreases with age and may be estimated by the equation:

$$Pao_2 = 109 - 0.41(\text{age in years})$$

Although emphasis is often placed on the degree of hypoxemia, the resulting tissue hypoxia and organ dysfunction are more important. The capacity of blood to carry O_2 to the tissues is determined by the arterial O_2-carrying capacity:

$$Cao_2 \text{ (mL } O_2/\text{min)} = 1.39(\text{Hb})(Sao_2) + 0.003(Pao_2)$$

where Hb is hemoglobin concentration (g%), Sao_2 is the O_2 saturation of hemoglobin (% sat), and 0.003 (Pao_2) is the contribution of the relatively small amount of O_2 dissolved in the blood. The Cao_2 is an important determinant of O_2 transport (Do_2):

$$Do_2 \text{ (mL } O_2/\text{min)} = Cao_2 \times CO$$

where CO is the cardiac output (L/min). Efficient O_2 delivery is also dependent on optimal regional blood flow to the organs and O_2 release from hemoglobin (Hb). The latter depends on the position of the O_2-Hb dissociation curve, with a right-shifted curve (resulting from $\downarrow$ pH, $\uparrow$ $Paco_2$, $\uparrow$ 2,3-DPG, $\uparrow$ temperature) favoring O_2 unloading to the tissues and a left-shifted curve (resulting from $\uparrow$ pH, $\downarrow$ $Paco_2$, $\downarrow$ 2,3-DPG, $\downarrow$ temperature) inhibiting O_2 release.

2. Acute symptoms of hypoxemia generally reflect inadequate O_2 delivery to specific organs and may produce organ dysfunction (Table 35–1). In normal individuals, acute hypoxemia will first be manifested by central nervous system dysfunction at a $Paco_2$ <55 mm Hg (1). Acute hypoxemia leads to a series of physiologic responses that increase O_2 delivery to tissues. With chronic hypoxemia, adaptive responses (eg, $\uparrow$ 2,3-DPG) improve O_2 off-loading at the tissue level, but other physiologic alterations can result in significant and sometimes irreversible organ dysfunction, especially in anemic individuals and those with reduced cardiac function.

B. Mechanisms of hypoxemia

(Table 35-2). The $Paco_2$ is determined by the inspired O_2 concentration (Fio_2), the amount of alveolar ventilation (Pao_2), and the matching of ventilation to perfusion within the lung.

1. **Ventilation–perfusion (V/Q) mismatch** is the most common cause of hypoxemia encountered in clinical practice and is the principal cause of hypoxemia in pulmonary embolism, pneumonia, asthma, and chronic obstructive pulmonary disease (COPD). Furthermore, V/Q mismatch contributes to hypoxemia in the acute respiratory distress syndrome (ARDS), cardiac pulmonary

543

Table 35-1. Effects of hypoxemia

Organ dysfunction	Mechanism	Manifestations
Pulmonary vascular	Pulmonary vasoconstriction (reversible) Structural remodeling of vascular smooth muscle and endothelium (irreversible)	Pulmonary hypertension
Right ventricular	↑ Pulmonary vascular resistance ↑ Right ventricular stroke work	Right ventricular hypertrophy Right sided S_3, heave Jugular venous distention Pedal edema, hepatic congestion Effort syncope Exercise intolerance
Left ventricular	Inadequate O_2 delivery to myo-cardium ↑ Myocardial O_2 demand ↑ Afterload (↑ SVR) ↑ Cardiac output ↓ Myocardial contractility	Myocardial ischemia Myocardial infarction Congestive heart failure Arrhythmias Tachycardia Exercise intolerance
Central nervous system (CNS)	Inadequate O_2 delivery to CNS	Euphoria, confusion ↓ Cognition ↓ Short-term memory ↓ Fine motor control Impaired judgment Headache, irritability ↓ Neuropsychiatric performance Coma (Pao_2 <30 mm Hg) ↓ Quality of life
Renal	Impaired free-water clearance	
Hematologic	↑ erythropoietin production	Erythrocytosis Hyperviscosity ↑ Pulmonary vasculature resistance ↓ Cerebral blood flow
Respiratory	↑ Minute ventilation ↑ Work of breathing (WOB) ↓ Respiratory muscle function	Tachypnea Dyspnea Exercise intolerance
Skeletal muscle	↓ O_2 delivery to muscles	Exercise intolerance Early shift to anaerobic metabolism
Nutrition	↓ Sao_2 during eating ↑ Energy expenditure (↑ WOB) Dyspnea while eating	Weight loss Skeletal muscle weakness Respiratory muscle weakness

Table 35-2. Summary of mechanisms of hypoxemia

Cause of hypoxemia	$(A-a)o_2$	$Paco_2$ (mm Hg)	Pao_2 breathing 100% O_2 (mm Hg)	$(A-a)o_2$ breathing 100% O_2
Hypoventilation	N	↑	>600	N
V-Q mismatch	↑	N↓↑	>600	↑
Abnormal diffusion	↑	N↓	>600	↑
Anatomic shunt	↑	↓	<<<600	↑
↓ Fio_2	N	↓	>600	N
↓ Cvo_2	↑	↓	Variable	↑

$(A-a)o_2$ = pulmonary alveolar to arterial O_2 difference; Cvo_2 = mixed venous oxygen content; Fio_2 = fraction of inspired O_2; N = normal; V/Q = ventilation–perfusion ratio.

edema, and interstitial lung disease. **The hypoxemia of V/Q mismatch corrects with supplemental O_2 administration. In uncomplicated exacerbations of asthma or COPD, only small increases in the F_IO_2** are therefore required to correct hypoxemia.

2. **Shunts** may be intracardiac (atrial or ventricular septal defects, patent foramen ovale, patent ductus arteriosus) or intrapulmonary (arteriovenous malformation, complete lobar atelectasis, cardiac or noncardiac pulmonary edema). Hypoxemia secondary to true anatomic shunting can be differentiated from other causes of hypoxemia by having patients breathe 100% O_2. This will not substantially increase the Pao_2 or reduce the alveolar-arterial oxygen gradient $[(A-a)o_2]$ in cases of anatomic shunt >50% of the cardiac output. When there is less flow through the shunt and V/Q mismatch coexists, supplemental O_2 will improve the Pao_2 by removing the component of hypoxemia due to the V/Q mismatch. In such cases, primary emphasis should be placed on reversing the pathophysiologic cause of the V/Q mismatch (eg, positive end-expiratory pressure in ARDS or chest physiotherapy and bronchoscopy in lobar atelectasis to remove mucous plugs).

3. **Hypoventilation** occurs when the patient is either physically unable to breathe (eg, respiratory muscle dysfunction from cervical spine injury, amyotrophic lateral sclerosis, Guillain-Barré syndrome, phrenic nerve injury, myasthenia gravis) or unable to initiate breathing (eg, central sleep apnea, narcotic or benzodiazepine overdose, cerebrovascular accident, metabolic alkalosis). The $Paco_2$ is always elevated and the $(A-a)o_2$ difference is initially normal. Persistent hypoventilation results in significant atelectasis and increases the $(A-a)o_2$ difference. The hypoxemia of hypoventilation is typically not severe and is exquisitely sensitive to correction by supplemental O_2. Simultaneous efforts should be made to correct the cause of hypoventilation or institute artificial ventilation.

4. In the presence of underlying lung disease (V/Q mismatch or shunt), **a reduced mixed venous O_2 content (Cvo_2) can contribute to hypoxemia.** The contribution of the lower O_2 content of blood flowing through the shunt (or area of reduced ventilation) reduces the overall O_2 content of the blood mixing in the left atrium. A fall in Cvo_2 results when peripheral O_2 extraction is increased or in states of decreased O_2 delivery (congestive heart failure, cor pulmonale, shock, anemia). Under these circumstances, efforts to improve the Cvo_2 (eg, ↑ cardiac output, ↑ Hb) can improve oxygenation.

5. **Reductions in diffusion** do not often contribute to significant hypoxemia in clinical practice. Diffusion limitations can occur when the pulmonary capillary transit time is too rapid for adequate diffusion of O_2 from alveolus to capillary (severe interstitial lung disease, moderate interstitial disease during exercise, high cardiac output states). Supplemental O_2 at high concentration can significantly improve the Pao_2 by increasing the O_2 pressure gradient between the alveolus and the capillary.

6. **At high altitude, the FIO_2** is reduced, leading to a reduction in PAO_2 and hypoxemia. This may be problematic for individuals with worsening lung disease, living at high elevations, or traveling by air. The FIO_2 in pressurized cabins of commercial airline flights is equivalent to 5000–8000 feet. The normal physiologic response of hyperventilation modestly improves the PaO_2, but this response is ineffective in patients with severe COPD or neuromuscular disease. Supplemental O_2 increases the FIO_2 and reverses the hypoxemia.

C. **Analysis of hypoxemia.** Categorization and analysis of hypoxemia may be simplified by using the alveolar air equation:

$$PAO_2 = (P_B - P_{H2O}) \times FIO_2 - Paco_2/R$$

where P_AO_2 is the alveolar O_2, P_B is barometric pressure, P_{H2O} is water vapor pressure (usually 47 mm Hg), F_IO_2 is the inspired O_2 concentration, and R is the respiratory quotient (usually 0.8) to calculate the alveolar-arterial difference

$$(A\text{-}a)O_2 = PAO_2 - PaO_2$$

Assuming normal barometric pressure, FIO_2 of 21%, and R = 0.8, the alveolar air equation can be simplified from

$$(A\text{-}a)O_2 = (760 - 47) \times 0.21 - Paco_2/R$$

to

$$PAO_2 = 150 - Paco_2 \times 1.25$$

The physiologic $(A\text{-}a)O_2$ is <10 mm Hg in normal subjects. Increases in this difference are found with aging.

To calculate the $(A\text{-}a)O_2$ using arterial blood gases obtained in a patient breathing room air (measured arterial blood gas values were PaO_2 82 mm Hg and $PaCO_2$ 40 mm Hg):

$$PAO_2 = 150 - 40 \times 1.25$$

$$PAO_2 = 100$$

$$(A\text{-}a)O_2 = 100 - 82$$

$$(A\text{-}a)O_2 = 18$$

An increase in the $(A\text{-}a)O_2$ suggests the presence of parenchymal lung disease.

II. **Diagnosis and monitoring of hypoxemia.** The main consequence of hypoxemia is tissue hypoxia, usually manifested as organ dysfunction or metabolic acidosis. Tissue hypoxia is difficult to assess directly, and diagnostic efforts should focus on identifying hypoxemia. The physical examination is unreliable in predicting hypoxemia because cyanosis occurs only when the SaO_2 is <75% to 85% (2) Direct measurement of PO_2 by analysis of arterial blood gas or indirect measurement of SaO_2 by pulse oximetry may be used to diagnose hypoxemia. Initial or baseline arterial samples of oxygenation are necessary to determine the adequacy of ventilation ($PaCO_2$, pH) and renal compensation.

A. **Arterial blood gases**
1. Arterial blood may be sampled by intermittent puncture, using a heparinized syringe, or via an indwelling arterial line. (3) The most commonly used puncture sites are radial, brachial, and femoral arteries. The arterial puncture procedure is safe, and pain, paresthesias, and bruising are the major side effects.
2. A decrease in arterial pulse after puncture is common, but this usually resolves spontaneously. Although Allen's test (reperfusion with release of ulnar artery compression) is recommended to assess arterial blood flow prior to puncture, many patients with a positive test will have an uncomplicated radial artery puncture.
3. **Blood gas measurement errors** occur when too much heparin remains in the syringe and mixes with the sample (falsely ↓ $PaCO_2$), the sample is not promptly placed on ice (falsely ↓ PaO_2), or there is a very high peripheral white

blood cell count (falsely $\downarrow$ Pa_{O_2}, "leukocyte larceny"). Calculated Sa_{O_2} values are often provided when an arterial blood gas is obtained. Given the uncertainty of the position of the Hb-O_2 saturation curve, these estimations are inferior to directly measured Sa_{O_2}.

B. **Pulse oximetry** provides a noninvasive and continuous method for assessing Sa_{O_2}. In certain settings (eg, operating rooms, intensive care units, transporting critically ill patients, invasive diagnostic procedures), oximetry can identify unsuspected hypoxemia.

    1. The pulse oximeter consists of a light sensor and two diodes that emit light of 660-nm (red) and 940-nm (infrared) wavelengths. These wavelengths are differentially absorbed by oxygenated Hb (HbO_2) and reduced Hb; the Sa_{O_2} is determined by the ratio of HbO_2/Hb (4). Most transmitted light is absorbed by soft tissue, skin, bone, and venous and arterial blood. With each arterial pulse, an absorption peak can be detected that corresponds to the Sa_{O_2}.

    2. Skin pigmentation and thickness minimally affect accuracy of measurement. In contrast, ambient light sources (surgical, fluorescent, or heating lights), nail polish (especially green, black or blue), intravascular dyes and pigments (bilirubin, indocyanine green, methylene blue), motion artifact, severe anemia (Hb <5 g/dL), and poor distal perfusion with cool extremities can reduce accuracy (5). The latter effect can be minimized by warming the extremity, instituting a vasodilator (ie, nitroglycerin ointment), or using a probe designed for use on the nose or ear.

    3. The normal Sa_{O_2} ranges from 95% to 99%. The relationship between Sa_{O_2} and Pa_{O_2} is governed by the Hb-O_2 dissociation curve. When the Sa_{O_2} is between 50% and 90%, the relationship is roughly linear with the estimated Pa_{O_2} (mm Hg) = Sa_{O_2} − 30. Under extremes of pH, Pa_{CO_2}, temperature, and positional changes in the Hb-O_2 dissociation curve disrupt this relationship, and the Pa_{O_2} is best determined by direct measurement. With a Sa_{O_2} <50%, saturation falls disproportionately faster than Pa_{O_2}, and direct measurement of the latter is indicated to assess hypoxemia. Oximeters are generally valid within a range of ±4%. A measured value of 96% may indicate saturations ranging from 92% to 100%, reflecting a Pa_{O_2} of 60–150 mm Hg. Accuracy falls significantly when the Sa_{O_2} is <70%.

    4. With increased levels of carbon monoxide or carboxyhemoglobin (CO-Hb), the Sa_{O_2} will be overestimated because CO-Hb has similar light-absorptive characteristics to HbO_2. In contrast, methemoglobin (Met-Hb) has absorptive characteristics between HbO_2 and Hb, resulting in a saturation of around 85%. Using a four-wavelength co-oximeter to analyze the blood, the contributions of CO-Hb and Met-Hb can be directly measured and the true Sa_{O_2} determined.

III. **Normobaric O_2 therapy in the acute setting** Guidelines for initiating O_2 therapy in the acute setting include a specific indication with well documented evidence of hypoxemia (or significant risk for hypoxemia), prescription of a specific dosage (flow rate or concentration), and monitoring the response to therapy with subsequent dosage adjustments based on objective measurements. O_2 should never be administered without an written order by the physician; lack of an appropriate order and/or proper notation in the nursing Kardex and discrepancies between the ordered and delivered F_IO_2 are often found to occur in the acute setting (6). O_2 therapy must be instituted prior to documentation of hypoxemia when strong clinical evidence of tissue hypoxia exists (shock, severe respiratory distress, CO poisoning) (7). Subsequent documentation of the Pa_{O_2} is essential to allow for proper titration of the dose.

A. **Supplemental O_2 is indicated in acute medical conditions when the Pa_{O_2} <60 mm Hg or the Sa_{O_2} <90%.** This most commonly occurs in the setting of **acute myocardial infarction** and **acute pulmonary diseases** such as exacerbations of obstructive airways disease, pneumonia, pulmonary embolism, episodes of congestive heart failure, acute atelectasis, and hypoventilation after drug overdose or other central nervous system events. Concern for tissue hypoxia and resulting organ damage are paramount. With the exception of hypercapnic COPD exacerbations, initiation of therapy is usually best with a high FiO_2 of between 40% to 100% to assure adequate Pao_2, and then titrating downward utilizing objective measurements. Mechanical ventilation may be required if the Pao_2 fails to correct or if ventilation decreases significantly ($\uparrow Pco_2$).

1. **Acute myocardial infarction (MI).** The use of supplemental O_2 is mandated in the setting of complicated MI with hypoxemia, and the Pao_2 or Sao_2 should be used to guide therapy. Mild hypoxemia is frequently present during the early course of an uncomplicated MI, and therapeutic or prophylactic use of low-flow O_2 (eg, 2 L/min) should be routine. No randomized controlled data exist to suggest improved outcome with routine use of high F_iO_2 for uncomplicated MI. Vasodilators, such as nitrates and calcium channel blockers, are used commonly in the peri-MI period. These agents can inhibit hypoxic vasoconstriction and worsen V/Q mismatch and hypoxemia. If hypoxemia worsens in the presence of these medications, the FiO_2 should be increased while the vasodilator is either discontinued or the dose reduced.

2. When **Hb is abnormal or tissue O_2 delivery is inadequate**, tissue hypoxia can occur in the absence of hypoxemia, with the Pao_2 >60 mm Hg and the Sao_2 >90% (normoxic hypoxia). Supplemental O_2 may marginally improve O_2 delivery.

   a. **Carboxyhemoglobinemia** produces tissue hypoxia for several reasons: a leftward shift in the Hb-O_2 dissociation curve, the inability of CO-Hb to bind and carry O_2, and a direct toxic effect of CO on the mitochondria. Administration of 100% O_2 decreases the half-life of CO-Hb from 320 minutes to 60 minutes and is the treatment of choice, unless hyperbaric O_2 is available. Use of hyperbaric O_2 can further reduce the half-life to 20–25 minutes. O_2 therapy independently increases O_2 delivery by increasing the amount of O_2 dissolved in blood.

   b. **Methemoglobinemia** produces tissue hypoxia because HbO_2 is decreased due to the exposures to nitrites/nitrates (nitroprusside), sulfa drugs, lidocaine or procaine, chlorate, phenacetin, or other drugs or toxins. The treatment is administration of 100% O_2 while the cause of methemoglobinemia is reversed.

   c. **Sickle cell crisis** produces tissue hypoxia because of sickling of erythrocytes in the peripheral circulation. Extreme sickling results in ischemia and pain. Although the clinical response to supplemental O_2 is variable, initial therapy with 100% O_2 is indicated while other therapies (eg, narcotics, hydration, exchange transfusion) are initiated.

   d. **A normal maternal Pao_2 of 60–65 mm Hg during pregnancy** is not associated with significant decreases in fetal oxygenation. However, concomitant reductions in the O_2 content of uterine artery blood because of low Hb or reduced cardiac output (reduced uterine artery flow) will result in diminished O_2 delivery to the fetus. Under these circumstances, supplemental O_2 should be given until the underlying cause for reduced O_2 delivery is diagnosed and treated.

   e. Anemia and reduced cardiac output during shock reduce O_2 delivery and require supplemental O_2. 100% O_2 should be administered to increase the O_2 content of arterial blood by about 10% in conditions with reduced cardiac output and by 25% to 30% in severe anemic states.

B. **Supplemental O_2 therapy is indicated in situations where hypoxemia is likely to occur.**

   1. **Postoperative supplemental O_2. General anesthesia**, by reducing functional residual capacity (FRC) and increasing V/Q mismatch, may lead to transient hypoxemia in the immediate postoperative setting. Thoracic and abdominal (especially upper abdominal) surgery results in atelectasis at the lung bases and reductions in FRC leading to V/Q mismatch and physiologic shunt. These effects are particularly important in obese, elderly smokers and in individuals with pulmonary disease; they may last for up to 1 week postoperatively. Treatment consists of low-flow O_2 therapy combined with lung expansion maneuvers (ie, incentive spirometry) and early ambulation. For nonabdominal/nonthoracic procedures in otherwise young and healthy subjects, O_2 therapy can

be stopped quickly. The more proximal the surgery is to the diaphragm, the greater is the chance of postoperative hypoxemia. The FiO_2 in all cases should be titrated through pulse oximetry monitoring.

2. Procedures using **conscious sedation** require supplemental O_2. Endoscopic procedures can result in hypoxemia because of sedative-related hypoventilation or through direct effects on V/Q matching. Hypoxemia frequently occurs during nonendoscopic procedures such as cardiac catheterization and coronary angioplasty. (8) Low-flow O_2 should be administered and titrated as above. Crash carts should be available in areas where conscious sedation is given in the event that emergent ventilatory support is required.

3. With a large or symptomatic **pneumothorax**, immediate aspiration of the thorax followed by tube thoracostomy is indicated. Smaller asymptomatic pneumothoraces can be treated by observation, and administration of supplemental 100% O_2 can create a pleural-to-arterial nitrogen gradient that increases the rate of pleural air absorption four times or more.

4. When sea-level dwellers rapidly ascend, a number of **high altitude disorders** may develop: acute mountain sickness (headache, lethargy, insomnia, nausea, dyspnea, fluid retention), high altitude cerebral edema (altered mental status, ataxia), and high altitude pulmonary edema. Although descent to a lower altitude constitutes definitive therapy, supplemental O_2 should be administered acutely. O_2 therapy may also be useful for chronic mountain sickness (headache, lethargy, dizziness, insomnia, cyanosis, polycythemia) when relocation to a lower altitude is not possible.

IV. **Chronic, outpatient, home (domiciliary) O_2 therapy**

A. **Long-term O_2 therapy should only be ordered for patients who have been on maximal medical therapy for at least 30 days prior to ordering O_2** (9). The HCFA considers O_2 to be durable medical equipment rather than a medication. HCFA requires physicians to complete a certification of medical necessity (HCFA Form 484), specifying the O_2 equipment and all elements of therapy. Documentation of the indication for O_2 and assessment of the response to therapy can be by arterial blood gas (preferred) or oximetry (performed by a qualified laboratory). O_2 should never be prescribed on an as-needed (prn) basis. (9)

1. The Nocturnal Oxygen Therapy Trial (NOTT) and the Medical Research Council (MRC) trial clearly demonstrated that continuous O_2 therapy has the best therapeutic effect in patients with COPD, with survival increasing in proportion to the number of hours per day that O_2 was administered. Thus, **continuous O_2 therapy is superior to nocturnal therapy, while both are better than no therapy.**

2. An O_2 prescription must specify the O_2 flow rate and number of hours per day O_2 will be given. The majority of patients will require ≤ 4 L/min to maintain a $Pao_2 \geq 55$ mm Hg.

3. Remember that the benefits deriving from the above recommendations have only clearly been demonstrated in patients with COPD; these data have been extended to imply similar benefits accruing to chronically hypoxemic patients with other pulmonary diseases.

B. The overwhelming majority of patients requiring long-term home O_2 (>30 days) have COPD (chronic bronchitis, emphysema), while substantially fewer have chronic interstitial lung disease (idiopathic pulmonary fibrosis), bronchiectasis (cystic fibrosis), or pulmonary vascular disease. The trend toward early hospital discharge has increased the number of patients with isolated acute pulmonary diseases such as pneumonia or pulmonary embolism who may require short-term (<30 days) home O_2 therapy.

1. Long-term O_2 therapy in hypoxemic patients with COPD improves survival and decreases hospitalization, although the mechanism remains unknown. NOTT compared 12 to 24 hours of O_2 and demonstrated a 50% reduction in mortality at 26 months (10). The MRC trial compared 15 hours with 0 hours of O_2 and demonstrated a reduction in mortality at 5 years (67% to 45%) (11).

2. In COPD, continuous O_2 therapy can lead to a modest yearly decrease in pulmonary artery pressures (11,12). Chronic (but not acute) therapy seems to im-

prove cardiac function at rest and with exercise (13,14). Acute therapy will reduce pulmonary artery pressures and resistance when hypoxic vasoconstriction is the principal pathogenetic mechanism. When pulmonary hypertension is due to permanent structural changes in the vasculature (primary pulmonary hypertension, scleroderma, interstitial lung diseases, emphysema) O_2 is of little benefit in decreasing the resting pulmonary artery pressure.

3. As hypoxemia worsens (Pao_2 <50 mm Hg), neuropsychiatric deficits develop in patients with COPD (15). Improvement in motor function, alertness, and general quality of life has been demonstrated with 6 months of continuous O_2 therapy (7,11).

4. Walking distance, exercise test performance, and endurance are also improved by O_2 therapy because more O_2 is delivered to the exercising and respiratory muscles, thereby improving ventilatory efficiency (minute ventilation per workload) and reducing perceived dyspnea. These benefits apply particularly to those with hypoxemic interstitial lung disease and COPD, where exercise leads to further desaturation (16–18).

5. **Improvement during sleep**
   a. In COPD and particularly in hypoxemic bronchitis, sleep is characterized by hypoventilation, increased V/Q mismatch, and rapid, shallow breathing, resulting in worsening hypercapnia and hypoxemia. Reductions in Sao_2 can occur during rapid-eye-movement (REM) sleep, even in the absence of true sleep apnea (19). With REM sleep, accessory and intercostal muscle activity decreases, placing the respiratory load on a diaphragm that may be dysfunctional secondary to hyperinflation. More than 25% of patients with COPD who are normoxic during the day demonstrate nocturnal hypoxemia, leading to pulmonary hypertension, cor pulmonale, cardiac arrhythmias, deteriorating sleep quality, and increased mortality (10,19,20). Supplemental O_2 at night prevents desaturation, blunts the rise in pulmonary pressures, improves hypersomnolence and morning headache, and may increase survival (21). If a sleep Pao_2 cannot be obtained in a patient with COPD on continuous O_2, the nocturnal flow rate should be empirically increased by 1 L/min above the resting continuous rate.
   b. Desaturation during sleep is less prominent with interstitial lung disease but frequently occurs with chest wall diseases (kyphoscoliosis) and neuromuscular diseases (muscular dystrophy) (22–24). In true obstructive sleep apnea, supplemental O_2 has a variable effect on the apnea but does increase the nadir desaturation; daytime hypersomnolence is not improved (25,26).

6. In COPD patients who stop smoking, long-term oxygen therapy reduces secondary **erythrocytosis**.

7. Supplemental O_2 decreases exercise-related dyspnea by improving respiratory muscle function, decreasing chemoreceptor activity, and reducing required minute ventilation (16,18). **Resting dyspnea**, in the absence of hypoxemia, is not improved by supplemental O_2.

C. **Indications for chronic O_2 therapy** The decision to prescribe O_2 depends on both the arterial blood gas (or Sao_2) and the clinical situation. Most patients with severe hypoxemia will have preexisting lung disease in addition to clinical and laboratory evidence of tissue hypoxia. Although the HCFA guidelines allow the Sao_2 to be used as a measure of hypoxemia, arterial blood gases should be used to document baseline hypoxemia for the reasons stated earlier. The medical therapy of the pathophysiologic mechanism responsible for hypoxemia should be optimized prior to the initiation of O_2 therapy. Patients should be educated about the proper use of O_2, especially since many have a tendency to use O_2 only during times of increased dyspnea. **O_2 delivered for <12 h/d has not been proven to be beneficial** (11,27).

1. **Resting ambulatory therapy. Continuous O_2** is indicated when the resting room-air Pao_2 is ≤55 mm Hg (Sao_2 ≤88%) or when the Pao_2 ≤59 mm Hg (Sao_2 ≤89 mm Hg) with P pulmonale noted on the electrocardiogram (P wave >3mm in leads II,III,aVF) in association with erythrocytosis (hematocrit >56%) or de-

pendent edema suggestive of cor pulmonale. When the $Pa_{O_2} \geq 60$ mm Hg or the $Sa_{O_2} >90\%$, O_2 can only be prescribed with compelling medical justification and documentation that other measures to improve function have failed.

2. **Therapy during exercise.** Noncontinuous O_2 can be given with exercise when dyspnea occurs with a $Pa_{O_2} \leq 55$ mm Hg or $Sa_{O_2} \leq 88$ mm Hg during minimal exertion. Studies in normoxic patients with COPD or interstitial lung disease indicated that exercise-related hypoxemia occurs primarily with a diffusing capacity of CO <50% to 60% of predicted values (28,29). Exercise testing with oximetry is recommended whenever hypoxemia is suspected as a contributing cause of exercise intolerance and dyspnea.

3. **Therapy during sleep.** Predicting which normoxic patients with underlying lung disease will desaturate during sleep has proven difficult. In the setting of pulmonary hypertension, daytime hypersomnolence, or cardiac arrhythmias, an overnight oximetry study should be performed and O_2 administered if the nocturnal $Pa_{O_2} \leq 55$ mm Hg or the $Sa_{O_2} \leq 88\%$. No firm evidence exists that O_2 therapy benefits patients with obstructive sleep apnea, and therefore it should be restricted to those patients who fail or cannot comply with other therapies such as continuous positive airway pressure. If O_2 is used, documentation of improvement with nocturnal O_2 therapy is mandatory.

V. **Special situations**

A. **Hyperbaric O_2 therapy** refers to the delivery of O_2 at pressures above sea level. About 300 chambers are available nationwide (30).

   1. **Physiology.** Hyperbaric O_2 therapy mechanically compresses gas so that more can be dissolved in blood. O_2-carrying capacity rises significantly with increasing Pa_{O_2} (at 3 atm, $Pa_{O_2} = 2000$ mm Hg) because of the substantial increase in dissolved O_2.

   2. Hyperbaric O_2 therapy is **indicated** for severe CO poisoning, decompression sickness, and air embolism. Additional indications include clostridial myonecrosis, necrotizing soft tissue infections, refractory osteomyelitis, acute traumatic crush injury, radiation tissue damage, thermal burns, anemia with extensive blood loss, and compromised wounds or skin grafts.

      a. **Decompression sickness** with manifestations ranging from extremity pain to cardiovascular collapse occurs during the ascent from diving, when nitrogen leaves tissues and forms intravascular bubbles. By using hyperbaric O_2 therapy at 3–6 atm, bubble size decreases and ischemia is reversed. Hyperbaric O_2 is also effective in treating the complications of high-altitude exposure when early descent is not possible.

      b. **Severe CO poisoning** occurs when the CO level is >25% and is manifested by unconsciousness, neuropsychiatric symptoms, and cardiac ischemia and arrhythmias. Hyperbaric O_2 therapy reduces the half-life of CO to 20 minutes from 5 hours at normobaric room air and 90 minutes at 100% O_2.

      c. **Systemic air embolism** can occur during diving, cardiopulmonary bypass, neurosurgery performed on a patient in the sitting position, dialysis, lung biopsy, central line insertion or maintenance, gynecologic procedures, thoracic trauma, or barotrauma due to mechanical ventilation. Arterial air embolic disease in the cerebral circulation produces the acute onset of central nervous system dysfunction including coma. Hyperbaric O_2 therapy (6 atm) can alleviate these manifestations by reducing air bubbles to ⅛th their original size.

   3. **Hyperbaric devices.** Multiplace units consist of large, walk-in chambers filled with compressed air that can accommodate up to 10–14 patients. O_2 is delivered via a tent, mask, or endotracheal tube. Monoplace units are small chambers filled with 100% O_2 and designed for use by a single supine patient.

   4. **Complications.** O_2 toxicity occurs more frequently when O_2 is delivered under hyperbaric conditions. At 2 atm, pulmonary toxicity can occur as early as 6 hours into therapy. Barotrauma occurs frequently, especially in air-filled cavities unable to equilibrate with the hyperbaric pressure (ie, sinuses, middle

ear). Pneumothorax or air embolism can occur in patients with underlying lung disease. At 3 atm, the risk of central nervous system toxicity with grand mal seizures is high.

B. Air travel is feasible for most patients with lung disease, including those with COPD. The minimal desired in-flight Pao_2 is ≥ 50 mm Hg. Commercial flights are pressurized to an altitude of approximately 5000–8000 feet, leading to a fall in P_AO_2 and subsequent hypoxemia. The normal physiologic response consists of hyperventilation, which moderately increases PAO_2 and improves the Pao_2 to 50–60 mm Hg. When the capacity for hyperventilation is impaired (respiratory muscle weakness, COPD), this compensatory mechanism is significantly limited. Sleep, sedation, anemia, and drying of secretions (due to the reduced humidity in the cabin) can further worsen hypoxemia by decreasing ventilation and increasing V/Q mismatch and the work of breathing (31).

1. No consensus exists on the criteria for supplemental O_2 during air travel. Estimated flight Pao_2 can be determined using hypoxic altitude simulation with hypobaric chambers or hypoxic gas breathing (patient breathes 15% O_2 to simulate the PAO_2 at 8000 feet).

2. Alternatively, regression equations have been developed for predicting the in-flight Pao_2 (32). In the absence of hypercapnia, a resting, sea-level Pao_2 ≥ 68 mm Hg indicates a 90% chance of a Pao_2 ≥ 55 mm Hg at 5,000 feet. If resting, sea-level Pao_2 is ≥ 72 mm Hg, 90% of patients will have a Pao_2 ≥ 50 mm Hg at 8,000 feet (33)

3. In hypercapnic patients, minute ventilation may not rise sufficiently to increase the Pao_2; additionally, supplemental O_2 may worsen the hypercapnia. These patients should avoid commercial air travel and use ground transportation or an air ambulance (31).

4. Patients already using supplemental O_2 should increase the flow rate by 1–2 L during the flight.

5. Commercial airlines require ≥ 48 hours advance notification of the patient's diagnosis and O_2 requirements (flow rate, duration, and whether intermittent or continuous). The latter can be estimated using the equation

$$FiO_2 \text{ (flight)} = FiO_2 \text{ (ground)} \times P_B \text{ (ground)} \div P_B \text{ (flight)}$$

Under most circumstances, a F_IO_2 of 30% should be adequate. The physician letter should include statements about the patient's fitness, stability, and safety for travel. The airline will provide the necessary equipment including masks and nasal cannula. Personalized equipment is prohibited on flights. The airline will not provide O_2 therapy for ground use at the patient's final destination (31).

VI. Monitoring of O_2 therapy is often inadequate (6,34). In one study, 20% of patients remained hypoxic after starting O_2 therapy because of inadequate monitoring and adjustment of liter flow (34) Under most circumstances, the goal of therapy is to increase the Pao_2 to a minimum of 60 mm Hg or the Sao_2 to 90%. Because of the shape of the O_2-Hb dissociation curve, further increases in Pao_2 lead to only small increments in O_2 delivery, while the risk of O_2 toxicity may rise substantially. Efforts to enhance O_2 delivery through optimizing Hb level and cardiac output may be more beneficial. Nevertheless, higher O_2 levels (Pao_2 ≥ 70 mm Hg, Sao_2 $\geq 94\%$) are often necessary in the setting of a myocardial infarction or evidence of organ dysfunction resulting from reduced O_2 delivery. Pulse oximetry is noninvasive and easily standardized and performed, and is therefore the modality of choice for monitoring O_2 delivery. **When the risk of worsening hypercapnia exists (hypercapnic COPD, neuromuscular disease, hypoventilation), arterial blood gas level should be obtained <60 minutes after any change in FiO_2.**

A. Inpatient monitoring of response to O_2. Although conclusive studies of the efficacy of oximetry monitoring are not available for medical inpatients, the following **general guidelines for inpatient monitoring** of patients with or at risk for hypoxemia are recommended.

1. **Continuous pulse oximetry** monitoring should be performed for patients who have (a) a critical or unstable airway or are (b) in intensive care units

(ICU), (c) unstable, (d) hypoxemic and undergoing treatment, (e) at risk for hypoxemia during hemodialysis, (f) intraoperative or in the immediate postoperative or postprocedure period, (g) mechanically ventilated, (h) at risk for hypoxemia and require inter- or intrahospital transport, (i) receiving conscious sedation while undergoing procedures associated with hypoxia or airway compromise (eg, bronchoscopy, gastrointestinal endoscopy, cardiac catheterization, liver or kidney biopsy). Continuous pulse oximetry should also be considered for patients in the following situations:

    a.   Admission to a regular ward with a history of previous hypoxemic respiratory failure (Pao_2 <60 mm Hg on room air).

    b.   Transferral from the ICU after treatment for respiratory failure or mechanical ventilation. (Exception: patients with stable Sao_2 for the previous 24 hours.)

    c.   Transferral to the ward after a procedure associated with hypoxemia or patients continuing to require conscious sedation.

    d.   **Continuous oximetry may be discontinued** if the Sao_2 has remained ≥90% or higher for 24 hours or for the duration specified by the ordering physician. Further intermittent monitoring is necessary for any subsequent changes in Fio_2 and discontinuation of O_2 as outlined below.

  2. **Intermittent (spot-check) oximetry** should be considered in the following situations:

    a.   Changes in the liter flow or concentration of O_2. Oximetry should be performed continuously for 1 hour and repeated 8 and 24 hours later.

    b.   Upon discontinuation of O_2 therapy, continuous oximetry should be performed for 1 hour and repeated 8 and 24 hours later.

    c.   For stable patients on continuous O_2 therapy, oximetry should be checked with the same frequency as the vital signs. When the Sao_2 is ≥90%, consideration should be given to reducing the Fio_2, using the oximeter to determine the optimal liter flow or concentration. O_2 should be titrated down by 1 L/min for nasal cannula or by 5% to 10% Fio_2 for masks, until the patient is able to breathe room air or the Sao_2 is <90%. A 20–30-minute stabilization period should be allowed between changes in the O_2 concentration and measurement of the Sao_2.

    d. O_2 requirements may increase with sleep and exercise, and patients on continuous O_2 should have oximetry performed at least once during these activities to assess the adequacy of therapy.

    e.   Patients on continuous home O_2 may not require oximetry monitoring when admitted to the hospital, if there is no change in the liter-flow rate. If the liter flow is changed or the reason for hospitalization involves a change in the cardiopulmonary status, oximetry monitoring should be considered according to the parameters discussed above.

B. **Monitoring O_2 requirements in outpatients**

  1. Approximately 95% of stable COPD patients will respond to 1–3 L/min O_2 (35). When higher flow rates are needed, the patient is probably not stable. Interstitial lung disease may require higher flow rates, especially during exertion. O_2 liter flow should be adjusted to achieve a Pao_2 ≥60 mm Hg or a Sao_2 ≥90%.

  2. Adjustments to liter flow in outpatients may be done using oximetry measurements. An arterial blood gas reading is always indicated when concern exists about concomitant hypercapnia. Oximetry is particular useful for monitoring the response to sleep or exercise.

  3. When home O_2 is prescribed after recovery from an acute illness, O_2 requirements should be reassessed at 1 and 3 months because 30% to 45% of patients will no longer require O_2 (35,36). This is not necessary when long-term O_2 therapy either has been started in a stable outpatient setting or had already been prescribed prior to the acute illness. Reassessment should occur every 6 months thereafter to assure a continued adequate response. An initial Pao_2 <40 mm Hg in a stable patient suggests that subsequent blood gases will not demonstrate sufficient improvement to allow for discontinuation of therapy.

VII. Complications of O_2 therapy

  A. O_2 toxicity. With the exception of hyperoxia-induced damage to retinal blood vessels in neonates (retrolental fibroplasia), O_2 toxicity in the lung is primarily manifested by injury to the alveolar endothelial cells with a loss of type I cells and proliferation of type II cells. Although O_2 toxicity is experimentally related to dose and duration of exposure, limited data in humans preclude offering definite guidelines on either the range of safe FIO_2 or the optimal duration of treatment. In general, a FIO_2 of 100% appears to be safe for 6 hours for normal lungs, while a FIO_2 >60% appears safe for 1–2 days and a FIO_2 <50% is safe for at least 2–7 days. Higher concentrations and longer durations seem to be better tolerated in acutely inflamed lungs; that is, acutely injured lungs appear to develop O_2 toxicity after longer exposures and higher concentrations of O_2 than normal lungs. However, a good general rule is always to use the lowest possible FIO_2, preferably <60%. **Because of the limited ability to noninvasively deliver high FIO_2, O_2 toxicity is principally an issue for patients on mechanical ventilation.**

   1. O_2 toxicity can take several forms. After about 6–24 hours of 100% O_2, a tracheitis with a reduction in mucociliary transport can occur, often manifested as chest pain. After 24 hours of 100% O_2, vital capacity falls as a result of nitrogen washout (**absorption atelectasis**). After 24–48 hours of 100% O_2 (or >3 days of 60% to 100%), an acute lung injury can occur that is indistinguishable from ARDS, with damage to alveolar type 1 cells and endothelium, as well as edema, inflammation, and hyaline membrane formation (exudative phase).

   2. Worsening hypoxemia, the development of shunts and infiltrates, and decreased compliance are the physiologic correlates of this pathology. A fibroproliferative phase ensues, followed by an irreversible fibrotic phase. Bronchopulmonary dysplasia, well described in neonates, may occur in adults. Unfortunately, no reliable methods can detect early O_2 toxicity. No effective therapy is available other than utilizing the lowest FIO_2 possible (37). Outpatients receiving O_2 rarely develop toxicity because of the low flows and concentrations used.

  B. O_2-induced hypercapnia. In the absence of hypercapnia, the risk of supplemental O_2 producing a significant rise in $Paco_2$ is minimal. With severe **COPD** and associated chronic hypercapnia, significant increases in $Paco_2$ can occur with administration of supplemental O_2. The mechanism of O_2-induced hypercapnia is primarily V/Q mismatch from relief of hypoxic vasoconstriction rather than suppression of hypoxic ventilatory drive (38). This risk can be minimized with carefully titrated low-flow O_2 to produce a Pao_2 of 60 mm Hg. When >2 L/min via nasal cannula are necessary, use of a Venturi mask limits the maximal FIO_2 delivered. The $Paco_2$ will generally rise in the first few hours of O_2 therapy, and close monitoring with arterial blood gases should be frequent over this time. A late rise in $Paco_2$ will occasionally occur, and therefore 6- and 12-hour arterial blood gas readings should also be performed. The life- and organ-threatening consequences of tissue hypoxia mandate that the correction of hypoxemia supersedes concerns over O_2-induced hypercapnia. The latter can be treated by invasive or noninvasive ventilatory support as necessary. The incidence of significant CO_2 retention among stable outpatients with COPD is far less than in acutely ill patients. In stable hypercapnic COPD, nocturnal O_2 does not significantly increase $Paco_2$ (39). With coexisting obstructive sleep apnea, significant increases in $Paco_2$ can occur, and careful monitoring is required (40).

  C. Neuromuscular disease with diaphragm dysfunction. Low-flow O_2 (0.5–2 L) can lead to profound increases in $Paco_2$ (mean, 28 Torr) and the need for emergent assisted ventilation in patients with preexisting hypercapnia who develop neuromuscular disease and diaphragm dysfunction. With nocturnal assisted ventilation to rest the diaphragm and other respiratory muscles, daytime supplemental O_2 will not produce significant $Paco_2$ increases (32).

  D. Local complications and physical risks

   1. **Airway drying.** At high flow rates (>4 L/min) humidification is mandatory to prevent desiccation of the nasal mucosa with resultant epistaxis and pain.

2. **Skin irritation.** Nasal prongs can irritate the nasal mucosa. The tubing can be wrapped with gauze dressing at contact points to prevent the dermatitis that is sometimes seen on the cheeks and ears. With masks, pressure injury can occur at the bridge of the nose. Gas flow escaping from the mask can also desiccate the ophthalmic mucosa.

3. **Airway irritation** can occur at high flow rates, leading to substernal chest pain, bronchospasm, and otalgia.

4. Face masks (especially tight-fitting continuous positive airway pressure masks) may increase the risk of **aspiration and airway obstruction** when a patient vomits. To protect the airway, eating should never be allowed while the mask is in place.

5. **Rebreathing.** Exhaled gas contains variable amounts of CO_2 that may be present within the face mask at the onset of the next inspiration. If insufficient flow exists to wash this out, the CO_2 will be rebreathed and cause an increase in dead space.

6. **Smoking for outpatients while receiving O_2 is absolutely prohibited because of the risk of fire.**

7. Transtracheal O_2 can be complicated by surgical emphysema, cellulitis, hoarseness, minor hemoptysis, catheter infection, increased cough, dislodgment of the catheter, and mucous plugging that obstructs airways.

8. **Drug interactions.** High concentrations of O_2 can precipitate lung injury in patients who have previously received bleomycin or been exposed to the herbicide paraquat. Under these circumstances, low-flow O_2 or the use of the Venturi mask to regulate the maximum FiO_2 delivered is recommended.

VIII. **O_2 supply and delivery systems**

A. **Supply systems**

1. **Stationary systems. The O_2 concentrator** uses a molecular sieve or polymeric membrane to remove nitrogen and water vapor from room air. The former can yield 85% to 90% O_2 at 1–4 L/min, while the latter provides 30% to 40% O_2 at 1–10 L/min. The concentrator is bulky and not very portable. Long tubing is used to allow the patient some mobility at home. A backup cylinder is required in case of power failure.

2. **Portable systems. H and K stationary metal cylinders** are large reservoir tanks that contain compressed gas at high pressure, capable of lasting 2–3 days running at 2 L/min. **D and E cylinders** are smaller containers that last for 3–5 hours at 2 L/min. Although cylinder weight exceeds 10 lb, these devices can be made portable by placing them on a stroller.

3. **Ambulatory systems. Liquid O_2** can be dispensed from a large cylinder (4–10 day supply at 2 L/min) to a smaller unit (Dewar flask) weighing <10 lb. This lightweight thermos-like device can be carried over a shoulder and allows increased patient mobility (up to 8 hours at 2 L/min).

B. **O_2 Delivery systems.** Careful consideration should be given to choosing the optimal device for delivering O_2. Selection of a particular system depends on patient comfort and the desired F_iO_2. Education about O_2 and the delivery system is critical, as approximately 50% of inpatients are noncompliant with therapy (eg, mask worn improperly or removed completely, flow meter inappropriately turned off) (6,34). With many delivery systems, the FiO_2 can only be estimated and may vary considerably.

1. **Delivered FiO_2 depends on the mix of 100% O_2 from the source and the amount of room air (FiO_2 = 21%) entrained.** The liter-flow rate from the O_2 source is determined by the O_2 regulator and can be measured with a flow meter and inspiratory reservoirs. The liter-flow rate of entrained room air is a function of the minute ventilation, inspiratory flow rate, and pattern of breathing. The final FiO_2 is determined by the relative proportion of each.

2. Delivery systems have been categorized as either **low-flow systems**, which entrain room air and low flow from an exogenous O_2 source to meet the volume and flow demands of the patient and maintain the Pao_2 >60 mm Hg, or **high flow systems** for situations in which needs can be met only with high-flow-rate devices and reservoirs.

a. **Low-flow delivery systems** are popular, inexpensive, readily accepted by patients, and well tolerated. The continuous O_2 flow is always less than the demand requirements, and therefore room air is entrained to make up the difference. When patients have a regular ventilatory pattern, these systems provide a FIO_2 that can be estimated (Table 35-3). When the breathing pattern is abnormal, variable amounts of room air are entrained, and the FIO_2 (for a given flow rate) may vary. With a rapid and deep breathing pattern, the FIO_2 will be low. In contrast, the FIO_2 will be high with a slow and shallow breathing pattern.

   i. **Nasal cannulas** are the least expensive, most convenient, and most commonly used means of delivering O_2. Nasal cannulas are comfortable and allow the patient to talk and eat. O_2 is delivered by polyethylene or plastic prongs at a rate of 1–6 L/min (controlled by a flow regulator and displayed on the flow meter), achieving a FIO_2 of 22% to 40%. As long as the nares are patent, efficacy is maintained for both oral and nasal breathing (41). There is no difference whether O_2 is delivered to one or both nares simultaneously, since the nasopharynx serves as a small O_2 reservoir (42). Because 70% of the respiratory cycle is expiratory, much of the delivered O_2 is wasted. Although both minute ventilation and inspiratory flow rate influence FIO_2, the FIO_2 increases about 3% to 4% per liter delivered as long as the breathing pattern is normal (see Table 35-3). The FIO_2 will not significantly increase when flows >6 L/min are used. Humidification is needed at flow rates >3 L/min (43).

   ii. **Simple face masks** with flow rates of 6–8 L/min are able to deliver a FIO_2 as high as 60% because the effective reservoir is increased by 100–200 mL. Large variations in FIO_2 occur as room air is entrained through holes in the mask or at its edges when the mask fits poorly. Flow rates >5 L/min are needed to wash out exhaled gas from the reservoir and prevent an increase in the dead space by the rebreathing of CO_2. In contrast to nasal cannulas, the mask must be removed for eating, drinking, expectoration, and effective communication.

   iii. **Partial rebreathing and nonrebreathing (reservoir) masks** employ a large (1000 mL) bag reservoir and high liter flow (>6 L/min) to deliver a FIO_2 in the 60% to 90% range. The bag fills with the first one-third of exhaled gas (containing minimal CO_2, high FIO_2) with the remainder exhaled through side ports of the mask. With the next breath, fresh gas from the wall is supplemented by gas from the reservoir. If the bag deflates completely during inspiration, insufficient gas will be available on the next breath, leading to the entrainment of room air and a reduction in delivered FIO_2. Conversely, if

Table 35-3. Estimated FIO_2 with various low-flow delivery systems

Device	Oxygen flow rate (L/min)	Estimated FIO_2
Nasal prongs	1	24
	2	28
	3	32
	4	36
	5	40
	6	44
Standard mask	6–8	40–60
Mask with reservoir bag	6–10	60–90

Note: The inspired oxygen concentration (FIO_2) may be lower or higher depending on the patient's minute ventilation, inspiratory flow rate, and pattern of breathing.

the reservoir remains completely filled during inspiration and expiration, the mask is probably loose and room air is entrained. The nonrebreathing mask has one-way valves that divert exhaled gas away from the reservoir, which is filled with 100% O_2 from the wall source. As with simple masks, the FiO_2 may vary with the patient's inspiratory flow rate and minute ventilation, and improper fitting reduces the delivered FiO_2 by allowing the entrainment of room air.

iv. **Shovel masks** are open, loose-fitting devices that may be more acceptable to patients with claustrophobia. Although high liter flows can be used, the FiO_2 is quite variable because of the large and variable volumes of entrained room air.

v. **Combination systems** use more than one modality, such as a nasal cannula and a nonrebreathing mask, to increase the delivered FiO_2 and provide some backup when the patient temporarily removes the mask to talk, eat, or expectorate.

b. **High-flow delivery systems** are more expensive and less well tolerated than low-flow systems. By employing high flow rates (often delivered by gas blenders with flows >100 L/min) and an inspiratory reservoir, higher and more reliable FiO_2 levels can be achieved (44). The delivered flow rate nearly always exceeds the patient's inspiratory demand. High-flow masks are bulkier and less comfortable than those used in low-flow systems and can become dislodged during sleep (45). When the high flow rate is generated with O_2 rather than room air, an O_2 bubble humidification system is needed.

i. **Venturi masks** take advantage of the Bernoulli principle to deliver high gas flows. The FiO_2 is regulated by adjusting the O_2 flow rate (3–15 L/min) and the size of ports in the mask (Ventimask) or tubing (Hudson mask) to adjust the amount of room air entrained. FiO_2 levels of 24%, 26%, 28%, 30%, 35%, 40%, and 50% can be accurately produced. These masks deliver reliable levels of FiO_2 and are particularly useful when hyperoxia must be avoided. Although the minimum FiO_2 may still vary, the high total-flow rate (exceeding patient demand) serves to reduce the need for additional entrainment of room air. Ventimasks are color-coded by flow rate. The Hudson mask requires adjustment of the size of the O_2 jet hole and flow rate. Entrainment of large volumes of moist room air may obviate the need to add humidification. At higher FiO_2 settings, total delivered flow may fall below the demands of the patient, with subsequent unregulated entrainment of room air and decrease in FiO_2. The principal use for the Venturi mask is in hypercapnic COPD, in which hyperoxia can be complicated by worsening hypercapnia and precise levels of FiO_2 must be delivered.

ii. **Continuous positive airway pressure masks** can yield a FiO_2 that approaches 100% by employing a tight-fitting nasal or full-face mask. These devices are confining and preclude eating, talking, or expectorating. An awake and cooperative patient is required to rapidly remove the mask if vomiting occurs.

iii. **Intubation and mechanical ventilation** via an artificial airway into the trachea allow accurate O_2 delivery with concentrations up to 100%. The delivery of large tidal volumes and positive end-expiratory pressure can independently raise PaO_2 by reversing the cause of hypoxemia, such as shunt or hypoventilation. By reducing respiratory muscle O_2 consumption, mechanical ventilation improves oxygenation by elevating the mixed venous O_2 content. A nonventilated patient with a tracheostomy can have a collar placed over the tube or a T tube directly connected to ensure high FiO_2.

c. **O_2-conservation systems.** In COPD, the majority of patients require only low-flow O_2 (1–3 L/min), and therefore nasal cannulas are used. The

O_2 requirements for patients with interstitial lung disease can be greater, and a face-mask system may be needed to deliver the higher flow rates. Several approaches have been taken to maintain Sao_2 at a reduced O_2 flow rate and therefore decrease costs and enhance patient utility. Proper use of these O_2-conservation systems requires consultation with a pulmonary physician and a respiratory therapist.

   i. **Reservoir systems.** The addition of a small reservoir to the nasal cannula system can deliver an early inspiratory O_2 bolus and allow the flow rate to be decreased by about 50%. The reservoir can cover the face in a mustache distribution or hang over the chest like a pendant.

   ii. **Electronic demand systems.** These devices have an electronic solenoid valve that provides a short pulse of O_2 early in inspiration, thus conserving wasted O_2 flow during expiration.

   iii. **Transtracheal O_2** When the necessary FiO_2 is very high or cosmetic concerns are limiting compliance with nasal cannula or masks, O_2 can be delivered through a small flexible catheter percutaneously placed between the second and third tracheal rings. The transtracheal catheter procedure, performed under local anesthesia by a pulmonary physician or an otolaryngologist, is reasonably safe and well tolerated. O_2 is delivered directly into the trachea, bypassing some of the dead space of the upper airway and using the trachea as a reservoir. Documented benefits include improved compliance, improved cosmetics (the catheter can be concealed under a scarf or shirt), lack of irritation to the nose, increased stability during exercise and sleep, decreased O_2 flow needs at rest and during exercise, fewer hospitalizations, and decreased work of breathing (46,47).

References

1. Anthonisen NR: Hypoxemia and O_2 therapy. *Am Rev Respir Dis* 1982;124:729–733.
2. Nicholson D: Cyanosis: five grams of history. *Respir Care* 1987;32:113–114.
3. Tobin MJ: Respiratory monitoring. *JAMA* 1990;264:244–251.
4. Schnapp LM, Cohen NH: Pulse oximetry: uses and abuses. *Chest* 1990;98:1244–1250.
5. Ralston AC, Webb RK, Runciman WB: Potential errors in pulse oximetry: effects of interference, dyes, dyshaemoglobins and other pigments. *Anaesthesia* 1991;46:291–295.
6. Small D, Duha A, Wieskopf B, et al.: Uses and misuses of oxygen in hospitalized patients. *Am J Med* 1992;92:591–595.
7. Fulmer JD, Snider GL: American College of Chest Physicians (ACCP)/National Heart, Lung and Blood Institute (NHLBI) conference on oxygen therapy. *Arch Intern Med* 1984;144:1645–1655.
8. Amar D, Greenberg MA, Menegus MA, Breitbart S: Should all patients undergoing cardiac catheterization or percutaneous transluminal coronary angioplasty receive oxygen? *Chest* 1994;105:727–732.
9. O'Donohue WJ: Prescribing home oxygen therapy: what the primary care physician needs to know. *Arch Intern Med* 1992;152:746–748.
10. Fletcher EC, Miller J, Divine GW, Fletcher JG, Miller T: Nocturnal oxyhemoglobin desaturation in COPD patients with arterial oxygen tensions above 60 mm Hg. *Chest* 1987;92:604–608.
11. Nocturnal Oxygen Therapy Trial Group: Continuous or nocturnal oxygen therapy in hypoxemic chronic obstructive lung disease. *Ann Intern Med* 1980;93:391–398.
12. Weitzenblum E, Sautegeau A, Ehrhart M, Mammosser M, Pelletier A: Long-term oxygen therapy can reverse the progression of pulmonary hypertension in patients with chronic obstructive pulmonary disease. *Am Rev Respir Dis* 1985;131:493–498.
13. MacNee W, Wathen CG, Flenley DC, Muir AD: The effects of controlled oxygen therapy on ventricular function in patients with stable and decompensated cor pulmonale. *Am Rev Respir Dis* 1988;137:1289–1295.
14. Timms RM, Khaja FU, Williams GW: Hemodynamic response to oxygen therapy in chronic obstructive pulmonary disease. *Ann Intern Med* 1985;102:29–36.

15. Heaton RK, Grant I, McSweeny AJ, Adams KM, Petty TL: Psychologic effects of continuous and nocturnal oxygen therapy in hypoxemic chronic obstructive pulmonary disease. *Arch Intern Med* 1983;143:1941–1947.
16. Dean NC, Brown JK, Himelman RB, et al.: Oxygen may improve dyspnea and endurance in patients with chronic obstructive pulmonary disease and only mild hypoxemia. *Am Rev Respir Dis* 1992;146:941–945.
17. Harris-Eze AO, Sridhar G, Clemens RE, Gallagher CG, Marciniuk DD: Oxygen improves maximal exercise performance in interstitial lung disease. *Am J Respir Crit Care Med* 1994;150:1616–1622.
18. Bye PTP, Anderson SD, Woolcock AJ, Young IH, Alison JA: Bicycle endurance performance of patients with interstitial lung disease breathing air and oxygen. *Am Rev Respir Dis* 1982;126:1005–1012.
19. Fleetham JA, Mezon B, West P, et al.: Chemical control of ventilation and sleep arterial oxygen desaturation in patients with COPD. *Am Rev Respir Dis* 1980;122:583–589.
20. Hagarty EM, Skorodin MS, Stiers WM, et al.: Performance of a reservoir nasal cannula (Oxymizer) during sleep in hypoxemic patients with COPD. *Chest* 1993;103:1129–1134.
21. Fletcher EC, Luckett RA, Goodnight-White S, et al.: A double-blind trial of nocturnal supplemental oxygen for sleep desaturation in patients with chronic obstructive pulmonary disease and a daytime PaO_2 above 60 torr. *Am Rev Respir Dis* 1992;145:1070–1076.
22. Donner CF, Braghiroli A, Ioli F, Zaccaria S: Long-term oxygen therapy in patients with diagnoses other than COPD. *Lung* 1990;168(suppl):776–781.
23. Sawicka EH, Branthwaite MA: Respiration during sleep in kyphoscoliosis. *Thorax* 1987;42:801–808.
24. Smith PEM, Calverley PMA, Edwards RHT: Hypoxemia during sleep in Duchenne muscular dystrophy. *Am Rev Respir Dis* 1988;137:884–888.
25. Gold AR, Schwartz AR, Bleecker ER, Smith PL: The effect of chronic nocturnal oxygen administration upon sleep apnea. *Am Rev Respir Dis* 1986;134:925–929.
26. Fletcher EC, Munafo DA: Role of nocturnal oxygen therapy in obstructive sleep apnea. *Chest* 1990;98:1497–1504.
27. Medical Research Council Working Party: Long-term domiciliary oxygen therapy in chronic hypoxic cor pulmonale complicating chronic bronchitis and emphysema. *Lancet* 1981;i:681–686.
28. Kelley MA, Panettieri RA, Krupinski AV: Resting single-breath diffusing capacity as a screening test for exercise-induced hypoxemia. *Am J Med* 1986;80:807–812.
29. Owens GR, et al.: The diffusing capacity as a predictor of arterial oxygen desaturation during exercise in patients with chronic obstructive pulmonary disease. *N Engl J Med* 1984;310:1218–1221.
30. Grim PS, Gottlieb LJ, Boddie A, Batson E: Hyperbaric oxygen therapy. *JAMA* 1990;263:2216–2220.
31. Gong H: Air travel and oxygen therapy in cardiopulmonary patients. *Chest* 1992;101:1104–1113.
32. Gay PC, Edmonds LC: Severe hypercapnia after low-flow oxygen therapy in patients with neuromuscular disease and diaphragmatic dysfunction. *Mayo Clin Proc* 1995;70:327–330.
33. Gong H Jr, Tashkin DP, Lee EY, Simmons MS: Hypoxia-altitude simulation test: evaluation of patients with chronic airway obstruction. *Am Rev Respir Dis* 1984;130:980–986.
34. Albin RJ, Criner GJ, Thomas S, Abou-Jaoude S: Pattern of non-ICU inpatient supplemental oxygen utilization in a university hospital. *Chest* 1992;102:1672–1675.
35. Timms RM, Kvale PA, Anthonisen NR, et al.: Selection of patients with chronic obstructive pulmonary disease for long-term oxygen therapy. *JAMA* 1981;245:2514–2515.
36. Levi-Valensi P, Weitzblum E, Pedinielli JL, Racineux JL, Duwoos H: Three-month follow-up of arterial blood gas determinations in candidates for long-term oxygen therapy. *Am Rev Respir Dis* 1986;133:547–551.
37. Denke SM, Fanburg BL: Normobaric oxygen toxicity of the lung. *N Engl J Med* 1980;303:76–86.
38. Sassoon CS, Hassell KT, Mahutte CK: Hyperoxic-induced hypercapnia in stable chronic obstructive pulmonary disease. *Am Rev Respir Dis* 1987;135:907–911.
39. Goldstein RS, Ramcharan V, Bowes G, et al.: Effect of supplemental nocturnal oxygen on gas exchange in patients with severe obstructive lung disease. *N Engl J Med* 1984;310:425–429.
40. Guilleminault C, Cummiskey J, Motta J: Chronic obstructive airflow disease and sleep studies. *Am Rev Respir Dis* 1980;122:397–406.
41. Gould GA, Forsyth IS, Flenley DC: Comparison of two oxygen-conserving nasal prong systems and the effects of nose and mouth breathing. *Thorax* 1986;41:808–809.

42. Petty TL, Nett CM, Lakshminarayan S: A single nasal prong for continuous oxygen therapy. *Respir Care* 1973;18:421–423.
43. Evans TW, Waterhouse J, Howard P: Clinical experience with the oxygen concentrator. *BMJ* 1983;287:459–461.
44. Banzuaye EA, et al.: Variability of inspired oxygen concentration with nasal cannulae. *Thorax* 1992;47:609–611.
45. Costello RW, Liston R, McNicholas WT: Compliance at night with low-flow oxygen therapy: a comparison of nasal cannulae and Venturi face masks. *Thorax* 1995;50:405–406.
46. Christopher KL, Spofford BT, Petrun MD, et al.: A program for transtracheal oxygen delivery. *Ann Intern Med* 1987;107:802–808.
47. Walsh GL, Morice RC, Putnam JB Jr,et al.: Resection of lung cancer is justified in high-risk patients selected by exercise oxygen consumption. *Ann Thorac Surg* 1994;58:704–711.

36   Home Care of the Respiratory Patient

Donna M. Poyant

I. Home oxygen
A. Diagnosis
1. An accurate cardiopulmonary diagnosis is required when a request for home oxygen (O_2) therapy is made. The most common pulmonary conditions that may require long-term O_2 therapy (LTOT) in the home or extended care facility are:
   a. Chronic obstructive pulmonary disease.
   b. Diffuse interstitial lung disease.
   c. Cystic fibrosis.
   d. Bronchiectasis.
   e. Pulmonary neoplasm.
2. Patients with the following medical illnesses may also be appropriate candidates for LTOT because of hypoxia-related symptoms:
   a. Pulmonary hypertension.
   b. Recurring congestive heart failure secondary to chronic cor pulmonale.
   c. Erythrocytosis/erythrocythemia.

B. The benefits of LTOT for the hypoxemic patient include improvements in survival, pulmonary hemodynamics, exercise capacity, and neuropsychologic performance (1–3).

C. Indications for LTOT (Table 36-1)
1. **Indications for continuous LTOT**
   a. Pao_2 ≤55 mm Hg measured at rest in the nonrecumbent position (1–6).
   b. Pao_2 56–59 mm Hg with evidence of organ dysfunction (secondary pulmonary hypertension, cor pulmonale, secondary erythrocytosis, central nervous system dysfunction) attributable to hypoxia (1–6).
2. **Indications for nocturnal LTOT**
   a. Pao_2 ≤55 mm Hg (or arterial blood oxygen saturation [Sao_2] ≤88%) during sleep, associated with organ dysfunction attributable to hypoxia (1–6).
3. **Indications for excercise LTOT**
   a. Pao_2 ≤55 mm Hg (or Sao_2 ≤88%) during exercise, with O_2 significantly improving objectively measured exercise capacity (1–6).

D. Problems associated with LTOT and their solution
1. **Unresolved hypoxemia**
   a. This is generally caused by inadequate O_2 supplementation. Hypoxemia should be documented with arterial blood gas measurements or by oximetry while the patient is breathing O_2 at the prescribed concentration or flow using the prescribed delivery system and/or source. If the degree of O_2 supplementation is insufficient, the flow rate and/or concentration may be increased. The mode by which the O_2 is delivered may also need to be changed (4,6).
   b. Poor compliance with O_2 prescription may be solved by patient education (4,6).
2. **Carbon dioxide (CO_2) narcosis.** Caused by reduced hypoxic ventilatory drive in response to an excessive flow rate or high concentration of O_2, CO_2 narcosis should be documented by arterial blood gas determinations; oxime-

Table 36-1. Indications and requirements for oxygen therapy

Clinical data	Oxygen requirement
Room-air resting Pao_2 ≤55 mm Hg	Continuous oxygen
Room-air resting Pao_2 56–59 mm Hg with signs of hypoxic organ dysfunction	Continuous oxygen
Room-air resting Pao_2 ≥56 mm Hg without signs of hypoxic organ dysfunction	Oxygen not required at rest
Room-air Sao_2 ≤88% during sleep with signs of hypoxic organ dysfunction	Oxygen during sleep
Room-air Sao_2 ≤88% with exercise in which oxygen significantly improves exercise capacity	Oxygen during exercise

try is not adequate because Pco_2 is not measured. An indwelling arterial line should be placed, and repeated Po_2 and Pco_2 measurements should be made while increasing amounts of O_2 are breathed. O_2 therapy should utilize the highest fraction of inspired oxygen (Fio_2) required to eliminate hypoxemia that does not result in CO_2 retention (4,6).

3. **Excessive costs**
   a. The use of **inappropriately high flow rates** that exceed the needs of the patient will result in excessive costs. Arterial blood gas and oximetry assessments should be performed to determine the lowest Fio_2 required to eliminate hypoxemia.
   b. **Inappropriate compliance** with a correctly written prescription resulting in indiscriminate increases in flow rate or Fio_2 will also result in higher than necessary costs. This problem can be reduced by patient education (4,6).
   c. **Improper selection of an O_2 delivery system** will generate excessive costs. The least expensive delivery method and source that meets the patient's needs should be used. O_2 concentrators should be used as first-line delivery systems, unless special circumstances pertain (eg, a highly mobile patient, noise or space concerns).

4. **Fire. O_2 supports combustion.** Patients should be instructed never to smoke in the presence of O_2. Those who continue to smoke in the presence of O_2 should be advised to always remove nasal cannulas while smoking. Signs warning of O_2 use and of potential fire hazard should be posted. All frayed electrical wiring should be replaced, and all electrical equipment in the immediate vicinity of O_2 use should be grounded. No petroleum-based products such as Vaseline should be used in the presence of O_2. Only water-soluble lubricants should be used. Liquid O_2 should be stored in a cool and well ventilated space (4,6).

5. **Nasal problems**
   a. Nasal irritation, dryness, occasional epistaxis, sore throat, rhinitis, and sinusitis are common symptoms due to insufficient humidification. O_2 can be humidified directly or commercial bedside vaporizers can be used to increase the amount of water vapor in the environment.
   b. Painful ulceration of the nares sometimes occurs in patients using nasal prongs. This condition may be treated by occlusion of one of the nasal prongs and alternating the open prong between nares.
   c. A lubricating ointment may be used to relieve nasal discomfort.

6. **Otic laceration or ulceration.** Otic lacerations or ulcerations may be caused by pressure from the nasal cannula. Padding the cannula with cotton, gauze, using foam "Oxy-Ears", or wearing the cannula more loosely may alleviate this problem.

   7. **Contact dermatitis** may be caused by sensitivity to polyvinyl chloride. Wrapping cannulas in hypoallergenic tape or trying another brand of cannula may help.
E. **Prescribing O$_2$**
   1. The following elements are needed prior to prescribing LTOT:
      a. **Diagnosis.** An accurate, current cardiopulmonary diagnosis.
      b. **Laboratory evidence of hypoxia.** Blood gas and oximetry results should show a requirement for O$_2$ and relief with therapy. O$_2$ should be given at a dosage sufficient to alleviate hypoxemia (Pao$_2$ >55 mm Hg) and/or the effects of hypoxic organ dysfunction.
      c. **Additional medical documentation** of hypoxemic organ dysfunction and improvement with O$_2$ (1–5).
   2. The O$_2$ prescription should contain information about:
      a. Method of delivery (nasal cannula, face mask, etc.).
      b. Flow rate in liters per minute (or in concentration for tracheotomized patients).
      c. Frequency of therapy. Hours per day, continuous, nocturnal, with exercise, etc.
F. **Method of delivery** (Table 36-2)
   1. **Nasal cannula.** The most common method of providing home O$_2$, the nasal cannula should be the method used whenever possible. Cannulas consist of two prongs that direct O$_2$ flow into the nares. The rate of O$_2$ flow must be spec-

Table 36-2. Oxygen devices

Device	Advantages	Disadvantages
Nasal cannula	Simple, inexpensive, comfortable Patient is able to eat and speak with it on	Can cause nasal irritation, otic lesions, contact dermatitis
Oxygen-conserving cannulas	Less oxygen is required Portable system will last longer, capable of delivering high-liter flows	Cosmetically apparent due to larger construction, heavier increasing chances of nasal and otic lesions Not humidified, increasing chance of nasal irritation Cannot be used with pursed-lip breathing
Oxygen-demand devices	Because it is used with a nasal cannula, the advantages are the same as above, as well as using less oxygen	Noisy, different flow patterns Patients must be tested individually for results
Transtracheal oxygen	Eliminates nasal and otic problems as well as contact dermatitis Conserves oxygen, improves exercise tolerance Improved patient appearance	Expensive Increased chance of infection at site Mucous balls
Oxygen to tracheotomy via entrainment device	Portable	Uses high-liter flow
Oxygen to tracheotomy via aerosol device	Delivers oxygen with humidification	Not portable F$_{IO_2}$ must be analyzed

F$_{IO_2}$ = fraction of inspired oxygen.

ified in the prescription; flow rates up to 6 L/min may be ordered. Flow rates >4 L/min will require additional humidification.

   a. **Advantages.** Nasal cannulas are simple and inexpensive and afford a high patient-comfort level; eating or talking is not impeded.

   b. **Disadvantages.** Nasal cannulas cause nasal irritation, otic lesions, and contact dermatitis in some individuals.

2. **Reservoir cannulas.** These O_2-conserving devices enable decreases in O_2-flow-rate requirements by delivering a bolus of O_2 early in the inspiratory phase of breathing. During exhalation, the reservoir expands and fills with dead-space gas removed from the reservoir by the continuous flow of gas from the O_2 source. At equilibrium, the reservoir contains gas that is nearly pure O_2. Early in inhalation, a high F_IO_2 bolus will thus be delivered to the patient. There are two types of reservoir cannulas: the O_2-conserving nasal cannula in which the reservoir is situated just below the nose and the O_2-conserving pendant with wide-diameter tubing and a reservoir situated at the level of the chest (6,7).

   a. **Advantages.** Since patients can be adequately oxygenated at lower flow rates, less O_2 is required; yearly O_2 savings can be between 50% and 75% (7). O_2 cylinders will last longer, resulting in fewer changes. If high flow rates are necessary to oxygenate the patient, reservoir cannulas can deliver flow rates greater than the 6-L/min limit of a standard cannula.

   b. **Disadvantages.** These devices are unsightly and can negatively affect appearance. In addition, the larger construction and increased weight cause more frequent nasal and otic problems than with the nasal cannula. Since reservoir cannulas must be used without humidification, the chance of nasal problems is further increased. The effectiveness of the reservoir device is reduced at low flow rates in patients who pursed-lip breathe, since exhaled air is needed to open the reservoir for the next bolus.

3. **Demand flow devices.** These devices sense the beginning of inspiration and trigger a solenoid valve that delivers a pulse of O_2. Precise timing allows the pulse to be delivered when most likely to reach the alveoli. Demand devices are available with specifically designed liquid O_2 portable and stationary units or as devices that can be added to cylinders. They can be pressure driven, flow driven, or pressure and flow driven (6,7).

   a. **Advantages.** These devices are similar to a standard nasal cannula but provide an O_2 savings of 50% to 86% at rest and possibly at exercise as well (7), allowing a cylinder or portable system to be used for increased lengths of time.

   b. **Disadvantages.** Patients need to be individually assessed while using the demand-flow system to determine the correct O_2 prescription and whether the noise and flow pattern generated by the device can be tolerated.

4. **Transtracheal O_2 delivery.** In this system, O_2 is directly delivered to the upper airway via a small, indwelling intratracheal cannula. Since O_2 enters the trachea directly during inspiration, O_2 waste is decreased. During exhalation, O_2 fills the anatomic reservoir of the upper trachea and nasopharynx, storing a bolus of O_2 for the next inspiration. Transtracheal O_2 delivery alters the normal breathing pattern and ventilatory requirements so that inspired minute ventilation and inspiratory time are reduced (6,7). Three systems, two percutaneous and one subcutaneous, are currently available:

   a. **Scoop system** (Transtracheal Systems, Englewood, Colorado). The Scoop delivers O_2 through a tracheal stent placed through a tract produced by a small percutaneous catheter that is later removed.

   b. **Micro Trache system** (Life Medical, Midvale, Utah). This System does not use a stent, and the transtracheal catheter is not removed for cleaning.

   c. **Johnson Intratracheal Oxygen Catheter** (ITO$_2$C, Cook, Bloomington, Indiana). This subcutaneous system uses a silicone rubber catheter inserted via the anterior chest wall, tunneled up to the trachea, and sutured in place.

d. **Advantages.** These systems conserve O_2 and eliminate contact dermatitis, as well as nasal and otic problems. Patient compliance is excellent, improved exercise tolerance is usually experienced, and patient appearance is not affected because the catheter can easily be concealed.

e. **Disadvantages.** The costs of the initial procedure and the replacement catheters are very high. Superficial skin and subcutaneous infections at the catheter insertion site are common side effects; other complications may also develop, the most serious of which is catheter plugging with thick mucus.

5. **O_2 delivery to tracheotomized patients.** Many tracheotomized patients require supplemental O_2; the devices already discussed are not suitable for these situations. Two common methods are used:

a. **Trach masks** with entrainment devices are designed to use a low flow from the O_2 source while drawing a large flow of room air to achieve a specific O_2 concentration. Preset concentrations include 24%, 28%, 31%, 35%, 40%, and 50% O_2. Higher liter flows may be required to achieve the higher O_2 concentrations. This device is generally used without humidification and is frequently used in portable systems. If necessary, the air the mask entrains can be humidified with an air compressor and nebulizer.

i. **Advantage.** It is portable.

ii. **Disadvantage.** It utilizes high O_2 flows to deliver high concentrations.

b. **Aerosol Trach masks** utilize an air compressor to deliver a room-air mist to which a liter flow of O_2 is bled in.

i. **Advantage.** It delivers O_2 containing humidification.

ii. **Disadvantages.** It is not portable, O_2 concentrations must be determined with an O_2 analyzer, and the air compressor is noisy.

G. **O_2 sources** (Table 36-3)

1. **Compressed O_2** is delivered using steel or aluminum cylinders containing 100% O_2 under very high pressures (1800–2400 psi at 70°F). A large volume of O_2 may be stored in a small space using cylinders. A regulator is required to convert the high tank pressure to a working pressure of 50 psi. The length of time a tank will last depends on the volume (size) of the cylinder, the pressure of the contents, and the flow rate at which gas is removed. Conversion factors are used to calculate how long the tank will last (1,4,6,8).

a. **Advantages.** Cylinders can be stored indefinitely without leakage or spoilage. Aluminum (E) cylinders are lightweight and used as a source of portable O_2, including use with O_2-conserving reservoir cannulas or demand systems.

b. **Disadvantages.** Steel cylinders are heavy and unwieldy and must be stored in a stand or secured for safety reasons. Replacement of the regulator requires more arm strength than many compromised patients have. Smaller (D) cylinders are available but require more frequent replacement.

2. **O_2 concentrators** use a molecular sieve to remove nitrogen from the air. Room air is pumped by a compressor to a sieve bed composed of sodium-aluminum silicate pellets. O_2 passes freely through the sieve, while CO_2, nitrogen, water vapor, and hydrocarbons are trapped. The gas leaving the sieve bed of the concentrator is >90% O_2; it is stored in a reservoir and then pumped through a flow meter to the patient. The most common flow rates available by concentrator are the 1–3-L/min and the 1–5-L/min ranges. At least one company produces a concentrator that can deliver up to 6 L/min. However, as the flow rate increases the delivered O_2 concentration generally decreases. Concentrators should deliver at least 90% O_2 over the entire rate range (1,4,6,8,9).

a. **Advantages.** A concentrator is generally less expensive than liquid O_2, and there is no need for routine deliveries, which is ideal for people living in remote areas. Some models are small and light enough to lift into a car, making travel easier and some models can be adapted to operate from a

Table 36-3. Oxygen delivery systems

System	Advantages	Disadvantages
Cylinders	Oxygen can be stored indefinitely Can be used with oxygen-conserving cannulas and demand valves Oxygen concentration constant	Heavy, must be stored securely Requires arm strength to change regulator; smaller, lighter sizes don't last long
Concentrators	Less expensive, no need for routine deliveries Good for someone living in a remote area Many have built-in alarms Some models are small enough to use for travel and can run off a car lighter	Requires electricity (needs reliable electrical power), filter changes, and regular maintenance Noisey Cost may be high in are with high energy costs Oxygen concentration declines as flow rate increases Limited flow rates available
Liquid	Extremely portable Little maintenance Oxygen concentration constant	Requires manual dexterity to transfill the portable Excess venting may pose a fire hazard Potential for skin burns from extreme cold temperatures Requires regularly scheduled deliveries Oxygen will escape when idle
Enrichers	Oxygen concentrators constant Because of lower concentration no risk of fire Does not require regular deliveries	Because of the lower concentration, must use higher flow rates to provide sufficient oxygenation; these higher flow rates may be uncomfortable for some patients Requires electricity, may be costly in high energy-cost areas Requires regular service

car cigarette lighter. Many models have built-in alarms to indicate malfunction and low O_2 concentrations. Concentrators can be supplied with a tubing length of up to 50 feet without affecting delivery.

    b. Disadvantages. Because concentrators require electricity, a backup cylinder should always be on hand. Patients living in areas prone to power outages should consider other sources of O_2. Concentrators are noisy and should be kept in a room not used for sleeping. These devices require the user to clean a filter, and regular servicing by a technician is necessary. Active persons will need an additional, separate portable O_2 source such as aluminum cylinders. Lastly, flow rates are limited and not high enough to meet the needs of some individuals.

    c. Cost is a factor in areas with high power costs, since electric bills will increase. The following calculation can be used to estimate the monthly costs to operate the concentrator:

$$\text{Monthly cost} = 1000 \text{ kW/d} \times \text{local cost per kW-hour} \times 30 \text{ d/mo}$$
$$= \text{power consumption of concentrator (W/d)} \times 30 \text{ d/mo}$$

3. Liquid O_2 systems. Liquid O_2 expands 860 times to become gaseous O_2, so much greater quantities of O_2 can be stored per unit of space as a liquid. Liquid O_2 is generated from dried, compressed air. The heat of compression is removed after cooling the air to a liquid ($-300°F$); after rewarming, the other gases revert to gaseous form sooner and are removed. This cycle is repeated until the remaining liquid is >99% pure O_2. Liquid O_2 is delivered in containers similar to thermos bottles at temperatures maintained at $-300°F$. Most liquid O_2 containers keep the O_2 at a pressure of 20 psi. O_2 flow is controlled by the selected size of the orifice or flow restrictor (1,4,6,8).

    a. Advantages. A smaller portable can be transfilled directly from a larger stationary reservoir, allowing superior portability for the active patient. The portable can be filled as frequently as needed and is not limited to a set number of cylinders per delivery schedule. Maintenance is minimal, consisting of emptying of condensate. Transfilling is simple but requires some manual dexterity.

    b. Disadvantages. Excess venting, especially in poorly ventilated areas or in warmer temperatures, increases ambient O_2 concentration and the risk of fire. Space is required for bottle storage; liquid O_2 should be stored in a cool, well ventilated part of the house at least 6 feet from any electrical outlets or open flames. Skin damage can occur from handling cylinders in which frost has collected around the vent. Dust or excessive ice may collect in or around the valve and prevent proper closing, thus allowing clouds of O_2 to vent into the air. If this occurs, the vendor should be immediately notified, and any sources of sparks or flames should be eliminated; the room should be left unoccupied until the reservoir empties. Liquid O_2 use requires regularly scheduled deliveries determined according to reservoir size and liter flow of use. Liquid O_2 reservoirs lose O_2 through condensation even when not in use, so unused reservoirs empty over time.

    4. O_2 enricher. An O_2 enrichment device consists of a compressor that creates a constant vacuum and draws air across a thin membrane. O_2 and water vapor are more permeable through the membrane than nitrogen, so gas concentrated to 40% O_2 can be obtained. Enrichers require higher flow rates (two to three times) to achieve the same blood gas levels as those achieved with 100% O_2 (6,8).

        a. Advantages. O_2 concentration remains constant regardless of flow rate, and gas is humidified because water vapor is not removed by the enrichment process. The delivered O_2 concentration is about 40%, and thus there is no fire risk, making enrichment a good choice in noncompliant smokers.

        b. Disadvantages. Enrichers require electricity; backup systems are necessary in case of malfunction or loss of electricity, and electric bills will increase. Some patients will find the high flow rates generated by enrichers uncomfortable. Enrichers are also noisy. They are rarely prescribed.

H. Patient education. For safe and effective use of home O_2 and for the improvement of compliance with the home O_2 prescription, the following elements should be included in the education of the patient:

    1. The reason for and expected benefits of O_2.

    2. The patient should clearly understand the O_2 prescription.

    3. The potential effects of not using O_2 as prescribed.

    4. The signs and symptoms of hypoxemia and hypercapnia and what to do if they occur.

    5. Safety precautions to follow when O_2 is used.

    6. The operation and maintenance of the equipment, as well as how to troubleshoot potential problems.

    7. Infection control measures to follow.

    8. Who, when, why, and how to call the appropriate person or organization when help is necessary.

I. Home monitoring

    1. The clinical status of the patient and the functional status of the equipment should be assessed routinely by the caregiver (4).

    2. Patients should be objectively assessed at least once a month by a respiratory care practitioner. Measurement of vital signs, chest physical examination, and oximetry should be routinely performed during home visits. All equipment should be tested and maintenance performed, and compliance with the O_2 prescription and with all safety and infection control measures should be assessed and documented in a log (4).

J. Personnel. Credentialed respiratory care practitioners should be utilized to assess the patient, initiate and monitor O_2 delivery systems, recommend changes in therapy, instruct the patient, and maintain communication with the caregiver (4).

K. Duration of need. Documentation of continued need for O_2 should be performed on a regular basis. Although those patients with chronic pulmonary diseases will usually continue to need O_2, those with acute diseases that resolve and those with chronic diseases that improve on therapy may need less O_2 with time. Other patients will need more O_2 when clinical conditions worsen. **Assessment of need** is made by arterial blood gas and oximetry measurements while the patient is receiving the amount of O_2 currently prescribed (1,4,5). The O_2 prescription should be modified as necessary. Assessments should be performed:

1. **Monthly** in the clinically unstable patient whose condition and medications are changing.
2. **Semiannually** in stable patients after an acute illness has resolved.
3. **Annually** in the stable chronic patient.

II. **Home mechanical ventilation**

A. Diagnosis. The disorders for which home mechanical ventilation may be required are listed in Table 36-4.

B. Goals of mechanical ventilation. The primary goals of mechanical ventilation are listed in Table 36-5.

C. Indications for home mechanical ventilation

1. Patients partially dependent on mechanical ventilation at night to reduce CO_2 and/or rest the diaphragm and nondiaphragmatic respiratory muscles.
2. Individuals completely dependent on mechanical ventilation for survival or improved quality of life.

D. Prerequisites for home ventilation

1. **Adequate physiologic and clinical stability.** Properly selected patients should not require major diagnostic studies or changes in therapy for at least 1 month.

Table 36-4. Disorders possibly requiring mechanical ventilation

Obstructive pulmonary disorders

End-stage chronic bronchitis and emphysema
Bronchopulmonary dysplasia
Cystic fibrosis

Restrictive pulmonary disorders

Interstitial pulmonary fibrosis
Kyphoscoliosis
Chest wall deformities

Sleep apnea syndromes

Central sleep apnea
Mixed central and obstructive sleep apnea

Neuromuscular disorders

Poliomyelitis
Muscular dystrophy
Amyotrophic lateral sclerosis
Myasthenia gravis
Spinal cord lesions
Phrenic nerve lesions
Undifferentiated neuromuscular disease

Table 36-5. Goals of mechanical ventilation

To extend life

To improve the quality of life

To reduce morbidity

To improve or sustain psychological and physical function

Cost benefit; reduction in inpatient stays (16)

      Patients are not anticipated to require frequent hospital admissions or emergency department visits (10–14).

2. **Patient and family readiness.** The patient should be motivated to live at home with mechanical ventilatory support in as independent and functional a manner as possible. The family unit should be assessed as to its emotional strength and willingness to meet the demands with which it will be faced (10–15).

3. **Financial support.** The cost of ventilator care in the home will depend greatly on the individual needs of the patient and family. Cost will be determined by the type of equipment and supplies used, the need for home care personnel, the resources available, and local economic factors (13–15).

4. **Physical environment.** Adequate space is necessary to accommodate equipment and supplies, as well as enough additional space for the patient to exit quickly if necessary. The area should safely meet al.l electrical needs (outlets for multiple pieces of equipment will be required). An intercom, buzzer, or bell for communication to others outside the room where the ventilator will be located is required. Removal of fire, health, and safety hazards from this location is paramount.

5. **Medical support.** An accessible primary care physician and consulting pulmonary physician are necessary in addition to quick access to the emergency medical system.

6. **Technical support.** A home care vendor with 24-hour respiratory care service and fast response time is necessary. An adequate stock of backup equipment and supplies should be available. Ongoing teaching and supervision should be provided with at least monthly home visits to assess patients and to check the equipment.

7. **Education** should be consistent with the level of understanding of all participants. Written instructions on use of the equipment should be given to the patient, including measurable performance objectives. Education should include hands-on demonstrations of how to use and maintain all equipment and should begin in the hospital setting with the exact equipment to be used in the home. The home respiratory care provider should participate in the educational process in the hospital and later in the home.

E. **Contraindications to home mechanical ventilation**
  1. Inability of the patient to make decisions or provide some measure of self-care.
  2. Lack of motivation to utilize home mechanical ventilation.
  3. Clinical instability
     a. FIO_2 requirement >40% to maintain PO_2 >60 mm Hg.
     b. Positive end-expiratory pressure requirement >10 cm H_2O to maintain PO_2 >60 mm Hg.
     c. Requirement for continuous nursing services and/or monitoring.
  4. Lack of a mature tracheostomy.
  5. An unsafe physical environment: fire, health, or safety hazards in the home.
  6. Lack of financial resources
     a. Lack of appropriate basic utilities.
     b. Insufficient heating, air conditioning, electricity, or handicap access.
     c. Insufficient access to or coverage by medical practitioners.
  7. Personnel limitations: inadequate number of skilled caregivers, including family members and/or visiting nurses (10–12).

F. Home ventilator prescriptions for respiratory care plan. A prescription should be written covering a 24-hour period with defined instructions for ventilator parameters and nonventilator requirements. The prescription should include:

1. **Ventilator parameters.** These include tidal volume, rate, mode, high pressure alarm/limit, low pressure alarm, inspiratory time or flow rate, sensitivity, and F_IO_2. All settings should be determined in the hospital and confirmed to be adequate utilizing measurement of arterial blood gases.

2. **Frequency/duration of ventilation.** Time on and off (day or night).

3. **Weaning instructions.** FIO_2, O_2 delivery device (cool mist, nasal cannula).

4. **Monitoring parameters**
   a. Daily by patient or caregiver. Confirm ventilator setting and pressure check circuit, assess resources (O_2, power, supplies), and perform patient assessment (secretions, dyspnea).
   b. Monthly by home respiratory practitioner. Measure F_IO_2 and exhaled tidal volume, assess equipment function, and assess patient by measuring the Sao_2, the frequency of suctioning, and adequacy of tracheostomy care;

5. **Maintenance schedule.** Ventilator circuit changes, filter changes, and cleaning.

G. Equipment requirements
1. Ventilator (two ventilators may be required depending on the length of time the patient can safely be off the ventilator).
2. A manual resuscitator.
3. Alternate power source (battery or generator).
4. O_2 supply (stationary and portable).
5. Multiple ventilator circuits.
6. Humidification system.
7. Suction equipment and supplies.
8. Artificial airway of appropriate make and size.
9. Aerosol (medication nebulizer and/or trach mist).

H. Complications of home mechanical ventilation
1. **Medical**
   a. Barotrauma.
   b. Hemodynamic instability.
   c. Airway complications.
   d. Respiratory infections.
2. **Mechanical**
   a. Equipment failure.
   b. Loss of utilities.
   c. Inadvertent changes in ventilator settings.
   d. Ventilator circuit leaks.
   e. Accidental disconnect.
   f. Accidental decannulation.
3. **Psychosocial**
   a. Depression, anxiety.
   b. Loss of resources (financial, caregiver).
   c. Change in family support.

I. Prevention of complications
1. A detailed discharge plan developed by a team should include the names and responsibilities of the physician, social service consultant, respiratory care practitioner, nursing service practitioner, the home care vendor, and family members. This clear delineation of lines of responsibility will help to avoid problems. The goals of home management should be realistic and clearly stated.
2. The patient and family should be educated in the medical and mechanical aspects of care as mentioned above.
3. Several demonstrations by the patient and caregivers to the hospital team should be made to assess their ability to independently initiate and perform all aspects of care prior to discharge, including the use of an Ambu bag.
4. Knowledge of all established emergency procedures (see below).
5. A social service assessment should be made prior to discharge, with continued planned follow-up.

6. To ensure that the residence is suitable and safe, a home visit by the respiratory care provider may be needed prior to discharge.
7. Dependable financial resources.

J. Emergency procedures
1. The patient should have a list of phone numbers for emergency assistance, including the phone numbers of the power company and the home care vendor. A clear plan of action in case of emergency should be written down.
2. **Loss of power.** Available emergency supplies include an Ambu bag, flashlight and fresh batteries, and an alternate power source for the ventilator and suction machine. Aerosolizable bronchodilators and saline should always be available.
3. **Mechanical failure.** All caregivers should receive training in troubleshooting. A second ventilator, manual resuscitator, backup O_2 tank, and metered-dose inhalers should be readily available.
4. **Tracheostomy tube.** The patient or a caregiver should be trained to change a tracheostomy tube.
5. **Medical emergency.** The patient and caregiver should be trained to continually assess the patient's condition and seek medical assistance early.

K. Types of home ventilators
1. **Positive pressure ventilators**
   a. The choice of ventilator should be determined by the clinical needs (F_IO_2) and goals (portability) of the patient, the abilities of the caregivers, and the physical environment (space, location) (16).
   b. The following ventilator characteristics are necessary for the home environment:
      i. The ventilator should be reliable and not require excessive or costly preventive maintenance.
      ii. The ventilator should provide a variety of choices of modes (assist/control, IMV, SIMV) of ventilation and allow patients capable of breathing spontaneously to do so.
      iii. The ventilator should have a system of alarms that monitors disconnection, leaks, loss of volume (pressure), high pressures, or ventilator malfunction.
      iv. The ventilator system should be simple to understand, use, and maintain.
      v. The ventilator should incorporate a humidification system with temperature alarms and shutoffs.
   c. Precautions
      i. The use of positive pressure can cause barotrauma.
      ii. Tracheostomies and tracheostomy tubes require preventive maintenance and frequent (bimonthly) changes.
2. **Noninvasive ventilatory support is an alternative or adjunct to positive-pressure ventilation.** Four noninvasive ventilatory modalities are available: negative-pressure ventilation, pneumobelts, rocking beds, and continuous positive airway pressure (CPAP), or bilevel positive-pressure ventilation (BiPAP).
   a. **Negative-pressure ventilation**
      i. A negative-pressure ventilator consists of a chamber encasing the thorax and a negative-pressure generator to create negative pleural pressure, mimicking normal ventilatory efforts. Chambers available include the full-body container ("iron lung"), the cuirass ("turtle shell"), the wrap ("raincoat"), or the pneumosuit (15). Three controls set the ventilator: the maximum negative pressure to be generated, the inspiratory time, and the expiratory time. Some of these devices use a cannula to sense inspiratory effort, which triggers an assist breath (6,8,16).
      ii. O_2 is administered exogenously via a nasal cannula. The effectiveness of these devices is dependent on the quality of the seal around the body or thorax. As with CPAP ventilation, a backup ventilator should be available in case of mechanical failure, and an alternate power source should be available in case of power failure.

       iii. **The care of these devices is simple.** The chamber should be wiped down with mild soap daily and disinfected as per specifications of the manufacturer. The negative-pressure generator should receive routine preventive maintenance. Wraps should be inspected for holes or tears.

        (a) **Indications.** Negative-pressure ventilation is useful in patients with neuromuscular disease, kyphoscoliosis, or central hypoventilation. Periodic ventilation with these devices may be helpful in patients with respiratory muscle fatigue who refuse intubation to rest the respiratory muscles.

        (b) **Contraindications.** Negative-pressure ventilation can cause airway obstruction in patients with obstructive sleep apnea.

        (c) **Advantages.** Tracheostomy is not required, so the risk associated with a tracheostomy tube is eliminated.

        (d) **Precautions.** Patients should be cautioned not to eat or drink while using the ventilator due to an increased risk of aspiration. Leaks result in decreased ventilation.

b. **Pneumobelt.** A pneumobelt is a bladder within a belt connected to a positive-pressure generator. The belt is attached around the abdomen, and inflation of the inner bladder compresses the abdominal contents, raising the diaphragm and causing exhalation. Upon deflation of the bladder, the diaphragm passively descends, increasing intrathoracic volume and causing gas to enter the airway. Patients should be sitting at a $\geq 75°$ angle for best results (6,8,16).

       i. **Advantages.** Care of the device is minimal; cleaning of the belt and preventive maintenance of the generator are necessary. Pneumobelts may be used to provide daytime ventilation in patients who do not have much intrinsic lung disease but require continuous ventilation.

       ii. **Disadvantages.** The pneumobelt does not respond to inspiratory efforts, and patients may find it difficult to synchronize with the device. Emergency alternative source of ventilation and power should be available for patients requiring continuous ventilation.

c. **Rocking bed.** This device is a motorized bed that rocks or rotates about an axis parallel to its width located half way up its length. The patient should be placed in the bed so that the diaphragm resides over the axis of motion. Rocking of the bed shifts the patient's abdominal contents, altering intrathoracic pressures and producing ventilation. The amount of ventilation is controlled by the rate and the pitch of the bed (6,8,16).

       i. **Indications.** Rocking beds work best in the patient with neurologic or neuromuscular disease who has diaphragmatic paralysis but some accessory respiratory muscle function and no pulmonary disease.

       ii. **Advantages.** The motion of the bed may assist in the mobilization of secretions. A tracheostomy tube is not required.

       iii. **Disadvantages.** Not much ventilation can be achieved, so some level of CO_2 retention may result.

d. **CPAP.** The indications for this mode of noninvasive ventilation include obstructive sleep apnea/hypopnea syndrome, Cheyne-Stokes respiration or central apnea, and snoring.

       i. **The pressure should be adjusted to the minimum level that restores ventilation, oxygenation, and uninterrupted sleep.** These improvements should be documented in various body positions (especially supine) and in rapid eye movement (REM) and non-REM sleep (17). In some patients, significant oxyhemoglobin desaturation may persist in spite of the elimination of apneas. Supplemental O_2 can be added to the CPAP system either directly into the side port of the mask or into the inspiratory flow through the tubing leading to the mask. Higher levels of O_2 will be required if the O_2 flow is not introduced into the mask itself (17).

ii. **Contraindications to the use of CPAP include** bullous lung disease and recurrent sinus or ear infections. One major complication is redness of the face associated with the interface (mask or nasal pillow) and usually due to wearing the mask too tightly, using a mask of the wrong size, having large cheeks (in which case, use a mask with flaps), or development of a contact dermatitis (in which case, use a hypoallergenic mask or nasal pillows, which have smaller contact surface area). A second complication is claustrophobia (nasal pillows may be better tolerated in such patients). A third complication is an inability to adjust to the pressure (in which case, a pressure ramp will allow the patient to fall asleep before the pressure increases to therapeutic level). A fourth complication is the development of a dry mouth, usually caused by air flowing past an open mouth (in which case, use a chin strap or a pass-over humidifier). Nasal steroid sprays and humidification may help nasal rhinitis. In some cases, a heated CPAP humidifier will help.

iii. CPAP devices use a blower to generate a bias flow ranging from 20 L/mim to 60 L/mim to deliver pressures of 2–20 cm H_2O at the mouth. To maintain a constant pressure throughout the respiratory cycle, the blowers reduce flow during expiration as the pressure rises and increase flow during inspiration as the pressure falls. To prevent rebreathing of CO_2, exhaled gases are vented through an expiratory valve placed near the mask or through a small hole in the mask that creates a minimal leak of about 10–15 L/min (17).

iv. Features to consider in the choice of a device. The pressure limit should be as high as 18–20 cm H_2O, and the patient should be able to program the device to start at a low pressure and then ramp up to the desired therapeutic level (ramping). The device should have an hour meter so that patient compliance may be monitored. The noise produced by the compressor should be minimal, and the device should be as portable as possible and should be able to use a D/C adaptor. In addition, humidification devices (purchased separately) should be available for the unit.

v. **Patient compliance** is greatest in those who experience symptomatic relief. The interface selection and fitting are important factors in continued compliance. Patients educated about their disease and the importance of therapy will be more compliant (18).

vi. **Follow-up** is recommended at regular intervals after institution of CPAP: at 1 month and every 3–6 months thereafter. Communication must be maintained with the home care therapist to assess compliance and difficulties. Routine follow-up testing should be done to confirm that the prescribed pressure level is being delivered by the device; this can be done by the home care therapist during each home visit. The therapist should also review and confirm patient understanding of the proper use, cleaning, and maintenance of all equipment during each visit (18).

vii. Preventive maintenance and servicing should always be performed per manufacturer's recommendations.

e. **BiPAP ventilation.** These ventilators are time cycled, positive pressure, and pressure limited and apply a higher pressure at the nose or mouth during inspiration than expiration. They require setting an inspiratory pressure, an expiratory pressure, a backup rate that can be delivered in the event that the spontaneous respiratory rate falls below the set rate, and a set inspiratory/expiratory ratio. Care is simple; the mask, hose, and headgear require cleaning with mild soap and periodic disinfection. Preventive maintenance of the ventilator should be done according to the manufacturer's guidelines (6,8,16).

i. **Indications.** BiPAP ventilation is useful in patients with obstructive sleep apnea who are unable to tolerate the high pressure levels needed to prevent obstruction (the lower expiratory pressure makes exhalation more comfortable). Central sleep apnea patients who have extended periods of apnea during which a backup rate can provide ventilation also may benefit from this device. CO_2 retention can be reduced in patients with obesity hypoventilation, chest wall deformities, and neuromuscular disease.

  ii. **Advantages.** The devices are quiet and simple to operate, and O_2 can be easily bled in. Many interfaces (masks, nasal pillows) are available, provided by a number of manufacturers.
  iii. **Disadvantages.** They cannot provide continuous ventilation. Facial irritation caused by the interface is a problem (in which case, providing an optional interface allows the patient to switch when one interface causes discomfort). Hypoallergenic masks may be used in patients with allergy to plastic materials. Humidification may be required if the patient complains of dryness or nasal irritation. Some patients will become claustrophobic from the nasal mask.

References

1. Fulmer JD, Snider GL: American College of Chest Physicians (ACCP)/National Heart, Lung and Blood Institute (NHLBI) national conference on oxygen therapy. *Chest* 1984;86:234–247.
2. Tarpy SP, Celli BR: Long-term oxygen therapy. *N Engl J Med* 1995;333:710–714.
3. Tarpy SP, Farber, HW: Chronic lung disease: when to prescribe home oxygen. *Geriatrics* 1994; 49:27–33.
4. Lewis D, Barnes TA, Beattie K, et al.: AARC clinical practice guidelines: oxygen therapy in the home or extended care facility. *Respir Care* 1992;37:918–922.
5. Levin DC, Neff TA, O Donoue WJ, et al.: Conference report: further recommendations for prescribing and supplying long-term oxygen therapy. *Am Rev Respir Dis* 1988;138:745–747.
6. Turner J, McDonald G, Larter N: *Handbook of adult and pediatric respiratory home care.* St Louis, Mo: Mosby-Yearbook 1994:242–267,273–284.
7. Hoffman L A: Novel strategies for delivering oxygen: reservoir cannula, demand flow, and transtracheal oxygen administration. *Respir Care* 1994;39:363–376.
8. Mcpherson SP: *Respiratory home care equipment.* Dubuque, Iowa: Daedalus, 1988:10–22, 51–67, 116–121, 123–143.
9. Oxygen concentrators: clinical and technical overview. *Health Devices* 1993;22:3–24.
10. Robart P, Make BJ, McInturff SL: AARC clinical practice guideline: discharge planning for the respiratory care patient. *Respir Care* 1995;40:1308–1312.
11. Robart P, Make BJ, McInturff SL: AARC clinical practice guideline: long-term invasive mechanical ventilation in the home. *Respir Care* 1995;40:1313–1320.
12. O'Donohue WJ, Giovannoni RM, Keens TG, Plummer AL: Long-term mechanical ventilation: guidelines for management in the home and at alternate community sites. *Chest* 1986;90:1S–37S.
13. Prentice WS: Placement Alternatives for long-term ventilator care. *Respir Care* 1986;31:288–293.
14. Make B, Gilmartin M: Rehabilitation and home care for ventilator-assisted individuals. *Clin Chest Med* 1986;7(4):679–691.
15. Clark K: Psychosocial aspects of prolonged ventilator dependency. *Respir Care* 1986;31:329–333.
16. Kacmarek RM, Spearman CB: Equipment used for ventilatory support in the home. *Respir Care* 1986;31:311–328.
17. American Thoracic Society: Indications and standards for use of nasal continuous positive airway pressure (CPAP) in sleep apnea syndrome. *Am J Respir Crit Care Med* 1994;150:1738–1745.
18. Ordal KL: Compliance pressure, a CPAP how-to. *J Respir Care Pract* 1995; 51–61.

Subject Index

A

Abdominal diseases, 437–441
Abnormal diffusion
  hypoxemia and, 545
Abnormal nasogastric tube placement
  image of, 5
Abnormal sweat
  cystic fibrosis and, 254
Abscess
  HIV-related, 432
  postobstructive, 390
  pulmonary, 386–390. *See also* Lung abscess
Absorption atelectasis, 554
Acanthosis nigricans
  lung cancer and, 132
Accelerated silicosis, 475
Acetazolamide
  obstructive sleep apnea and, 320
Acid-base status, 32
Acid-fast bacilli stains
  TB and, 150
Acid maltase deficiency, 339–341
Acquired immunodeficiency syndrome (AIDS)
  coccidioidomycosis and, 168
  cryptococcosis and, 169, 170
  histoplasmosis and, 166, 167
  nocardiosis and, 174
  pneumothorax and, 211–212
  sporotrichosis and, 172
Acquired myopathic disorders, 341–343. *See also* Inherited myopathic disorders
  complications, 343
  diagnostic approach, 341–342
  differential diagnosis, 341
  etiology, 341
  pathogenesis, 341
  symptoms, 341, 342
  treatment, 342–343
  types of, 342
Acromegaly, 453
Actinomycosis, 172–173
  diagnosis, 173
  pathogenesis, 173
  sulfur granules and, 173
  symptoms, 173
  treatment, 173
Acute airway obstruction
  acute respiratory failure and, 301
Acute asthma
  symptoms, 68. *See also* Asthma
Acute chest pain
  pneumothorax and, 207
Acute hypersensitivity pneumonitis, 187–189
  allergic bronchopulmonary aspergillosis and, 188
  complications, 189
  diagnostic approach, 188–189

differential diagnosis, 188
  etiology, 187
  laboratory tests and, 189
  Monday-morning fever, 187
  pathogenesis, 187
  physiology, 187–188
  specialist referrals, 189
  symptoms, 187
  treatment, 189
Acute lupus pneumonitis
  systemic lupus erythematosus and, 448–449
Acute myocardial infarction
  oxygen therapy and, 547–548
Acute pancreatitis, 440–441
Acute pulmonary exacerbation, 257–259. *See also* Cystic fibrosis
  lab testing, 257
  symptoms, 257
  treatment, 257–259
Acute pulmonary histoplasmosis, 165
Acute respiratory failure, 296–305. *See also* Chronic respiratory failure
  causes, 300–302
  definition, 296
  diagnostic tests, 300–302
  endotracheal intubation, 299
  etiology, 299, 300–302
  hypoventilation and, 304
  hypoxemia and, 298–299
  oxyhemoglobin dissociation curve and, 297
  physiology, 296–298
  specialist referrals, 304–305
  symptoms, 296
  treatment, 299–304
Acute severe dyspnea
  emphysema and, 232
Acute silicosis, 475–476
Acute status asthmaticus
  complications, 80
Acute steroid myopathy, 342
Adenocarcinoma, 130
Adenoid cystic carcinoma
  image of, 14
Adenoidectomy
  obstructive sleep apnea and, 319
Adenopathy
  sarcoidoses and, 176
Adenovirus, 123
Adult respiratory distress syndrome
  acute respiratory failure and, 300
  drug-induced, 407–409. *See also* Drug-induced pulmonary disease
  pancreatitis and, 441
Aeroallergens
  inhaled, 56. *See also* Allergy
Aerobic pneumonia
  empyema and, 390–391

575